Nursing in Today's World

TRENDS, ISSUES & MANAGEMENT

8th Edition

Nursing in Today's World

TRENDS, ISSUES & MANAGEMENT

Illustrations by
Tomm Scalera

Janice Rider Ellis, RN, PhD
Professor of Nursing
Director of Nursing Education
Shoreline Community College
Seattle, Washington

Celia Love Hartley, RN, MN
Professor Emerita
College of the Desert
Palm Desert, California
Curriculum Consultant
Camano Island, Washington

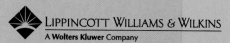
LIPPINCOTT WILLIAMS & WILKINS
A Wolters Kluwer Company

Philadelphia • Baltimore • New York • London
Buenos Aires • Hong Kong • Sydney • Tokyo

Acquisitions Editor: Margaret Zuccarini
Managing Editor: Barclay Cunningham/Helen Kogut
Editorial Assistant: Carol DeVault
Senior Production Editor: Sandra Cherrey Scheinin
Senior Production Manager: Helen Ewan
Managing Editor/Production: Erika Kors
Art Director: Carolyn O'Brien
Design Coordinator: Brett MacNaughton
Interior Designer: Joan Wendt
Cover Designer: Melissa Walter
Manufacturing Manager: William Alberti
Indexer: Angie Wiley
Compositor: TechBooks
Printer: RR Donnelley, Crawfordsville

8th Edition

9 8 7 6 5 4 3 2 1

Library of Congress Cataloging-in-Publication Data

Ellis, Janice Rider.
  Nursing in today's world: trends, issues, and management / Janice Rider Ellis, Celia Love Hartley ; illustrations by Tomm Scalera.— 8th ed.
     p. ; cm.
  Includes bibliographical references and index.
  ISBN 0-7817-4108-4 (alk. paper)
  1. Nursing.   2. Nursing—Practice—United States.   I. Hartley, Celia Love.   II. Title.
  [DNLM: 1. Nursing—trends—United States.   2. Delivery of Health Care—trends—United States.
3. Ethics, Nursing—United States.   4. Legislation, Nursing—United States.   5. Licensure, Nursing—United States.
WY 16 E47n 2004]
RT82.E45 2004
610.73—dc21   2003044664

Reviewers

Janet L. Andrews, RNC, PhD, WHNP
Associate Professor
Georgia College and State University
Milledgeville, Georgia

Mary Ann Cosgarea, RN, BSN, BA
Nurse Administrator/Coordinator
Portage Lakes Career Center
W. Howard Nicol School of Practical Nursing
Green, Ohio

Betsy Frank, RN, PhD
Professor, Department of Baccalaureate and
    Higher Degree Nursing
Indiana State University School of Nursing
Terre Haute, Indiana

Karen F. Gapper, RN, MSN
Associate Professor
Queensborough Community College,
    Department of Nursing
Bayside, New York

Rebecca Gesler, RN, MSN
Associate Professor
Saint Catharine College
Saint Catharine, Kentucky

Nancy Hinzman, RNC, MSN
Associate Professor of Nursing
College of Mount St. Joseph
Department of Nursing
Cincinnati, Ohio

Paula A. Olesen, RN, MSN
Associate Degree Nursing Program
    Director
South Texas Community College
McAllen, Texas

Alice Rasmussen, RN, BSN, MSN
Nursing Coordinator and Health Science
    Department Chair
Lake Michigan College
Benton Harbor, Michigan

Carolyn R. Tuella, RN, EdD
Chairperson
Bloomfield College
Bloomfield, New Jersey

Bernadette Wise, RN, MSN
Associate Professor of Nursing
Iowa Lakes Community College
Emmetsburg, Iowa

Preface

The eighth edition of *Nursing in Today's World: Trends, Issues, and Management,* like the previous editions of this textbook, focuses on the nonclincal aspects of the professional nursing role. Much of this content is just as critical to practicing safely as is competence in the performance of clinical skills. Nursing continues to experience significant changes as it responds to the transformation occurring in the health care delivery system. As those adjustments and modifications have taken place, we have endeavored to keep the content of this textbook in tune with the times, revising and updating each chapter with the latest information and related Internet resources. Additonally, we have made every effort to be responsive to suggestions provided by our readers. Thus, the eighth edition includes two new chapters devoted to the topics that surround the leadership and management role of the nurse. And we have retained in a concise and readable format the content that is basic to a textbook that has the nursing profession as its focus. Here is what you will find.

Text Organization

From the onset, we have attempted to design a textbook that can provide a flexible approach to instruction with the intention that each chapter be able to stand alone with references occurring throughout that will lead the reader to related content appearing in other areas of the book. This goal has been maintained so that content can be reordered if so desired. For example, those of you who prefer a chronologic approach to the development of nursing as a profession, are encouraged to adapt your use of the various chapters to match this preference. If you prefer to study the origins of nursing first, that section of this text (Chapter 4) can be read and deliberated before studying the first three chapters. Similarly, some content areas might be combined or perhaps eliminated if it appears elsewhere in the curriculum of your program.

The textbook is organized to four major units of study.

- Unit I: Economic and Political Aspects of Health Care Delivery

We believe that if students are to gain an appreciation of nursing's place in the health care delivery system, it is best facilitated by gaining an understanding of how the health care delivery system functions and what forces impact its operation. Thus the text begins with an overview of economic and political aspects of health care delivery, including such information as how it got to where it is today, how it operates, how it is financed, and how it is politically influenced. Of particular application to nursing is Chapter 3, which is devoted to the relevance of the politial process to nurses, including information describing how one can become informed. It also outlines a variety of ways in which nurses can affect the political process. This chapter also includes a discussion of the many nursing organizations, why so many exist, and the major focus of each.

- Unit II: Appreciating the Development of Nursing as a Profession

Chapters 4, 5, and 6 focus on nursing itself. By understanding the early origins of nursing and it's challenges as a profession, and by exploring the various educational avenues providing entry into the profession of nursing, students will be better prepared to participate in the various nonclinical activities and discussions that are part of nursing. Students will learn about the development of the profession and the challenges to that professional standing. The various educational paths that prepare graduates for registered nurse licensure are presented. Issues discussed include the controversy that exists regarding the form of educational preparation deemed most appropriate for entry-into-practice, the implementation of differentiated practice, and whether continuing education should be mandatory or voluntary.

- Unit III: Legal and Ethical Responsibility and Accountability for Practice

This area of study comprises four chapters. It begins with a focus on legal and ethical accountability and includes a discussion of the credentials found among health care providers, tracing the history of credentialing in the United States and leading to an exploration of the legal issues facing today's nurse. Also incorporated into this unit is a chapter devoted to ethics that provides a foundation for ethical decision making, including a broad discussion of various bioethical issues that impact nursing and nursing practice. The bioethical chapter will challenge students as they consider the many facets related to stem cell research, gene therapy, and the human genome project.

- Unit IV: Career Opportunities and Professional Growth

This section of *Nursing in Today's World* focuses on career opportunities and professional growth and includes two new chapters devoted to the leadership and management role of the professional nurse. It begins by exploring the various employment opportunities available to nurses today and provides valuable information related to seeking, applying for, and resigning from a nursing position. This is followed by a discussion of the workplace and includes a discussion of organizations, their purpose and function, as well as the topic of collective bargaining as it applies to nursing. The final two chapters discuss the leadership/management role of the nurse. Following a discussion of the various forms of leadership, practical suggestions for team building, motivating others, dealing with conflict, and managing change provide the student with critical information needed to effectively perform in a leadership role.

Pedagogical Features

- Learning outcomes introduce each chapter to guide learning efforts
- Key terms used in the chapter discussion are listed
- Critical thinking activities interspersed throughout each chapter help students critically process possible application of the content
- "Situations" in selected chapters provide examples of real-life experiences to assist students in understanding difficult concepts presented in the chapter.
- Key concepts summarize each chapter

Special Features

All of the illustrations in this eighth edition of *Nursing in Today's World* have been redrawn to provide eye-catching and provocative interpretation of concepts presented in each chapter. The cartoon feature, always a hallmark of this text, has been redone in full color; the illustrations complement the easy reading style and logical approach of this textbook. We hope you will appreciate the humorous aspects that can accompany your commitment to nursing.

Instructor's Resources

An Instructor's Resource CD-ROM is available to faculty adopting this text. This invaluable resource tool includes:

- Instructor's Guide
- Computerized Test Generator
- Image Bank—includes all illustrations from text.
- Power Point Slides with basic lecture outlines

Instructor's Guide

This invaluable resource manual includes:

- Chapter overviews
- Situations to Foster Clinical Thinking that provide additional clinical thinking tools
- Gaming in the classroom
- Student Review Sheets with Matching, Discussion/Essay, Fill-in-the Blank/Short Answer, True/False, and Multiple Choice questions to assess student learning.

In addition to all of the above resources, instructors and students may access the ***connection*** Web site, *http://connecton.lww.com./go/ellis8e*. Here, faculty will find lesson plans that have been developed to facilitate classroom teaching.

Students can find WebQuests, Web Resources, content updates, and printable Student Review Sheets for every chapter that include learning activities (short answer, true-false, fill in the blank and multiple choice questions) in a chapter work sheet format.

Your Input is Welcomed

We continue to appreciate the comments and suggestions of colleagues, friends, and students. We encourage you to review this text critically and advise us of ways in which we can make it better meet classroom needs. We thank the many educators who continue to select *Nursing in Today's World* as the textbook for your class. In this competitive market, we know there are many texts from which to choose. We appreciate your support and strive to bring to you the book that will continue to meet your needs.

Special Acknowledgments

We are always appreciative of the help and support that we enjoy from the fine staff at Lippincott Williams & Wilkins, particularly that of our editor Margaret Zuccarini and her editorial assistants. We have enjoyed working with Tomm Scalera, who is new to this edition of the textbook, and is responsible for capturing our concepts in the colorful illustrations. We want to express our special gratitude and appreciation to our respective husbands, Ivan and Gordon, for their continued support and encouragement during the development of another edition of the text. Their willingness to let deadlines take precedence over home or social activities and their assistance with household duties and errands has allowed us to meet publication deadlines.

Janice Rider Ellis
Celia Love Hartley

Contents

Economic and Political Aspects of Health Care Delivery

A significant part of the economic and political life of any nation relates to the health care available to its people. The percentage of a country's gross national product devoted to health helps to demonstrate the values of the society and may also serve to point out those areas where problems exist. Another significant economic indicator is how those finances are distributed across the society: which aspects are given priority, who has access, and how decisions are made. Concerns about who delivers care, credentials of the care provider, the knowledge and skills they possess, and their availability are other important aspects of the system. Similarly, there is concern about those who have difficulty obtaining health care because they lack insurance or geographic accessibility.

Because of the importance of this topic, the first unit in this text provides you with a basic overview of the health care delivery system in the United States. Beginning with the part of the system with which you are probably most familiar—those settings that employ nurses—content expands to include some of those less commonly understood. The specific characteristics of these settings—their roles in health care, the roles of nurses in these settings, the colleagues with whom nurses work, and alternative health care resources—are the focus of the first chapter in the unit.

The second chapter in this unit discusses the financial aspects of the health care delivery system. Because this topic is much too complex to discuss in detail in a single chapter, an overview must suffice. After gaining an understanding of the various players in the system, you should find it easier to analyze specific issues as they arise—issues related to access to the system, finance, power, and control.

The unit concludes with a discussion of the political process—how it affects nursing and how nurses can affect it. An understanding of the various aspects of the health care delivery system can be relevant to your professional experience.

1

Understanding the Health Care Environment

LEARNING OUTCOMES

After completing this chapter, you should be able to:

1. Identify the various ways of classifying health care agencies and explain how these classification systems differ in their focus.
2. Describe the ownership, types of services offered, and usual length of stay in various health care facilities.
3. Discuss the roles that registered nurses perform in hospitals, long-term care facilities, and community agencies.
4. Analyze how the nurse could use knowledge of the health care system when teaching clients and planning for continuity of care.
5. Compare the approach to the client/resident care between acute care hospitals and long-term care facilities.
6. Describe the roles of the various health care providers and analyze how these roles affect the relationships between providers.
7. Analyze how issues related to education, credentialing, and scope of practice of health care occupations affect individual providers and clients within the health care system.
8. List the major categories of complementary/alternative health care and identify major issues that surround the use of these therapies.
9. Describe ways in which you could use your knowledge of complementary/alternative therapies when working with clients.

KEY TERMS

Accreditation	Continuing care retirement community (CCRC)	Primary care provider
Acute care		Primary health care provider
Alternative health care	Herbal medicine	Proprietary agency
Alternative therapy	Homeopathy	Skilled nursing facility (SNF)
Ambulatory care	Hospital	
Assisted-living facility	Long-term care facilities	Subacute care
Community mental health centers	Naturopathy	Tertiary care hospital
	Nonprofit	Therapeutic touch
Complementary health care	Nursing homes	Transitional care
Complementary therapy	Outpatient care	

Health care is an exciting and rewarding field but also a challenging one due to the issues that surround it. The entire health care system reverberates with change. The roles of nurses in this system consistently are expanding and changing. You can function more effectively within this system if you understand the various health care agencies and their services, the roles that nurses perform in those agencies, and the colleagues with whom you work (Fig. 1-1).

As **complementary** and **alternative health care** practices grow in popularity with the public, health care providers are challenged to understand these diverse approaches and to work effectively with clients who choose those resources. To help you with this task, we discuss complementary and alternative health care options.

CLASSIFICATION OF HEALTH CARE AGENCIES

The health care industry is so large, so diverse, and so complex, that it is not easily understood. Generally, agencies providing care are classified according to one of three ways: length of stay, ownership, or type of service. These classifications are somewhat arbitrary, and any agency may be placed in more than one classification. With the systemic changes that are occurring, one large entity may exist that includes multiple lengths of stay, different types of service, and different ownership patterns. Therefore, understanding these categories is useful because they are used to plan for services, to describe institutions, and to allocate funding. Your understanding can also be used to guide clients and families through what sometimes seems a maze of confusion in the health care system.

Classification According to Length of Stay

One way of classifying in-patient agencies is according to the average length of time patients remain in the facility; that is, the *length of stay*. In-and-out care, short-stay, traditional acute care,

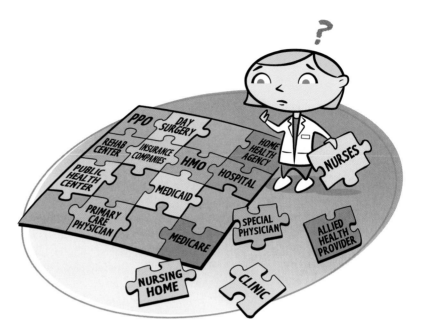

FIGURE 1-1   The many aspects of health care in the United States.

and long-term care are terms that reflect the average length of stay in a facility. Table 1-1 outlines the various definitions of care according to length of stay.

Classification According to Ownership

The second method of classifying health care agencies is according to *ownership*. Agencies may be classified as governmental or public, proprietary or nonprofit.

TABLE 1-1.	HEALTH CARE INSTITUTIONS CLASSIFIED BY LENGTH OF STAY
LENGTH-OF-STAY	**DESCRIPTION**
In-and-out care	Contact with client is measured in minutes vs. hours. Typical examples are office visits, emergency department visits, and therapy sessions.
Short-stay	Provides care to patients who suffer from acute conditions or require treatments that require less than 24 hours of care and monitoring. Diagnostic tests or minimally invasive surgery are examples.
Acute care	Traditionally occurs in hospitals where patients stay more than 24 hours but less than 30 days. Stays are shortened since the advent of managed care and DRGs.
Long-term care	Provides care to residents for the remainder of their lives; care also includes services to patients with limited recovery needs, functional losses, chronic disease, mental illness, or major rehabilitation, which may range from 30 to 90 days.

GOVERNMENT-OWNED FACILITIES

Public or government agencies, which receive some tax support for capital or operational costs, may be owned and operated by federal, state, or local governments. The federal facilities usually serve the needs of a special group, such as veterans, military personnel, Native Americans, or inmates in federal prisons. State mental facilities and **hospitals** operated by the state are also governmental institutions. Cities, counties, and hospital districts may operate acute care and long-term care agencies and public health departments.

PROPRIETARY AGENCIES

Proprietary agencies (also known as for-profit) are investor owned and operated. Proprietary agencies are commonly part of a corporation owned by stockholders. Some small nursing homes or group homes are owned by one or more individuals. In proprietary agencies, the original capital costs are provided by the owners and investors, with profits from the institution providing a return on the money invested by these same individuals. Historically, some proprietary hospitals were owned and operated by a small group of physicians, but over the years many of these have been sold to community groups or to corporations. Recently, there has been a significant trend toward the acquisition of health care enterprises by investor-owned corporations and the formation of multiunit, for-profit systems. Examples include Columbia/HCA Healthcare Corporation, based in Nashville, and Humana Incorporated of Louisville. Each of these groups owns more than 80 hospitals and operates several others. Although not true for the country as a whole, there are areas in which most hospitals are proprietary. In the long-term care field, Beverly Enterprises and Hillhaven Corporation are examples of corporations that own and operate many nursing homes across the country.

NONPROFIT AGENCIES

Voluntary, or **nonprofit**, agencies are those operated by nonprofit groups such as universities, religious organizations, fraternal groups, and community boards. More than 50% of the nation's short-term hospitals and most of the large medical centers fall into this classification. Original capital costs are obtained in a variety of ways, but most often through donations. Community fund-raising campaigns raise money for building, capital start-up costs, and special projects. One current concern is the purchase of nonprofit agencies by profit-making corporations. Communities often believe their interests and contributions are discounted in these large business mergers.

The term "nonprofit" may be misleading. All facilities must have income sufficient to meet the current costs of the care provided, to maintain facilities and services, and to plan for capital improvement and development. However, facilities that are classified as nonprofit must put any income in excess of that needed for maintenance and operation to work in the facility as improvement or growth rather than distribute it to stockholders. In the past, charitable care was supported through some of this excess income earned by nonprofit agencies, as well as being supported by special fundraising efforts of these organizations. Today this may present a challenge for nonprofit institutions since various price controls affect their ability to use a profit margin in this way.

Classification by Type of Care

Health care agencies may also be classified according to *type of care* provided. Many agencies provide more than one type of care.

ACUTE CARE

Acute care refers both to a type of care and a length of stay. The term *acuity*, when used to describe a client's condition refers to the seriousness and rate of change that is occurring. Higher acuity means that the illness is more serious and/or changing more rapidly. Individuals with major surgery, trauma, newly developing illness, and exacerbations of chronic disease may all need acute care because of the high acuity of their conditions. Their conditions are serious, subject to rapid deterioration and require highly skilled patient care. Acute care has a high concentration of professional care providers from a variety of disciplines. The physician is expected to visit daily to manage the rapid changes that may occur. In large hospitals, resident physicians may be available 24 hours a day to respond to problems and emergencies. Registered nurses (RNs) are always in charge of patient care and are present 24 hours a day.

LONG-TERM ACUTE CARE

Long-term acute care represents a relatively new type of care setting. Hospital costs continue to rise, and there is pressure to discharge patients and limit traditional hospital stays. Patients with wounds that need specialized care for healing, individuals on extended ventilator support, individuals needing dialysis who remain unstable, and other patients may need such high levels of on-going care that the traditional nursing home will not admit them. However, their conditions are not changing rapidly. Funding for nursing homes is based on a system designed to take into account the traditional nursing home client, not this high-demand client. Corporations responded by developing long-term acute care hospitals, funded differentially to take into consideration the significant cost of caring for patients needing a high intensity of care but whose conditions are not changing rapidly. These facilities must meet the requirements established by the Center for Medicare and Medicaid Services (CMS) for long-term care facilities regarding documentation, standards of care, and various processes. They must also meet some standards related to acute care and often are accredited by the same agency that accredits traditional acute care hospitals.

SUBACUTE CARE

Subacute care is a type of service that may be offered in a special unit of a hospital (where it is sometimes termed **transitional care**) or in a long-term care setting. This care is seen as a "middle ground" between the high level of care provided clients in the acute care hospital and the care provided to more traditional long-term care clients. The typical length of stay in short-term subacute units is up to 30 days. Some units focus on intermediate lengths of stay, usually ranging from 31 to 90 days, when clients may recover enough to be discharged to home or their conditions stabilize so that their needs can be met in a nursing home.

SKILLED NURSING CARE

Skilled nursing care provides health care related to skilled rehabilitation services, observation and assessment of the patient's condition, patient teaching and training, direct skilled nursing services (such as tube feedings), and management and evaluation of the patient's care plan (Hawryluk, 1999). People who need close monitoring during and after hospitalization and those progressing toward independent care are recognized as having skilled nursing needs. An RN must be in charge of the care. The designation of skilled care originated in Medicare and Medicaid legislation and has been adopted by insurers and managed-care providers. The assumption is that *all* hospital care requires skilled nursing care but that only *some* long-term care requires skilled nursing. Long-term acute care and transitional care qualify as providing skilled nursing services. Skilled nursing care also may take place in nursing homes designated as **skilled nursing facilities**, often referred to as **SNFs** (pronounced "sniffs") and in the home. Reimbursement for skilled nursing care provided outside the hospital depends on careful documentation by the care provider of the specific skilled nursing tasks required by the patient.

CUSTODIAL CARE

Custodial care refers to care focused on meeting deficits in multiple areas of daily living. Although the individual may have some routine health care concerns, the reason for admission is the need for assistance with activities of daily living (ADLs). Unfortunately, people often associate this term with a low level of care that does not require special educational preparation to plan or deliver. Even though maintaining function and preventing decline in a person with multiple deficits requires a broad background of nursing knowledge and careful attention to details of care, there is limited recognition of the difference that skilled nurses can make to individual well-being. As a result, reimbursement pays for only limited RN oversight. Custodial care may take place in private homes, group homes, large institutions, and nursing homes. Understanding the difference between custodial care and skilled care is important when funding is considered. Medicare and health insurance plans do not cover custodial care; costs must be borne by the individual unless that individual is eligible for some type of public assistance.

HOSPICE CARE

Hospice care is by definition multidisciplinary, providing medical, nursing, social work, a variety of therapies, and spiritual support for individuals who are dying and for their families and friends. Hospice care may be provided either at home or in a hospice facility. The focus is symptom management, comfort, and individual autonomy in determining what care will be provided. Additionally, hospices usually provide bereavement counseling and support to family and care providers.

REHABILITATION CARE

Rehabilitation is designed to support restoration of function, the ability to complete ADLs, or to engage in an occupation (vocational rehabilitation). The multidisciplinary team, including physicians, nurses, therapists, psychologists, social workers, and vocational counselors, creates the most effective approach to rehabilitation. Most rehabilitation clients also have skilled nursing care needs. Active rehabilitation is considered skilled care for reimbursement purposes.

AMBULATORY CARE

Ambulatory care also is referred to as **outpatient care**. Traditionally, ambulatory care focused on individuals who came for visits (in-and-out care) to clinics or primary care offices. This is still the major focus of ambulatory care. In fact, clinic locations are expanding into schools, workplaces, and senior communities. Today's ambulatory care, however, includes a wide variety of diagnostic and treatment services that fall within the short-stay category.

Day surgery centers provide an ever-increasing percentage of all surgical procedures. Presurgical care on a day before surgery also may be provided and can include assessment, laboratory tests, and preoperative education. On the day of surgery, the patient arrives at a scheduled time, which may be as early as 5:00 AM, for preoperative care before surgery. The pace in these preoperative units is rapid, with patients being admitted, treated, and discharged in a continuing process throughout the day.

Medical treatment services, originally established for those in the hospital, gradually have expanded to include services for outpatients. Physical therapy, occupational therapy, respiratory therapy, and other treatments support health care for whole segments of the community. Special outpatient units provide chemotherapy, dialysis, parenteral nutrition, antibiotic therapy, intervention radiology, and other medical treatments.

Sophisticated *diagnostic services* are provided as ambulatory care. Admitting individuals to hospitals to have major diagnostic procedures is rare today. Some diagnostic services occur in hospital departments, others occur in physician offices. Individuals may provide self-care for all preparation, including enemas, medications, and dietary restrictions. After brief periods of post-procedure monitoring, patients are sent home with instructions for self-care.

HOME CARE

Home care encompasses nursing care, therapies, personal assistance and household chores. Traditionally, home care agencies were independent organizations, but the number of hospitals offering *home care services* (including hospice home care) is growing as hospital stays have been shortened or eliminated. Home services may operate as independent departments, in conjunction with other services, or through a contractual relationship with a home care agency. Just as with long-term care facilities, home care agencies often are restricted in the care for which they will be reimbursed by definitions of skilled care and by specific mandated limitations on number of visits.

Critical Thinking Activity

Recall the last time that you needed health care. Categorize the place where you received health care in regard to length-of-stay, ownership, and type of care provided. Describe those characteristics of the care setting that formed the basis for your decisions regarding classification.

UNDERSTANDING TODAY'S HOSPITAL

The modern hospital is often viewed as the hub or center of the health care delivery system and as central to the health care of a community, although more and more care is moving into community settings. A primary characteristic of hospital care is its focus on the current problem, rapid assessment, stabilization or treatment, and then discharge to home care or to long-term care.

In addition to supplying health care to clients, hospitals also provide education to a wide variety of health care workers and to the community. In many cases, they also serve as centers for research and its dissemination. Hospitals are using their status and position in health care to enter into cooperative agreements and alliances with other types of health care providers, insurance companies, and even other hospitals. To better understand the hospitals of today, you will find it useful to look at their history and development in Chapter 4.

Inpatient Versus Outpatient Care

Two terms used frequently to describe today's modern hospital services are *inpatient care* and *outpatient care*. Individuals are termed "inpatient" when they have been admitted for the purpose of staying 24 hours or longer. The outpatient comes to the hospital for services but is expected to stay less than 24 hours.

INPATIENT SERVICES

Hospitals provide inpatient care in a variety of departments that are commonly designed around the acuity or seriousness of the patient's condition. These units compose what most people think of when they use the designation "acute care hospital" (Table 1-2). Nurses work in all of these service departments, coordinating the nursing care for individual clients, managing the care environment, delegating and supervising care provided by others, and providing direct skilled care.

Many hospitals have had empty beds because of shortened lengths of stay and the shift to outpatient procedures. In an effort to use costly resources effectively to generate income, hospitals have developed transitional care and rehabilitation units that provide long-term care services, often closing some units and converting them to areas offering these other types of care. A transitional care or rehabilitation unit allows a hospital to discharge an individual from acute, inpatient care in a timely fashion because the next level of services is guaranteed to be available. Reimbursement is based on long-term care guidelines, and the care must meet long-term care standards for skilled nursing care. Even rehabilitation stays are becoming shorter. Inpatient rehabilitation services may be provided for only a brief period of time, followed by outpatient rehabilitation services.

OUTPATIENT SERVICES

Many diagnostic and treatment procedures, surgeries, and emergency health needs are treated as outpatient care. The outpatient goes through an admission process, has a procedure performed or care delivered, is determined to be ready for home care, and subsequently is discharged.

Sometimes an outpatient is retained for observation beyond the standard 24 hours. Although this individual may be moved to a conventional hospital room, admission as an inpatient may never occur and the person may be discharged as an outpatient with an extended

TABLE 1-2.	HOSPITALS CLASSIFIED BY MIX OF SERVICES
TYPE	**SERVICES**
General or community hospital	Medical, surgical, obstetric, emergency, and diagnostic, plus laboratory services
Tertiary care hospital	Referral centers for clients with complex or unusual health problems such as level 1 trauma, major burns, bone marrow transplant, and research-based oncology, in addition to standard care
	Part of a large medical center associated with a university. Serves a wide geographic area.
Specialty hospital	Offers only a particular type of care (ie, psychiatric, pediatric)

stay. The distinction between the categories of inpatient and outpatient is important in regard to both billing and discharge to a nursing home. Both Medicare and Medicaid are billed differently for outpatient care than for inpatient care. Medicare payments for nursing home care after hospitalization require that the person be admitted as an inpatient with a minimum 3-day hospital stay. When these conditions are not met, Medicare payment is denied. Patients and their families may not understand this distinction and how it affects the bills they receive and their eligibility for some types of reimbursement. Nurses must understand that different rules may apply and refer patients and families to appropriate sources for accurate information as they help patients to plan for needed care after discharge.

Mix of Hospital Services

Hospitals are often referred to by the mix of traditional inpatient services that are offered. Not every hospital offers each of the services mentioned earlier, but more are becoming part of a corporate entity that provides all of these services The terms most commonly used to describe the mix of services are the general or community hospital, the **tertiary care hospital**, and the specialty hospital (see Table 1-2).

Other Services

Hospitals may offer a wide variety of other services that are not directed solely at client care, such as hospitality units or education for health professionals. Day procedures and early discharge for inpatient care may present travel difficulties for individuals who live a long distance from a major care center. To facilitate care for these patients and their families, some hospitals have developed hotel-like services, often termed *hospitality units.* To be present for the morning surgery appointment, the patient scheduled for day surgery may plan to arrive the day before and stay overnight at a hospitality unit. A family member can stay in the unit during the individual's hospitalization. After discharge, both the patient and the family member may stay one or more days before traveling home. Although the cost of staying in a hospitality unit usually is not covered by insurance, it is often less expensive than staying at a nearby hotel or motel and is much more convenient. Additionally, if an emergency occurs, the patient in a hospitality unit has care immediately available.

The education of health care providers is an important function of many hospitals. Although the number of hospital-based schools of nursing offering diplomas has been decreasing steadily, some are well supported and expect to continue operation. There are also hospital-based programs for respiratory therapy, dietetics, and other health-related occupations. Many hospitals serve as clinical laboratory sites for individuals enrolled in colleges and universities that provide education for health care professionals.

Graduate medical education includes all the residency programs for physicians preparing for independent practice. Residents receive a salary from the hospital and are responsible for providing services in return. Residents augment the services of primary physicians, who are often referred to as the *attending* or *staff physicians.* Residents often provide the majority of medical services for individuals who are part of the medically underserved in a community, consulting with the staff physician in charge as needed. Part of the funding for residency programs comes from money made available through Medicare reimbursement policies.

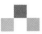

THE LONG-TERM CARE FACILITY

Long-term care is the term applied to any of the different care settings that involve coordination of the entire multidisciplinary team to provide counseling, nursing care, rehabilitation, nutritional support, social services, and sometimes special education programs over months to years. Managing a positive living environment is as important as managing health problems for long-term care residents. **Long-term care facilities** include nursing homes, assisted living centers, adult care homes (also called board and care homes), chronic disease hospitals, psychiatric hospitals, and group homes for those with developmental disabilities. The majority of long-term care facilities are nursing homes that care primarily for the elderly.

The Nursing Home Today

The **nursing home** is the care facility most often associated with long-term care. Although nursing homes suffer from negative images of the past and not all meet appropriate standards for care, they do offer a far different environment than they did 10 years ago. Nursing homes in the United States provide care and a positive living environment for individuals who have the greatest number of deficits in ADLs and who need ongoing nursing care. Just as in the acute care hospital, the nursing home is expanding services beyond those traditionally associated with nursing home care.

WHO ARE THE RESIDENTS?

Although most of the elderly live in community settings, many will spend their last years in a nursing home. Approximately two thirds of the residents are women, reflecting the longer life span of women and the greater likelihood that a woman's spouse will precede her in death. Typically, nursing home residents range in age from 65 to older than 100, with an average age of about 84. The number of individuals requiring nursing home care is expected to steadily increase based on the increasing numbers of elderly. According to the 2000 census, the number of people 80 to 84 increased since the 1990 census by 26%, those 90 to 94 increased by 45%, and those over 100 increased by 35% (The Herald, 2001).

HEALTH SERVICES IN NURSING HOMES

The majority of residents in nursing homes remains there because of major deficits in self-care abilities and the need for ongoing care that is custodial in focus rather than treatment oriented. Maintenance of function, independence, autonomy, and rehabilitation are all goals for nursing home residents. Residents are concerned with the living environment and the health care environment.

Units designed for the cognitively impaired provide facilities constructed without barriers to mobility and without the need for restraints. Facility design and alarm systems prevent residents from wandering away. A unit for the cognitively impaired has special approaches to care delivery that decrease stress and reduce the potential for catastrophic reactions such as hostile, angry outbursts. Reality orientation is used for those who might benefit from this therapy. Validation therapy and reminiscence also are planned to provide a supportive and rich environment. Staff development assists caregivers in responding appropriately to the special challenges of working with the cognitively impaired.

Some nursing homes have entire wings for individuals receiving posthospital convalescent care in subacute units. These individuals are admitted with a specific planned stay of 14 to 30 days. During this time, the individual is aided in restoring functional abilities and planning for self or family care. Rehabilitation is a major focus of some subacute units. This might include physical therapy for the person with a hip replacement or speech therapy after a stroke. The goal is to enable residents to return to independent living in the community.

The level of autonomy expected of nurses in nursing homes where physicians visit monthly is often surprising to those who have always worked in acute care hospitals, where physicians visit patients daily and resident physicians are available when needed. In nursing homes, the individual may be a permanent resident and the nurse may be charged with managing both quality of life and quality of care. Additionally, nurses in these settings must manage care conducted by a variety of assistive personnel and work effectively with an interdisciplinary team.

FUNDING NURSING HOME CARE

The cost of nursing home care is a concern for many because it often exceeds $5,000 per month, depending on the care needs of the individual and the geographic location of the nursing home. Medicare pays for only a limited number of days for individuals who meet specific criteria regarding hospitalization and who need skilled care or rehabilitation rather than custodial care. Some individuals have long-term care insurance that will pay part of their costs. Although this type of insurance is fairly new, more and more individuals are purchasing policies, which are available through a number of organizations. The personal financial resources of most individuals may be exhausted by a prolonged nursing home stay. State-administered public assistance in the form of programs such as Medicaid and Medi-Cal pays for nursing home care when an individual's personal financial resources have fallen below a certain state-determined level. As the number of elderly individuals requiring nursing home care has risen, these costs are becoming a serious budget concern in most states.

REGULATION OF NURSING HOME CARE

Nursing homes are among the most regulated of all health care settings. Because the federal government pays for some of the care, there are federal regulations affecting nursing homes across the country. Starting primarily with the Federal Budget Act of 1987 (OBRA 87), government regulations mandate specific assessment tools; planning processes; standards of care, including the use of restraints and psychoactive medications; documentation systems used; and evaluation tools. Data are collected according to a standardized minimum data set (the MDS). State regulations may place additional constraint on nursing homes. Nursing homes are visited by a survey team that is responsible for assuring adherence to regulatory standards. The results of nursing home surveys are public documents and must be displayed in each facility in a place accessible to the public and to residents who wish to review them. Nursing home survey results may be seen on the Medicare Web site at *www.medicare.gov/ Nhcompare/Home.asp.*

Critical Thinking Activity

Use the Web site to investigate a nursing home in your community. Find out its average length of stay, the types of services it offers, and its type of ownership. Analyze the quality of care provided as represented through the nursing home survey. Compare this facility with two other nursing homes in your geographic area.

Assisted-Living Facilities

The **assisted-living facility** provides care for those needing help with up to three ADLs. In an assisted-living arrangement, the resident can maintain maximum independence and use a shared decision-making model to decide when additional help or support is needed. Husbands and wives reside together and may often bring their own furniture and belongings to create a homelike atmosphere. Those who are able to perform any ADLs are seeking the less costly and more independent and flexible living found here. Assisted-living facilities have been much less regulated than nursing homes. As these facilities admit more impaired individuals or as individuals living in them want to "age in place," concerns are being raised about the quality of care provided. Increasing regulation is expected. The Joint Commission on Accreditation of Healthcare Organizations has begun a voluntary accrediting process for assisted-living centers (West, 2000).

CARE IN ASSISTED-LIVING FACILITIES

In an assisted-living facility, all instrumental ADLs such as shopping, cleaning, meal preparation, and laundry are provided. A resident is expected to have some mobility (even though it may require a walker or a cane) and to eat in a dining room except if the person is temporarily ill. Residents also are expected to manage their own medication and health needs, although they may be assisted with remembering to take medications. Assistance is provided with bathing, dressing, and other personal care as needed. Most care is provided by unlicensed assistive personnel. Nurses may be employed in a supervisory capacity and may plan for care. One area of controversy is the level of assistance with medications and health needs that can be provided by unlicensed, unregulated personnel. Some states are authorizing delegation of selected nursing tasks (for residents of assisted living), such as giving oral medications, to appropriately trained assistive personnel.

When the ability to perform ADLs is lost, transfer to a nursing home is required by regulation. For some individuals, the transitions from independent living to assisted living and from assisted living to nursing home care are smooth ones, thus avoiding the transition or relocation stress that impacts well-being. This is particularly true when multiple levels of care are available in the same retirement living setting. (See discussion of continuing care communities below.) For others, this change triggers serious stress.

FUNDING ASSISTED LIVING

Assisted living is not supported with Medicare funds and therefore does not have to meet the stringent regulatory standards of federal legislation. Public assistance, in the form of Medicaid, Medi-Cal, or other programs, may provide some support for assisted living when the alternative would be expensive nursing home care for which the state would be responsible. However, this is not true in all jurisdictions. Most assisted living is paid for by the individual or family.

Retirement Communities

Retirement communities, which continue to grow, may be self-contained towns, retirement villages, retirement subdivisions, retirement residences, or continuing-care retirement communities. The basic retirement complex is designed to provide the environment for self-care and may support independence longer than would a regular house or apartment. Home care services are provided to those in retirement communities in the same way that they are provided to those in regular homes or apartments.

Continuing care retirement communities (CCRC) provide a variety of levels of independent living and care to residents based on each resident's need. Most residents enter the community to reside in a retirement apartment and then move within the community to an assisted living section and from there to a convalescent or nursing home center. Services such as occupational therapy, physical therapy, and dental care also may be available as home care or for those in the convalescent center. The aim is for people to reside in the setting that provides maximum autonomy and independence while assuring that needs are met. There is data to suggest that residents of continuing care retirement communities maintain better health and require less nursing home care than the general population (Fonda, Clipp, & Maddox, 2002). A major limiting factor is the cost of such communities to the individual residents. While originally there was no governmental financial assistance available in these residences, in some states Medicaid will provide support in assisted living if it prevents admission to the more costly nursing home setting.

Rehabilitation Centers

Rehabilitation centers typically focus on a specific health care problem just as rehabilitation units in acute care hospitals do. For example, there are centers for those with spinal cord injuries and other centers focusing on head injuries or cerebral vascular accidents. Although many of these agencies prefer nurses who have taken advanced courses in rehabilitation nursing, many employ nurses with different backgrounds, such as those who have worked in a nursing home focused on rehabilitation principles.

AMBULATORY CARE SETTINGS

Ambulatory care has long been provided in offices, clinics, and the day-procedure units of hospitals. Some ambulatory care is provided in settings where people work and go to school. Providing care where people routinely spend their days rather than requiring them to go to a different site for health care often results in more effective use of health services. Some ambulatory care settings rely heavily on the skills of RNs while others focus on medical care and physician assistants.

Primary Care Offices

The health care provider contacted initially by clients who seek health care is considered a **primary care provider**. Today the federal government considers general practitioners, family practice specialists, pediatricians, internal medicine specialists, and obstetricians as primary care physicians. Physician assistants and nurse practitioners also are recognized as primary care providers. The primary care provider is the mainstay of basic care for most individuals.

One of the major changes in health care has been the decrease in the number of solo practice offices and the growth of group and organizational practices. In 1996, for the first time, more physicians were employed in group practice settings than in solo practice offices. Advanced practice nurses and physician assistants also are working in many of these group practice settings. Other RNs in these settings may have responsibility for triage, assessment, teaching and providing direct care. Nursing roles in ambulatory care are expanding as the need for cost-effective use of physician time is modifying practice patterns.

Walk-in Clinics

Walk-in clinics treat clients with emergent conditions that do not require the high-technology resources of the emergency room. Walk-in clinics may be referred to as immediate care facilities, urgent care centers, or emergent care centers and are usually open during extended hours that include evenings and weekends, in addition to the traditional Monday through Friday office hours. Walk-in clinics have grown in popularity as people have found it increasingly difficult to gain access to traditional health care settings because of personal time constraints.

Many walk-in clinics have gradually added services such as sports physical examinations for school-age children, pelvic examinations and Pap tests for women, and routine immunizations. Some are beginning to act as primary care settings, advertising the willingness of staff doctors to become "family doctors." Walk-in clinics have relatively small nursing staffs, often employing only one RN during a shift; therefore, each nurse must have a wide variety of skills and be able to function with a high degree of autonomy. Some settings do not use RNs in direct care; they are hired in these settings only to supervise other clinic staff members and may oversee more than one facility. Licensed practical nurses may be employed in ambulatory care to collect data, carry out specific treatments, and give medications.

COMMUNITY AGENCIES

Agencies providing care in the community include public health agencies, home care agencies, and home hospice care.

Public Health Agencies

Public health departments are operated as agencies of the government. In general, the focus of health departments has been on broad community issues, communicable diseases, and infant and child health. Public health nurses originally did a great deal of individual family visiting, but today fewer funds are available for visits. As a result, public health nurses now focus on individuals who are high risk and whose health affects the entire community, such as those with tuberculosis. Public health nurses responsible for community health issues are required to have a baccalaureate degree in nursing; however, some agencies operate a variety of clinics (such as immunization clinics) in which RNs with an associate degree or diploma provide teaching and direct care services.

Home Care Agencies

Home care agencies, such as the traditional visiting nurse services and the proprietary home health care companies, provide a broad spectrum of care that may include nursing care, personal care assistance, minor housekeeping, physical therapy, occupational therapy, speech/language therapy, and respiratory therapy for individuals in their homes. Teaching family and caregivers is a large part of the home care professional's responsibility. The focus of home care agencies is broad. It ranges from providing short-term visits for clients who need assistance after a hospital stay or acute illness to assisting clients who will need ongoing home care for years, such those requiring dialysis or ventilator support in the home. This care may require nursing care for 8- to 12-hour shifts in the home or episodic visits that last from 15 to 60 minutes.

Hospice Home Care

The goal of *hospice care* is to assist the individual in living as he or she wishes until death. It has gained momentum as a way to provide maximum quality of life to terminally ill people. Multidisciplinary teams may include physicians, nurses, clergy, occupational and physical therapists, home health aides, social workers, and volunteers. The members of multidisciplinary teams work with both the hospice patient and the family or other caregivers. Nurses provide special skills in symptom management for physical problems such as pain, nausea, anorexia, and constipation and psychosocial support for end-of-life events and issues. Nurses are usually responsible for the management and coordination of hospice care.

Community Mental Health Centers

Community mental health centers were established to allow individuals with psychiatric problems to remain in their communities and to end the poor care found in large state mental institutions. Services may include individual counseling and therapy, group or family counseling, evaluation, and referral. For those who must be hospitalized, the community mental health center provides follow-up care that facilitates early discharge. These centers usually employ a variety of mental health workers including psychiatrists, clinical psychologists, social workers, marriage and family counselors, psychiatric nurses, and community workers.

Many psychiatric care providers hoped that psychiatric clients who remained in their communities on an outpatient basis, with family and community ties intact, would have more successful treatment outcomes. Another hoped-for advantage of community mental health centers was that people would seek help more readily when it was available in the community. Unfortunately, community mental health centers have not been funded adequately to meet the many and varied needs of individuals with mental health problems. Mentally ill clients often are eligible for care only when they become acutely ill and not for care that can maintain their health. Some people are not eligible for help because of the complex rules and regulations governing funding. Others do not continue with prescribed treatment and thus relapse; legal constraints do not allow involuntary treatment. Although recognition of the rights of the mentally ill has been important, there also is concern that society expects mentally ill people to make rational decisions about their own best interests when, in fact, they are not mentally capable of understanding the consequences of their actions. The entire area of community mental health has many problems and challenges.

Critical Thinking Activity

Identify an agency in your community that offers home health care. Investigate the services offered by this agency. Compare these with the list of possible services offered by home care agencies mentioned in this chapter. If the lists do not match, analyze the factors in your community that may be responsible for the difference.

Day Care Centers for the Elderly

Elder day care centers provide care for elderly people who cannot safely be alone throughout the day. Each day clients are transported to the center by a family member or a van operated by the center. At the center they receive a variety of social and health services that enable them to continue to live in their own home or a family member's home. Various maintenance and rehabilitative services usually are available, including exercise classes, medication education and supervision, recreational activities, mental health care, and an opportunity to interact with other people. Some centers provide "drop in" or intermittent services for clients who need only one aspect of the program. Other centers provide care each day for clients who need continuing supervision while family members are at work or school. The nursing role in these settings may vary considerably. Some settings have advanced practice nurses who plan care and work with families. Others have RNs who provide medication supervision, assessment for ongoing health problems, and who may lead groups in reminiscence, reality orientation, or validation therapy. LPNs may be hired to give medications and carry out specific treatments.

Ambulatory Care Dialysis Centers

Individuals with chronic renal failure who need ongoing renal dialysis may be managed by home dialysis or by dialysis performed in a dialysis center. A dialysis center provides an environment where the individual who does not have a family care provider or a home dialysis assistant can go two to three times a week for dialysis. Nurses in dialysis centers must have high-level skills because clients with renal failure who need in-center dialysis usually have the most complex problems and coexisting illnesses. Both LPNs and RNs may be employed in these centers.

COLLEAGUES IN HEALTH CARE

Hundreds of different types of health care workers have been identified in the United States. Various providers exist because they meet the needs of our society in some way. It is not within the scope of this book to discuss each of these occupations individually. Table 1-3 provides

TABLE 1-3.	AN OVERVIEW OF COMMON HEALTH CARE OCCUPATIONS	
OCCUPATION	**EDUCATIONAL REQUIREMENTS**	**ROLE**
Dentist Title: Doctor of Dental Surgery (DDS) American Dental Association *www.ada.org*	Bachelor's degree followed by 4-year Doctor of Dentistry program Specialty postgraduate programs available	Provide primary care of the teeth and mouth Prescribe medications related to care of teeth and mouth Perform some health screening, such as blood pressure monitoring, and examine the mouth and throat for tumors or disease and refer to a physician.
Diagnostic Imaging Technologist Titles: Radiologic Technologist (RT) American Society of Radiologic Technicians *www.asrt.org* Sonography Technologist Society of Diagnostic Medical Sonography *www.sdms.org* Nuclear Medicine Technologist Society of Nuclear Medicine Technology *www.snm.org*	2-year hospital-based certificate Associate degree Bachelor's degree in Radiology/ Diagnostic Imaging Technology	Perform radiography, radiation therapy, nuclear medicine, sonography, mammography, CT, magnetic resonance, dosimetry, and cardiovascular interventional technology
Nutritionist or Dietitian Title: Registered Dietitian (RD)	Bachelor's degree plus 6 months–1 year of internship to become a registered dietitian	Plan for the special dietary needs of client populations Work with individual clients in planning appropriate diets and teaching nutrition to meet specific needs
Dietetic Technician Title: Dietetic Technician Registered (DTR) American Dietetic Association *http://www.eatright.org*	Associate degree in dietetic technology	DTR—plan menus and adjust diet plans for individuals in institutional settings, under the supervision of the RD
Occupational Therapist Title: Occupational Therapist Registered (OTR or OT) Title: Occupational Therapy Assistant (OTA) American Occupational Therapy Association (AOTA) *www.aota.org*	Bachelor's or master's degree in occupational therapy Master's degree required after 2007 Associate degree in occupational-therapy assisting	Assist the client in restoring fine-motor skills and performing ADLs Perform treatment, including exercise, the making of splints and assistive devices, and identify ways to modify the environment to make the performance of ADLs possible Analyze work environments to determine ergonomic hazards and identify ergonomically sound conditions and practices. Provide diversional activities (such as crafts or games) appropriate to the client's strength, ability, interest, and physical or psychosocial goals OTA—carry out exercises and treatment plans under the direction of the OT

(*continued*)

TABLE 1-3.   **AN OVERVIEW OF COMMON HEALTH CARE OCCUPATIONS (*Continued*)**

OCCUPATION	EDUCATIONAL REQUIREMENTS	ROLE
Optometrist Title: Doctor of Optometry (OD) American Optometric Association *www.aoanet.org*	Bachelor's degree, followed by 4 years of optometry school	Examine vision and prescribe eyeglasses and contact lenses, low-vision aids, and vision therapy Examine, diagnose, treat, and manage diseases and disorders of the visual system, the eyes and associated structures, as well as diagnose related systemic conditions in states with an expanded scope of practice
Pharmacist Title: Registered Pharmacist (RPh) American Pharmaceutical Association (APhA) *www.aphanet.org*	Previously: Bachelor's degree in pharmacy Requirement beginning 2001: Bachelor's degree in science followed by Pharmacy Doctorate (PharmD) program	Dispense drugs, manage drug therapy, consult with physicians, recommend therapy, assist with monitoring therapy, provide consultation for nurses, and teach clients Perform clinical work in a hospital or other patient care setting
Physical Therapist Title: Registered Physical Therapist (PT)	Bachelor's degree in any field with specified pre-requisites, followed by Master's degree program in PT or doctoral program in physical therapy (DPT)	Restore normal function of large muscle groups, bones, and joints Perform treatments, including exercise, heat and cold therapy, electrical stimulation, and the use of other physical agents Teach the client to use crutches, prostheses, and other assistive devices Teach individuals about safe exercise, provide direction for exercise fitness, and help individuals with health problems to gain maximum function
Physical Therapy Assistant Title: PTA American Physical Therapy Association *www.apta.org*	Associate degree in applied science	PTA—carry out treatment plan under direction of PT
Physician Title: Medical Doctor (MD) *www.ama.org* Doctor of Osteopathy (DO) *www.aoa-net.org*	Bachelor's degree followed by 4-year medical school, followed by 1–4 years of residency	Diagnose and treat disease, including prescribing medications, providing treatment, and performing surgery Plan and order all diagnostic tests and procedures Refer for therapies by other health care providers Manage admission and discharge to any health care facility

TABLE 1-3.	AN OVERVIEW OF COMMON HEALTH CARE OCCUPATIONS (*Continued*)	
OCCUPATION	**EDUCATIONAL REQUIREMENTS**	**ROLE**
Podiatrists (formerly called chiropodists) Title: Doctor of Podiatric Medicine (DPM) American Podiatric Medicine Association (APMA) *www.apma.org/*	Bachelor's degree followed by years of 4-year podiatry medicine program. Two thirds of the states require an additional year of residency before licensure is allowed.	Care for corns, bunions, and toenails Prescribe and fit corrective shoes and arch supports Perform surgery on the feet, such as correcting deformities and removing bunions and small tumors. Treat wounds of the feet.
Respiratory Therapist Title: Registered Respiratory Therapist (RRT)	Associate degree in respiratory therapy	Provide direct care related to respiratory treatments and the use of respiratory devices Give inhaled medications Provide client teaching related to respiratory care procedures
Speech, Language, Hearing Therapist Titles: Registered Speech/ Language Pathologist (RSLP) Speech/Language Pathology Assistant (SLPA) Audiologist American Speech, Language, and Hearing Association *www.asha.org*	Bachelor's degree followed by Master's degree in speech/language pathology Associate degree in speech/language pathology	Assess and plan treatment for rehabilitation needs in speech and language function and swallowing difficulties Serve as a consultant to health care team regarding communication strategies and methods to support swallowing Work with clients, carrying out treatment plans under the direction of the SLP SLPA—provide speech/language treatment under the direction of the RSLP Measure hearing ability, identify hearing disorders, provide rehabilitative services, assess amplification devices and instruct in their care, provide training in speechreading, and serve as consultants to government and industry on issues concerning environmental, noise-induced hearing loss

an overview of the education and licensure for some of the more common health care providers. The discussion below focuses on some of the issues related to the health care professions.

Roles of Health Care Workers

With the many types of health care workers, some concerns have been how those roles are defined, how education or training is provided, and how the role is regulated. Although the major health occupations provide academic education with legal licensure and a defined

Display 1-1   ORGANIZATIONS PROVIDING ALLIED HEALTH ACCREDITATION

1. Accreditation Council for Occupational Therapy Education
2. Commission on Accreditation of Allied Health Education Programs (CAAHEP has 17 separate committees on accreditation; each focuses on a different allied health area.)
3. Joint Review Committee on Educational Programs in Nuclear Medicine Technology
4. Joint Review Committee on Education in Radiologic Technology
5. National Accrediting Agency for Clinical Laboratory Sciences

scope of practice, many of the allied health workers have much less defined roles. For some health care occupations there are differences in regulations and requirements from state to state. One of the major Pew Reports in the 1990s focused on the need for a more clearly described and uniform regulation of health care professionals across the country (O'Neil, 1993). National organizations that provide **accreditation** for allied health educational programs serve to provide standardization of some occupations (Display 1-1).

With a shortage of licensed health care workers in areas such as nursing (Beyers, 2001), and laboratory sciences (Hansen & Laventy, 2001), some employers are advocating for short term training of unlicensed assistive personnel (UAPs). These individuals may be used beyond their knowledge and skills.

Even within professions, increasing specialization has sometimes created conflict over expertise and territory. Pressure from insurers has mandated a decreased use of specialty physicians and mandated that more care stay within the perview of the general practice physician. In five states (New Mexico, Hawaii, Georgia, Illinois, and Tennessee) clinical psychologists may now obtain authority to prescribe medications, a treatment modality formerly limited to physicians and certain advanced practice nurses (Inner turmoil, 2002). This decreases the need for referral to another mental health care provider. Psychiatrists feel that this change decreases the access of clients to the most highly educated person. When nurse anesthetists can be reimbursed independently, more facilities hire those nurse specialists, which decreases the demand for anesthesia physicians. Even within hospital units, some facilities eliminated positions for clinical nurse specialists who were prepared at the master's degree level and assigned their duties to less-well-prepared nurses. Those with greater education argue that the patient loses when the provider has a lesser background. The education, regulation, and use of all health care workers will continue to be an issue in the coming years (Fig. 1-2).

Health Care Worker Supply

There is a short supply of qualified individuals in some health occupations such as nursing, pharmacy, and dental hygiene. There are also geographic shortages, with inner cities and rural areas having the greatest deficit. Within nursing, the aging of the nursing workforce is contributing to the shortage (Fig. 1-3). Another aspect is the lack of care providers

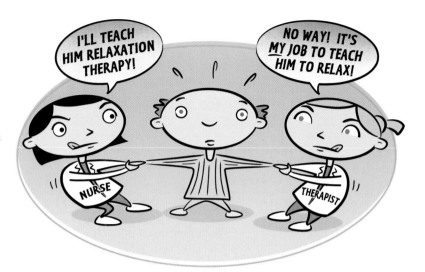

FIGURE 1-2 Overlapping roles and unclear boundaries between health care occupations can lead to conflict.

that share the ethnic background of some patient populations. This may pose special difficulties for both the client and the care provider when the two are unable to communicate effectively. To better meet the needs of all clients, many programs are in place that strive to increase diversity among health care providers. As the health care workforce changes, some clients must alter their perspectives to adapt to a wider diversity in health care providers.

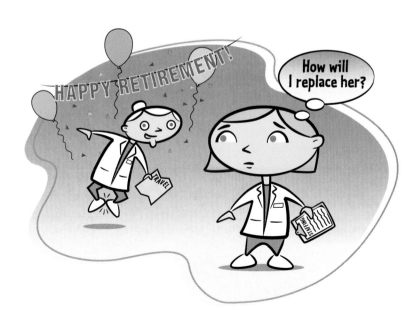

FIGURE 1-3 The aging of the nursing workforce will affect the supply of nurses.

Access to Primary Health Care

The **primary health care provider** furnishes entry into the health care system. These physicians, nurse practitioners, and other providers are licensed in all states and are authorized to treat illness and prescribe drugs. The cornerstone of many managed health care plans is an emphasis on the primary health care provider as the "gatekeeper" for the system (see earlier discussion of a primary care provider). The primary provider implements health maintenance activities that prevent the need for more expensive care. This individual provides referral to more specialized care when it is needed and must often receive permission for referral or for items of higher cost. The belief has been that this would prevent health care consumers from needless focus on higher cost diagnostic tests and specialists. One large managed care company (Aetna) announced in 2002 that it would remove this requirement (Coile, 2001). They identified that there was no significant change in the use of specialists or diagnostic tests with this plan and that there was a significant cost to the extensive record-keeping and management necessary to document that this requirement was met.

Lack of access to primary care has been one of the health care problems for individuals residing in rural areas, economically disadvantaged areas in large cities, and those on welfare programs. Often it has resulted in delaying care until the problem is more complex and requires greater resources to resolve. In urban areas, the lack of access to primary care has often resulted in the inappropriate use of emergency room services for routine illnesses. To meet the needs of society, there is pressure to increase the number of professionals who are authorized to deliver primary care.

Interdisciplinary Teamwork

As the health care system has grown more and more complex, it is clear that it is impossible for one individual, educated to a specific role, to manage all aspects of care. This has led to an increasing emphasis on collaborative work that will provide the benefits available through the expertise of different professions. Interdisciplinary teamwork has always been part of hospice care—physicians, nurses, social workers, therapists, home health aides, and pastoral staff all bring their unique insights to the client's care. The current regulations for long-term care require that there be interdisciplinary collaboration in planning for resident care.

In 1995 in a report titled "Critical Challenges: Revitalizing the Health Professions for the Twenty-first Century," the Pew Health Commission emphasized the importance of interdisciplinary care. Their report further focused on the need for students in health profession programs to begin working in interdisciplinary teams while still students to move effectively into this mode as practitioners. Many nursing programs responded to the Pew Report by developing increased opportunities for nursing students to be involved in interdisciplinary health care.

COMPLEMENTARY AND ALTERNATIVE HEALTH CARE

The National Center for Complementary and Alternative Medicine (NCCAM, 2002) has defined this field as "those healthcare practices and medical practices that are not currently an integral part of conventional medicine" (*http://nccam.nih.gov/health/whatiscam,* 2002).

This definition focuses on what alternative care is *not* more than what it *is*. Part of that definition occurs because of the broad range of health care practices included in this category. The list of health care practices considered complementary and alternative (CAM) is constantly shifting as some are proven safe and effective and enter mainstream practice, others are proven of little value or even harmful and fade from use, and still others emerge.

Major Types of Complementary and Alternative Medicine

As of 2002, the NCCAM has categorized complementary and alternative medicine (CAM) into five domains for the purpose of discussion and study. (This is a change from the former eight domains previously used.) These include alternative medical systems, mind–body interventions, biologically-based treatments, manipulative and body-based methods, and energy therapies. See Tables 1-4 and 1-5.

Specific alternative care providers may use more than one type of treatment in their practice. Additionally, there are many areas of overlap between conventional medical practice and CAM. The major types of alternative care available are described briefly in the following sections.

ALTERNATIVE MEDICAL SYSTEMS

Alternative medical systems represent complete systems of theory and practice that approach health care differently than the traditional Western biomedical approach. The most recent efforts to clarify understanding of complementary and alternative medicine have classified the many different approaches into traditional indigenous systems and unconventional Western systems of medicine (NCCAM, 2002). Each of these systems uses a variety of specific therapies.

Traditional Indigenous Systems. In indigenous medicine, there are complete systems of explanation for health and illness. The therapies chosen are based on these theoretic systems of belief. Often termed *folk medicine,* these traditions usually are handed down by word of mouth and are used to treat common health problems. Indigenous medicine practitioners use a variety of approaches to health care, often combining herbs, food, and traditional ceremonies.

TABLE 1-4. ALTERNATIVE MEDICAL SYSTEMS	
SYSTEM	**EXAMPLES**

Traditional Indigenous Systems	Traditional Oriental medicine
	  Qi gong
	  Acupuncture
	  Herbal medicine
	  Oriental massage
	Ayurvedic medicine
	Native American medicine
	Other folk medicine systems
	(Mexican, South American, etc.)

Unconventional Western Systems	Homeopathy Naturopathy

TABLE 1-5.	TYPES OF COMPLEMENTARY AND ALTERNATIVE THERAPIES
CLASSIFICATIONS	**SPECIFIC THERAPIES**
Mind–Body interventions	Relaxation exercises Hypnosis Meditation Dance Prayer Visualization Biofeedback
Biologic-based therapies	Herbal medicines Special diets Food supplements Vitamin therapy Biologic substances, such as bovine and shark cartilage
Manipulative and body-based healing	Chiropractic Massage therapy Reflexology

Energy therapies	Bioelectromagnetic (BEM) applications to the body
	  Radio-frequency hyperthermia
	  Radio-frequency diathermy
	  Magnets
	  Nerve stimulators
	Biofields—Manipulations of energy fields originating within the body
	  Reiki
	  Therapeutic touch

Little is understood about many of the herbs used, but some have demonstrated therapeutic effects while others may be questionable.

Some indigenous systems are quite formal in approach, with individuals studying and serving apprenticeships before practice. These include traditional oriental medicine and Ayurvedic medicine. Traditional oriental medicine may include the use of qi gong (a form of energy therapy), oriental massage, acupuncture, and herbs. Ayurvedic medicine, a traditional system from India, has existed for more than 5,000 years and has a specific theoretic and therapeutic focus on imbalance in the individual's consciousness. Lifestyle interventions are the major form of Ayurvedic preventive and therapeutic treatment. There is one Ayurvedic hospital in North America.

Other folk systems are more informal. In a given ethnic group, certain people may be designated as healers or as having special knowledge and ability regarding illness. The advice of such a person may be sought instead of the advice of a physician. Native American cultures may use a shaman. Mexican Americans may use the services of a *curandero,* or healer. A system of understanding hot and cold disorders and foods that help to balance heat and cold in the body is part of this folk tradition. NCCAM points out that "other traditional medical systems have been developed by Native American, Aboriginal, African, Middle Eastern, Tibetan, Central and South American cultures" (NCCAM, 2001). To work most effectively with a client who uses folk medicine, you need to investigate the specific beliefs and resources that the client is using.

Unconventional Western Systems of Medicine. Unconventional Western systems of medicine originated in Western society but did not find general support. Some individuals continued to practice in the theoretic precepts of these systems and some have re-emerged as the public looks for alternatives to conventional medical care.

Perhaps the most common of these unconventional systems is homeopathy. **Homeopathy** is based on the belief that exposure to extremely small quantities of either the substance causing an illness or a related substance will stimulate a cure. Of course, this principle is also the basis for immunization and allergy desensitization. The application of this principle to other diseases, however, has not been accepted by the medical community. The dilutions used in many homeopathic remedies are so great that a dosage may contain only a few molecules of a substance. Homeopathy was popular in the early 20th century but fell into disrepute as standard medical research advanced. There is currently a resurgence of interest in this approach to therapy, and some new research is being done. Homeopathic practitioners once again are offering an alternative to standard medical care.

Naturopathy gets its name from the natural agents used in treating disease, such as food, exercise, air, water, and sunshine. The naturopathic physician treats people by recommending changes in lifestyle, diet, and exercise, and the use of vitamins and herbs. For many, this is a successful form of treatment. Naturopathic physicians follow a prescribed course of study that includes clinical experiences with clients and results in the doctor of naturopathy (ND) degree. Naturopathy is licensed in some states.

MIND–BODY INTERVENTIONS

Mind–body interventions seek to control physical processes through the mind's capacities. In addition, they treat emotional concerns. Increasingly, mind–body interventions are being incorporated into standard health care practice. Traditional psychotherapy, a well-established part of standard health care, is a mind–body approach to health. The use of prayer, support groups, yoga, meditation, relaxation, biofeedback, and visualization are all mind–body therapies.

Relaxation exercises, hypnosis, and meditation are examples of controlling physiologic stress responses through mental processes. Relaxation exercises, breathing techniques, meditation, and visualization are used to reduce anxiety, reduce blood pressure, and lessen the body's response to stressors. These techniques also are designed to prevent stress-related problems from developing; for many people, they are part of a plan to increase health and well-being. These techniques also are suggested for the management of specific health problems and may be used in conjunction with traditional medical treatment.

Every major religion of the world responds in particular ways to those who are ill. A well-established way for supporting an ill person is through the prayers of others who care. Nurses recognize that spiritual distress has a significant impact on a client's ability to move toward wellness. Supporting the individual's quest for spiritual solace and healing has been a part of the mission of many health care agencies that were established by religious bodies. The separation of prayer and spiritual care from other health care is a modern phenomenon.

Visualization may be used to help children manage painful medical procedures. Suggestions regarding healing and postoperative recovery are used in the operating room by some anesthesiologists and surgeons. The anesthesiologist may talk to the patient who is still anesthetized, suggesting that pain will be minimal, nausea will not occur, and recovery will be

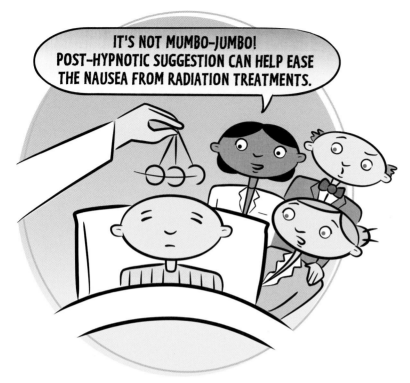

IT'S NOT MUMBO-JUMBO!
POST-HYPNOTIC SUGGESTION CAN HELP EASE
THE NAUSEA FROM RADIATION TREATMENTS.

FIGURE 1-4 Alternative health care is moving more and more into mainstream practice.

rapid. This is similar to posthypnotic suggestion. Hypnosis has been used in other illnesses for symptom relief (Fig. 1-4).

Biofeedback is a specific mechanism to assist individuals to alter physiologic responses through mental processes. The machines used for biofeedback provide visual or auditory feedback of physiologic parameters such as blood pressure or galvanic skin response. By observing these parameters, the individual learns to change the underlying physiologic process. Some individuals with migraine headaches use biofeedback control over circulation to abort migraine attacks rather than taking medications.

Mind–body interventions in general allow people to participate actively in their own care. People often are changed emotionally and psychologically in the process of treating illness or disease. A big advantage of the mind–body therapies is that they are safe and economical and can be used easily in conjunction with other therapies.

BIOLOGIC-BASED THERAPIES

Biologic-based therapies include **herbal medicine**, special diets, food supplements, vitamins, and specific biologic substances such as bovine and shark cartilage.

Herbal medicines are plant products that are used to treat almost all illnesses. We know that plants often have active ingredients that affect the human body. Digitalis, for example, was originally a dried leaf of the foxglove plant. (Digitalis drugs are now synthesized in the laboratory.) It was indeed a potent and effective medication when used as an herb, but dosage was not accurate and little scientific information existed regarding its effects. As research into plant products continues, our understanding of the efficacy of herbs is increasing. Many herbalists in the United States are Asian Americans who received their training in herbs during an apprenticeship with an experienced herbalist. Many naturopathic physicians also use herbs.

It is wise to recognize the potential problems as well as the potential benefits of the use of herbal medicines. Individual plants may vary in their concentration of active chemicals. This makes accurate and stable dosage of herbs difficult. Sometimes the active ingredient may have potent side effects. For example, many individuals have used herbs that contain ephedra. Ephedra acts as a stimulant, dilates bronchioles, and decreases appetite. Therefore, it has been used for the herbal treatment of fatigue, asthma, and obesity. It also raises blood pressure, increases pulse rate, and creates feelings of tension and anxiety. These side effects have been severe enough to precipitate stroke and cardiac problems in some individuals.

At present, there are no laws regulating the potency or purity of herbs sold in the United States. Because herbs are not considered drugs, there are no regulations regarding testing for efficacy or safety as there are with drugs that must be approved by the Food and Drug Administration (FDA). Thus, information about safety may only be available after problems have arisen and been reported with enough frequency to come to the attention of authorities. Some countries such as Germany have regulated herbal medications for many years. Canada is currently considering regulating herbs.

Many herbs are imported from around the world. Rules and regulations regarding accurate labeling and content purity may not be as strict in some developing countries as they are in the United States. This means that some herbs that are sold may contain contaminants. Serious illnesses and even deaths have been traced to contaminants in herbal medicines. Herbs may also interact with prescription and over-the-counter medications, altering the effect or increasing side effects.

Clients taking herbal medicines should be encouraged to share this information with their health care provider. They also should be encouraged to question carefully the sources of the herbs that they take. These actions might help clients avoid potentially harmful interactions with prescribed medications or other adverse effects.

Biologic treatments include a variety of substances not approved as medical treatment by the Food and Drug Administration. These products have been developed by individuals and organizations and are often sold as food supplements rather than as medicines. Cartilage products from sharks, cattle, sheep, and chickens are being used to treat both cancer and arthritis. Peptide fractions derived from human blood and urine, called antineoplastons, are being used to treat cancer. Coley's toxins are killed cultures of bacteria that have been used for treating cancer. Apitherapy is the use of honeybee venom to treat rheumatic diseases, dermatologic conditions, chronic pain, and cancer. Research on the efficacy of these treatments is costly, and sponsors willing to bear that cost are hard to find. Some small studies are being funded with federal grants.

The health food movement in the United States is extraordinarily popular. Countless books are written and innumerable products are produced for this market. One of the appeals of this approach to health care is that it focuses on everyday, natural resources as opposed to science and technology. Poor dietary practices are common in the United States, with many individuals eating far more fat than is recommended and neglecting fruits, vegetables, and whole grains. Many people achieve better health by paying attention to good nutrition.

Medical research is beginning to identify some benefits of using food and vitamins in therapeutic ways. We have long known that many individuals who develop type 2 diabetes later in life may be able to manage their blood sugar through dietary control. The role of antioxidants in decreasing cell damage and the effect of certain phytochemicals contained in cruciferous vegetables in preventing bowel cancer are just two examples of the theoretic benefits of nutrients.

There are hazards in this approach to health care, however. Megadoses of vitamins may prove toxic. Some nutrients interact with medications, decreasing their effectiveness. Individuals who choose to avoid all traditional medical care and rely on unsubstantiated claims about the therapeutic effects of nutrients may suffer a deterioration in health.

All health care professionals need to support and encourage healthy dietary practices. Often it is possible to assist clients who rely on the use of nutrients for health care by becoming knowledgeable about the research regarding nutrition, accepting what clients believe helps them (as long as it is not detrimental to their well-being), and keeping an open mind. When you are willing to acknowledge the validity of some aspects of their preferred approach to health care, these clients may be willing to combine more conventional medical care along with their nutritional approaches.

MANIPULATIVE AND BODY-BASED TREATMENTS

Manual healing is the physical manipulation of the body to achieve health goals. Perhaps the most commonly known type of manual healing is chiropractic. Manual healing also is found in massage therapy and reflexology. Massage therapy uses both fixed and movable pressure and holding by the hands and sometimes the forearms, elbows, and feet. There is evidence that these techniques affect the musculoskeletal, circulatory–lymphatic, and nervous systems. Reflexology is massage of the feet to activate points on the feet that correspond to other body parts or systems.

Chiropractic care is based on the theory that disease is caused by interference with nerve function. It uses manipulation of the body joints, especially the spinal vertebrae, in seeking to restore normal function. The chiropractor also may use other treatments commonly associated with physical therapy, such as massage and exercise. There are definite differences among chiropractors. Some state that there are illnesses that cannot be treated through manual healing and do recommend that certain clients seek conventional medical care. Others believe that all illnesses may be treated by chiropractic methods and do not refer clients for conventional medical care. A major concern is that some clients may have more serious illnesses that may be missed altogether or not recognized in time to be given optimal medical attention. Another problem with chiropractic care is the use of chiropractic treatments on infants and young children in place of immunizations and other well-child services.

Many people with joint and muscle strain and tension find that chiropractic treatments relieve discomfort and support effective functioning. The Agency for Health Care Policy and Research recommends chiropractic treatment as a useful option in specific circumstances for relieving pain discomfort in acute back pain (ACHPR, 1994, *www.ahrq.gov*).

ENERGY THERAPIES

The use of energy therapies (sometimes referred to bioelectromagnetic [BEM] therapies) is based on the understanding that electrical phenomena are found in all living organisms. There are magnetic fields that extend from the body, which can be measured and may be affected by external forces. The mechanisms by which the electromagnetic fields occur in the body, how these can be changed, and the effects of such changes are under study. Many modalities have been used for years without clear studies of their effectiveness. Some believe that bio-electromagnetics may be a unifying theory explaining why such widely diverse therapies as acupuncture and homeopathy produce results.

Some energy therapies are based on applying external energy to the body. There are thermal applications of BEM therapy in the form of radio frequency hyperthermia and radio frequency diathermy. Nonthermal applications include magnets and nerve stimulation. One common application is the use of magnets to relieve musculoskeletal problems. Magnetic insoles for shoes and magnets to be worn on the body are sold widely.

There are also methods used to manipulate the interior biofields of the individual. These include **therapeutic touch** and reiki. Both of these practices are based on a system of changing the energy fields without applying external energy forces to the body.

Understanding the Use of Complementary and Alternative Health Care

The use of complementary and alternative health has been steadily increasing in the United States (Eisenberg, Ettner, Appel, Wilkey, Van Rompay, & Keesler, 1998). For many clients with chronic conditions, mainstream medical care offers few options. Long-term treatments with medications often produce their own iatrogenic (treatment-caused) health problems, some of which are as troubling to the individual as the original disease process. A common response to these problems has been to add more medications and more treatments, each with its own potential adverse effects. Mainstream health care providers often give little attention to the problems of daily living that are of greatest concern to the individual. Stress and anxiety also add to the burden of these clients. For clients with acute health conditions, certain treatments or medications may produce unpleasant or harmful side effects. Clients often are looking for alternative treatment methods that do not appear to have the same potential for harm.

Some alternative therapies have been available for many years, and there are people who believe that they have been significantly helped by these approaches. Unfortunately, traditional health care providers often have dismissed these therapies without investigating them thoroughly. On the other hand, few alternative therapies have been formally researched, and proponents often rely on undocumented reports of effectiveness.

Research into alternative therapies now is supported by the federal government but only in a small way compared to other research. The federal government has an Office of Alternative Health Care and a Web page of references, the National Center for Complementary and Alternative Medicine. (See list of Web sites.) More attention is being paid to the responses of individuals. Concern about the role of stress in illness has prompted an increased openness to nonmedical methods of managing stress. The possibility of alternative care practices working in a complementary fashion with traditional medical care is gaining wider acceptance. Often these **complementary therapies** are used to address the whole person and not simply the disease.

Part of the appeal of alternative health care is the caring and personalized response that clients often receive. People who have been intimidated by businesslike clinics and made to feel unimportant by impersonal professionals may find that the warm, concerned, accepting atmosphere of the nonconventional setting meets many personal needs. The fact that stress and anxiety play a major role in any health problem may help explain why many people are helped by therapies that may not be based on sound scientific knowledge.

To learn more about any specific therapy, or to research alternative and complementary therapies for any condition, you can use the CAM Citation Index found on the Web site of the National Center for Complementary and Alternative Medicine (see references). You may also use MEDLINE at the National Library of Medicine to research various therapies.

ASSISTING CLIENTS WHO CHOOSE ALTERNATIVE HEALTH CARE

Many people who support conventional methods of health care have long ignored or repudiated the value of unorthodox health care traditions. We must recognize that complementary and alternative health care practices have persisted because people have found them to be valuable. Acknowledging health care alternatives and working cooperatively with them is usually much more productive than trying to oppose them.

The NCCAM suggests a five-step process for the consumer considering a particular **complementary** or **alternative therapy**. This process has a heavy emphasis on careful information gathering.

First the individual should assess the safety and effectiveness of the therapy in relationship to his or her own condition. One of the difficulties is finding accurate safety and efficacy data. Web sites and other sources of information need close scrutiny to determine the qualifications and bias of the sponsoring individual or group. The NCCAM Web site (*www.nccam.nih.gov*) has Fact Sheets regarding some specific therapies and additional links to research reports and scientific papers. Research reports may also be found through PubMed, the National Library of Medicine's online access (*www.ncbi.nlm.nih.gov/PubMed*). All complementary and alternative therapies are classified there under the Medical Subject Heading (MeSH) of "complementary therapies." The University of Pittsburgh Health Sciences Library System maintains an Alternative Medicine Homepage (*www.pitt.edu/~cbw/altm.html*) that provides links to additional information sites on the Web.

The second step is to examine the expertise of any therapy practitioner. Whether this person is a physician or another type of provider, determine whether there is appropriate education and licensing if that is required. Some consumer organizations will direct individuals to reliable practitioners in the community. The client might also want to talk with others who have had experience with the practitioner in question. Clients should not hesitate to ask the practitioner about education and credentials. The Center for the Health Professions at the University of California, San Francisco, have published a template by Dower, O'Neil, and Hough (2001) for asking questions about an alternative health care provider. These are summarized on the Center's Web page.

Service delivery is the third aspect the client should investigate. How many patients are seen per day? Where is the therapy available and what barriers does that pose? Are there standards for safety, privacy, and confidentiality in place?

A fourth consideration is the cost of the therapy. Part of this is investigating what coverage may be obtained from an insurance carrier. Are the costs clear? How are payments made? Some unscrupulous practitioners collect large sums of money before any service and then may not provide what was promised.

The fifth step is to discuss this proposed treatment with a regular health care provider. The interaction of any traditional treatment and a complementary or alternative treatment may or may not pose a problem. Many health care providers support the use of various complementary therapies.

Things that the health care provider must also consider are such issues as client choice, informed consent, and the ethical principles of beneficence and nonmaleficence (see Chapter 9). As complementary and alternative therapies move into the mainstream, greater accountability to the public is essential.

Critical Thinking Activity

Identify a specific form of complementary or alternative therapy. Do a literature search regarding this therapy. Review the information available in other sources. Analyze the information to determine whether the data supporting the use of this therapy are weak, moderate, or strong. Provide a rationale for your determination.

KEY CONCEPTS

- The various types of health care services are differentiated by the needs of the client being served and range from specific specialized services to skilled care to custodial care.
- Many different types of agencies provide health care services, including long-term care settings, acute care hospitals, ambulatory care centers, home care agencies, and health care businesses. There are a wide variety of nursing roles in these different settings. Health care agencies are classified according to length of stay, mix of services provided, and ownership of the agency.
- Acute care facilities center around the work of the traditional hospital, which has become a hub for health care in most communities.
- Long-term care facilities provide many types of care. Nursing homes provide care for those without the ability to manage activities of daily living and who need ongoing care. Assisted-living centers provide fewer services. Rehabilitation centers assist the individual in returning to a maximum level of independence.
- Ambulatory care settings provide care on an outpatient basis. This care may range from simple office calls for common illnesses and health promotion activities such as immunizations to the performance of ambulatory surgery.
- Home health agencies offer a wide variety of care services that may include traditional public health services, high-intensity skilled care in the home, and rehabilitation services. Home care agencies offer services within the home that assist individuals in avoiding institutional care settings when they are unable to complete their own activities of daily living.
- Changes in the health care delivery system are creating many problems that affect health care workers. Among these are issues related to primary care, accreditation of health professional education programs, and the future of health professional education and licensure.
- Alternative health care is growing in popularity. Some types of alternative care are being used along with traditional medical care as complementary therapies. Understanding the different types of alternative health care services, why people choose alternative health care, and how you may assist people who seek this care will form a foundation for more effective relationships with clients.

RELEVANT WEB SITES

Agency for Healthcare Research and Quality (AHRQ—formerly Agency for Health Care Policy and Research: Practice Guidelines [AHCPR]) *www.ahrq.gov*

Alternative Medicine Home Page. Folk Library of the Health Sciences, University of Pittsburgh provides links to Internet information regarding alternative health care: *www.pitt.edu/~cbw/altm.html*

American Pain Society: Policies and Recommendations on Pain Management: *www.ampainsoc.org*

Joint Commission for the Accreditation of Healthcare Organizations (JCAHO): *www.jcaho.org*

National Center for Complementary and Alternative Medicine: Federal Government database of scientific articles and abstracts: *http://www.nccam.nih.gov*

National Guideline Clearinghouse: *www.guideline.gov/index.asp*

National League for Nursing Accrediting Commission: Nursing Education Accreditation Standards and Criteria: *www.nlnac.org*

National Library of Medicine, MEDLINE data base search through PubMed: *ncbi.nlm.nih.gov/PubMed*

REFERENCES

Beyers, M. (2001). Nursing workforce: A perspective for now and the future. *JONAS Healthcare Law, Ethics, & Regulation 3*(4), 109–113.

Coile, R. C. (2001). Competing in a "consumer choice" market. *Journal of Healthcare Management 46*(5), 297–301.

Dower, C., O'Neil, E., Hough, H. (2001). Profiling the professions: A model for evaluating emerging health professions, Center for the Health Professions, University of California, summary retrieved from the World Wide Web at *www.futurehealth.ucsf.edu* on April 20, 2002.

Eisenberg, D. M., Ettner, R. B., Appel, S., Wilkey, S., Van Rompay, M., & Keesler, R. C. (1998). Trends in alternative medicine use in the United States, 1990–1997: Results of a follow-up national survey. *Journal of the American Medical Association 280,* 1569–1575.

Fonda, S. J., Clipp, E. C., & Maddox, G. L. (2002). Patterns in functioning among residents in affordable assisted living housing facility. *Gerontologist 42*(2), 178–187.

Hansen, K. & Laventy, D. (2001). Laboratory personnel shortages. *Clinical Laboratory Sciences 14*(3), 130.

Hawryluk, M. (1999). Final rule clarifies coverage issue. *Provider 25*(10):33–34.

Healthcare demand soars. (October 3, 2001). *The Herald*, p. A9, Everett, WA.

"Inner turmoil," *Scientific American 287*(1):25–26, 2002.

National Center for Complementary and Alternative Medicine (NCCAM). (2002). Major domains of complementary and alternative medicine, retrieved from the World Wide Web at *www.nccam.nih.gov/fcp/classify/* on February 23, 2002.

O'Neil, E. H. (1993). Health professions education for the future: Schools in service to the nation. San Francisco: Pew Health Professions Commission.

Pew Health Profession Commission. (1995). Critial challenges: Revitalizing the health professions for the twenty-first century. San Francisco: UCSF Center for the Health Professions.

West, B. (2000). Assisted living gains accreditation option. *Provider 26*(11), 53–54.

2

Health Care Finance and Control

LEARNING OUTCOMES

After completing this chapter, you should be able to:

1. Describe different means for financing health care.
2. Describe actions taken by the federal government that have influenced the financing of health care and the function of the system.
3. Discuss the various approaches to managing costs in the health care delivery system, including changing patterns of payment and controlling providers.
4. Analyze the issues related to access to health care, including types of barriers and indicators of access.
5. Discuss the mechanisms being used to measure and assure quality in organizations and agencies that are delivering health care.
6. Analyze the use of power by regulatory agencies, payers, providers, and consumers in the health care system.
7. Explain continuing concerns regarding the effective use of health care and concerns about changing the system.

KEY TERMS

Acuity

Capitation

Case management

Case mix

Comorbidity

Cost containment

Diagnosis-related groups (DRGs)

Disease manager

Entitlement

Fee-for-service payment

Health maintenance organization (HMO)

Independent practice association (IPA)

Insurance

Intensity measures

Joint Commission on Accreditation of Healthcare Organizations (JCAHO)

Key indicators

Long-term care

Managed care

Medicaid

Medicare

Medicare intermediary (carrier)

Medigap insurance

Minimum data set (MDS)

Outcome measures

Point-of-service plan

Power

Preferred provider organization (PPO)

Primary care provider

Prospective payment

Prospective payment system (PPS)

Quality indicators (QI)

Resource utilization groups (RUGs)

Third-party payer

Skilled nursing care

Vertically integrated systems

Throughout the world, the concern over health care has everyone's attention. In most of the industrialized world, with the exception of the United States, health care is seen as a right or an **entitlement** of every citizen. Based on this right, health care in most industrialized countries is operated by governmental systems that provide universal health care coverage. In some countries, such as Sweden and the Netherlands, there is strong centralization of financing and control. In other countries, such as Canada and Germany, systems are controlled regionally through provincial authority. These governmental systems are successful in accomplishing overall health outcomes such as low maternal–infant mortality, high immunization rates, and reduction of preventable deaths. The problems found in these systems are related to the high cost of providing health care and subsequent attempts to control those costs. The delay before receiving care may be long and some care, especially care that is very costly such as dialysis, may be rationed. Because of these situations, private medical care that is paid for by individuals also may be available to those with sufficient income.

In developing nations, health care may be limited or almost nonexistent. Some care may be paid for by the government and some by private means, but there are not enough individual nor institutional providers to meet the needs of the population. The available resources may not meet the standards that those in more affluent countries have come to expect. Hospitals may lack adequate safe water and sanitation. Ordinary supplies such as dressing materials and sterile needles may be unavailable. Drugs may be in short supply, and diagnostic and laboratory testing may be nonexistent. Health care outcomes in these countries tend to be poor, especially regarding infant and child mortality. The World Health Organization (WHO) is most active in these developing nations, trying to improve health outcomes through immunization, sanitation, and other public health programs.

In the United States, health care has not been accepted as a right for the whole society. Therefore, no mechanism exists to build a coordinated health care system. Much of the complexity found in the U.S. health care system relates to the variety of mechanisms for funding and controlling health care. Although the United States has ready access to the most sophisticated medical technology and expertise, deficiencies are seen in some of the key measures of population health. Some individuals have access to the most effective health care in the world, while others have no health care access except in cases of emergency, when hospitals are required by law to provide care.

This chapter explains the various organizations and agencies responsible for health care financing and control in the United States, and how that affects the availability of health care and access to it. Understanding this aspect of the health care system can enable you to be a more effective participant in it.

FINANCING HEALTH CARE FOR INDIVIDUALS

Currently, there are many different approaches to financing health care for individuals in the United States. Personal payment, charitable care, **insurance** plans, **health maintenance organizations (HMOs),** and a variety of government programs are all forms of health care financing. Agencies such as insurance companies and government programs that pay providers for health services provided to individuals are termed **third-party payers** (Display 2-1). Increasingly, decisions about an individual's health care are made by a combination of the patient-consumer, the provider, and the payer rather than by any one of them alone.

Personal Payment

Originally, health care was paid for each time it was provided. Although the payment was usually in cash, in a more rural society payment sometimes extended to barter, with garden produce, chickens, and eggs traded for medical care. Individuals who did not have the means to pay for a doctor or hospital visit often did not receive needed care.

Today most individuals still pay for health care but often in indirect ways that make them less aware of the specific costs. Health insurance premiums may be deducted from a paycheck,

Display 2-1   APPROACHES TO FINANCING HEALTH CARE

- Personal payment
- Charitable care
- Health insurance plans
- Health maintenance organizations
- State-administered health plans
- Federal government programs

or an employer may pay premiums directly, considering them part of employee compensation. Most health insurance plans require the subscriber to pay a deductible (a portion of the bill), which may be computed for each service or may be an aggregate for the year. The size of the deductible that is the individual's responsibility has been increasing in many insurance plans, giving people greater incentive to use services wisely.

Charitable Care

Charitable care has played a significant role in the history of health care. The earliest hospitals were religious institutions that provided health care as a form of ministry and as a charitable service. Some large charitable groups still provide a great deal of care for people who are unable to pay, such as the Shriner's Children's Hospitals. Although these hospitals do collect insurance and payment from those who can afford care, they also raise money for the purpose of providing high-level care to children in need.

During the 1970s and 1980s, federal funds were made available through the Hill-Burton Act for hospital construction. Hospitals constructed with these funds accepted an obligation to provide some charitable care in their communities. As these obligations expired, concern about what was happening in emergency care led to legislation that requires hospitals to provide emergency care regardless of an individual's ability to pay.

Historically, some money for charitable care was raised through donations. As insurance became more widespread, hospitals often supported charitable care by charging paying clients more than the cost of their care and using the excess income to offset the costs of charitable care. However, as negotiations for lower health care costs for managed care continue and regulations have limited Medicare reimbursement, hospitals are experiencing a decreased ability to provide charitable care without severe financial difficulties. (Medicare is discussed more fully later in this chapter.)

Individual physicians also have provided forms of charitable care. Only rarely did people directly ask physicians for charitable care; rather, the physician often did not pursue the payment of a bill that could not be paid by a family. Physicians and other care providers also have provided charitable care by volunteering their time at "free" clinics. Many people who could not afford care simply did without because they did not want to ask for charity.

Health Insurance Plans

Starting in the 1930s, insurance companies gradually began to pay a greater share of medical fees. The basic framework of insurance coverage is that of shared risk of having high cost health care needs. Individuals pay for coverage whether or not they incur health care costs; when an insured individual requires health care, the insurance pays for that care. Thus the individual has a stable health care cost without the risk of incurring high costs that are difficult to meet from ordinary income and the insurance company stays financially solvent because more money is coming in than is going out.

Historically, health insurance was for hospital care and related services only. Outpatient visits, immunizations, costs of drugs, and other such benefits were not covered by insurance policies. One disadvantage of this system was that consumers had no incentive to reduce their use of services; they paid the same regardless of their needs or use of the system. People sought to have care delivered on an inpatient basis to obtain reimbursement. Another disadvantage was that individuals often neglected preventive health care that had to be paid for out-of-pocket. Health insurance policies now cover many preventive services, outpatient costs, and some prescription costs.

At the heart of the process of setting insurance rates and specifying coverage is identifying what will be covered, determining the risk (probability) of health services being needed for different groups of individuals, and projecting the costs of care. The more heterogeneous the group, the more likely that the average cost for those in the plan will mirror the population average, and therefore, insurance costs will be kept reasonable for all. Limitations on coverage that eliminate individuals with high probability of needing services (such as the elderly diabetic) protect insurance companies from the risk of excessive costs. When high-risk individuals are excluded from insurance, it lessens the cost for low-risk subscribers within the plan, but leaves those who are most in need of assistance without the benefit of insurance.

Most insurance companies are private profit-making companies owned by stockholders. They provide service to policyholders in return for insurance payments and create profit for stockholders in the company. Aetna is an example of a nationwide for-profit insurance company that primarily provides plans for employers to offer to groups of employees.

Nonprofit insurance companies are established within different legal regulations. They are "owned" by those who have insurance policies. All profits from the company are theoretically used to enhance the company or to decrease the cost of the insurance. Additionally, the nonprofit companies have certain benefits in terms of taxes. The "Blues" (Blue Cross and Blue Shield companies) originally were established as not-for-profit organizations.

Legal regulations place restrictions on the rate setting, investments, and general management of nonprofit companies that do not apply to private profit-making companies. This has limited their ability to grow in size and compete for some types of business. In some areas of the country, Blue Cross and Blue Shield have asked regulatory authorities for permission to convert from nonprofit to profit-making status and to sell stock in the company (and have changed their names in the process). In some states, courts have required that these corporations provide remuneration to their communities in return for this change in status. In other states, these changes have occurred without public input.

As the cost of health care has increased, insurance premiums also have increased greatly. An additional public concern is that health insurance is unobtainable for individuals with existing health problems and often economically beyond the means of those who are not insured as part of an employee group. Legislation to require insurance companies to cover everyone has passed in some jurisdictions and is being considered in others. One of the responses by insurance companies to this legislation is to withdraw from selling insurance in the state that requires insurance companies to insure anyone who seeks coverage. The insurance companies argue that individuals do not carry insurance when they are well; when faced with illness, they purchase insurance, receive reimbursement far in excess of any premiums paid, and then drop coverage when they are well.

Although insurance companies originally focused on paying for health care, they now are involved in establishing standards for care, evaluating care, and negotiating charges. They are active participants in all areas of health care and, because of the economic power they wield, have great influence. Insurance companies determine whom they will pay and what procedures they will reimburse. Thus, insurance companies can and do limit health care choices.

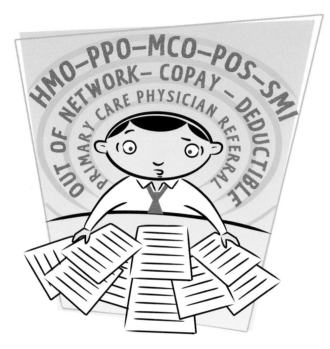

FIGURE 2-1 Health care insurance plans are complex and often confusing to the ordinary consumer.

All insurance plans have written rules regarding notification, acceptable providers, and precisely when and how reimbursement will occur. Sometimes these rules result in a denial of payment. Many people have expressed concern about the process of reviewing and denying insurance claims (Fig. 2-1). Realistically, the foremost goal of most health insurance plans is to return a profit to investors. Providing good health care to an individual is a means to that end and not the focus of effort.

Federal legislation, the Health Insurance Portability and Accountability Act (HIPAA), was passed in 1996. Title 1 of that act focuses on measures that assist in maintaining health care insurance coverage for those who change or lose their jobs. (See *http://aspe.hhs.gov/ admnsimp/pl104191.htm* for the full text of the Act.) The Center for Medicare and Medicaid Services maintains a Web site (*http://cms.hhs.gov/hipaa/*) with consumer information regarding the protections provided by this federal legislation to allow people to maintain coverage when they change jobs. This legislation also has provided tax incentives for those purchasing **long-term care** insurance. (The HIPAA legislation had additional provisions regarding patient health records' privacy that will be discussed in Chapter 8, Legal Responsibilities for Practice.)

Most elderly individuals who receive Medicare also pay for supplemental insurance to cover the part of the health care bill for which Medicare does not pay. This is commonly referred to as **Medigap insurance**. (See discussion of Medicare later in the chapter.)

Health Maintenance Organizations

Health maintenance organizations originated as an alternative to traditional insurance plans and were nonprofit in nature. Although traditional insurance plans paid for care when subscribers were ill, HMOs were the first to provide payment for care aimed at preventing illness.

Health maintenance organizations provided well-child care, prenatal care, immunizations, gynecologic examinations, and other preventive services when insurance companies did not provide these services.

Because the HMO receives the same income (except for modest copayments) whether a client requires extensive care or very little care, there is a built-in incentive to emphasize preventive care and avoid costly hospitalization. A flat charge per month covers routine preventive health care, care for illness, hospitalization and, in some instances, prescription costs, outpatient care, and other services. HMO-enrolled individuals are often responsible for a copayment (meaning the client pays a part of the bill). Copayments support part of the cost of care and give the consumer an incentive to use services wisely.

Health maintenance organizations are currently characterized by many differing patterns of finance and governance. Some are operated by insurance companies; some are private profit-making organizations; some are nonprofit organizations; and still others are consumer owned and operated. Many newer HMOs operate as business entities that manage the financial aspects of health care and, through financial management, access to services.

Health maintenance organizations are also characterized by differing patterns of providing health services. Primary health care providers may be employed by an HMO and receive a fixed salary. In some cases, a group of primary health care providers, termed an **independent practice association** (IPA), may contract with an HMO to provide services for a preset fee per individual in the program. HMOs also may employ many other health care workers, including nurses. In some HMOs, clients have a choice of care providers; in others they do not. HMO plans that allow an individual the option of going outside of the plan for services that the plan does not or will not provide are called **point-of-service plans**. Usually the subscriber is eligible for some reimbursement of costs for these outside services, but by a greatly reduced amount.

Health maintenance organizations were the first type of health plan to provide managed care. The concept of managed care has broadened considerably and now includes many types of health plans. Managed care is discussed in detail later in this chapter.

Health maintenance organizations have been in existence in the United States for more than 50 years, but their growth in number was slow until federal legislation in 1972 and 1974 created economic incentives to start new HMOs. Because HMOs traditionally had lower health care costs than conventional fee-for-service systems, the federal government subsidized the creation of new HMOs and encouraged employers to offer HMOs as alternatives to traditional health insurance plans. Federal subsidizing of HMOs also helps to contain costs in all health plans as a result of competition.

People on Medicare now have the option of joining HMOs. Under such circumstances, Medicare makes a single payment for each individual Medicare recipient directly to the HMO, and the HMO provides all care without the individual needing to purchase additional Medigap insurance. The amount per individual was calculated as an average of the expenses incurred by Medicare recipients for all costs. The original Medicare HMOs advertised "no copays" and "full prescription coverage" to attract new members. The HMOs expected to be able to provide this through carefully managed care that would decrease the use of costly services. However, most HMOs in operation today have a copayment fee and assess some charges for prescriptions.

Beginning in 1998, a crisis occurred in Medicare HMOs. Many plans found that overall costs were greater than anticipated. The savings managed care had successfully demonstrated when caring for a broad range of ages did not materialize when they were working with the older population who tend to have more chronic illnesses and more serious health problems. They could not sustain all the promised benefits within the Medicare payments. These HMOs refused to renew their contracts to provide Medicare-HMO services. This left many elderly individuals with difficult choices to make as they returned to conventional Medicare plus Medigap Supplemental Insurance. These conventional plans often did not provide outpatient pharmacy coverage, thus greatly increasing the costs of health management for the individual.

State-Administered Health Plans

States may operate a variety of health care resources for residents. All states manage some type of insurance plan for workers injured on the job. These workers' compensation plans may be managed as a state monopoly or may be contracted to private insurance companies. Employers are required to pay premiums based upon statistical information about covered injuries and hazards in various job categories. An individual injured on the job is assured of receiving care paid for by the workers' compensation plan.

Some states administer health insurance plans on a wider basis. Hawaii assures universal health care coverage for its residents. Minnesota has been a leader in attempting to provide health services for all its residents. The state of Washington has developed an insurance plan called the Basic Health Plan for working individuals who earn too much money to be eligible for tax-supported health care, but who do not have incomes high enough to afford regular insurance. Unfortunately, this plan, which is subsidized by tax revenue, cannot accommodate all who are eligible.

The federal government also provides funds through the Medicaid programs that are administered by the states and matched with state funds. Included in this funding are the costs of health care for families on public assistance and support of nursing home care for those who have exhausted their personal financial resources. In 1999 the federal government provided a mechanism for states to enlarge their Medicaid programs so they could enroll children from low-income families who did not qualify for Medicaid and who would otherwise be without health care coverage. This Children's Health Insurance Plan (CHIP) represents the first time that the United States has supported health care as a right for all children. Not all states have agreed to participate in the plan because it requires their financial contribution and provides for some federal control of the program.

Most states support state mental hospitals and public health services. Additional public health services may be supplied through county and city governments. Hospitals designed to provide care for those who are indigent may be operated by the city (such as New York City hospitals) or by the county (such as Cook County Hospital in Chicago).

Federal Government Programs

The federal government in the United States is deeply involved in health care financing. Federal programs cover the elderly, the poor, federal workers, the military, veterans, and Native Americans and Native Alaskans. Some individuals are concerned about governmental involvement in our health care system. When all of these programs and agencies are considered together, it is clear that, for good or ill, the federal government already controls many aspects of health care.

MEDICARE AND MEDICAID

In 1965, after years of effort and testimony by many health-related groups (including the ANA), and with widespread public support, an amendment to the Social Security Act was passed. Title XVIII of the act, which was termed **Medicare**, provided payment for hospitalization (Part A), and insurance that could be purchased to meet physicians' fees and outpatient costs (Part B), for people over age 65 and certain others who were receiving Social Security payments. Participation in Medicare Part A is automatic for those on Social Security, whereas participation in Medicare Part B is optional and a premium is deducted from the social security check to pay for Part B. Medicare Part A pays only for acute hospitalization and a limited amount of rehabilitative care that may occur in a nursing home. Medicare does not pay for any long-term or custodial care in a nursing home. Part B reimburses for physician care and outpatient services based on a fixed schedule of payments.

Medicare is administered through a federal agency called the Center for Medicare and Medicaid Services (CMS), formerly called Health Care Financing Administration (HCFA), which uses contracted insurance companies termed **Medicare carriers** or **Medicare intermediaries** to process claims (*http://www.cms.gov*). Payments from Medicare do not cover the entire cost of the care provided. The amount authorized is determined by CMS. Medicare then pays a fixed percentage of that authorized amount. The individual pays the remaining percentage of the authorized amount. If the provider charges more than the authorized amount, that portion of the fee is not recoverable from either Medicare or from the patient.

Title IX of the Social Security Act, which was termed **Medicaid**, provides funds for health care for those dependent on public assistance and certain other low-income individuals. Costs for Medicaid are shared between the federal government and each state. Each state is responsible for administering Medicaid: the state determines eligibility and level of coverage. Payments from the federal government to the states are administered by CMS. Benefits vary greatly among states. California's plan, called Medi-Cal, historically has been one of the most comprehensive. As health care costs rise, there has been great pressure to cut this program. To avoid federal control, a few states have not participated in the Medicaid program. Some states, such as Oregon, have requested waivers from CMS's usual regulations governing Medicaid and Medicare to allow experimentation with different plans that might help to control costs.

The complexity of filing claims with Medicare and also with an insurance company designed to supplement Medicare coverage is confusing for many people. Even when claims are filed by the provider, they may be denied payment if they do not conform to specific rules and regulations. Often elderly people accept an initial denial of payment for the claim as the final decision and do not pursue the matter further. There is a high rate of reconsideration when denials are appealed; therefore, it is often wise to encourage clients to appeal a denial of payment.

Medicare and Medicaid are important health care resources, but they have not been without problems. Costs have been much greater and have been rising faster than anticipated. There has been a great deal of publicity about instances of abuse, and even fraud, associated with these two programs. The goals of providing cost-effective health care to the elderly and the indigent through these programs have yet to be achieved.

The Medicare bill contains many provisions that have made a significant impact on nursing. A definition of **skilled nursing care** in the original bill was narrow and excluded many important aspects of care necessary to maintaining the health of clients. Through later efforts and testimony, nursing organizations were instrumental in convincing legislators to recognize that the definition of skilled nursing was critical. As a result, a Senate subcommittee asked the ANA to study skilled nursing care to provide background data for the Senate. Amendments to the Medicare/Medicaid Act of 1972 encouraged study of alternative ways of providing health care to contain costs. These alternatives included the use of nurses in expanded roles and the use of HMOs.

Amendments to the Medicare/Medicaid Act were also responsible for mandating review and evaluation of health care. This was done in the interests of cost control or containment. Institutions must review records of Medicare/Medicaid clients and compare them with specific criteria for care. Many insurance companies have followed this pattern and required review and evaluation of care of their clients.

In 1982, the 97th Congress revised Medicare to prevent the serious financial deficits in the system that escalating costs could potentially create. The revisions increased the premium for Part B of Medicare (the optional portion that provides for out-of-hospital and physician care) and also increased the deductible that the individual must pay for covered service. The system of payment was changed to prospective payment based on diagnosis-related groups (DRGs). (See the discussion on patterns of payment later in this chapter.) The planners who revised Medicare also included a new mechanism for reimbursing hospice care.

In 1993, more changes, restrictions, and controls were instituted in the Medicare system: the payroll deduction for Medicare (paid by all employed individuals regardless of income level or age) was increased; the length of stay was shortened; and rehabilitation and convalescent services moved from acute care environments to newly created subacute units in long-term care facilities and in hospitals. Many procedures that previously required an inpatient stay became outpatient services.

The growing number of elderly, the rising costs of medications, supplies, and wages, and the widespread use of costly, highly technical therapies all have contributed to escalating health care costs. As the "baby boom" generation moves into retirement years, this will further strain the financial resources of the system. Despite these concerns, Medicare and Medicaid have provided health care dollars and services to many people who would otherwise have done without.

Critical Thinking Activity

What changes are occurring in the health care systems in your community? Are some hospitals growing or merging? Are some facilities changing their focus? Have any health care providers had economic difficulties or even closed? Have new providers established facilities? Analyze how these changes may affect nursing practice.

MILITARY HEALTH CARE

The military branches of the Defense Department operate hospitals and clinics and also finance health care through civilian health providers in an extensive program known as TRICARE (*http://www.tricare.osd.mil*). This program has three different options for those under age 65. TRICARE Prime is a managed care plan (the required plan for active duty military personnel); TRICARE Extra is a preferred provider plan; and TRICARE Standard is a fee-for-service option that costs the individual more but allows for greater choices. TRICARE for Life is a program coordinated with Medicare for retired military personnel and their dependents.

OTHER FEDERAL HEALTH CARE PROGRAMS

The U. S. Department of Health and Human Services provides direct health care services to identified underserved populations. Through the Health Resources and Services Administration (HRSA) it provides "643 community and migrant health centers, and 144 primary care programs for the homeless and residents of public housing" (DHHS, 2002). Another agency, the Indian Health Service (IHS), operates "37 hospitals, 60 health centers, 3 school health centers, 46 health stations and 34 urban Indian health centers" (DHHS, 2002).

The Department of Veterans' Affairs operates many clinics, hospitals, and nursing homes for veterans. These are found across the country. For those who are eligible for care from the Veterans' Administration (VA), benefits are comprehensive. The VA is engaged in a major effort to improve services to veterans. Information on the VA's Strategic Plan 2000–2006 is available at *http://www.va.gov/*.

PATTERNS OF PAYMENT

Understanding the various methods of paying for health care services can help you understand what is happening in the organizations and agencies involved in the health care system. The following discussion covers those most commonly used methods of paying for health care services.

Fee-for-Service Payment

Fee-for-service payment means that each time a service is provided, a fee is generated and then billed to the care recipient. The more services provided, the more fees charged. This was the traditional method of charging for health care in the United States. Initially, private individuals paid almost all fees. When insurance companies began assisting with payment, the individual's bill was sent to the insurance company and to the client. The insurance company then paid the amount established in the policy (for example, 80%) and the client was required to pay the rest.

As costs rose, insurance companies began setting a standard for reimbursement. Under this system, if a policy stated that a company reimbursed at 80%, this meant 80% of a fee that the insurance company determined was reasonable. If the provider charged more than the "reasonable" fee, the client was responsible for the excess, in addition to 20% of the "reasonable" fee. Insurance companies usually set these fees based on statistical analysis of prevailing fees in a geographic area. In a time of rapid inflation, providers complained that there was often a serious discrepancy between the fee used for calculating benefits and the actual fees being charged. This standard fee still provided for paying a fee for each service rendered.

Prospective Payment

A **prospective payment** is a fixed reimbursement amount for all the care required for a particular surgical procedure, an illness, or an acuity category. This reimbursement amount is determined in advance of the provision of service. The predetermined amount is paid without regard to actual services required or the costs of those services in individual situations. Thus, the same payment is made whether the person is healthy and has an uncomplicated hospital stay or whether the person is in poor health and has complications that increase the cost of care or the length of the hospital stay.

Prospective payment is designed to provide an incentive for hospitals to control costs. Prospective payment has accomplished this as hospitals began to monitor the use of high cost testing and pharmaceutical products and to limit the length of stay. Another advantage to payers in a prospective payment system is that costs are predictable. The system transfers the burden of risk (the probability that an individual may require extraordinary services) from the payer to the provider. Several specific types of prospective payment are in place that have particular significance for nurses. These are Diagnosis-Related Groups (DRGs) and Resource Utilization Groups (RUGs).

DIAGNOSIS-RELATED GROUPS

The first major change in the method of payment for health care services began on October 1, 1983, when the federal government stopped using a fee-for-service reimbursement system for Medicare, and introduced a prospective payment system using **diagnosis-related groups (DRGs)** to determine the payment for each Medicare client admitted to the hospital. This change was designed to stop the spiraling costs of Medicare and to correct inequities that made the costs of care in one facility very different from those in another facility.

The method of determining the rates to be paid in the Medicare prospective payment system—the creation of DRGs—resulted from a computerized analysis of costs that had been billed for hospitalized individuals in the past and a determination of an average length of stay. This analysis led to the formation of categories of medical diagnoses that require similar treatment and for which costs are similar. Each category (or DRG) has a name and number; for example, DRG 236 is "fracture of the hip and pelvis." In addition, a decision was made to increase the payment for care when another illness or condition is present. This second condition is termed a **comorbidity**. Thus, a person with heart failure whose basic DRG is "fractured hip" is designated "fractured hip with congestive heart failure." A hospital receives greater reimbursement for providing service to this person because care is more complex and costs are higher. Hospitals also receive additional amounts for cases that are determined to be "outliers." An outlier is a case in which the client's length of stay significantly exceeds the average. The number of days needed to qualify a case as an outlier is predetermined. For example, the average length of stay for DRG 236, "Fractured hip and pelvis," is 6.2 days, but the stay must reach 29 days for the case to be considered an outlier. Pressure is placed on all providers to assure that the patient is discharged within the average length of stay upon which payment is based.

Most hospital costs are included in the DRG reimbursement. The actual DRG reimbursement amount is calculated each year by CMS through a complex formula that considers the area of the country in which the care was provided (eg, Northwest, Southeast), the urbanization of the area (eg, rural, suburban), and the type of care required. Some hospital costs still are reimbursed separately. In the past, the separate reimbursements included costs for medical education of resident physicians and research conducted by the hospital. These were reimbursed because the federal government supports the need for research and medical education and also acknowledges that the resident physicians provide care to Medicare and Medicaid recipients. However, pressure is mounting to stop this as a separate payment. Private physicians bill and are paid independently, but some suggest that when these services relate to hospital care, they should be included in a single rate for the entire hospitalization and care. The American Medical Association has vigorously opposed this.

Most of the controversy surrounding the implementation of DRGs has not been concerned with the incentives for cost control, or the prospective reimbursement system itself, but, rather, how the payment amounts are determined and how the system is being administered. A concern continues that clients reportedly are discharged after much shorter stays, when they are still in need of care (the "quicker and sicker" concern—clients are discharged quicker and feeling sicker). Because the method of calculation of payments was based on costs before the system was implemented, providers in some areas of the country receive significantly higher payments for the same DRG than do others. For example, payments in the Southeast are greater than those in the Northwest. Providers in the areas with lower reimbursement express concern that they cannot continue to provide care and remain economically viable with the current reimbursement.

Hospitals with a large population of extra-high-risk clients (eg, the very elderly or poor) have expressed concern that discharging a client for convalescence in a home with a caring family, good food, and a clean environment is much different from discharging a client to an impoverished environment. Many believe the individual situation should be considered when determining regulations for length of stay. The proponents of shortened stays point out that shortened stays are effective cost-containment measures. They argue further that a client's lack of a support system is a social problem and that hospitalization cannot be used to solve social problems. Alterations and modifications of the system will continue, but the basic prospective plan is not expected to change.

RESOURCE UTILIZATION GROUPS

Resource utilization groups (RUGs) are the categories used to determine prospective payment for nursing home clients. Each RUG represents a group of residents who require a similar amount of care and thus will be similar in the cost to support that care each day. Unlike the hospital prospective payment, which is a flat amount for the entire hospital stay, the prospective payment for nursing home care is a fixed daily rate. This daily rate must include all the services, including medications and treatments, that a resident needs. The actual daily rate of reimbursement to the nursing home is the average of the RUGs for all residents. This is often referred to as the **case mix**.

The basis for determining to which RUG a nursing home resident will be assigned for reimbursement purposes is the comprehensive **minimum data set (MDS)** prepared by the registered nurse (RN). This assessment must be transmitted electronically to the appropriate center for review and payment categorization. If the assessments are not completed accurately or are not submitted in a timely manner, the resident automatically is assigned to the lowest reimbursement RUG category. The facility is then unable to recover the difference between the lowest RUG and the actual RUG to which the resident is eventually assigned. Reassessments are required at specified intervals. These reassessments are used to reassign the resident to a RUG.

The use of a **prospective payment system (PPS)** for long-term care—that is, a fixed reimbursement for all the care provided—was phased in over 2 years beginning in 1997 with the first pilot groups. The PPS has created great consternation throughout the nursing home industry because payments to nursing homes have dropped precipitously since its implementation.

The nursing home industry is lobbying for changes in the reimbursement plan because they believe that low reimbursement is undermining their ability to provide appropriate care. The costs of compliance are high, the reimbursements are lower, and there are more restrictions on such items as the provision of therapy services. Many nursing homes have reduced staff, have changed practice patterns, and have made other adjustments to adapt to the decrease in reimbursement. One unintended result of the move to PPS for the nursing home has been the refusal of nursing homes to admit high-cost residents. For example, an individual with an extensive wound that requires intensive wound care with expensive products might cost more per day for care than the highest RUG category allows. In the past, it was possible to bill separately for the expensive dressings and topical agents used. When this is not possible, the facility may refuse to admit the patient. This actually may increase costs for the payer, because patients remain in the high-cost hospital if no long-term care facility will admit them.

OTHER PROSPECTIVE PAYMENT SYSTEMS

In addition to Medicare and Medicaid, many states are adopting systems similar to DRGs, and some private insurance carriers are now using these basic concepts in their cost-control efforts through prospective payment. These prospective payments are often the result of negotiations between health care agencies and the insurance companies. Although the specific amounts and the totals of what is included may differ, some of the same concerns regarding the adequacy of payments remain.

Capitation

Capitation is yet another way of determining payment within the health care system. In a capitated system, a fee is paid to a provider organization for each person (each "head," thus the term) signed up for the plan whether or not that person uses any health care services. Global capitation refers to the inclusion of all services, both inpatient and outpatient, including physician costs in the capitated amount. Capitation may also be limited and only include outpatient and physician costs.

Capitation shifts an even greater share of the risk of providing costly health care from the third-party payer to the provider organization. Providers in a capitated system have an incentive to guide individuals to low-cost outpatient services or other care environments rather than to the acute care hospital. A goal of this payment system is to encourage preventive services that may make high-cost interventions unnecessary. Thus, in a capitated system you may find that services such as mammograms, immunizations, stop-smoking clinics, and back-injury classes do not have any copayments attached, or the copayments may be quite low. Health maintenance organizations were the original capitated systems.

A criticism of a capitated system is that when the provider is at risk for providing care, there may be an unconscious (or even deliberate) attempt to deny medically necessary care to keep costs down. In some capitated systems, consumers have complained that they were unable to obtain services they believed were medically necessary.

COST CONTROL IN HEALTH CARE

Because health care costs continue to rise, cost control is a major focus of the health care system of today. Many factors are contributing to the rising costs of health and many different strategies have been used to attempt to limit the rate of increase.

Understanding Increasing Costs

Many factors contribute to the rising costs of health care (Display 2-2). One important factor in cost increase is the price of new technology. New, more sophisticated diagnostic and treatment devices are developed each year. The rising cost of technology affects every area of the health care field, from the cardiac care unit to the laboratory.

An increasing population needs a greater number of facilities, and the construction of new care facilities also contributes to rising costs. In addition, existing facilities often require modifications. More space is needed for new technologies both at the bedside and in many hospital departments. Computer systems are used more often for documentation of care. Bedside computers that enable documentation to be done at the point of care decrease the amount of time required for "paperwork." More offices and conference rooms are needed. The regulations governing hospital construction also have become more stringent, requiring more fire-safety and infection-control measures, and protection against environmental hazards. These factors combine to make the "per bed" cost of new hospital construction or remodeling increasingly expensive. Additionally, decreases in the length of hospital stay and the move to outpatient services have left many hospital beds unused on a fluctuating basis. Unoccupied hospital beds create a major drain on organizations, because large sums of capital investment are tied up and not returning any income.

The average length of hospital stay for standard diagnoses has decreased steadily. The typical client in today's hospital is discharged rapidly to convalesce at home or in a long-term-care

---

Display 2-2   CONTRIBUTING FACTORS IN RISING HEALTH CARE COSTS

- Price of new technology
- Construction of new facilities
- Higher survival rates, leading to greater need for costly intensive or long-term care
- Growing population of elderly adults requiring health care
- Rise in salaries for health care workers
- High costs of drugs and health-related equipment

facility, leaving behind only the acutely ill. Many clients who would have died quickly in earlier years live through a crisis but require long and intensive care. All of these factors make the acuity level of a client today much greater. This in turn requires more intensive observation and care and the use of more specialized equipment.

The population as a whole is growing older and, statistically, the elderly have an increased incidence of all chronic illnesses. A greater percentage of the population requires health care on a regular basis and may depend on medications, treatments, and therapies for continued functioning.

Until recently, the salaries of health care workers (except for physicians) were far below those of the general society. To remedy this, for a time, salaries of health care workers rose more rapidly than the general inflation rate. Physicians also had an increase in income greater than the relative inflation rate until the mid 90s, when changes in the system began to affect income levels for physicians.

Companies that manufacture health-related devices and drugs reportedly have some of the highest profits in any industry. These companies justify their profits as appropriate relative to the risk and cost involved in research and development; however, some critics believe these companies take advantage of the public's dependence on their products. For example, recent evidence indicates that drug companies spend more on advertising than they do on research. For those health insurance plans and HMOs providing prescription coverage, the costs of prescription drugs are cited as a key reason for premium increases. The public has expressed concern that drug companies sell identical drugs in other countries for far less money than the drugs cost consumers in the United States. Drug companies state high costs in the United States are essential to support continued drug research, which is very costly. One of the realities contributing to this situation is that other countries place price controls on drugs and the United States does not.

Lack of competition in the health care field is one factor that may contribute to higher costs. Although physicians continue to be primary gatekeepers in the system, the advent of other **primary care providers**, such as nurse practitioners and nurse midwives, has offered alternative and less costly care for many routine problems, and for normal life processes such as pregnancy and childbirth. However, there has been opposition to allowing these practitioners to operate in collaborative rather than dependent or subsidiary roles.

As health care costs have continued to rise, third-party payers have used several methods to control costs, including changing patterns of payment, controlling the actions of providers, and other techniques (Fig. 2-2).

Critical Thinking Activity

Choose a patient. Make a list of all the therapies, medications, diagnostic tests, and surgeries or procedures that this patient has received. Research the cost of these therapies and the daily rate for hospital care in your area for one day. Research the DRG reimbursement for that diagnostic group. Compare the reimbursement with the costs being incurred for this individual patient. Identify ways that nurses could reduce the costs involved in this patient's care.

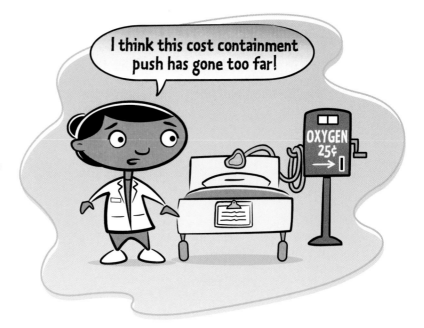

FIGURE 2-2   Federal regulations put pressure on hospitals to limit the rapid rise of health care costs.

Strategies for Cost Control

Third-party payers and government and public agencies all have used different strategies to control costs.

LIMITING HOSPITAL COSTS

With the changes in payment, hospitals have developed many mechanisms to limit costs. Because federal regulations limit the reimbursement to hospitals, physicians are asked to judge carefully the necessity of diagnostic studies and costly procedures for hospitalized patients. Physicians sometimes are asked to consult with a pharmacist before prescribing certain high-cost drugs to determine whether a low-cost therapeutic alternative exists. For example, although the latest aminoglycoside antibiotic might be effective, an inexpensive first-generation cephalosporin antibiotic also might be effective, while costing 90% less. There is great pressure on physicians to discharge patients by the average length of stay to assure that costs remain within the established prospective payment amount. Physician practices are monitored and they have even been threatened with denial of hospital privileges if their patients consistently stay beyond the expected length of stay. Many physicians are upset about these cost-containment measures because they may interfere with the physician's independent decision-making about what care is needed and when.

To add new high-cost equipment or additional client care facilities, a health care institution may be required to apply for a certificate of need from the state. This establishes that there will not be unnecessary duplication of services in an area and that a need for them exists. For example, if every hospital purchased magnetic resonance imaging (MRI) equipment that was used to only one fourth or one third of its capacity, the cost per use would have to be higher to cover the investment and maintenance costs than if the device were used to capacity.

In many states, nonprofit hospitals must make application for rate increases. In their applications, they must document all the factors contributing to the need for an increase. Hearings are held, and permission for rate increases is given only when the evidence indicates that all possible economies are being observed. Private, profit-making hospitals are not held to these rules.

PREFERRED PROVIDERS CONTRACTS

In an attempt to contain costs, third-party payers such as insurance companies, HMOs, and managed care organizations sometimes negotiate with providers of health care to supply certain kinds of care at an agreed-upon, usually lower, price. The third-party payers then provide incentives for clients to use these "preferred providers." These incentives may include the waiver of all or part of copayments by the insured, or coverage of additional conditions or situations.

Preferred provider organizations (PPOs) may be hospitals, nursing homes, corporations employing care providers, or groups of care providers who have cooperated to negotiate more successfully with third-party payers for these special contracts. The advantage to the provider is the assured number of clients and the guaranteed income. In a time of competition in health care, this may be a significant advantage. Each PPO operates independently without government regulation; therefore, the exact structure and contractual arrangements are independently determined.

MANAGED CARE

Managed care refers to any system in which the use of health care services is controlled and monitored carefully to ensure that policies are followed, that neither too much nor too little care is provided, and that costs are minimized. Owens (1995, p. 5) identifies managed care more specifically as "a system to control the cost of health care by using a select group of providers who have agreed to a predetermined payment, with the clinical interventions being managed via utilization and/or a case management process." A managed care plan may be controlled by the payer (such as an insurance company), may include both payers and providers, or may be a business entity that serves only as a go-between. HMOs always have acted as managed care systems. Many of the current health plans referred to as HMOs are in reality managed care systems that do not focus on health maintenance at all.

In a managed care system there is always someone assigned to the role of "gatekeeper." This person monitors and restricts the use of services by the client. In most managed care plans the primary physician is expected to serve as the "gatekeeper." The physician sees the client first and then determines whether referral or diagnostic services are needed. In some managed care systems, the primary physician has decision-making authority. However, in many managed care systems, the actual gatekeeper is a plan manager who must be consulted regarding the use of services. A written request may be required before the client receives permission for a referral. This may result in delay or denial of needed care and is one source of consumer dissatisfaction with some managed care plans.

Many managed care decisions about individual clients are made based on a set of predetermined protocols for treatment. The original protocols were developed by physicians, based on broad statistical patterns. Thus the protocol may not be responsive to individual differences. These protocols often are administered by plan employees who are not health care providers. Physicians express dismay over a mechanism that allows a nonphysician who has never seen a client to make critical decisions about the care needed and to deny any individualization of the plan.

Managed care usually requires that care be authorized or approved for payment before it is provided. Clients identify the required approval of any type of care as a major problem. A managed care plan may not approve or pay for care that it considers nonessential. If a health care provider and a plan consultant disagree about which type of treatment is appropriate, the client often feels caught in the middle. This situation frequently occurs in emergency care. Even when approval is granted, the process may have been long and frustrating for the client and physician involved.

In some managed care plans, a subscriber who needs emergency care and is outside the appropriate service area is subject to what is called the standard of the "prudent consumer." This means that if a prudent layperson would consider the symptoms an emergency, the plan will pay for care. Thus, if a person with chest pain goes to an emergency room, the plan pays even if the chest pain turns out to be esophageal reflux. Some plans created a standard related to the final medical diagnosis. A plan with this standard would pay for an individual who visited the emergency room with chest pain only if the final diagnosis were myocardial infarction, but would not pay if the final diagnosis were esophageal reflux. This approach caused such public consternation that legislation was enacted in some areas that required any kind of health plan to cover emergency care based on the "prudent consumer" model.

Some plans require that an individual travel to a designated hospital when an emergency is not life-threatening. Thus, one consumer was denied payment for a fractured ankle sustained while skiing because it was not life-threatening and because the injury was treated in the skiing community rather than back home in the consumer's designated hospital.

Managed care controls extend to such matters as the medications that can be prescribed. A managed care company may have a specific formulary of drugs for which it has negotiated purchase at low prices. For many conditions, there are clear therapeutic equivalents and medication restrictions are not a concern. For the person with a chronic health condition who has been stabilized on specific medications, however, moving into a managed care plan can pose a real threat to health maintenance if the plan will not approve the client's current drugs.

All of these actions are designed to hold down costs. Managed care plans that originally focused on health maintenance and keeping relatively healthy people healthy showed great promise for controlling health care costs. However, as managed care has encompassed people with serious chronic illnesses, controlling costs has become more difficult.

CASE MANAGEMENT

Case management is a technique used to efficiently move an individual requiring major health services through the system. This results in more effective use of services and lessens cost. According to the Case Management Society of America (CMSA), case management is "a collaborative process which assesses, plans, implements, coordinates, monitors, and evaluates options and services to meet an individual's health needs through communication and available resources to promote quality cost-effective outcomes" (CMSA, 2002). Case managers most commonly are assigned to high-risk clients, such as those with chronic illnesses or major traumas, who will require rehabilitation. In some settings, the case manager specializes in a particular group of high-risk clients, such as those with diabetes, and is referred to as a **disease manager**.

The case manager is an experienced health professional with knowledge of available resources who oversees or monitors a case to ensure that necessary care is instituted promptly and is provided in the most cost-effective setting. Nurses have often assumed the role of case manager. In this role, the nurse monitors the care as it is provided, ensuring that appropriate referrals are made, that changes in the plan of care are instituted appropriately, and that the care follows established standards. Because of their understanding of the whole person, both physiologically and psychosocially, and their understanding of how the system works, nurses are particularly well suited to this role. The CMSA provides a system for certifying professional case managers.

Case managers may operate within only one part of the system; for example, managing cases from admission through discharge in a nursing home or hospital. These managers are often referred to as internal case managers. Some may manage cases across all phases of care from outpatient through hospitalization, rehabilitation, and back to outpatient. These individuals are termed external case managers. At their best, case management systems ensure that delays in patient transfer or breaks in communication do not occur, and that costs are minimized through efficiency. Case managers often act as advocates for clients in the system. Physicians sometimes object to what they see as the interference of the case manager in a decision-making process that previously included only the client and the physician.

VERTICALLY INTEGRATED HEALTH CARE SYSTEMS

Organizations contracting to provide managed care also are expanding their own control through the development of **vertically integrated systems**, that is, those that provide every level of health care service. A vertically integrated system may have contracted physicians, laboratories, a hospital, a subacute facility, a rehabilitation facility, and a home care agency. This allows the contracting organization to offer managed care corporations a package that provides care at all levels for each enrolled member of the managed care plan for a capitated fee. The contracting organization then has an incentive to control costs by decreasing the use of high-cost services and more effectively using low-cost alternatives. It is also in a better position to negotiate with the managed care system about reimbursement. As large systems develop in this manner, hospitals become a cost center rather than a revenue center. This merging of systems is resulting in the closure of hospitals in many communities.

A more recent development has been the splitting off of subsidiaries that were added to large health systems. For example, in late 1999 Columbia/HCA and Tenet, two of the largest health systems in the United States, announced that they were going to divest the corporations of the physician practices that had been purchased in the last 10 years. Their announcement indicated that they had found the system lacked the expertise to manage physician practices and that they were unable to manage costs and create profits as they had originally expected (Kirchheimer, 1999).

USING ACUITY MEASURES TO DETERMINE COSTS

Health care providers who are negotiating contracts and planning care need very accurate data regarding the specific cost of each service. One way of trying to understand and control these costs is through the development of **acuity** measures. Acuity in this context refers to the severity of illness and the rapidity of change in the client and thus the intensity of medical and nursing care and other therapies required.

Various ways of measuring acuity in both acute and long-term care settings have been devised. Most systems use categories that reflect the different types of care needed. Each category is assigned a numerical value on a scale of 1 to 4 (or on a similar scale). All applicable category values are summed and compared with a standard. For example, an acuity measuring system might have one category reflecting the need for assistance in personal hygiene. As a person needs more assistance, more points are assigned. Another category might reflect the amount of time needed for monitoring vital signs: the more time required, the more points assigned. Each category is assigned an appropriate number of points, and the total is computed. The points identified for an individual client are then compared with a standard and the client is assigned an acuity level. Clients with the fewest points are level 1 and require the least care. Those with the most points are level 4 and require the most care. Each system in use has its own scale for determining acuity. Acuity values are sometimes called **intensity measures** because they reflect the intensity of care needed.

In some settings, acuity levels or intensity measures are used as a mechanism for determining the staffing needs of a client care unit. Acuity levels also are used as a means of billing for the level of nursing care needed, and are reflected in a variable rather than flat charge for the nursing portion of a client's room charge. It also has been suggested that prospective reimbursement might be based on acuity level rather than on medical diagnosis because acuity levels reflect the real impact on resources more accurately than do medical diagnoses. The RUGs developed for prospective reimbursement in long-term care are essentially an acuity measure based on the nursing assessment.

INCREASING THE AVAILABILITY OF LOWER COST PROVIDERS

Because physicians are the most costly health care providers, increasing the use of nonphysician primary care providers (such as nurse practitioners and physician assistants) has been used to decrease health care costs. The use of nonphysician providers relies on the ability to obtain reimbursement for the care these individuals deliver.

One attempt to increase the availability of nonphysician care has been the movement to obtain legislation requiring that government agencies and third-party payers pay the nonphysician (eg, the nurse practitioner) who provides primary care service. The traditional pattern required that payment always be made to a physician, who in turn paid the nonphysician provider. Progress has been made in regard to third-party reimbursement for nurses in primary care; however, this continues to be a problem and a major thrust of political pressure by nurses.

CHANGING FEE STRUCTURES

In addition to reducing payments through prospective payment systems, the federal government has sought to control costs for Medicare and Medicaid by establishing higher deductibles (the portions that individual clients must pay) and by limiting the fees that the government will pay. Because the elderly and the poor are often unable to pay these deductible amounts, they become liabilities for health care providers, who cover these costs by collecting higher fees from those who do pay their bills. Hospitals, physicians, and pharmacies argue that as more limits have been imposed, the limited reimbursement no longer covers the actual costs of care. This jeopardizes the entire system. Medicaid costs also have been contained by tightening eligibility requirements, which shuts more people out of the health care system.

CONTROLLING FRAUD AND ABUSE

As Medicare and Medicaid have become a larger and larger part of the financing for the health care system, fraud also has become a larger problem. The Health Insurance Portability and Accountability Act of 1996 (HIPAA) created a federal Health Care Fraud and Abuse Control Program. This program coordinates federal, state, and local law enforcement activities in fighting health care fraud and abuse. Information on preventing Medicare fraud is available at the Medicare Web site *www.medicare.gov/fraudabuse/overview.asp*.

OTHER COST-CONTAINMENT MEASURES

In medical facilities, personnel now are asked to be more cost conscious. Cost consciousness involves such ordinary measures as being conservative with telephone use, canceling meal trays when clients are discharged, and using expensive supplies with care. Nursing personnel also must be aware of the tremendous cost of any complication or additional length-of-stay. Preventing complications and getting clients ready for early discharge have become a major focus of care. Care pathways specify care and identify outcomes for each day of hospitalization with the goal of assuring that resources are used wisely.

All of these efforts at reducing costs have affected the health care system in areas other than **cost containment**. They have affected decision-making processes, power structures, the kinds of care provided, and the ways that individual health care providers practice. Concerns about cost continue to exert pressure for change in the system.

Critical Thinking Activity

What cost-control measures have you seen in places where you have had clinical practice? Analyze the effects of these cost-control measures on client care.

ACCESS TO HEALTH CARE

Access to health care refers to the individual's ability to obtain and use needed services. Access can be an economic, geographic, or sociocultural issue.

Economic Access

Creating access for those who are economically disadvantaged requires a broad approach that encompasses not only access to health providers and hospitalization, but that also addresses other factors that affect health. In addition to providing a family with a prescription, for instance, a provider must determine whether there is a way to fill that prescription. It is not enough to prescribe a special diet without learning whether or not that individual has the necessary knowledge and resources to follow that diet.

Coverage by third-party payers impacts economic access. As more small businesses find their health care benefit costs escalating, they may eliminate these benefits. Individuals and families whose incomes are marginal may be unable to purchase insurance because of the high cost of individual policies. Although giving people an incentive to use services wisely is the stated goal of raising deductibles and copayments, the result for some families may be the delay or avoidance of timely care.

Some individuals are unable to obtain health insurance because of preexisting illnesses. These are often the people who are most in need of health care services. Another group concerned about being denied insurance coverage are those with the potential for serious health problems. As genetic testing for potential health problems has become more widespread and the information gleaned from it more exact, insurance companies have used the results of these tests as a basis for denying coverage to healthy individuals. As more tests become available, this issue is cause for growing concern, especially as it relates to access to health care (see Chapter 10, Bioethical Issues in Health Care).

Geographic Access

Geographic access to health care is a special concern for those in rural areas. As changes have occurred in the health care system, small rural hospitals have found themselves unable to compete or to manage financially. This has led to the closure of some small rural hospitals. When a rural hospital closes, area residents lose emergency room care, hospital access, and diagnostic services. The need to travel to receive health care especially affects the elderly and poor (Reif, DesHarnais, & Bernard, 1999).

Communities without hospitals find it more difficult to recruit physicians and other primary care providers. Historically, most health care providers have preferred not to work in areas that lack hospitals available to provide diagnostic and treatment services; consequently, rural communities found it difficult to recruit health care providers. Many medical schools, with the support of both federal and state funds, developed programs to encourage medical students and residents to consider family practice as a specialty and practice in a rural location. Although successful in increasing the number of physicians entering rural practice, in some states they were unable to keep up with the number leaving rural practice.

Geographic access may be a concern for those in urban areas as well. Economically depressed areas of large cities have fewer health care providers, thus forcing the residents of those areas to travel long distances, often using inconvenient public transportation, to receive health care. The Healthy People 2000 Report (DHHS, 1990) recommended that health care services be made available in locations such as work sites and schools to improve access.

Access to health care also is affected by whether all services are available in one location. It is common for individuals to be required to visit several geographically separate locations to receive all needed health care. Some organizations now offer all health services in one geographic location. A single health care site makes it unnecessary for an individual to go to one location to see a primary provider, to another to see a specialist, to still another for diagnostic tests, and to yet another location for procedures. This makes efficient use of the client's time, lessens the likelihood that the client will fail to follow through with recommended procedures, and simplifies communication between providers.

Sociocultural Access

Sociocultural differences also affect access. When individuals feel uncomfortable in a setting because of their socioeconomic status or because their cultural background and beliefs are not respected, they are reluctant to use the services provided. Making care culturally accessible may mean having available in the care setting translation services, materials in multiple languages, and care providers who understand and are sensitive to cultural differences.

Access to health care is discussed in more detail later in this chapter, in association with key indicators of system effectiveness.

ACCREDITATION OF HEALTH CARE INSTITUTIONS AND AGENCIES

To maintain quality in health care institutions and agencies, a variety of standards and processes to enforce those standards have been established. Meeting the standards of a state governmental agency is termed approval or *certification*. Meeting the standards of a nongovernmental agency is usually designated as *accreditation*. Health care institutions are often both certified by a governmental body and accredited by a nongovernmental agency. In some instances, governmental bodies accept accreditation as the equivalent of governmental standards and do not require an additional approval process. Approval by a specific organization may be required for an agency to receive some types of third-party payment. Therefore, accreditation is important for the agencies involved.

Governmental Approval

Institutions and agencies providing health care usually must be approved by the governmental agency, often a department of health, in the state where they are located. Approval may take the form of state licensing, which usually focuses on maintaining minimum standards to safeguard public health. For some agencies, this meets their needs.

Medicare/Medicaid Certification

Those agencies that seek Medicare or Medicaid funding must meet specific federal standards and be Medicare certified in addition to meeting the basic state standards. For example, Medicare certifies nursing homes as meeting Medicare standards. The Medicare standards relate to many aspects of care. By designating those to whom payment will be given, Medicare effectively exerts control. Because the costs of private care are so high, most people choose to receive care where it can be reimbursed. When care is not reimbursable, individuals may make other choices.

Health care institutions and agencies also may seek accreditation from nongovernmental bodies that set standards for high quality and provide guidelines to assist in developing policies and procedures. Medicare and Medicaid have granted several of these nongovernmental agencies what is called *deemed status*. This means that the standards of the agency are "deemed" to equal or exceed the Medicare standard. Therefore, a health care agency that has been accredited by the voluntary process described below may be "deemed" to meet the standards set by Medicare and Medicaid and is not required to pursue an additional Medicare certification process.

Joint Commission on Accreditation of Healthcare Organizations

Hospitals, nursing homes, and related organizations may seek accreditation from the **Joint Commission on Accreditation of Healthcare Organizations (JCAHO)**. This nonprofit, voluntary organization originally was established by the American College of Surgeons and the American Society of Internal Medicine to set standards for hospital care. Today's organization has a board of directors with members from many health care and public occupations. The standards of the organization are comprehensive and involve evaluating the structural aspects of institutions, policies and procedures, and the outcomes of care provided. JCAHO has deemed status for federal programs. In the past, assisted living settings have not had a standard accreditation, and, in many states, little regulation. The Joint Commission began providing accreditation for assisted living facilities in 2001.

Community Health Accreditation Program

The Community Health Accreditation Program (CHAP) is an organization that was established to provide a voluntary accreditation system for community health and home health agencies. This is a peer-reviewed process governed entirely by community health agencies with public representation. CHAP has deemed status for Medicare and Medicaid certification.

National Committee for Quality Assurance

The National Committee for Quality Assurance (NCQA) reviews and evaluates HMOs. It is a relatively new, independent nonprofit organization developed by the HMO industry. NCQA has established a set of statistical measures called Health Plan Employer Data and Information Set (HEDIS). This information is available from their Web site at *www.ncqa.org*. These data provide a standard set of information that both employers and consumers can use to compare and evaluate HMOs. Included in the HEDIS data set are nine indicators of quality, seven of which are related to processes and two of which are related to outcomes. Most of these data relate to prevention and not to the effective diagnosis and treatment of illness.

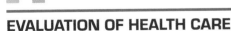

EVALUATION OF HEALTH CARE

A variety of evaluation mechanisms are used within the health care system. Some involve evaluating agencies providing care and others involve evaluating client outcomes.

Peer Review and Quality Assurance

The first systematic evaluation of health care services was established through the Professional Standards Review Organization set up by Medicare and Medicaid. As part of the 1982 revisions of Medicare, the evaluation process was altered to require that hospitals contract with an external medical review organization, called a Utilization and Quality Control Peer Review Organization (abbreviated PRO). These organizations were established through competitive bidding for contracts awarded by the Secretary of Health and Human Services. Most of the PROs are statewide in scope and are required to have a substantial number of physicians represented in the organization to set standards and review care effectively.

Evaluation may include preadmission, preprocedure, concurrent, or retrospective (after discharge) reviews. The purpose of the reviews is to determine whether care given was necessary and whether it was given in the appropriate manner. For example, the reviews have resulted in an increase in the number of outpatient surgeries (day procedures) performed, and a subsequent decrease in the number of inpatient surgeries. These changes have resulted in significant economic savings. The PRO also is required to evaluate outcomes of care to ensure that the changes made do not jeopardize clients.

Outcome Measures

Outcome measures refer to actual health results in the clients and communities served. Outcomes now are measured in relationship to hospitals, long-term care facilities, and the population as a whole. Some outcomes have been designated **key indicators**, also termed **quality indicators (QI)**, which are specific, measurable aspects of health care that show the effectiveness of the system as a whole and indicate whether access to services is available. These are major factors in changes health care institutions are undertaking.

HOSPITAL HEALTH CARE OUTCOMES

The federal government compiles statistics related to hospital health care outcomes. These include infection rates and morbidity and mortality rates associated with specific hospitals and procedures. In 1995, the federal government began releasing these figures to the public. These government statistics may be helpful in evaluating some aspects of care. One result of outcome studies has been the recommendation that only hospitals that perform a specified number of highly technical surgeries (for example, cardiac surgeries) each year should offer those procedures. Hospitals that perform fewer procedures per year have higher complication and mortality rates.

In the early 1990s, the Agency for Health Care Policy and Research created the Healthcare Cost and Utilization Project (HCUP) to identify a set of items that could be used as indicators of quality of care and community access to care. They identified three groups of quality indicators: prevention quality indicators, inpatient quality indicators, and patient safety quality indicators. Since their beginning, these quality indicators have been refined through the use of extensive data banks maintained by the DHHS.

The prevention quality indicators consist of "ambulatory care sensitive conditions," hospital admissions that evidence suggests could have been avoided through high-quality outpatient care or that reflect conditions that could be less severe, if treated early and appropriately

(AHCPR, 2002c). The inpatient quality indicators reflect "quality of care inside hospitals and include inpatient mortality; utilization of procedures (such as hysterectomy) for which there are questions of overuse, underuse, or misuse; and volume of procedures (such as cardiac catheterization) for which there is evidence that a higher volume of procedures is associated with lower mortality" (AHCPR, 2002a). The patient safety indicators are adverse outcomes for hospitalized patients that reflect an adverse event that is preventable such as falls and nosocomial infections (AHCPR, 2002b). The first two sets of indicators are now online.

Many health care agencies are constructing their documentation systems to collect data that demonstrates performance in relationship to these quality indicators. This is enlarging the purpose of documentation from a focus on the individual client to a focus that includes system concerns.

INDIVIDUAL INSTITUTIONAL OUTCOMES MEASUREMENT

Individual institutions also are establishing ways to measure the outcomes of the care they provide. *Outcomes* here refers to data such as the number of clients admitted with a fractured hip who had uncomplicated recoveries leading to effective rehabilitation and the number of clients who had complications or did not recover. Knowledge of outcomes is essential for planning and, increasingly, for effective marketing. Often data have been collected but are scattered among many different records and are difficult to retrieve. Because data only become valuable for planning when they are organized in a useful framework for analysis, health care agencies have moved rapidly to the computerization of data and the implementation of standardized protocols for data collection.

One of the standardized tools hospitals use to monitor outcomes is called the clinical pathway. This is also referred to as a critical path, a care map, or an anticipated recovery path. The clinical pathway describes the optimum progression through the system of the individual with a particular health problem. By establishing the desired outcome for day 2 of the postoperative client with a fractured hip, it is possible to determine when an individual client is not meeting the desired outcome. The advantage for the individual is that care can be modified immediately to address the problem. The advantage for the system is the ability to aggregate data across all clients and examine what is working well and what needs to be changed.

LONG-TERM CARE QUALITY INDICATORS

Quality indicators also are used in long-term care as part of the regulatory process. CMS has identified 11 areas of care in which they specified 24 quality indicators. CMS states that these 24 indicators represent common conditions and items that are important to residents. These quality indicators serve as the focus for the state surveyors. Long-term care facilities are being encouraged to track these indicators themselves and use them as a focus of improvement (Gold, 1999).

NATIONAL HEALTH INDICATORS

In 1992 the Department of Health and Human Services and the Public Health Service published Healthy People 2000, National Health Promotion and Disease Prevention Objectives. The purpose of this document was to establish national goals to serve as a focus for health promotion and disease prevention activities by individuals, organizations, and the federal government. Achievement of these benchmarks could indicate the overall health status of the

Display 2-3 OUTCOMES FROM *HEALTHY PEOPLE 2010*

A. Health and Disease Outcomes
   1. General physical well-being
   2. Infant mortality
   3. Death rates from preventable causes
   4. Disability-free survivorship
   5. Self-reported health status
   6. Sexually transmitted diseases
   7. HIV
   8. Cancer
   9. Low birth weight
   10. Cardiovascular disease (CVD)
   11. Asthma or chronic obstructive pulmonary disease (COPD)
   12. Hip fractures or osteoporosis
   13. Injury
   14. Diabetes
   15. Disability days

B. Preventive Health Behaviors
   1. Unintended pregnancies
   2. Immunizations
   3. Tobacco use
   4. Physical activity
   5. Alcohol use
   6. Substance abuse
   7. Appropriate body weight
   8. Nutrition

C. Mental Health
   1. Psychological status

D. Health System Access
   1. Physical accessibility
   2. Poverty
   3. Health literacy
   4. Education levels

E. Ecologic
   1. Air quality
   2. Iatrogenesis
   3. Firearm death and injury rates
   4. Violence
   5. Homelessness
   6. Motor vehicle accident death and injury rates

population being served. Unfortunately, achievement of these benchmarks has been a far more difficult task than originally envisioned.

In an effort to continue moving forward, the Healthy People 2010 project was developed. Five sets of indicators of the overall health of the population of the United States have been developed. These include health and disease outcomes (such as the incidence of specific preventable diseases), preventive health behaviors (such as the percentage of individuals who smoke), mental health indicators (such as psychological status), health system access (such as physical accessibility of health resources), and ecological indicators (such as firearms injuries and deaths). The specific indicators and measurable criteria for tracking the nation's progress are being refined through consultation with many interested groups (Display 2-3).

POWER IN THE HEALTH CARE SYSTEM

Part of trying to understand any system involves examining some of the unique sources of power and authority within it. If we define **power** as the capability of doing or accomplishing something, then understanding how power is distributed and used in the health care system can help us to function more effectively. Sources of power unique to the health care system are the authority to decide who may enter and leave the system, who may practice in it, and how funding is controlled.

Regulatory Power

The primary regulatory agencies in health care are governmental bodies. These agencies administer licensing laws that govern who is allowed to practice and which institutions are allowed to provide care. Other agencies approve or accredit institutions that educate personnel for health care and licensing, or approve those that provide services. Through regulation these agencies have a profound effect on how institutions operate.

The accrediting bodies (such as JCAHO, CHAP, and NCQA, as discussed earlier in this chapter) all have power to stimulate change in the system. If you have the opportunity to be in an institution when accreditation visitors are present, you will note that every aspect of the physical plant, the policies and procedures, and the competence of staff are examined. Preparing for an accreditation visit stimulates the agency to self-evaluate and correct any deficiencies.

Third-Party Payer Power

Because they represent the financial interests of large groups of people and control payments for services, third-party payers have the power to demand changes in the health care system. When they were first established, these agencies did not see their role in health care as anything beyond a financial relationship. As health care costs rose, these agencies began looking for ways of controlling costs to maintain their competitive place in the insurance market. They have set increasingly rigid criteria for payment for services. The standard rates set for payment for procedures have tended to place some restraints on charges (although actual fees often are slightly ahead of payment schedules). By determining whom they will pay for services, insurance companies reduce the choices available to those who carry insurance—and subscribers usually must select from the choices available if they wish to be reimbursed. Third-party payers therefore exert a more powerful influence over institutions and care providers than do individual subscribers.

Physician Power

Physicians historically had almost unlimited power within the health care system. They determined who entered the system and when. They decided if and when other services and personnel would be used, and they determined when clients would leave the system. As other agencies and professionals in the health care system have obtained some power and independence, the overall power of the physician has diminished.

As a group, physicians have opposed changes that would disperse power in the system, arguing that they are the most educated and knowledgeable of all health care providers and that their professional judgment should be accepted. Those favoring increased distribution of power have argued that more competition, more choice for consumers, and input from a greater variety of health care providers and from consumers will make the system more balanced and more responsive. Despite changes, physicians are still powerful in the health care system.

Consumer Power

The sources of power previously discussed present problems for the client because the client is excluded from them. Clearly, the client is involved in only the most basic aspect of entry into the system: determining that he or she needs care. The client cannot enter any institution without the express approval of a physician. The client has no control over who becomes a primary care provider, and, with the advent of HMOs and PPOs, may have limited choice in selecting providers. Funding usually is controlled by third-party payers, and the client is often powerless to determine who will be paid, how much will be paid, and when payments will be made.

Consumers do have rights in the health care system. These are stated in different ways by different institutions and groups, but all revolve around the recognition of the health care consumer as an individual with the ability and right to be self-determining. As a general rule, consumers are not aware of their rights, and even when they are aware, they may be reluctant to take advantage of them. Consumers are in a particularly vulnerable position in the health care system. Because they depend on those in the system for life itself, they are often reluctant to complain or request changes for fear of offending those on whom they depend. When consumers try to exert power in the system, they may meet with resistance. Consumers are most often effective in exerting power in the system by working in groups and through established committees and agencies.

A health care consumer bill of rights was passed by the U. S. House of Representatives in 2001 and forwarded to the Senate. The Senate has not yet acted on this bill. When they do, it is expected that there will be some changes, and therefore both houses of Congress will need to confer to reach a compromise. Most of the areas of conflict involve rights related to financial aspects of care and whether consumers should have the right to sue a health plan for adverse consequences of denial of care.

Nurse Power

Nurses commonly have had limited power in the health care system, a situation that has its roots in many of the traditional aspects of nursing. These are discussed in Chapter 4. Change may not occur as rapidly as desired, and nurses often are frustrated because of their inability to influence the system. Many new graduates are especially distressed to learn that, as individuals, they cannot affect the system. Somehow they expect that if they speak with a voice of reason and act in the best interest of their clients, others will respond positively. This may not happen. Nevertheless, things are changing in nursing. We discuss these issues throughout this text. Nursing organizations are working to provide nurses with a voice at higher decision-making levels in health care. By understanding the political realities and the ways in which decisions are made, and by working together to speak with a united voice, nurses can increase their power in the system (see Chapter 3). Nursing education programs increasingly try to educate nurses to act as client advocates and agents of change (see Chapters 6 and 14).

Collective bargaining and shared governance have provided nurses with mechanisms for demanding recognition of the importance of their role and for being participants in decision-making processes (see Chapter 12).

Critical Thinking Activity

Nurses are actively seeking power in the health care system. Consider the roles of nurses in the facilities with which you are familiar. How might nurses in these settings increase their power?

IMPLICATIONS FOR NURSES

Nurses have continuing interest and concern in the direction in which health care moves. Nurses are most concerned about client well-being in the midst of a powerful system. As pressures to change increase, nurses continue to speak out for consumers. Who will help consumers cope with their health problems and those of their families? Who will assist them in negotiating the various parts of the health care system? Will the individual identities and unique needs of consumers be addressed, or will each person be treated as the mythical "standard client" (Fig. 2-3)?

There are a variety of implications for nurses in the current cost-control environment. The availability and accuracy of documents that reflect the acuity level and multiple problems of a client when records are audited for compliance is essential (determination of acuity level is discussed earlier in this chapter). The need for discharge planning is always present but is more critical as the length of stay becomes shorter. A longer length of stay significantly increases the costs to the hospital; therefore, nursing actions that prevent complications, avoid inappropriate scheduling, and facilitate early discharge are important. Nurses in home health agencies and long-term care facilities are caring for clients with complex nursing needs. A major concern is whether the reimbursement system provides adequate funds for quality nursing care to be delivered.

Another important concern of nurses is whether that aspect of health care that we call "nursing," with its focus on the individual, will be maintained. Will the pressures for demonstrating cost-effectiveness result in a loss of caring because it is not always quantifiable? Will the system recognize the critical thinking skills and abilities of nurses as well as their technical skills? Will many educated and skilled nurses be replaced by unlicensed assistive personnel? The future poses many as yet unanswerable questions!

There are ongoing concerns in the health care system relating to the actual use of health care services by the public and to the structure of the system itself. The impetus for change continues to grow. Several states already have instituted efforts to create a more coordinated health care system for their citizens. In recent years, the U. S. Congress considered several bills for health care reform, but none passed. No one can predict the details of the future system with certainty, but we have tried to point out the major changes now occurring and the directions in which the new health care system is moving. Nurses need to remain

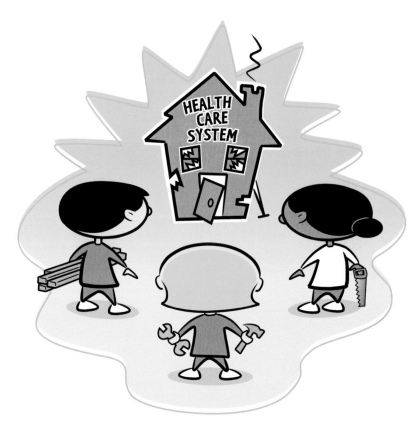

FIGURE 2-3   The pressure for change in the health care system continues to grow.

knowledgeable and involved in the political processes involved as changes are proposed in the health care system.

Critical Thinking Activity

Identify clients you have encountered from a variety of social, cultural, and economic backgrounds. Given these clients' needs and backgrounds, what type of practitioner would best meet their needs for primary care? What barriers might they meet in trying to gain access to primary care? What might you do to assist these individuals?

KEY CONCEPTS

- The financing of health care is complex and involves personal payment, insurance companies, HMOs, preferred providers, and governmental systems, each of which operates differently.
- Through control of financing, third-party payers exert control over all aspects of health care.

- Cost increases have created stress in the health care system. Understanding the basis of these increases is essential for planning to contain costs.
- Mechanisms for controlling costs and improving patterns of care have been instituted. These have included changing methods of payment, controlling health care providers, and managing care. The federal government has played a major role in the development and implementation of these mechanisms.
- Access to health care must be considered in terms of economic, geographic, and sociocultural access. A major concern in the system is those who do not have access.
- Quality of care is maintained by a wide variety of mechanisms. Institutions and agencies providing care receive oversight in the form of governmental approval and accreditation by certifying organizations.
- Quality is evaluated through peer review and the use of outcome measures, including key indicators and individual patient outcome standards.
- Power is exerted in the health care system by those who control finances, those who control access, and those with special knowledge. Traditionally, nurses and consumers have enjoyed little power in the system. Both are working to gain recognition and to affect more significantly the way the system functions.
- There are many implications for nurses in the financing and control of health care, including cost control, the well-being of the client, the effective use of health care resources, and changing the health care system.

RELEVANT WEB SITES

Agency for Health Care Quality and Research (AHCQR): *www.ahcpr.gov*
Center for Medicare and Medicaid Services (CMS), Administering Medicare and Medicaid: *www.cms.hhs.gov*
Department of Health and Human Services (DHHS): *www.hhs.gov/agencies*
Department of Veteran's Affairs (VA): *www.va.gov*
Foundation for Accountability (FACCT): *www.facct.org*
Joint Commission on Accreditation of Healthcare Organizations (JCAHO): *www.jcaho.org*
Medicare Information for the Consumer: *www.medicare.gov*
National Committee for Quality Assurance (NCQA): *www.ncqa.org*
TRICARE, Health Care for Military and their Dependents: *www.tricare.osd.mil*

REFERENCES

Agency for Health Care Policy and Research. Inpatient Quality Indicators. Available at *http://www.ahcpr.gov/data/hcup/inpatqi.htm*. Accessed August 4, 2002a.
Agency for Health Care Policy and Research (AHCPR). Patient Safety Indicators. Available at *http://www.ahcpr.gov/data/hcup/inpatqi.htm*. Accessed August 4, 2002b.
Agency for Health Care Policy and Research. Prevention Quality Indicators. Available at *http://www.ahcpr.gov/data/hcup/prevqifact.htm*. Accessed August 4, 2002c.

Case Management Society of America. *www.cmsa.org/meminfo/*. Accessed July 8, 2002.

Department of Health and Human Services (DHHS), Health Insurance and Portability Act, Available at *http://cms.hhs.gov/hipaa/*. Accessed August 4, 2002.

Department of Health and Human Services (DHHS), HHS Agencies, accessed at *www.hhs.gov/agencies/*, July 8, 2002.

Department of Health and Human Services (DHHS). (1990). Healthy People 2000: National Health Promotion and Disease Prevention Objectives, (DHHS Publication No. PHS 91-50212). Washington, DC: U.S. Government Printing Office.

Gold, M. F. (1999). Rewriting the book on quality (special section). *Provider 25*(7), 2–4.

Health Insurance and Portability and Accountability Act of 1996, Available at *http://aspe.hhs.gov/admnsimp/pl104191.htm*. Accessed August 4, 2002.

Kirchheimer, B. (1999). Cutting the docs loose. *Modern Healthcare 29*(36), 2.

Owens, C. (1995). *Managed care organizations*. New York: McGraw-Hill.

Reif, S. S., DesHarnais, S., & Bernard, S. (1999). Community perceptions of the effects of rural hospital closure on access to care. *Journal of Rural Health 15*(2), 202–209.

Vickery, K. (1999). JCAHO issues assisted living accreditation principles. *Provider 25*(6), 16.

3

The Political Process and the Nursing Profession

LEARNING OUTCOMES

After completing this chapter, you should be able to:

1. Explain why it is important for nurses to be knowledgeable about and involved in the political process.
2. Discuss seven ways you might influence the political process.
3. Describe ways in which the current U.S. federal government is involved in health care.
4. Discuss common state legislative concerns.
5. Discuss common local political concerns.
6. Explain the reasons for the existence of the large numbers of nursing organizations.
7. Identify the major purpose of each specialized organization presented in the chapter.
8. Analyze the ways that nursing organizations seek to affect the health care delivery system and the political processes that control it.
9. Explain how politics is relevant to your participation in organizations.

KEY TERMS

Accreditation

Allocation of resources

Authorization act

Conditions of participation

Department of Health and Human Services (DHHS)

Hatch Act

Lobbying

Nurse Practice Act

Nurses Strategic Action Team (N-STAT)

Occupational Safety and Health Act (OSHA)

Omnibus Budget Reconciliation Act (OBRA)

Political action committees (PACs)

Politics

Tricouncil for Nursing

Whistleblower

Politics is the way in which people in any society try to influence decision making and the **allocation of resources**. Because resources (money, time, and personnel) are limited, it is necessary to make choices regarding their use. There is no perfect process for making optimum choices, because whenever one valuable option is chosen, some other option must be left out. Politics is a part of every organization and a part of government at every level. In a democratic society, all individuals can choose to be involved at some level in this decision-making process. This chapter presents the political process, discusses some of the current issues in regard to political decisions, and describes how you can play a role in the political arena and in nursing organizations.

RELEVANCE OF THE POLITICAL PROCESS FOR NURSES

Nurses always have been involved in politics. Florence Nightingale used her contacts with powerful men in government to obtain supplies and the personnel she needed to care for wounded soldiers in the Crimea (Woodham-Smith, 1983). Hannah Ropes was able to fight incompetence and obtain decent care for wounded Civil War soldiers because she understood who the influential people in Washington were and who would be receptive to her efforts on the soldiers' behalf (Lienhard, 2002.) Isabel Hampton used the buildup and excitement of the World's Fair and Columbian Exposition to bring together nurse leaders to form the first nursing organization.

Modern times are no different. With many voices competing to be heard in the decision-making circles of any nation, the person who understands power and politics is the one most likely to obtain the resources needed to accomplish desired ends.

Health care is costly, and public dollars can be and are spent in many ways to provide health care. What part of the federal budget should be allocated to health care? What part of the state budget? The local governmental budget? Of the money allocated, what part should be used for preventive health programs? What part for research? What part for care and treatment? What part for education? What diseases or conditions should be targeted for investigation? Who should receive those dollars? Where can more dollars be obtained? These questions are answered by legislation and by administrative decisions of governmental agencies.

Decisions also must be made in health care agencies. What positions will be funded? What equipment purchased? What programs should be adopted and which of the current programs should be dropped? These questions are answered by committees, managers, and governing boards.

Nursing organizations are confronted with similar questions. What is the role of the organization? Should resources be spent on benefits for members? On activities relevant to the nursing profession as a whole? On activities related to general health care? In the political arena? How can nurses affect decision making? What is the individual's role as a nurse in the organization? These questions may be answered by representative assemblies, committees and commissions, and elected officers.

Knowing where the decision making occurs, who makes the decision, and being familiar with how you can influence that process is critical. Each governmental entity, agency, and organization has its own mechanism for operating. However, they have many similarities that can help you plan your activities.

Your practice as a nurse is controlled by a wide variety of governmental decisions. One of the most basic is the **Nurse Practice Act** of your state. In that document, nursing is defined legally, and the scope of nursing practice is outlined. This document affects what you do each day that you practice. All of the philosophic discussions about the role of the nurse must return to the reality of the nurse's role as legally defined in the state's practice act. Do you care what that role is now or what changes are made in it? Does it make any difference to you what education that law requires, or if that law requires continuing education? Answering "yes" to any of these questions emphasizes the relevance of the political process for you.

Many decisions are made in the various nurses' organizations. These organizations speak for nurses in many settings. Are you happy with the way they are spending funds paid in dues? Do you agree with all of the public statements they make? Do you support their mechanisms for decision making? Are you happy with the image of nurses and nursing the public receives from these organizations? Do you care what these organizations do with their resources? The political process is an important part of their functioning, too.

Critical Thinking Activity

Identify a current health care issue in your state or province. Investigate that issue and form a position that you can support with data. Examine your position for personal biases.

INFLUENCING THE POLITICAL PROCESS

You can have an effect on such things as what health care legislation is submitted, the content of the legislation, and what legislation is passed. However, this does not happen without effort and action. Historically, women have been less active in politics than men. This has been the result of a variety of societal factors. Gradually, women are assuming a more active role in politics: more are running for and being elected to office, more work with policy-making bodies, and more vote. Because more than 90% of nurses are women, this changing social climate is important to nursing. All women, but nurses in particular, have demonstrated increasing political awareness.

Each person must determine his or her own level of personal involvement, but there is, in the broad realm of the political process, a way for everyone to find a suitable role. Some of these ways are outlined here and in Display 3-1.

Becoming Informed

To become informed about legislation and health care, you need to learn about the sources of information available. Each source of information is valuable to you but should be weighed based on its known biases. Even the most objective-sounding report can be biased, not only in what is reported, but also in what is not reported. Identifying the groups that support and the groups that oppose a particular viewpoint might help you to recognize bias. Typically, do those

Display 3-1 **INFLUENCING THE POLITICAL PROCESS**

- Become informed through a variety of sources.
- Vote for candidates or ballot issues that reflect your concerns.
- Vote for officers within professional or political organizations.
- Express your opinions through letters or in public forums.
- Communicate directly with legislators and public officials.
- Work for or contribute to nonlobbying nursing organizations or political action committees.
- Work for or contribute to candidates who represent your views.
- Testify before decision-making bodies.

groups take a liberal or a conservative stand on issues? Determine whether a group and its members would tend to gain or lose personally by the passage of proposed legislation. Are special interest groups voicing an opinion? When biases are evident, it is advisable to obtain information from groups with divergent viewpoints. Decisions must be based on firm factual data.

Once you are informed about the current issues in legislation or in an organization, you are better prepared to form personal opinions about them and to try to influence the outcome of the political process. A wide variety of resources are available.

NEWS MEDIA

Your daily newspaper or weekly news magazine can be an excellent source of information about significant legislation being proposed, when an issue is controversial or of widespread interest. When you rely on the newspaper for information, however, you sometimes learn of legislation only after it has already been passed.

Television and radio news reports are usually quite brief and give only an overview of a particular piece of legislation being introduced. This overview may be helpful in alerting you to something that you will want to study more intensively. Some television programs, such as those on public television, do discuss issues in depth. In an attempt to meet the Federal Communications Commission (FCC) rules regarding equal time, these programs usually make an attempt to present both sides of any issue.

SPECIALIZED PUBLICATIONS

Professional journals usually devote some space to current legislative issues. This is done routinely in *American Journal of Nursing* and in *The American Nurse*. When major issues are being debated, other nursing periodicals often contain articles of interest. The journals of other health care professions also may carry information regarding current issues. Newsletters and journals of organizations that have a political focus provide information on what they see as current issues. These organizations include consumer groups such as Common Cause, political groups such as Young Democrats and Young Republicans, and nonpartisan groups such as the League of Women Voters. Magazines directed to special interest groups such as *My Generation* for the 50–55-year-old or *Modern Maturity* for those 50 plus, carry articles related to political issues that would be of particular interest to that group.

Copies of legislation are usually available through your congressional representatives (for federal matters) and your state representatives (for state matters). Along with copies of the legislation, a legislator may send other informational material. Government agencies affected by proposed legislation also may provide information about its potential effects, although they are not allowed to try to influence legislation (Display 3-2).

INTERNET WEB SITES

Internet Web sites are an increasingly useful source of information. Federal legislation can be found at *http://thomas.loc.gov/*, a site maintained in the public interest by Congress. In most states, the text of bills being introduced is available on a governmental Web site, where you can read the bill on the computer or print the document to read. State sites can be accessed by linking from a national Web site: *http://lcweb.loc.gov/global/state/stategov.html*. Nursing and health care organizations that maintain Web sites often have a site devoted to political issues affecting members of the organization or relevant issues that affect health care. The ANA maintains a legislative Web site at *http://nursingworld.org/gova/*. Many news organizations (television stations, newspapers, and magazines) maintain Web sites with information on current issues. Any of these sites may provide links to still more sites that provide useful information. Materials may be read while online or the materials can be downloaded for later use.

ORGANIZATIONAL MEETINGS

Nursing organizations and other health-related organizations sometimes hold open meetings to present and discuss legislative issues. Often, knowledgeable speakers can help you to understand what is being proposed and the potential effects of a proposal. These organizations also may sponsor e-mail networks to get out information on important pending legislation. Nursing organizations can be excellent sources of information because they often are in touch with legislators and legislative staff.

Voting

Your individual vote on a ballot issue is significant, although it is a common practice to belittle the importance of the individual vote in any election. Recent major elections in this country, however, have demonstrated how important every vote can be. One of the unfortunate statistics in the United States is that only a very small percentage of eligible people are registered voters. Nurses, as a group, represent a high percentage of all people who vote. When legislators hear statistics such as "1 in 17 women voters is a nurse," or "1 in every 44 voters is a nurse," they pay attention to the opinions of nurses. Although you cannot vote directly on legislative issues, you can vote for candidates whose positions you support on initiatives and referendums and who share your values. Absentee ballots are always available for those who cannot be present at their polling place on the day of an election. These ballots must be requested well in advance of the election, however.

Voting for officers in organizations may be ignored by a large majority of members. They look at the ballot, cannot identify those running for office, and therefore do not vote. Most organizations do make an attempt to introduce members to the various candidates. If you do not know the candidates, you can seek information about them by reading their prepared

HOUSE	CONSTITUENT	SENATE
Representative introduces bill. Clerk of the House refers it to appropriate committee.	Start with your letter-writing campaign urging representatives and senators to cosponsor the legislation.	Senator introduces bill. Clerk of the Senate refers it to appropriate committee.
Committee chair refers bill to a subcommittee, which holds hearings to examine arguments for or against the bill.	Write to each subcommittee member. Place special emphasis on members from your state.	Committee chair refers it to a subcommittee, which holds hearings to examine arguments for or against the bill.
Subcommittee holds a 'mark-up' session to discuss and vote on the bill. A majority vote in favor moves the bill to full committee.	Request that your local paper print an article you've written. Meet with the paper's editorial board to urge its support.	Subcommittee holds a 'mark-up' session to discuss and vote on the bill. A majority vote in favor moves the bill to full committee.
Full committee reviews subcommittee hearing record and may hold additional hearings. A mark-up session is held and if the bill is approved it is reported to the full House.	Meet with your representative and senators in their home district offices. Send a copy of your paper's editorial to every member of the full committee.	Full committee reviews subcommittee record and may hold additional hearings. A mark-up session is held and if the bill is approved, it is reported to the full Senate.
Prior to the House vote, the Rules Committee sets the rules on length of debate and whether amendments are allowed.	Keep up your media campaign with letters to the editor, and call congress members' Washington offices to check their voting plans. Urge your friends to do the same.	Prior to the Senate vote, senators must unanimously agree to a time limit. There are seldom-used parliamentary maneuvers to get around this.
The bill passes if a majority approves it. / A bill can be expedited under 'suspension of the rules.' Suspension bills bypass Rules Committee, require a two-thirds vote for passage, and cannot be amended.	Let conference committee members know whether you prefer the House or the Senate version. Ask your representative and senators to lobby the conference committee.	The bill passes if a Senate majority approve it.

Differences in House and Senate versions of bills are resolved in a conference committee comprised of senators and representatives from the bill's original committee.

| House votes on conference report. | | Senate votes on conference report. |

When conference report is approved by both House and Senate, the bill goes to the President. If President vetoes, a two-thirds vote of both House and Senate is required to override.

statements of position and learning about their previous activities. Those elected to office usually determine the direction and priorities of an organization. If you are contributing your dues dollars, you want to have a voice in choosing those who are entrusted with making the decisions.

Shaping Public Opinion

Public opinion does influence the actions of legislators and regulatory bodies. As a registered nurse (RN), you can help to shape public opinion; your judgment about matters that affect health care can help others make their own decisions. Share the knowledge you have gained through your personal experience and research. Do not be afraid to state your own position, although you must be prepared to support your position with evidence if you want to be considered a thoughtful health care professional. Certainly, you will not want to make every social occasion an opportunity to share political positions, but you should take advantage of opportunities that arise to present your concerns to others (Fig. 3-1).

Another means of shaping public opinion is writing a letter to the editor of a newspaper or news magazine. These letters are read by many people. The following suggestions will maximize your chances of appearing in print:

- Carefully follow the instructions provided by the publication for letters to the editor. These usually will refer to length, signature, address, and telephone number.

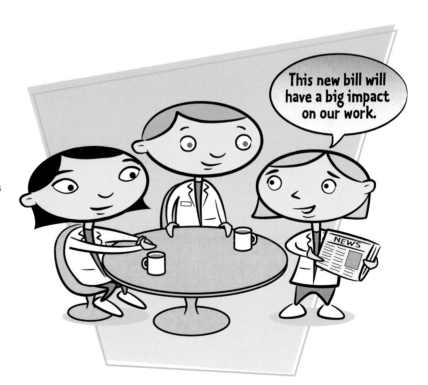

FIGURE 3-1 Sharing your opinions is one avenue of political involvement.

- Clearly present your opinion with well-reasoned arguments.
- Including personal experiences that illustrate health care concerns can be useful; however, you must be careful that health care examples do not violate the confidentiality of clients or divulge confidential information regarding your employer.
- Avoid personal attacks on others.

Within an organization, you may also influence opinion and action by clearly presenting reasoned arguments. You can discuss issues with other members, attend meetings, and voice your opinion. Remember that a viewpoint supported by strong, reasoned judgment and rationale will be better received than a simple statement of opinion.

Communicating With Legislators and Officials

Legislators are affected by the views of their constituents. The legislator's staff reviews letters sent to a legislator; views are tabulated, and letters with significant opinions or information are directed to the legislator for individual consideration. Although some groups encourage members to sign form letters or postcards, personal letters always have the greater impact.

Concern regarding the rules and regulations of a specific department of government can be addressed to the officials of that department. It is possible for officials to become insulated from the effects of their decision making. Communication from concerned citizens can be as important to them as it is to legislators. Letters to officials should reflect the same care and professional viewpoint as letters to legislators to be most effective.

A carefully written personal letter reflecting thoughtful and informed opinions on an issue that a person is competent to evaluate will receive the most attention from any governmental person or department. As an RN, you have expertise in an area of health care and can provide a valuable viewpoint. Identify yourself as an RN in your letter and outline why you are concerned about the issue in question. Legislators often appreciate personal anecdotes from your practice (with identities concealed, of course) that underscore your point. The names and addresses of your congressional representatives and of your individual state representatives are available online from the American Nurses Association (ANA). Go to *www.nursingworld.org* and link to "*CapitolWiz.*" This page connects you to a list of members of Congress, their names, and addresses. Additional information about effective communication with legislators is provided by the ANA on its Web site regarding "Governmental Affairs" at *http://nursingworld.org/gova/.*

Many governmental agencies, both legislative and regulatory, have e-mail addresses that allow you to send messages electronically. As the "information highway" becomes more widely accessible, using this form of communication has become easier. E-mail has the advantage of being extremely timely. Although you may have e-mail access at your place of work, your employer may not allow you to use it for political activity. If you are employed by a government entity, such as a public health department, the law prohibits you from using governmental resources such as e-mail for political activity. Members of the U.S. Congress may be e-mailed by linking through the *www.nursingworld.org* Web site identified above. That Web site also gives you information about the legislative process. An e-mail message should be composed as carefully as a letter. One important point is to include your full name and home address in your e-mail. Staff members review the address, forward only those messages that are personally identifiable, and especially note those from a congressperson's own district. Do remember that e-mail is public. You should not say things on e-mail that you would be uncomfortable with presenting in public.

Telephone calls can be made to the legislator's office. Staff members keep a record of all calls, and the positions of callers are noted. To call a member of Congress, contact the U.S. Capitol Switchboard at (202) 224-3121, and ask for the individual's office. In some states, a toll-free number is maintained for calls to state legislators during the legislative session. You will be asked to leave a message. Be sure to identify yourself fully, including both name and address. State the bill or issue about which you are calling and clearly state your position.

Visiting congressional or state representatives also is an effective means of expressing your concerns. One of the best ways to arrange to speak with congressional representatives and senators is to contact their local offices. Through these offices you may receive assistance in arranging your visit. They may also help you to arrange other interesting and valuable activities, such as attending committee hearings, taking tours, and visiting Congress in session. Appointments should be made well in advance, as representatives and senators often have busy schedules. If your time is limited, you may have to modify your expectations and meet with a staff member who will relay your concerns. Plan carefully for your visit. It is helpful to write out concerns and questions. Be sure to leave time for answers to the questions that you pose. Even when you disagree with the position taken by your legislator, be polite and present your concerns calmly. Rudeness will result in the legislator's unwillingness to listen to what you have to say.

Some legislators hold public meetings (often referred to as "town hall" meetings) in their legislative districts for the purpose of hearing from their constituents. These meetings can be both an opportunity to learn about issues and the legislators current position and to give input in regard to issues of concern to you. If you bring written materials to support your viewpoint, these may be given to the legislator and further reinforce your position.

These same activities may be useful in working within an organization. Those elected to office do not know the views of members unless communication occurs. For communication to be effective, you must know when and where boards meet, how to get information to board members, and the names of those responsible for specific aspects of the organization's operations.

Critical Thinking Activity

Identify a political issue about which you feel strongly. Write a letter to a governmental official that provides a sound rationale in support of your position.

Group Action

The political process in the nursing profession takes many forms. Nurses can be involved as individuals, but they are far more effective when they work in groups. Because nursing is the largest single health care occupation, nurses have many votes. For this reason, legislators pay attention to positions held by groups of nurses.

NONLOBBYING NURSING ORGANIZATIONAL EFFORT

Most traditional nursing organizations are nonprofit groups and therefore are limited in their political activity. The major role of nonprofit groups in politics involves testifying to facts, organizational positions, and concerns in the health care arena. The ANA has an office in Washington, DC, and tries to keep the nursing profession informed about legislative matters of importance in health care. The ANA also provides experts in the nursing profession who testify before congressional and regulatory groups about proposed legislation.

The **Tricouncil for Nursing** is a collaborative effort of the ANA, the National League for Nursing (NLN), the American Organization of Nurse Executives (AONE), and the American Association of Colleges of Nursing (AACN). It represents the interests of nursing practice, research, and education. By working collaboratively, these organizations have strengthened the voice of nursing and its visibility in Washington, DC. This coalition has become the trusted spokesperson for nursing. Legislators rely on the information it provides and recognize it as a united voice for the nursing profession (Fig. 3-2).

The ANA organized the **Nurses Strategic Action Team (N-STAT)** to provide nurses with a means to mobilize quickly to influence legislative policy. This organization promotes grassroots involvement in legislative issues, meets with members of Congress, and organizes letter-writing and telephone campaigns. It involves thousands of nurses. You can

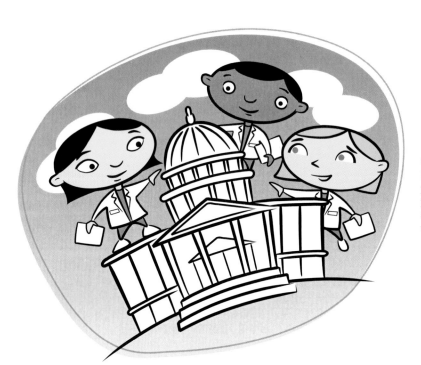

FIGURE 3-2 Nurses may lobby to get desired legislation passed by visiting legislators, by presenting information and arguments about the bill, and by writing letters.

imagine that receiving thousands of letters about a single topic might get the attention of a legislator.

Another effort by the ANA to inform nurses about legislative issues is the regular publication on its Web site of *Capitol Update: The Legislative Newsletter for Nurses*. This publication brings the latest in legislative concerns to your attention on a regular basis throughout the year.

The Nurses' Coalition for Legislative Action is a group of 28 nursing specialty organizations that works to support the positions of its member organizations at the federal level. Specialty nursing organizations have joined this coalition to bring a larger voice to the support of issues that affect nursing specialty practice. Like the Tricouncil, the focus is on information gathering for member organizations and on testifying regarding education, research, and practice issues in nursing.

Most state and district nurses' associations have legislative committees that monitor legislative and regulatory actions in their areas. They may provide educational events for nurses regarding current issues, and testify at hearings concerning health-related issues. They also may seek to mobilize letter-writing or telephone campaigns.

POLITICAL ACTION COMMITTEES

Lobbying is the process of attempting to influence legislators to take a particular action. The law differentiates lobbying from providing general information and places restrictions on who can lobby. Nonprofit groups such as the ANA can provide information but cannot take direct action on behalf of specific candidates or partisan issues. To take a more active role in seeking the passage of desired legislation, the defeat of undesired measures, and the election of particular candidates, groups form organizations called **political action committees** (often referred to as **PACs**). These organizations are registered as political action groups and are free to try to affect the political process. They are not considered nonprofit organizations because their funds are used for political purposes; therefore, donations to them are not tax deductible.

The ANA political action organization is titled the ANA-Political Action Committee (ANA-PAC). ANA-PAC actually lobbies for the passage or defeat of bills and supports candidates for public office. Since the 1976 federal elections, ANA-PAC has raised funds to support candidates for the Senate and the House of Representatives based on their expressed and demonstrated stands on key health issues, such as health care reform proposals, funding for nursing and biomedical research, extension and funding of nursing education, and third-party reimbursement for nurses. Not all candidates endorsed by ANA-PAC were supported financially because of the limited funds available. Candidates' successes are attributable to many factors, but the effect of nursing support has been demonstrated. Many state nursing associations also have political action organizations. These groups serve the same function on the state level as ANA-PAC does on the national level. Many candidates actively seek the endorsement of nursing organizations that are perceived as influential with voters.

Although these nursing political action groups have not grown rapidly in size, their growth has been steady. In addition, nurses are gaining more sophistication in their approach to the political process. Through their combined financial contributions, nurses can significantly help a candidate or issue. All of these factors have resulted in nurses gaining increased power in the political sphere. There is still a long way to go before nurses have the same kind of power that is wielded by those in labor, education, and medicine, but change is occurring.

Critical Thinking Activity

Contact your state nurses' association and find out if your state has a political action organization. If it does, contact that organization and ask what the current issues are in the state. Investigate those issues.

OTHER POLITICALLY IMPORTANT GROUPS

Many organizations in addition to those specifically related to nursing are concerned about health and social issues. Some are official lobbying groups; others provide information resources. Groups such as Common Cause (a consumer lobbying group), AARP (formerly the American Association of Retired Persons), the League of Women Voters, and even church organizations often act to affect the political process. You may support these groups simply by donating money for their needs or by being actively involved in their work.

Testifying for Decision-Making Bodies

Many decisions affecting nursing and health care are made by committees and commissions at various levels of government. These decision-making bodies often hold hearings to gather information before decisions are made. As a nurse, your testimony may have particular value when certain areas of health care are considered. A nurse may testify as either an official representative of an organization or as an independent individual.

You may learn of opportunities to testify through announcements in the newspaper and through professional publications. In general, you must register in advance to testify. In some instances, there is registration at the door before a meeting begins, but for more formal situations, you will have to notify the committee in advance that you wish to testify.

If you have an opportunity to testify, be sure to make your position clear so that the decision makers know whether you speak for yourself or for a larger group. Keep your testimony brief and concise. Prepare your testimony ahead of time (with copies for committee members), but try to avoid simply reading a statement. A less formal presentation is usually more interesting for the listener. Be prepared with sources for any facts or figures you present and explain any technical terms you use. Find out whether there is a time limit for each testimony. If you are given a time limit, make sure that you present your most important arguments and facts first. Most committees will accept written testimony if you cannot be there in person, but the personal presentation is usually more effective.

Individual Support for Legislation and Candidates

You may choose to personally support a specific piece of legislation by contributing money for publicity and campaigning or by working on a committee that is striving for the passage of a proposal. Funds are needed for printing and distributing literature, newspaper ads, and television and radio announcements. Workers may be needed for secretarial tasks, to contact people in a door-to-door campaign, and to speak on behalf of the issue.

Supporting a candidate for public office is accomplished in the same way. In our political system, the reality is that those who have actively supported a candidate during an election campaign are listened to more closely when decisions are being made. Working for a candidate is one way to make your view known. It is also an excellent way to gain firsthand knowledge of the political process. Both time and money are valuable to every candidate. Supporters may sponsor a coffee hour, post political signs, contribute money, assist with mailing, or visit door-to-door distributing campaign literature.

Working in Policy-Making Agencies

Nurses have been appointed to major administrative positions in state and federal health agencies and to the staffs of several senators and representatives. In these roles, they have major policy-making responsibilities. Knowledgeable nurses may be appointed to task forces that study health care concerns and recommend regulatory or legislative action. The Robert Wood Johnson Foundation has provided 1-year fellowships for nurses to study policy in Washington, DC. Nurses who complete these fellowships have the skills and abilities to be effective in influencing health care policy. Nurses have a promising future in the health policy arena.

Seeking Election to an Office

Those elected or appointed to an office, whether in a local nursing organization or the U.S. Congress, have considerable power to affect outcomes. Leaders in nursing organizations help to shape the direction and efforts of those organizations. Legislators have power to affect significant regulations and spending plans. Nurses in several states have been effective in shaping health policy by seeking and being elected to office as members of their state legislatures. Eddie Bernice Johnson, elected as a congresswoman from Texas in 1994, was the first nurse to hold an elective federal office. In the 1996 elections, four nurses were candidates for congressional seats, and of these, three were elected to office. As women in general have become more politically visible, nurses are a part of this growing political trend.

Limitations on Your Political Activity

If you are an employee of any governmental agency, such as a public health department or the Veterans Administration, your political activity is subject to restrictions that do not apply to the general public. Restrictions applying to federal government employees are defined in the **Hatch Act**. Prohibited activities are mainly those that have to do with supporting a particular political party by being an officer or party spokesperson. The Hatch Act also prohibits any political activity on the part of a government employee, on behalf of a party or in support of legislation that could be construed as representing his or her government agency.

The Hatch Act does not interfere with a private citizen's right to support parties and candidates financially, to join political parties, to work for or against measures that will appear on a ballot, or to participate in nonpartisan (ie, not connected with a political party) elections as a candidate. Each state has its own version of the Hatch Act. If you are employed by a governmental agency of any kind, you should investigate the limitations that your employment may place on your political activity.

THE FEDERAL GOVERNMENT'S ROLE IN HEALTH CARE

Federal legislation has affected nursing and health care in important ways. If you understand key concepts of the federal government's involvement in health care and how federal legislation has affected health care delivery, you will be more effective in the political arena.

Federal Agencies Related to Health Care

The federal government operates in the health care field in complex ways. Literally dozens of federal agencies are involved with health care in some way. The **Department of Health and Human Services (DHHS)** is a cabinet-level administrative unit of the federal government with four major service divisions (Display 3-3).

The Public Health Service, which includes the Centers for Disease Control and Prevention (CDC) is one agency with which you should already be familiar. The National Institutes of Health (NIH), the Food and Drug Administration (FDA), the Health Resources Administration (HRA), and the Center for Medical and Medicare Services (CMS) are all part of the DHHS. This agency has tremendous impact through its rules and regulations and the projects it funds.

Display 3-3   **MAJOR SERVICE DIVISIONS OF THE DEPARTMENT OF HEALTH AND HUMAN SERVICES**

Office of Human Development Services
Administration on Aging
Administration for Child, Youth, and Families
Administration for Native Americans
Administration for Public Service

Public Health Service
Centers for Disease Control and Prevention
Food and Drug Administration
Health Resources Administration
Health Services Administration
National Institutes of Health
Alcohol, Drug Abuse, and Mental Health
  Administration

Social Security Administration
Systems
Governmental Affairs
Family Assistance
Hearings and Appeals
Operational Policy and Procedure Assessment

Health Care Financing Administration
Health Standards and Quality Bureau
Bureau of Quality Control
Bureau of Program Operations
Bureau of Program Policy
Bureau of Support Services
Office of Child Support Enforcement

The Federal Budget Process

Because funding is a driving force in all decision making, you will find it useful to understand something of the federal budget process. The availability of government funding for each federal program depends on two separate legislative actions. The first action is the **authorization act**. This is a bill, passed by both the House of Representatives (where any revenue bill must originate) and the Senate, that describes a program and outlines the rules under which funds for the program can be expended. It also sets a ceiling on the amount of money that can be provided. It is under these authorization acts (often referred to by the "title" of the section of the authorizing act) that funds are dispensed for all the health-related activities described in this chapter.

The second necessary legislative action is the appropriations act. The appropriations process establishes the federal budget and the specific amounts of money appropriated for actual spending for each previously authorized program. Both the House and the Senate pass a budget appropriations act. Then a joint House and Senate committee meets to achieve a compromise that both will accept. The final result is called the "**Omnibus Budget Reconciliation Act**" (**OBRA**), which includes the compromises the budget committee has worked out between the House and Senate versions of the budget. Each budget act—for example, OBRA 1997—is identified by the year in the title. The amount appropriated for any program cannot exceed the amount originally authorized, but it can be, and often is, less. This is sometimes confusing because two monetary amounts, the authorized amount and the budgeted (or appropriated) amount, may be reported in connection with the same act.

The budget act also may place restrictions on the people and organizations receiving federal funds. It is under this authority that the federal government sets standards for nursing homes that receive reimbursement through Medicaid and Medicare. The rules and regulations for nursing homes, called the "**conditions of participation**," included in OBRA 1987 (the budget reconciliation act for 1987) were extensive. These rules and regulations did not take effect until October 1, 1990. This allowed the affected organizations to begin the process of change to meet the new requirements.

Historically, a third factor has affected the amount of money available for a specific federal program: the participation of the executive branch of government in decisions regarding how and when available funds will be spent. If money that has been authorized and appropriated has not been spent by the end of a budget period, it is lost. This money then must be reauthorized and reappropriated. The executive branch has used this mechanism to withdraw support for programs it opposes.

Funding for Nursing Education and Research

Beginning in 1964, the federal government provided funding to support nursing education through what was first titled the Nurse Training Act, later called the Nurse Education Act, and signed by President Bush in 2002 as the Nurse Reinvestment Act. In the 1960s and early 1970s, the funding was generous and included money for buildings, classroom renovation, equipment, faculty education and development, and student scholarships and traineeships. As the shortage of nurses abated and priorities changed in Washington, DC, the amount of funding gradually declined. The current nurse shortage once again resulted in political pressure by nursing organizations for the designation of funds for nursing education. The latest Act provides funds for scholarships and loan repayments for students and for encouraging the development of Magnet Hospitals (ANA pushes . . . 2002).

Every 2 years, when the biennial budget is passed, nurses try to rally congressional support for additional funding for nursing education. With the current nursing shortage, more groups are supporting nursing efforts to increase support for nursing education. Legislators are more open to discussions of the major needs of nursing. However, budget deficits at all levels of government arrived at the same time as the need for funds for nursing has increased. The passage of the Nurse Reinvestment Act of 2002 was welcomed by the entire health care community as a victory for health care in regard to budget priorities.

A major advance for nursing research in the 1980s was the addition of a National Institute for Nursing Research (NINR) to the other major divisions of the National Institutes of Health. Nurses and nursing organizations lobbied long and hard for legislative authorization for this institute. It is now a major financial source of nursing research dollars. Nursing groups continue to lobby for increases in the appropriation for the NINR.

Occupational Safety and Health

The **Occupational Safety and Health Act (OSHA)** mandates actions and prescribes safety equipment to improve the health and safety of the working environment. Many people think that the rules and regulations created by OSHA are too cumbersome. Nevertheless, concern for the safety of the working person is of considerable importance to nurses. Occupational injuries create major health problems for the adult population. They are costly not only in terms of health and personal loss but also in terms of lost productivity. Nurses also are affected by the provisions of OSHA in their own work environments. They, too, are subject to injury and accident on the job. The safety concerns of nurses in the workplace are discussed in Chapter 11.

Nurses in occupational health nursing also are involved in OSHA through educating workers about job safety. In some situations, safety precautions are time consuming and uncomfortable, and workers may be tempted to ignore them. Nurses may be able to help workers understand the importance of following health and safety regulations. Occupational health nurses also assist management in planning to make the environment safe and in establishing appropriate procedures for treating injuries.

OSHA regulations have required health care employers to provide the equipment, supplies, immunizations, and education to enable the implementation of CDC recommendations for "universal" precautions. The antiregulatory stance of Congress since 1994 has been reflected in the failure of OSHA to upgrade infection-control requirements to the CDC recommendation for Standard Precautions.

More recently, OSHA has been investigating the effects of repetitive strain injuries, among which are back injuries in health care workers. Funds for National Academy of Sciences research related to the link between repetitive motions and workplace injuries were included in the 1999 fiscal year appropriation. OSHA regulations regarding prevention of this type of injury were developed but not implemented during the Clinton presidency. These regulations were rescinded by the new Congress after President Bush took office. Based on Congressional and administrative opposition to creating more regulations, efforts to decrease musculoskeletal injuries have remained voluntary. The ANA is one organization working with interested members of Congress to develop a bill that will achieve bipartisan support for requiring the establishment of ergonomic standards (The Upright Fight, 2002).

Another occupational concern to nurses is needlestick injuries. OSHA has mandated that all health care agencies have in place a blood-borne pathogens prevention program. This includes both training for behaviors of staff and what are termed "engineering" controls. Engineering controls are the use of safe equipment that does not rely solely on the action of the individual to maintain protection. The FY 1999 appropriations bill included a requirement that employers record all injuries from potentially contaminated needles and other sharp instruments. The CDC, in November 1999, changed its recommendation to include the use of safe needles (NIOSH, 1999, *www.cdc.gov/niosh*). In 2000, the federal Needlestick Safety and Prevention Act was passed. This requires that hospitals provide safer devices to prevent needlestick injury. Several states have introduced needle safety legislation.

A current safety concern of health care workers is violence in the workplace. Nurses in psychiatric settings have long recognized the hazards they face in working with aggressive, violent, and sometimes out-of-control clients. Emergency rooms are sites where the violence of society spills over into the health care setting. Even obstetric units may encounter violence by family members. Nurses are asking that OSHA mandate health care workplaces to provide safety from violence. (See Chapter 11 for a further discussion of violence in the workplace.)

Nursing Home Regulations

OBRA 1987, the federal budget bill passed for 1987, contained regulations that for the first time mandated a national standard for quality of care in nursing homes receiving federal money through Medicare or Medicaid. Although the provisions of this act were set to take effect in October 1990, there were delays because of legal challenges to the requirements and because of the extra time that was needed to establish monitoring mechanisms. This is not unusual when legislation requires difficult and costly implementation. Therefore, some of the provisions of OBRA 1987 took effect as late as 1994. Despite earlier concerns, it is now clear that these regulations have positively affected the care environment in nursing homes. The use of restraints has decreased, resident rights are more effectively supported, and basic care needs are being identified and met. More recently, the budget bill for 1999 established a prospective payment system for skilled nursing facilities that resulted in decreased payments from Medicare and Medicaid.

THE STATE GOVERNMENT'S ROLE IN HEALTH CARE

Many issues that vitally affect the health care arena are decided at the state level. Because the health care issues in each state are different, only some general areas of concern are outlined here.

State Agencies and Health Care

State institutions range from those that care for the mentally retarded and the mentally ill to penal systems and institutions of higher education. Health care is a consideration in all of these settings. When budgets are planned, topics as diverse as immunization and contraception may be part of the debate. Nurses often can advocate for those who are unable to speak for themselves about their own health care needs. Sometimes nurses who work in these settings are unable to deliver quality care because of severe budgetary deficiencies. All nurses can support efforts to provide quality health care in such settings.

Nurse Practice Acts

Nurse practice acts are being discussed and revised in many states. This process is long and difficult and requires intense political effort by nurses to avoid creating problems for the profession. One current concern related to placing the act before a state legislature for action is the pressure to lessen the standards or allow unlicensed assistive personnel to perform more nursing tasks. Another concern is the implementation of multistate licensure. (See Chapter 6 for further discussion of licensure laws.)

State Legislative Concerns

Some of the major workplace concerns of nurses are emerging as topics of state legislation. The ANA has identified nine major state-level legislative issues of importance to nurses (see Display 3-4). In some states legislation has already been passed in regard to some of these issues. Concerns about the nurse's vulnerability when unsafe care is part of an institution's practice have led to efforts toward achieving whistleblower protection. A **whistleblower** is a person who reports to authorities the wrongdoing of individuals in their own work setting or the organizations in which they are employed. The state of New Jersey was the first to pass legislation that protects from retaliation health care employees who refuse to participate in or who report unsafe practices. The federal government encourages whistleblowing to reveal fraud in the Medicare and Medicaid programs and posts a complaint form on its Web site (Centers for Medicare and Medicaid Services, 2003).

An example of the concerns of nurses is the use of safe needles or protected devices for blood drawing and parenteral medication administration. These devices are being manufactured and do dramatically decrease the incidence of needlestick injury; however, they cost a great deal more than the needles they replace. For example, in one setting, a needle that cost 34 cents was replaced with a needleless connector that cost $1.74. When computed systemwide, that is a tremendous increase in cost. However, nurses are pointing out that the cost of surveillance and care of those who sustain needlestick injuries also must be added to the cost of using needles. What is the cost of a case of hepatitis C? Of hepatitis A? Of HIV?

Many of the state level issues are those that relate to increasing workplace satisfaction, such as prohibition of mandatory overtime, nursing staffing systems and ratios, and violence

---

Display 3-4

STATE-LEVEL LEGISLATIVE CONCERNS IDENTIFIED BY ANA

- Prohibition of mandatory overtime
- Nurse staffing systems and ratios
- Nursing workforce data collection
- Nursing education incentives
- Ergonomics
- Needlestick injury prevention
- Nursing quality indicators
- Violence in the workplace
- Whistleblower protection

in the workplace. Improving working conditions is an important aspect of addressing the nursing shortage. These issues will be discussed in greater detail in Chapter 11.

LOCAL POLITICAL CONCERNS

The budgetary process always seems to be at the root of most political and legislative concerns. Because only a limited amount of money is available, budgets always are developed through a series of compromises. To gain one objective, it is sometimes necessary to recognize that funds will not be available for achieving another. In most communities, budgets for public health departments, school nurses, and so forth are developed over a period of several months. Hearings are often held, at which members of the public may ask questions and address issues. Nurses often have found that involvement at this planning stage is most rewarding. Determining priorities for health care is essential, and nurses can speak with authority on these matters. Nurses actually employed in a public department undergoing review may be limited in making their views known because of regulations governing their action in the political sphere. For this reason, it is significant that nurses outside of government institutions recognize the importance of community health. It is not only the practice of the public health nurse that is affected by the priorities of the agency. For example, a nurse who is employed in a hospital may wish to refer a discharged patient to a public health nurse for follow-up, only to find that, owing to changes in the ordering of priorities, home visits for the identified purpose are no longer being made.

In many communities, decisions about the allocation of federal money are made at the local level. Recent Congressional actions have been toward enhancing state and local control through creating large block grants where priorities would be decided locally. Support for alternative health care centers, blood pressure screening, and senior citizen centers may depend on whether those who are knowledgeable about the benefits of these services are willing to voice their advocacy in local decision-making bodies.

HEALTH CARE REFORM

Financing health care for all citizens has been the focus of many efforts for health care reform. When these efforts failed at the national level, the drive for providing health care moved to the state level. As each state debates these issues, common questions recur, including:

- Do people have a right to health care?
- If there is such a right, what level of health care can people expect to receive? Routine preventive services? Surgery and hospitalization for all conditions? Or treatment only for serious life-threatening conditions?
- Should catastrophic illnesses, transplantation, and experimental treatments and medications be included?
- What about fertility-enhancing services? Should contraceptive costs be covered? Should abortion services be included?

- How can health care be transformed into an effective, coordinated system?
- How will changes in the health care system be financed?

These are difficult philosophic and ethical questions, and there are no simple answers.

Nursing's Agenda for the Future

The ANA, the NLN, and 60 other nursing organizations cooperated in developing Nursing's Agenda for the Future, which addresses the nation's need for nursing care. Ten areas of concern are addressed in this document: leadership and planning, delivery systems/nursing models, legislation/regulation/policy, professional/nursing culture, recruitment and retention, economic value, work environment, public relations/communications, education, and diversity. For each of these areas, the Agenda contains objectives and strategies to move toward those objectives. (Trossman, 2002.) The current focus is on "action plans" developed by nursing organizations and groups that will implement the strategies. In addition to combating the current nursing shortage, these action plans will move the profession forward, creating a desired future for nursing within the health care system. (See the ANA Web site for complete information on Nursing's Agenda for the Future.)

Critical Thinking Activity

Identify an aspect of health care reform that concerns you. Analyze the various proposals currently before Congress or your state legislature regarding that specific concern. Rank the proposals in order of your preference, providing rationales for your decision making. In a small group, hold a discussion in which you share your analysis of the various proposals.

NURSING ORGANIZATIONS

A student once said that it seems that every time nurses identify a problem, their first action is to form a new organization. Although this may be something of an exaggeration, it contains a bit of truth. When you first learn about the great number of nursing and nursing-related organizations, it all seems confusing and their purposes and functions may seem duplicative.

The existence of a large number of diverse organizations for nurses is, in many ways, a reflection of nursing itself. The profession offers a wide variety of employment opportunities to its members, with distinct and varied contributions and interests in health care. When nurses become committed to a particular specialty group, they have a tendency to want to advance the purposes and interests of the people working in that area. For example, operating room nurses have more in common with other operating room nurses, in terms of interests and concerns, than they have with nurses working in hospice care. Likewise, nurses involved in hospice care would probably prefer to share concerns with one another than to discuss them with critical care nurses. With more than 2.2 million nurses in the United States, it is understandable that there are many different areas of nursing interest, and therefore many different nursing organizations.

The formation of a large number of nursing organizations has resulted in concern regarding the overlapping of function and interrelationships among some of the organizations. Unfortunately, there has often been a spirit of competition rather than cooperation among these groups in the past. Because nurses traditionally have not had high incomes, joining more than one organization has not been a desirable option for economic as well as philosophic reasons.

Nursing organizations recently have made a concerted effort to promote cooperation. Nurses are better informed about the various organizations and receive better salaries than in the past. However, these facts have not resulted in significantly greater participation by professional nurses in their organizations. Some people specifically do not join because of philosophic differences, but many nurses seem to be apathetic and do not recognize the importance of nurses acting together. Some, because they are combining a job with family and home responsibilities, feel they do not have the time or energy to become involved. Nurses need to recognize the potential for power that they possess as a group. As the nation moves toward health care reform, this has never been a more critical issue.

Critical Thinking Activity

Do you believe that there are too many nursing organizations? Give the rationale for your answer. If you could develop a method for reducing the number of nursing organizations, what criteria would you suggest be used to support the continuation of existing groups? Provide the rationale for each criterion you suggest.

American Nurses Association

The ANA, the professional association for RNs, had its origins in a meeting of nursing leaders at the World's Fair in Chicago in 1890. Through their suggestions and efforts, the alumnae organizations of 10 schools of nursing sent delegates in 1896 to form a committee to organize a professional association. The resulting organization was called National Associated Alumnae of the United States and Canada. The name was changed in 1899 to the Nurses' Associated Alumnae of the United States and Canada. In 1901, Canada was dropped from the title because the state laws of New York (where the organization was incorporated) did not allow for representatives from more than one country. The name "American Nurses Association" was adopted in the United States in 1911; Canadian nurses formed their own organization at that time.

The ANA has been identified as the organization for RNs. As such, it has always had as its primary interest the concerns of the nurses it represents. Throughout history, the organization has been active in issues relating to licensure (see Chapter 7), collective bargaining (see Chapter 12), nursing education (see Chapter 6), and a host of other concerns facing nurses and nursing.

MEMBERSHIP

The ANA membership comprises the 50 state nurses' associations and the three territorial constituent units. State nurses' associations (SNAs) comprise the district nurses' associations (DNAs). The individual nurse belongs to the ANA through the SNA. Before 1982, when the federation model was adopted, individual nurses were members of the ANA. The change to membership through the SNAs was made because it was thought that SNAs would be able to recruit more members and have greater control. However, there has not been an increase in membership. Each state is free to establish its own membership plans; however, membership is limited to RNs. The only exception to this rule is the admission to membership of some new graduates who have not yet passed the licensing examination.

It is regrettable that fewer than half of the RNs in the United States participate in the ANA. Those who do participate are often the leaders in the nursing profession. One reason for the low level of membership is the high cost of membership. Annual dues to the national association and the state and district associations are paid together, and in most parts of the country they are more than $300 combined. Another reason nurses have for not joining is a lack of time to participate in activities. Many nurses have the dual responsibilities of job and home and feel that they have no time left for involvement in a professional organization. Other nurses do not see how the benefits available through membership in the association are personally valuable. Some explain that they are just not interested in the issues and concerns of the organization. Finally, some nurses do not join because they do not agree with the position of the ANA on major issues; this has been especially true with regard to the role of the SNAs in collective bargaining and with regard to some of the ANA's positions on nursing education.

Those who are active in the ANA believe that its work is severely hampered by the low level of membership. The number of members limits the funds of the organization. Because some specific programs, such as the collective bargaining programs, are costly to the state association, there has been a strong move to require nurses to belong to the association if it serves as a bargaining agent. In some states, the state association has set a specific percentage of an agency's staff that must be members before they will become the bargaining agent for the nurses in that agency.

A current controversy involves differing views regarding the purpose of the professional organization. Many nurses believe that the organization primarily should be concerned with what it can do for the individual nurse. Others believe that a truly professional approach focuses on what the individual nurse can contribute to the profession through the organization. Some think that the organization should be a more vocal advocate in the realm of economic security while others do not see this as an appropriate focus for the professional organization. Another point of controversy is the organization's stand on political issues.

In 1995, the California Nurses Association experienced a great deal of internal turmoil because of a perceived lack of support from the ANA regarding the massive changes being created by health care reform (Costello, 1995). As a result, the CNA delegate assembly voted to withdraw from the ANA and to establish itself as an independent "international" organization. This enabled the CNA to keep all of the dues in the state for its own purposes, but it also deprived CNA members of a voice and opportunities at the national level. Some nurses who did not support the separation of the CNA from the ANA joined ANA affiliate organizations in bordering states during the dispute. The ANA tried to resolve the problems but was unsuccessful; instead, it subsequently established another organization called ANA-California. ANA is encouraging nurses in California who are interested in being part of the national organization and its efforts to join this new organization. Subsequently, a similar situation arose in Massachusetts, resulting in the withdrawal of the Massachusetts Nurses Association from the ANA.

ACTIVITIES AND SERVICES

The ANA is referred to many times throughout this book. As a professional association, it has been involved in all the issues that nursing has confronted. There has not been universal support in the nursing community for all of the activities that the ANA has championed or for the stands that it has taken. In any group as large as nursing, it is perhaps inevitable to have a wide range of viewpoints.

Advancement of the Profession. The ANA supports work on policies related to the profession as a whole, such as the Code of Ethics for Nurses (ANA, 2001). The ANA also supports research on topics related to the profession itself, such as historical patterns of licensure.

One of the most significant services the ANA offers to members is certification through the American Nurses Credentialing Center. Recognition for expertise in a particular area usually is granted based on demonstration of knowledge through testing and clinical practice, although the criteria for certification vary among specialties.

Legislative Activity. The ANA is extensively involved in legislative activity. The organization often represents the profession in testimony before Congress on numerous issues affecting nursing. The need to be geographically closer to legislators to have greater participation in legislative efforts was the major reason for the relocation of the ANA offices to Washington, DC in 1992. The organization provides testimony for or against legislation that will affect the profession, either directly or indirectly: legislative topics include funds for nursing education, collective bargaining issues, concerns for higher education, and human rights issues. It also testifies on health-related issues affecting the general public, such as the quality of care in nursing homes and health care reform. A newsletter, Capitol Update, is published monthly and provides information to the reader about issues currently being addressed in the Capitol. Capitol Wiz is available on the ANA Web site, *www.nursingworld.org*.

Collective Bargaining. An activity that has a major impact on the economic welfare of nurses is the organization's support of collective bargaining. This is also one of the most controversial services of the ANA. The SNAs are the official bargaining representatives in most instances (see Chapter 12). In 1999, the ANA restructured to create an arm titled United American Nurses that will represent nurses in workplace issues and provide a forum for the collective bargaining sections of the state associations.

Other Resources and Services. In addition to its activities, the ANA provides direct services to members. These include access to a group professional liability insurance plan and group insurance for health, disability, and accident coverage. From time to time the ANA also provides access to group travel arrangements and purchasing discounts.

Through its educational services, the ANA produces and distributes a wide variety of nursing educational materials, such as films, as well as a biennial report entitled "Facts About Nursing." This report provides basic statistical information that is used by many organizations and individuals. Reports of committees and commissions and special studies supported by the ANA also are published.

The American Nurse is the official publication of the ANA; official announcements of ANA business are published in this paper. The paper also contains current news relevant to nursing and health care, editorials, letters, and classified advertisements. The *American Journal of*

Nursing is the official journal of the organization. It is published monthly and contains some current news, but its major focus is professional articles. It is published by Lippincott Williams & Wilkins, but retains autonomy over its own content.

The ANA also publishes many pamphlets and informational resources of value to nurses. A complete list of publications is available at the ANA Web site and in print from the organization. The ANA Web site continues to expand the content available and now includes the Online Journal of Nursing, continuing education programs, and the many documents and position statements produced by the ANA.

Organizations Related to the ANA

Because it is an official professional association, the ANA is related to other organizations in unique ways. These organizations operate autonomously, but are closely tied to the ANA.

INTERNATIONAL COUNCIL OF NURSES

The International Council of Nurses (ICN) is the international organization for professional nursing, with membership consisting of national nursing organizations. The ANA, as a constituent member of the ICN, sends delegates to its convention and participates in its activities. The ICN is interested in health care in general and nursing care in particular throughout the world. It works with the United Nations, when appropriate, and with other international health-related groups, such as the International Red Cross.

The ICN concerns itself with such issues as the social and economic welfare of nurses, the role of the nurse in health care, and the roles of national nursing organizations throughout the world and their relationships to their governing bodies. The primary governing body of the organization is the Council of National Representatives, which meets biennially.

The ICN has representatives from 104 national nurses' organizations. The Council of National Representatives governs the organization, which consists of all the presidents of the member organizations. Activities of the organization are carried out by its Board of Directors, the officers, volunteer nurse members of constituent organizations, and employed staff, including an executive director. The ICN maintains headquarters in Geneva, Switzerland.

Every 4 years a quadrennial congress is held. This meeting is open to all nurses and to delegates from the national organizations. Concerns addressed at recent congresses focused on such issues as career ladders, educational standards, research, human rights, and nursing's role in the planning of a national health policy.

AMERICAN NURSES FOUNDATION

In 1955, the ANA established the American Nurses Foundation (ANF) as a tax-exempt, non-profit corporation for the purpose of supporting research related to nursing. It is independently financed and self-governing. The Board of Trustees is composed of members of the Board of Directors of the ANA, other nurse members, and non-nurse members from other health-related fields and from the public. To accomplish its varied objectives, the ANF solicits gifts and contributions from individuals and organizations. These gifts are tax deductible.

The ANF maintains a three-pronged approach to supporting research. The first objective is to conduct policy analyses to provide nursing leaders and public-policy makers with the information they need for decision making. The second objective is related to developing "nurse scholars" who engage in study of such areas as journalism and public policy. Support is directed toward independent study, research, and doctoral and postdoctoral work for these nurse scholars. The third objective is to facilitate the research and educational activities of ANA. This includes providing consultation and funding for groups in the ANA that wish to initiate projects.

AMERICAN ACADEMY OF NURSING

The ANA established the American Academy of Nursing (AAN) in 1973 as an honorary association in the ANA. The Board of Directors of the ANA chose the original members. The AAN is now an independent organization, and new members are selected by those currently in the AAN. Those elected to the AAN are called fellows and may use the title "Fellow of the American Academy of Nursing" (FAAN). The purpose of this organization is to recognize nurses who have made significant contributions to the profession of nursing.

National Student Nurses' Association

The National Student Nurses' Association (NSNA) is a professional organization for students in schools of nursing and was started in 1952. Although it works with the ANA, it is a fully independent organization, run and financed by nursing students. It sponsors its own annual convention.

Although the NSNA is an autonomous organization, it has close ties with the ANA. Members of the NSNA serve on selected committees in the ANA, speak to the House of Delegates at the ANA convention to provide a student viewpoint, and work together with the ANA regarding current issues.

Each state has a state nursing student association that operates in the same relationship to the state professional organization as the NSNA does to the national organization. State conventions and workshops are held in many states. State issues are addressed by the state association in the same way that national issues are addressed by the NSNA. Local nursing student organizations may or may not exist in individual schools of nursing. These local organizations may be closely tied to the state and national groups, or they may be independent. It is possible for an individual student to join the state and national student nurses' organizations even if no local counterpart exists.

A major project of the NSNA is "Breakthrough into Nursing," which is designed to recruit and maintain the enrollment of minorities in schools of nursing. The project has enlisted nursing students to speak to minority teenagers to interest them in nursing early in their scholastic careers, and to act as preceptors and tutors to increase the retention of minority students when they enroll in schools of nursing.

The NSNA often is asked to testify before congressional committees when issues relevant to nursing education are being considered. In this role, the organization becomes the public voice for all nursing students.

In 1975, the NSNA developed a Student Bill of Rights, which was updated in 1991. This document carefully balances the rights of students with the responsibilities of students. It supports the view of students as competent adults who are engaged in an educational program. The rights that are outlined relate to educational programs, to the rules and policies of an institution, and to freedom in personal life and decision making (Display 3-5).

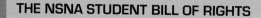

Display 3-5 THE NSNA STUDENT BILL OF RIGHTS

Bill of Rights and Responsibilities for Students of Nursing

An NSNA Student Bill of Rights and Responsibilities was initially adopted in 1975. The following updated version was adopted by the NSNA House of Delegates in San Antonio, Texas (1991).

Students should be encouraged to develop the capacity for critical judgment and engage in a sustained and independent search for truth.

The freedom to teach and the freedom to learn are inseparable facets of academic freedom: students should exercise their freedom in a responsible manner.

Each institution has a duty to develop policies and procedures that provide and safeguard the students' freedom to learn.

Under no circumstances should a student be barred from admission to a particular institution on the basis of race, creed, sex, color, national origin, handicap, or marital status.

Students should be free to take reasoned exception to the data or views offered in any course of study and to reserve judgment about matters of opinion, but they are responsible for learning the content of any course of study for which they are enrolled.

Students should have protection through orderly procedures against prejudiced or capricious academic evaluation, but they are responsible for maintaining standards of academic performance established for each course in which they are enrolled.

Information about student views, beliefs, political ideation, or sexual orientation which instructors acquire in the course of their work or otherwise, should be considered confidential and not released without the knowledge or consent of the student, and should not be used as a basis of evaluation.

The student should have the right to have a responsible voice in the determination of his/her curriculum.

Institutions should have a carefully considered policy as to the information that should be a part of a student's permanent educational record and as to the conditions of this disclosure.

Students and student organizations should be free to examine and discuss all questions of interest to them, and to express opinions publicly and privately.

Students should be allowed to invite and to hear any person of their own choosing within the institution's acceptable realm, thereby taking the responsibility of furthering their education.

The student body should have clearly defined means to participate in the formulation and application of institutional policy affecting academic and student affairs, eg, through a faculty–student council, student membership or representation.

The institution has an obligation to clarify those standards of behavior that it considers essential to its educational mission, its community life, or its objectives and philosophy.

Disciplinary proceedings should be instituted only for violations of standards of conduct formulated with significant student participation and published in advance through such means as a student handbook or a generally available set of institutional regulations. It is the responsibility of the student to know these regulations. Grievance procedures should be available for every student.

As citizens and members of an academic community, students are subject to the obligations that accrue to them by virtue of this membership and should enjoy the same freedoms of citizenship.

Students have the right to belong or refuse to belong to any organization of their choice.

Students have the right to personal privacy in their living space to the extent that the welfare and property of others are respected.

Display 3-5   **THE NSNA STUDENT BILL OF RIGHTS (*continued*)**

Adequate safety precautions should be provided by nursing programs, for example, adequate street lighting, locks, and other safety measures deemed necessary by the environment.

Dress code, if present in school, should be established with student input in conjunction with the school director and faculty, so the highest professional standards are maintained, but also taking into consideration points of comfort and practicality for the student.

Grading systems should be carefully reviewed periodically with students and faculty for clarification and better student faculty understanding.

Students should have a clear mechanism for input into the evaluation of nursing faculty.

National Student Nurses' Association, 1991. Available at http://www.nsna.org/pubs/billofrights/ *Accessed March 7, 2003. (Reprinted by permission of the National Student Nurses' Association)*

National League for Nursing

Another major nursing organization is the National League for Nursing (NLN), which was established in 1952 and is often referred to as "The League." Its history and background are discussed in Chapter 4. The NLN identifies its mission as "The National League for Nursing advances quality nursing education that prepares the nursing workforce to meet the needs of diverse populations in an ever-changing healthcare environment." (NLN, 2002). The goals of the organization focus on five areas: (1) nursing education development and improvement, (2) faculty development, (3) nursing education research, (4) data collection, and (5) assessment and evaluation.

MEMBERSHIP

The NLN offers membership to individuals and agencies. It is unique among nursing organizations in offering membership and participation to consumers, to non-nursing members of health care teams, and to institutions concerned with nursing service and nursing education, as well as to nurses.

ACTIVITIES AND SERVICES

The NLN works in a complementary, rather than competitive, manner with the ANA. Whereas the ANA speaks as the official voice of nurses, the NLN seeks to unite the interests of nursing with those of the community in support of excellence in nursing education.

Assessment and Evaluation Services. Until 1982, the NLN produced the licensing examination for the state boards of nursing. Although it no longer has this responsibility, it does have a large testing service that produces standardized assessment tests to be used in the nursing program admission process, achievement tests for various levels in a program that can be used by a program for evaluation, the NLN mobility examinations (which are used to provide advanced placement credit), and diagnostic examinations for those preparing for the NCLEX examinations.

Program and Professional Development. The NLN sponsors continuing education workshops and conferences throughout the country, often repeating a workshop in different locations to spare nurses and others the expense of travel. Subjects are determined in consultation with members and are geared to current needs and interests. Curriculum, research, accreditation, testing and evaluation, student recruitment and retention, political awareness and health care legislation, and a nurse executive series are regular subjects for continuing education. The constituent leagues, which are grouped by regional assemblies, also offer workshops designed to meet the interests of particular areas of the country.

Division of Research. When any group needs figures on nursing education, it cites data gathered by NLN's Division of Research. The division is a primary provider of statistics on nursing education, and each year surveys all schools of registered and practical nursing for enrollments, admissions, and graduations. It also conducts a yearly survey of newly RNs regarding the characteristics of their employment. Every 2 years, the nurse-faculty census is taken; every 3 years, data are gathered on men and minorities in schools of nursing.

Career Information and Publications. The career information service answers thousands of inquiries about nursing education that arrive each year by mail and by telephone. The NLN Web site contains information for individuals interested in exploring nursing careers.

Through its journal, *Nursing Education Perspectives*, and a newsletter, *NLN Update* (both available on the Web), members are kept informed about current issues. Sometimes NLN spokespersons offer testimony on legislation or rulings significant to the organization. The NLN publishes many texts and references about curriculum, ethics, public policy, nursing administration, long-term care, and other topics of interest to nursing. It also produces educational videos.

National League for Nursing Accrediting Commission

Many students are aware of **accreditation** that provides standards and criteria against which nursing programs can be evaluated. The NLN Accrediting Commission (NLNAC) accredits nursing programs of all types: practical nursing, diploma nursing, associate degree nursing, and baccalaureate and higher degree programs. Initially, nursing accreditation was performed by the National Nursing Accrediting Service, which merged in 1952 with other groups to form the NLN. After the merger, the NLN provided accreditation of nursing programs. In the 1990s, the Department of Education (DOE), which provides approval for accrediting bodies, required the NLN to develop a new structure that clearly separated the accreditation process from the rest of the organization. This was part of the new framework that the DOE established for voluntary accreditation and included many additional regulatory features. Beginning in 1997, the separate but related organization, the NLNAC, assumed accrediting responsibilities formerly carried out by the NLN (Fig. 3-3).

National Council of State Boards of Nursing

Although it is not a nursing organization like those previously discussed, our discussion would not be complete without mention of the National Council of State Boards of Nursing, Inc. (NCSBN). This organization was formed in 1978 to replace the Council of State Boards that had been part of the ANA. The purpose of this organization is to provide a forum for the

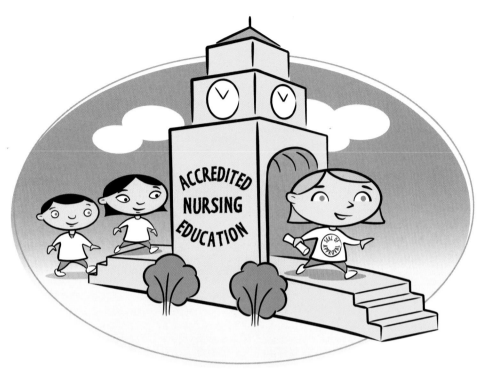

FIGURE 3-3   Accreditation is designed to help ensure that the desired outcomes of education are achieved.

legal regulatory bodies (whatever their particular state titles might be) of all states to act together in the development of the licensing examinations, and in other matters of common concern. There is one delegate to this council from each state agency. The actions of this council are particularly important because its membership represents the legal authority for the control of nursing education and nursing practice.

Although each state agency must operate within its own laws, it does have authority to establish many specific rules and regulations. Working together, the state boards hope to promote uniform standards for the nursing profession. One of the agenda items they have addressed is the development of a Model Nurse Practice Act. Much energy has gone into the development, validation, and establishment of computerized testing for the licensing examination for both registered and practical nursing. Currently the organization is studying the methods used to approve and license advanced practice nurses and the concerns associated with multistate practice.

Organizations Representing Licensed Practical Nurses

Two nursing organizations are concerned primarily with advancing the interests of practical (vocational) nurses. These two organizations are the National Federation of Licensed Practical Nurses (NFLPN) and the National Association for Practical Nurse Education and Service (NAPNES).

The National Federation of Licensed Practical Nurses (NFLPN) is one of the professional organizations for practical nurses. Founded in 1949, its membership is limited to licensed practical and vocational nurses. The NFLPN has assisted the ANA in some activities, and actively supports the need for the practical nurse in health care. State and local groups of the NFLPN are active in educational issues affecting the LPN, and have supported the associate degree as the appropriate educational preparation for the responsibilities of the LPN in the current health care system.

The National Association for Practical Nurse Education and Service (NAPNES) was organized as the Association of Practical Nurse Schools in 1941. Its purpose was to address the needs of practical nursing education. The name was changed in 1942 to the National Association for Practical Nurse Education; in 1959, it added "and Service" to that title. The official publication of the organization is *The Journal of Practical Nursing*, which has been published since 1951. It also publishes a newsletter, *NAPNES Forum*, that keeps members alert to activities of the organization. Membership is open to licensed practical/vocational nurses, practical/vocational nursing students, faculty, directors, and others interested in promoting the purposes of the organization. It was the first organization to provide accreditation for practical nursing programs, although that role now rests with the NLNAC.

North American Nursing Diagnosis Association

The North American Nursing Diagnosis Association (NANDA), established in 1982, is open to individuals as well as group members. The purpose of this group is to work toward uniform terminology and definitions to be used in nursing diagnosis and to share ideas and information regarding this topic. Members identify and research problems nurses manage, prepare documentation, and submit these to NANDA to be included in the consideration process. Committees then review the problems. Those that meet the basic criteria for nursing diagnoses are submitted to the membership. Defining characteristics are identified, and conditions that form the etiology or are related to the development of the diagnosis are identified. A national convention held every 2 years is the final forum for the debate and discussion of proposed new nursing diagnoses. The general outline of the taxonomy (classification system) was established by a group of nursing theorists and then accepted by the organization.

American Organization of Nurse Executives

According to their Web site, the American Organization of Nurse Executives (AONE) is the "national professional organization for nurses who design, facilitate, and manage care" (available at *www.aha.org/resources/AboutAone.html*). This organization provides the forum for nurses with managerial and executive responsibility to work collaboratively both with other nurses in similar roles and through the organization with other organizations. AONE is one of the members of the Tricouncil for Nursing, which serves as an information resource for legislative and governmental personnel.

Clinically Related Organizations

Some of the earliest specialty organizations were related to specific clinical practice areas of nursing. A major focus of these organizations now is continuing education related to a particular nursing specialty. Most groups also have some mechanisms, such as certification, for recognizing achievement in the field. One of the earliest specialty organizations, founded in 1941, was the American Association of Nurse Anesthetists, a group of approximately 24,000 members, of whom 40% are men.

Specialty organizations also include groups that began as auxiliaries to specialty physicians' organizations, such as AWHONN: Association of Women's Health, Obstetric and Neonatal Nurses. This organization was started for nurses affiliated with physicians who were "fellows" of the American College of Obstetricians and Gynecologists. As more members joined and nurses became more active, groups such as this one became autonomous.

The overlapping purpose and actions of the Councils on Practice of the ANA and the corresponding specialty organizations have caused some concern. One attempt to promote a more cooperative effort was the creation of the Nursing Organization Liaison Forum (NOLF), which operates as a forum in the ANA.

One of the newest nursing organizations is the National Alliance of Nurse Practitioners (NANP), organized in 1986. Its purpose is to promote the health care of the nation by promoting the visibility, viability, and unity of nurse practitioners. Its activities focus on advancing the role of the nurse practitioner in the health care delivery system. Issues related to the reimbursement of nurse practitioners are of major concern to this organization.

Groups Related to Ethnic Origin

As the movement for self-determination and preservation of identity arose within ethnic groups in the United States, nurses within various ethnic groups began to unite to achieve a greater voice in health care. Some ethnic groups are nationally organized; others are organized on a more local level. As these groups have become stronger and more organized, their interests have included the recruitment and support of nursing students from the particular ethnic groups they represent. These ethnic groups also encourage their members to become more politically involved in nursing and nursing leadership.

Honorary Organizations

Sigma Theta Tau is an international organization established in collegiate schools of nursing to recognize those with superior ability and leadership potential, and those who have made important contributions to nursing. Candidates may be asked to join during the senior year of a baccalaureate program, or any time thereafter. Sigma Theta Tau has established a nursing library at its headquarters in Indianapolis that has reference abilities to support advanced scholarship; the organization also provides the first online nursing journal that can be accessed by computer. Local chapters may maintain funds to support individual research projects, hold research conferences, and recognize those who have made significant contributions to nursing.

Alpha Tau Delta is a professional nursing fraternity. Students who are enrolled in baccalaureate nursing programs and demonstrate scholarship and personality characteristics in line with the organization's professional goals are eligible for membership.

Religiously Oriented Organizations

The National Council of Catholic Nurses and the Nurses' Christian Fellowship (primarily a nondenominational Protestant group) were organized to assist nurses in sharing concerns and integrating their work and their religious beliefs. These two organizations place special emphasis on meeting a patient's spiritual needs and on dealing with ethical issues.

Educationally Oriented Organizations

Since the 1960s, there has been a great deal of change and development in nursing education as it has moved from the hospital into the educational setting. During this time, there has been an increased emphasis on educational methods, curriculum development, and research.

In several major geographic regions of the United States, educational organizations extending membership to schools of nursing, members of the state boards of nursing, and other interested individuals were developed to promote interstate and interinstitutional cooperation in seeking pathways to improved nursing education and scholarship. These organizations are the Western Institute of Nursing (WIN), the Council on Collegiate Education for Nursing of the Southern Regional Education Board (CCEN/SREB), the New England Organization for Nursing (NEON), the Midwest Alliance in Nursing (MAIN), and the Mid-Atlantic Regional Nursing Association (MARNA).

The National Organization for the Advancement of Associate Degree Nursing (NOAADN) has four purposes: to speak for associate degree nursing education and practice; to reinforce the value of associate degree nursing education and practice; to maintain endorsement of RN licensure from state to state for the associate degree nurse; and to retain the RN licensure examination for graduates of associate degree nursing programs. Membership is open to individuals, states, agencies, and organizations.

The American Association of Colleges of Nursing (AACN) was formed to assist collegiate schools of nursing in working cooperatively to improve higher education for professional nursing. Membership is limited to deans and directors of programs that offer a baccalaureate degree in nursing, with an upper-division nursing major, and that are part of a regionally accredited college or university.

In 1996, this organization instituted planning to become an accrediting organization for baccalaureate and higher degree programs in nursing. A related organization, the Commission on Collegiate Nursing Education (CCNE), was formed to provide accreditation. This organization began accrediting activities in 1999. Thus, there are now two separate specialized accreditation organizations for baccalaureate and higher degree nursing programs. The development of two organizations for accreditation of these programs has created concerns in some areas of nursing that it may create competition rather than foster cooperative efforts for excellence in nursing education.

Miscellaneous Organizations

The American Assembly for Men in Nursing was formed by those who believed that, as a minority in the profession, men needed to speak about issues with a united voice. The membership has expanded to include women who are concerned about gender issues in nursing. The organization has addressed the issue of discrimination toward men in nursing and seeks to present nursing as a profession in which both men and women can contribute and excel.

Nurses House, Inc. provides assistance for nurses in need. It originated from a bequest in 1922 from Emily Bourne, who donated $300,000 to establish a country home where nurses might find needed rest. As the need for this residence decreased, supporters of this endeavor sold the estate and invested the proceeds. Income from the investment and funds donated by nurses (and friends of nurses) are used to provide guidance and counseling for nurses with emotional and chemical dependency problems, encouragement to homebound nurses, and temporary financial assistance to nurses who are ill, convalescing, or unemployed. Nurses House seeks members and donations to assist in continuing these activities.

The Gay Nurses' Alliance was an outgrowth of the movement of homosexual individuals to be accepted without having to disguise their sexual orientation. This group primarily has focused on the issue of gay rights. They also provide a forum for gay individuals to address the difficulties they may face in the nursing profession.

Critical Thinking Activity

As a new graduate, assume you have $400 per year to spend on membership in a nursing organization. In trying to decide which organization to join, how would you go about learning the focus of several groups that have attracted your interest? What process could you use to ensure that you are joining the group that best serves your needs? Which organization would you join? Provide a clear rationale based on both economic and professional reasons for your choice.

KEY CONCEPTS

- Because scarce resources are allocated through the political process, nurses will find that understanding this process is essential to influencing the health care system.
- Every individual nurse has many opportunities to affect the political process. This can be done simply by keeping informed, by voting, or by trying to shape public opinion. Communicating with legislators and officials can be done as an individual or as part of a group. Testifying presents issues of importance, and individual support can be given to those running for office. You may even decide to run for a public office.
- The federal government is active in health care through many existing agencies in the Department of Health and Human Services and in other branches of government. The federal budget process affects the health care services available through the many legislative acts affecting health care.
- A political process is part of any large organization, and nursing organizations are no exception. Understanding the political process can help you participate more effectively in a large organization.
- The variety of organizations in nursing is often confusing to the new nursing graduate and to the public. These organizations represent the nursing profession as a whole, as well as special interest groups within nursing.

- The American Nurses Association, whose membership is open to RNs only, provides the voice of professional nursing. Actions of the ANA are directed toward nursing practice issues, economic welfare of nurses, and broader issues of health care.
- The National Student Nurses' Association addresses the interests and needs of nursing students. As a fully autonomous organization, the NSNA membership is open to nursing students only.
- Another major nursing organization is the National League for Nursing which, historically, has championed better nursing education. Membership is open to individuals and agencies interested in nursing. The NLNAC, a subsidiary of the NLN, provides for the accreditation of all types of nursing programs throughout the United States.
- Two nursing organizations exist expressly to serve the needs of licensed practical (vocational) nurses. These groups are the National Federation of Licensed Practical Nurses and the National Association for Practical Nurse Education and Service.
- Organizations also exist that represent specialty groups in nursing. Members usually are drawn together by their common interests and concerns. The organizations provide continuing education and, in some instances, certification.
- Some organizations, such as Sigma Theta Tau, are honorary in their focus. These groups strive to bring recognition to nurses and nursing.
- A wide variety of other organizations meet the special needs of their membership. This may relate to social interests, ethnic background, or other common denominators. Two very active and prominent organizations are the Association of Nurse Executives (AONE) and the American Association of Collegiate Nursing Programs (AACN), which represents baccalaureate and higher degree programs and provides accreditation for those programs through its subsidiary the Council on Collegiate Nursing Education (CCNE).

RELEVANT WEB SITES

American Association for History of Nursing (AAHN): *http://www.aahn.org*
American Nurses Association (ANA), general site: *www.nursingworld.org*;
    Government/legislative information: *http://nursingworld.org/gova/federal/gfederal.htm*
American Nurses Association/American Journal of Nursing/Lippincott Williams & Wilkins:
    www.nursingcenter.com
Centers for Disease Control and Prevention: *www.cdc.gov*
Directory of Nursing Organizations: *http://directory.com/Health>Nursing>Organiza-
    tions>North America>United States* (or Canada)
Library of Congress: Access to current legislation in the "Spirit of Thomas Jefferson":
    http://www.thomas.loc.gov/
National League for Nursing: *www.nln.org*
National League for Nursing Accrediting Commission: *www.nlnac.org*
National Student Nurses' Association: *www.nsna.org*
U.S. Congress Handbook (address and links): *www.congress-handbook.com*

REFERENCES

American Association for History of Nursing (AAHN). Hannah A. Ropes [On-line]. *http://www.aahn.org/gravesites/ropes.html.* Accessed March 7, 2003.

American Nurses Association. (2002). Hill Basics: Communications Tips. [On-line]. Available: *http://nursingworld.org/gova/federal/politic/hill/gcomtips.htm.* Accessed August 8, 2002.

American Nurses Association. (2001) Code of Ethics for Nurses with Interpretive Statements. Washington, DC: ANA Publications.

"ANA lobbying team named in top 100." (1998). Washington Watch. *American Journal of Nursing, 98*(2), 16.

"ANA pushes Nurse Reinvestment Act through Congress." (2002). *The American Nurse, 34*(4), 3.

Capitol Update. (1999). *Appropriations (Health), 16*(20), 1.

Centers for Medicare and Medicaid Services. Fraud reporting form. [On-line]. Available: *http://cms.hhs.gov/forms.* Accessed March 7, 2003.

Costello K. (1995). ANA weak on protecting nursing practice. *California Nurse, 91*(8), 4, 16.

Lasswell H. (1986). *Politics: Who gets what, when, how.* New York: Meridian Books.

Lienhard, J. H. (2002). Engines of our ingenuity: Episode 867-Hannah Ropes. [On-line]. Available: *http://www.uh.edu/engines/epi867.htm.* Accessed August 8, 2002.

National League for Nursing. (2002). "Our Mission". Available at *www.nln.org/aboutnln/ourmission.htm.* Accessed August 16, 2002.

NIOSH Alert: Preventing needlestick injuries in health care settings. November 1999. DHHS (NIOSH) Pub # 2000-108. [On-line]. Available: *www.cdc.gov/niosh.* Accessed June 24, 2000.

Tanner, C. A. (1996). Accreditation under siege. *Journal of Nursing Education, 35*(6), 243–244.

Trossman, S. (2002). Envisioning a brighter future. *American Journal of Nursing, 102*(7), 65–66.

The Upright Fight. (2002). Washington Watch. *American Journal of Nursing, 102*(7), 24.

Woodham-Smith, C. (1951). *Florence Nightingale.* New York: Atheneum. (1983 reprint of 1951 edition).

See the following regular publications for current information:

American Journal of Nursing, Washington Watch (a monthly column)
The American Nurse. Kansas City, MO: American Nurses Association, monthly newspaper
See also the official publication of your state nurses association.

Appreciating the Development of Nursing as a Profession

The purpose of Unit II is to provide an understanding of the events that resulted in nursing developing into the profession it is today. Gaining knowledge about the history and development of nursing helps the individual who is just starting a caring career to better appreciate and interpret the things that presently are occurring, and thus move into the future more comfortably. Learning about the history and development of the profession can help you to appreciate the heritage of the discipline and the events that resulted in nursing offering the opportunities and challenges that it provides today. This unit begins with a history of nursing that describes its growth from early times, to an era when preparation for nursing existed as apprentice-type training, to a profession that now encompasses doctoral and postdoctoral education.

Many believe that nursing is a young profession. Some note that there has always been nursing in some form. Others question whether nursing should be considered a profession at all. These debates are considered in this unit. Some of the studies that were conducted about nursing are described and their impact on the development of the profession is discussed.

The educational processes by which we prepare nurses continue to experience change, modification, and refinement in response to changes that are occurring in the health care delivery system. The various routes to educational preparation for a nursing career are discussed, including a history of the different avenues. You will learn about some of the individuals who made significant contributions to the profession. The unit concludes with a discussion of the future of nursing education.

4

Exploring Nursing's Origins

LEARNING OUTCOMES

After completing this chapter, you should be able to:

1. Discuss the major health care practices of early civilizations.
2. Explain how the development of nursing as a profession has been influenced by three historical images of the nurse and by the "Dark Ages" of nursing.
3. Describe Florence Nightingale's contribution to and impact on nursing and its development.
4. Analyze the impact wars have had on the development of nursing education.
5. Discuss the development of the early nursing schools.
6. Describe the characteristics of early nursing programs.
7. Identify the first organizations created by and for nurses and discuss the purpose of each.
8. Discuss the history of hospitals and long-term care facilities in the United States.
9. Analyze the factors that influenced the development of health care facilities and the importance of each.

KEY TERMS

Almshouse	Materia medica	Poorhouses
Ancient cultures	Military influence	Reformation
"Dark Ages" of nursing	Monastic orders	Religious image of the nurse
Deaconesses	Nursing home	
Ebers papyrus	Nursing organizations	Servant image of the nurse
Florence Nightingale	Order of Virgins	
Folk image of the nurse	Order of Widows	Training for nurses
Hospital(s)	Pesthouses	Uncommon women

There is no particular date or time period when nursing came into being. Nursing, as we know it today, may go back less than 150 years. The early origins of nursing, like those of medicine, are intertwined with the ancient civilizations and cultures of the world, with little written reference to nursing from 500 B.C. to 476 A.D. Our best speculations regarding their origins necessarily must be tied to our knowledge of the many and varied cultures that existed in the past, and to the contributions that these cultures left for future generations. They reflected the events and developments (or lack of same) that characterized each period in history. In this chapter, we will review some of the various cultures and historical events that have contributed to the development of nursing as a profession.

HEALTH CARE IN ANCIENT CULTURES

The life of primitive societies and **ancient cultures** was necessarily a nomadic one. Well-defined groups, built around the nucleus of family relationships, wandered in search of food, warmth, and an environment that supported life. Solidarity among these scattered groups, organized for the convenient management of human affairs, existed for purposes of mutual protection. Anthropologists believe that primitive groups originated in Africa and migrated across the world. Ice ages in the northern latitudes drove these groups back to the warmer climates found around the Mediterranean Sea, in India, and in China, where civilizations developed. Historians suggest that the movement of early tribes radiated from the interior of Europe and Asia toward the warm shores of the Mediterranean Sea, India, and China (Jamieson & Sewall, 1944). From either perspective, it is believed that early cultures developed around these areas.

The regions around the Mediterranean Sea were thought to occupy the center of the earth, with all areas to the east known as "eastern" and all those to the west known as "western" (Donahue, 1996, p. 28). The sophistication of health care practices varied considerably from one culture to another, and were based largely on the ingenuity of the group. Consistent among most of them were strong beliefs in the power of gods, with sickness and suffering attributed to the presence of evil spirits. These evil spirits were dealt with in many ways, including noisy incantations and dances, making offerings and sacrifices, and working with medicine men who worked their "magic" to drive away the demons (Kalisch & Kalisch, 1995). The health care practices of some of the early cultures are highlighted in Table 4-1.

Egypt

While other cultures were settling along the Indus, Euphrates, and Tigris Rivers, the ancient Egyptians settled in the long, narrow valley that lay along the banks of the Nile River. The Egyptian community, considered to be much more advanced than others of the region, had by the year 5000 B.C., developed stone implements to facilitate work. The creation of the wheel and cart followed, and soon animals were domesticated to help with heavy burdens. A system of irrigation increased the productivity of the fertile soil.

Treating disease was considered the responsibility of priests. The Egyptians, like the people of all early cultures, looked on natural phenomena as the work of the gods. Health and security meant keeping the gods happy. Sickness reflected the presence of some evil spirit in

TABLE 4-1.	HIGHLIGHTS OF HEALTH CARE PRACTICES OF SELECTED EARLY CIVILIZATIONS
SOCIETY	**CONTRIBUTIONS**
Egypt	Provided the earliest medical records; included more than 700 classified drugs
	Developed system of community planning that helped avoid public health problems
	Established strict rules regarding cleanliness, food, drink, exercise, and sexual relations
Palestine	Developed Mosaic Code, which included an organized method of disease prevention
	Isolated people with communicable diseases, differentiated clean from unclean
	Established rules that forbade eating meat past the 3rd day after slaughter
Babylonia	Skilled mathematicians and astrologers; beliefs based on numbers and movement of the stars
	Believed illness a punishment for sin and used incantations and herbs for purification with surgery more advanced than internal medicine
	Developed Code of Hammurabi, which perhaps represents the first sliding scale for payment based on class
Assyria	A warlike group whose laws were severe and who made frequent use of death penalty
	Believed in good and evil spirits and in many gods. Ill health was a punishment for sin.
Persia	Followed the preaching of Zoroaster, who introduced the concept of two creators: one good, one evil
	Established early schools for priest-physicians, from which evolved three types of physicians: those who healed by the knife, those who healed with herbs, and those who healed through exorcism
Greece	Society heavily steeped in mythology, animal sacrifice, and faith in the power of gods
	Placed much emphasis on healthy bodies; founded the Olympic games
	Built beautiful temples where learning and healing occurred
	Built institutions to care for sick and injured called *xendochium; iatrion* were built to offer ambulatory care
	The home of Hippocrates, born about 400 B.C., who became known as the Father of Modern Medicine
Rome	Borrowed medical practices from the countries they conquered; physicians were often slaves
	Clung to gods, superstition, and herbs when faced with illness
	Practiced fairly advanced hygiene and sanitation with emphasis on bathing
	Women enjoyed more independence that in other comparable societies
India	Civilizations highly developed, with systems of sanitation, bathrooms, public baths, and other amenities
	Vedic age (1500 B.C.) characterized by worship to Brahma, which resulted in segregation of society into castes
	Emphasized hygiene and prevention of sickness and described major and minor surgery, children's diseases, and diseases of the nervous and urinary system. Advanced surgery and materia medica.
	Buddhism emerged about 500 B.C. with an advanced understanding of disease prevention, hygiene and sanitation, medicine and surgery. Prenatal care emphasized for mothers and public hospitals constructed staffed with nurses (mostly men).

TABLE 4-1.	HIGHLIGHTS OF HEALTH CARE PRACTICES OF SELECTED EARLY CIVILIZATIONS (*Continued*)
SOCIETY	**CONTRIBUTIONS**
China	Followed the teachings of Confucius; patriarchal rule dominated with emphasis on whole family; women considered vastly inferior to men
	Developed concept of yin and yang and had elaborate materia medica, using many drugs still used today
	Developed acupuncture skills still in practice today, studied circulation, and developed approach to examination: look, listen, ask, feel
	Baths used for reduction of fever, bloodletting to release evil spirits from the body
The Americas	Sun god of particular significance; health viewed as a balance between man, nature, and the supernatural
	Rites, ceremonies, herbal treatments, charms, and perhaps human sacrifice contributed to healing practices
	Medicine men (first known as shamans and later as priests) were responsible for curing ills of body and mind
Arabia	Populated by nomadic people who lived a difficult life in the hot, dry desert. Muhammad, born about 570 A.D., developed the religion of Islam that worshipped the god Allah. His teachings established, strict rules of living, dictating habits of cleanliness, eating, and human interaction. Elevated the position of women.

possession of the sufferer (Kalisch & Kalisch, 1995). To regain health, these evil spirits had to be driven out through a variety of rites.

The oldest medical records so far discovered and deciphered are those from Egypt, dating back as far as 3000 B.C. Early records, sometimes in the form of hieroglyphics, were carved in stone or written on papyrus. Dr. Ebers of Germany purchased one of the books in 1874. It became known as the **Ebers papyrus** and is considered to be the best of the Egyptian medical books (Jamieson & Sewall, 1944). These books outline surgical techniques and methods of birth control, describe disease processes, and suggest remedies The Egyptians developed an elaborate pharmacopoeia that classified more than 700 drugs.

A system of community planning was developed that helped to avoid public health problems, especially those related to diseases transmitted through water sources. Egypt is credited with being one of the healthiest of the ancient countries, perhaps because of the progress it made in the fields of hygiene and sanitation. The Egyptians developed strict rules regarding such things as cleanliness, food, drink, exercise, and sexual relations. They also established a "house of death," which was located at a site away from civilization. Mummies that have survived to the present day clearly show that the Egyptians were skilled in wrapping and embalming their dead. It is also believed that they were accomplished in dentistry, often filling teeth with gold. Out of this culture came the first physician known to history, Imhotep (2900 B.C.–2800 B.C.). He was recognized as a surgeon, an architect, a temple priest, a scribe, and a magician.

Although women in ancient Egypt received more respect than women in other Eastern countries, it is not clear whether nurses existed as such. Women most likely worked in the temples, along with priest-physicians, holding the rank of priestess or serving as midwives or "wet nurses."

Cultures of the Fertile Crescent

Several cultures made their homes in a crescent-shaped strip of land that extended from the Persian Gulf on the east to the Mediterranean Sea on the west. Known as the Fertile Crescent, this area enjoyed a warm, hospitable climate and rich soil, and benefited from the water provided by three great rivers: the Tigris, the Euphrates, and the Jordan. The Fertile Crescent often is referred to as the "cradle of civilization." Because the cultures that settled there were often warlike and took possession of land by conquering the empire in power, the boundaries of these early societies sometimes overlapped.

PALESTINE

The Hebrews made their home in the western end of the Fertile Crescent in a region that included what is now Israel, as well as some of the surrounding area. The land was mountainous, with narrow, gorge-like valleys that lacked the adequate rainfall and the richness of minerals found in other areas. The society of the Hebrews was primarily an agricultural one, as people learned to cultivate olive trees, grains, and vineyards.

The Hebrews are credited with more democratic sharing of knowledge than any of the other ancient civilizations because of their emphasis on reading of the scriptures. Possibly, the Hebrews gained much of their knowledge of health from the Egyptians, who, according to Hebrew scripture, held them captive for many years.

Under the leadership of Moses, the Hebrews developed a system of laws called the Mosaic Code. This included an organized method of disease prevention through the isolation of people with communicable diseases and differentiation of clean from unclean. The code addressed every detail of personal, family, and public hygiene.

Hebrew culture recognized one god who had power over life and death. From this belief evolved the role of the priest as supervisor of medical practices related to cleansing and purification. Priest-physicians took on the function of health inspectors. The writings of the early Jewish rabbis taught that visiting the sick was a duty, even if the sick were not Jews. Thus, religion, law, and medicine combined to control public health with the responsibility for enforcement given to the priest-physician, although kings ruled the country.

Bible scriptures, such as Leviticus 7:16–19 and 19:5–8, which forbade the eating of meat past the 3rd day after an animal was slaughtered, were no doubt written because of the effects of the warm climate and lack of refrigeration. Similarly, Mosaic and Talmudic regulations regarding the slaughtering of animals, which included requirements for examination and inspection to check for diseases of the internal organs, were in keeping with the advanced sanitary ordinances of Hebrew society.

BABYLONIA

At one time known as Mesopotamia, Babylonia was located in the southern part of present-day Iraq, although its borders differed from those of the modern country. Each city was an autonomous community governed by a divine ruler and a priest-king. Women had little esteem in Babylonian society, with their role being primarily domestic, not unlike other cultures of the time.

The Babylonians are credited with being skilled mathematicians and astrologers. Many of the beliefs of the Babylonians were based on their study of nature, their belief in the

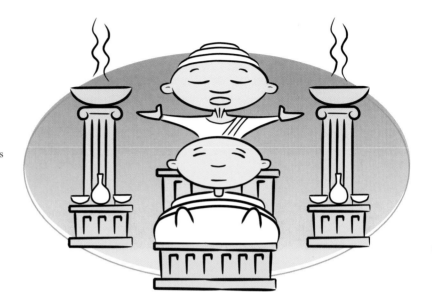

FIGURE 4-1 In many early societies the practice of medicine involved the use of magical formulas that drove away demons that possessed the body.

potency of numbers, and their observations of the movement of stars and planets. The division of the year into months, weeks, days, hours, and minutes is said to have originated with the Babylonians (Donahue, 1996).

The Babylonians believed illness to be the punishment for sin and for displeasing the gods. Purifying the body brought about a cure, usually by incantations and the use of herbs. Temples, in which the purification occurred, became centers of medical care (Fig. 4-1). Preventive medicine consisted of doing what it was believed the gods desired. Babylonia is the source of the second oldest surviving medical records (Nutting & Dock, 1935). In Babylonian culture, surgery was more advanced than internal medicine, which concerned itself primarily with banishing demons and avoiding evil spirits.

The Code of Hammurabi was developed in 1900 B.C., by Hammurabi, King of Babylonia. The principal source of our knowledge of this code is a stone monument found in 1901 and preserved today in the Louvre in Paris. This code, which may represent the first sliding scale for fee payment, divided the public into three classes. Those classified as "gentlemen" were expected to pay their surgeons in silver coins rather than in goods or services. A surgeon who bungled an operation on a "gentleman" risked paying a heavy price; the surgeon might have his hands cut off if the surgery was not successful. This puts the malpractice rates absorbed by physicians today in a different light.

ASSYRIA

The history of the Assyrians began around 2300 B.C. (Jamieson & Sewall, 1944). This nation was centered in the northern part of present-day Iraq, and, as it conquered other nations, extended into what is now Syria and southern Iraq. After ceaseless warfare, the Assyrians took possession of Babylonia. The Assyrians are characterized as a hardened, warlike group whose one supreme god was a "god of battles." Their instruments of war were said to be stronger than those of other cultures. The Assyrians were the first to use weapons made of bronze.

Their laws were severe, with mutilation and death inflicted on those who failed to follow the heavy mandates. Early Assyrians believed in good and evil spirits, in magic and superstition, and in many gods. Like many other early cultures, they also believed that ill health was a punishment for sin and that evil spirits could occupy a person's body. The practice of medicine developed around these religious beliefs as the Assyrians practiced only magic and empirical medicine consistent with their superstitions (Donahue, 1996).

Persia

Persia, one of the most extensive empires of the Near East, was located in what is now modern-day Iran and, at one time, extended throughout the Fertile Crescent. The Persians' quest for territory and power resulted in their conquest of much of that area. They believed in Zoroaster, a prophet who lived about 600 B.C. and wrote the sacred books of Persia. His writings introduced the world to the concept of two creators—one good, and one evil—and to the sacred elements of fire, earth, and water. The writings of Zoroaster also introduced the concept of immortality as a mental state. The Persians adopted the cultural practices of the lands they conquered, including many of the medical and surgical practices of Egypt. They established early schools to prepare priest-physicians, from which evolved three types of physicians: those who healed by the knife, those who healed with herbs, and those who healed through exorcism.

Greece

Greek civilization developed on a peninsula that extended into the Mediterranean Sea from the southeastern part of Europe. The ancient Greeks are remembered in part for their worship of gods and goddesses and for their emphasis on healthy bodies, which led them to found the Olympic games. In Greek mythology, Asklepios (sometimes spelled Aesculapius or Asclepius), son of Apollo, was taught the healing arts by Cheiron, a wise centaur. Asklepios usually is represented as carrying a staff, to show that he traveled from place to place, around which is entwined a serpent, representing wisdom and immortality. Some people believe that when the army medical services fashioned the caduceus, the symbol of the medical profession, the staff and serpent that were incorporated into the symbol came from this legend.

Exquisite temples, located on beautiful sites, were built as shrines to Asklepios; these temples became social and intellectual centers as well as places to obtain cures. The curative process usually began with animal sacrifice and continued through various purifying rituals. In addition to these shrines, two other institutions, the xenodochium and the iatrion, offered care to the sick in ancient Greece. At first offering care to travelers, the xenodochium later provided care to people who were sick and injured. This may have been the forerunner of the city or county hospital as we know it today. The iatrion was a facility offering ambulatory care and would correspond to our outpatient clinics.

It is rather surprising that from this society, so heavily steeped in mythology, animal sacrifice, and faith in the power of the gods, came the Father of Modern Medicine. Hippocrates was born about 400 B.C. on the island of Cos. He stressed natural causes for disease, treated the whole patient with a patient-centered approach to care, and introduced the scientific method of solving patient problems. His teaching emphasized the necessity of accurate observations and careful record keeping. Rather than attribute ill health to an infliction by the gods, Hippocrates believed that health depended on equilibrium existing among the mind, the body, and the environment. From his philosophy evolved the humoral theory of disease, which has lasted for centuries.

Many other early physicians came from Greece, although some eventually practiced their skills in Rome after the Roman Empire conquered Greece. Some physicians, such as Aristotle (who distinguished arteries from veins), Galen (a physician to the gladiators and renowned medical writer who is credited with demonstrating that arteries, when opened, always gush blood), Asclepiades (who helped establish medicine in Rome and proposed an atomistic approach to disease), and Pedanim Dioscorides (whose *De Materia Medica* contained descriptions of more than 600 herbal preparations) made such significant contributions to medicine that their names are remembered today (Kalisch & Kalisch, 1995).

Rome

At one time, the Roman Empire was quite extensive, stretching across the entire northern border of Africa and Egypt as well as southern and central Europe. The medical advances of the ancient Romans fell short of those of the Greeks. Medical practices often were borrowed from the countries the Romans conquered, and the physicians from those countries were made slaves who provided medical services to the Romans. Although the Romans clung to gods, superstition, and herbs when faced with disease, their hygiene and sanitation were fairly well advanced. Their genius found its best expression in the area of public hygiene rather than in medicine per se. Many homes were equipped with baths and cleanliness was valued. The Romans also constructed public baths.

Roman society was divided into two classes: the patricians, an affluent and privileged group; and the plebeians, who represented the poor or lower class and were denied citizenship. Patrician women in Roman society had more privileges than women of similar economic status in other ancient cultures. Women were quite independent and were allowed to own property, appear in public, and campaign publicly for causes they believed should be advanced. They could even entertain guests and sit with them at the table.

India

Located in the southern part of the Far East, India was essentially isolated by mountains from other parts of the ancient world. People who migrated from central Asia in ancient times traveled through the mountain passes. Excavations indicate that the first civilizations in India (3000–1500 B.C.) were highly developed, with systems of sanitation, bathrooms and public baths, and other amenities. The Vedic age began in 1500 B.C. and was characterized by worship of the eternal spirit Brahma. Brahmanism (also known as Hinduism) was to become a major religion in India, out of which developed the stratification of Indian society into four different castes and the concept of sacrifice to satisfy gods. Sources of information about health practices come from the Vedas, a sacred book of Brahmanism dating back to 1600 B.C. and considered by some to be the oldest known written material. Medicine, as described in the books of *Ayur Veda* (or the Veda of Longevity), emphasized hygiene and prevention of sickness and included discussions of major and minor surgery, children's diseases (including inoculation against smallpox), materia medica (the drugs and other remedial substances used in medicine), and diseases of the nervous and urinary systems (Nutting & Dock, 1935; Jamieson & Sewall, 1944). Their practice of surgery may have been the most highly developed of any ancient culture.

Siddhartha Gautama, who lived about 500 B.C., was a Hindu ascetic who, at age 29, left his wife and child to find salvation and to develop a more intimate relationship with the spiritual. He attained a state called "enlightenment," declaring himself Buddha and offering a new religious philosophy that came to be known as Buddhism. Buddhism emerged as the major religion of early India, although some would consider it more a moral discipline than a religion. Buddha aspired to bring peace and contentment (nirvana) to all, which he believed could be achieved by freeing the self of all desires and worldly things. During the Buddhist period, under the rule of King Asoka, India developed an advanced understanding of hygiene and sanitation, disease prevention, medicine, and surgery. The importance of prenatal care to both mother and infant seemed well understood and practiced. Buddhism disregarded the caste system of the earlier religion, and made education and the right to peace possible for everyone. Public hospitals were constructed during this time, and some vital statistics were collected. These hospitals were staffed with nurses whose qualifications were similar to those expected of today's practical nurses. The main difference was that, in almost all cases, Indian nurses were men. In rare instances, old women were permitted to assume this role. Donahue (1996) states that three main qualities of character were required of these attendants: high standards, skill, and trustworthiness.

China

Ancient China was located far to the northeast of India, across the range of the Himalaya Mountains and, like India, was cut off from the Mediterranean world. The Chinese are thought to have come from central Asia around 3000 B.C. (Jamieson & Sewall, 1944). Chinese civilization developed along the banks of the Yellow River. In approximately 500 B.C., the Chinese scholar Confucius began to teach a moral philosophy that addressed government, education, and one's obligation to society. Several hundred years after his death, his philosophy, which included service to the community and respect for authority, became the basis for education and government in China. Within this philosophy, patriarchal rule dominated, and emphasis was placed on the value of the family as a unit. Women were considered vastly inferior to men; the number of sons she could produce determined a woman's value. A daughter was always severed from connection with her family of origin when she married; her obligations and loyalties were automatically transferred to the family of her husband. Although young married women were treated almost as slaves, old women were received with love and given a position of high esteem in families. Ancestor worship attained great importance.

Great emphasis was placed on the value of knowledge in solving life's problems. The early Chinese established the philosophy of the yang and yin. The yang represented the active, positive, masculine force of the universe, and the yin represented the passive, negative, feminine force. The Chinese believed that these two forces operated in contrasting and complementary ways. Both forces flow through the body. Health practices based on this philosophy focused on prevention, and good health was believed to result from a balance between the yang and the yin, a concept that still influences some alternative medical practices.

China's medical knowledge extends far back in history. Dissection was performed in China before 2000 B.C. The development of elaborate **materia medica** was of major significance; many of the drugs used by the Chinese in ancient times, such as ephedrine, are used in modern medicine. The Chinese developed acupuncture skills that continue to be practiced today. They also studied the circulation and emphasized the behavior of the pulse. Principles of examination were based on the following guideposts: "look, listen, ask, feel." Baths were used for the reduction of fever, and bloodletting was used as a method of helping an evil spirit escape from the body.

The Americas

Early civilization in the Americas may have begun 10,000 or even 20,000 years ago (Donahue, 1996). It is thought that early inhabitants probably came from Central Asia, gaining access across a land bridge over the Bering Strait into Alaska. Like other early tribes, they were nomadic, wandering in search of food and shelter. Several groups, including the Mayas, Incas, Aztecs, and Toltecs, developed a high degree of civilization.

The sun god was particularly important to these cultures. Rites, ceremonies, herbal treatments, charms, shields, and, in some instances, human sacrifice, contributed to healing practices. Health was a balance among man, nature, and the supernatural. Nature was considered a power. Power centers, sacred places where the spirits and alleged "gods" resided were considered sacred and holy and therefore, to be respected (Lake-Thom, 1997).

Medicine, pharmacy, nursing, religion, and magic often were not viewed as separate entities. Medicine men (known first as shamans and later as priests) were responsible for curing ills of both the body and the mind, and disease was believed to result from displeasing the gods.

Little is known about the role of the nurse in these early civilizations, although the status enjoyed by Indian women was good and American Indians made significant contributions to modern-day medicine and medical practice. The Aztecs in particular had hospices for the care of the ill, used minerals as drugs, soporifics to decrease pain, and assisted women with childbirth (Donahue, 1996).

Critical Thinking Activity

Given the lack of organized nursing, how do you believe the people of the early cultures received care? Who do you think provided that care? How did they know what to do? From whom did they learn it?

HISTORICAL PERSPECTIVES OF NURSING

Writings about early health care make little or no mention of nursing or nurses. One might assume that a family member, particularly the wife or mother, provided needed care. Health practices varied depending on the level of development of a society. Ritualistic ceremonies and worship of gods were common and various individuals in the culture assumed the role of healer. Each primitive society had its own curative agents, taboos, and practices; some were more advanced than others. A sound theory of disease was absent from most early cultures.

Although ancient cultures developed medicine as a science and a profession, they showed little evidence of establishing a foundation for nursing, with the possible exception of the male attendants in early Buddhist hospitals in India, and of midwives, who had an established role in several cultures. It was not until the early Christian period that nursing as we think of it today began to develop.

Muriel Uprichard identifies three heritages from the past that impeded the development of nursing as a profession. They are "the **folk image of the nurse** brought forward from primitive times, the **religious image of the nurse** inherited from the medieval period, and the **servant image of the nurse** created by the Protestant-capitalist ethic of the 16th to 19th century" (Uprichard, 1973, p. 24). Whether they hampered progress, these concepts of the nurse have certainly had an impact.

The Folk Image of the Nurse

Since the time of the first mother, women have carried the major responsibility for nourishing and nurturing children, and caring for elderly and aging members of the family. It is difficult to pinpoint a particular time or place for the beginning of nursing as we know it. It is reasonable to assume those early tribes and civilizations required health care. It is also reasonable to assume that in those tribes and civilizations were people who demonstrated adeptness and a special interest in meeting the needs of those who were sick, injured, or bearing children. These "nurses" received their education largely through trial and error, by advancing those methods that appeared to be successful, and by sharing information. Superstition and magic played a significant role in treatment; folklore abounded, and a close relationship existed between religion and the healing arts.

Nursing skills primarily evolved from trial and error. For example, while planning a diet for the family, an astute woman would have noticed that eating certain foods resulted in episodes of diarrhea and vomiting, whereas eating other herbs, roots, and leaves had a soothing effect on the body. Families developed recipes that were handed down from generation to generation; effective treatments and cures were recorded and shared. This practice continued for many years. The following is listed as a treatment for croup in a family medical book published in its 213th revision in 1885.

> Roast a large Red Onion well, squeeze the juice out, and sweeten it with Honey until it becomes a thick syrup; then add 2 drops of Spirits of Turpentine. This may be given to a child of six months or a year old, in the course of the day. Do not allow the child to go out in the wet or damp air (Gunn, 1885, p. 1149).

This folk image of the nurse emphasizes that the nurse is simply a caring person who uses ordinary common sense to help the sick person and seemed to place this responsibility on the women in the household.

The Religious Image of the Nurse

The first continuity in the history of nursing began with Christianity. Christ's teachings admonished people to love and care for their neighbors. With the establishment of churches in the Christian era, groups were organized as orders whose primary concern was to care for the sick, the poor, orphans, widows, the aged, slaves, and prisoners, all in the name of charity and Christian love. Christ's precepts placed women and men on parity, and the early church made both men and women deacons, with equal rank. Unmarried women had unprecedented opportunities for service. Although these opportunities represented positive changes, they also fostered certain limitations. Because nursing developed an image closely tied to religion and religious orders, strict discipline was expected. Absolute attendance to the orders of persons of higher rank (eg, priests or physicians) was demanded. This view of nursing as requiring a strict obedience, a sense of religious devotion, and an altruistic setting aside of one's own needs has also affected nursing. Nurses were thought to be so devoted to patients that worldly concerns such as salary and working conditions were of no consequence.

THE DEACONESSES

The **deaconesses** of the Eastern Christian Church represent one group of particular significance to the history of nursing. Required to be unmarried or widowed, these women were often the widows or daughters of Roman officials, and thus had breeding, culture, wealth, and social position. The deaconess, like the deacon, was ordained, and, as a church official, worked on an equal basis with the deacon. These dedicated young women practiced "works of mercy" that included feeding the hungry, clothing the naked, visiting the imprisoned, sheltering the homeless, caring for the sick, and burying the dead. Often cited as the earliest counterparts to the community health nurses of today, the deaconesses carried a basket (a forerunner of the contemporary visiting nurse's bag) when they entered homes to distribute food and medicine. Phoebe, frequently referred to as the first deaconess and first visiting nurse, is often mentioned in books about nursing history. She carried Paul's letters and cared for him and many others. In the Epistle to the Romans, dated about 58 A.D., reference is made to Phoebe and to her work.

THE WIDOWS AND THE VIRGINS

Two other groups—the **Order of Widows** and the **Order of Virgins**—shared many common characteristics with the deaconesses and carried out similar responsibilities. Members of the Order of Widows may never have been married. It seems that the title of widow was used to designate respect for age. Those who were married, however, took vows never to remarry if widowed. The Order of Virgins emphasized virginity as essential to purity of life, and virgins were ranked as equals to the clergy. Because these women often visited the sick in their homes, they are often mentioned along with the deaconesses as being the earliest organized group of public health nurses. The movement peaked in Constantinople in about 400 A.D., when a staff of 40 deaconesses lived and worked under the direction of Olympia, a powerful and deeply religious deaconess. The influence of the deaconess order diminished in the 5th and 6th centuries, when church decrees removed clerical duties and rank from the deaconess.

Although the position of deaconess originated in the Eastern Christian Church, it spread west to Gaul (an ancient region in Western Europe consisting of what is now mainly France, Belgium and a section of northern Italy) and Ireland. In Rome, women who served in comparable positions were known as matrons. Active during the 4th and 5th centuries, these Roman matrons held independent positions and had great wealth, which they contributed to charity and to nursing. Among these Christian converts were three women who contributed

Display 4-1   ROMAN MATRONS

Fabiola

Fabiola, a charming and beautiful young woman, was born into an influential and wealthy Roman family. Growing up in a lavish home, she enjoyed a happy social life. However, her marriage to a worthless gentleman resulted in divorce. She married a second time and was no happier in her second marriage. Under the influence of Marcella, she converted to Christianity and, after the death of her second husband, began her career of charity. Fabiola's new beliefs made marriage after divorce a sin. She publicly acknowledged this, committed her life to charitable work, and in 390 A.D. built the first public hospital in Rome, described as a *nosocomium*. Here she cared for the sick and poor, whom she gathered from the streets and highways, personally washing and treating wounds and sores that repulsed others. Later in her life she is said to have built a hospice for strangers at Ostia, a seaport of Rome. St. Jerome tells of some of her work and her attributes in his writings. She died about 399 A.D., and scores of Romans are said to have attended her funeral to show their respect for her.

Marcella

A Roman woman of means, Marcella made her luxurious home into a monastery for women. Here other matrons such as Fabiola and Paula became involved in Christian study. Much inspiration came to them through a great friend and teacher, St. Jerome. Marcella devoted her life to instruction, charitable work, and prayer and became recognized as an authority on interpretation of biblical passages. She assisted St. Jerome in his translation of the Hebrew prophets. During the sack of Rome, her home was invaded by warriors, who expected to find valuables stored there. When they found little more than a bare building, they whipped Marcella, hoping she would reveal the hiding places of riches. After the assault she is said to have fled to St. Paul's church, which was nearby. There she died as a result of her injuries.

St. Paula

Learned, wealthy, and broken-hearted by the death of her husband, Saint Paula was also a scholar of Marcella. She is said to have assisted St. Jerome (whose lifetime exceeded that of all the women with whom he associated) in the translation of the writings of the prophets. St. Paula traveled to Palestine and devoted a fortune to the establishment of hospitals and inns for pilgrims travelling to Jerusalem. In Bethlehem she organized a monastery, built hospitals for the sick, and developed hospices for pilgrims, where tired travelers and the ill received care. Some credit her with being the first to teach nursing as an art rather than a service. She had a daughter, Eustochium, who joined her mother in the adoption of Christianity, and with her expressed its ideals through charitable work.

significantly to nursing. Their stories are told in Display 4-1. Later, the deaconess movement, suppressed by the Western Church, became all but extinct.

THE ROLE OF THE MONASTIC ORDERS

The **monastic orders** also developed during this period, including the order of Benedictines, which still exists. The monasteries played a large role in the preservation of culture and learning, as well as in offering refuge to the persecuted, care to the sick, and education to the uneducated. By joining a monastic order, young men and women were able to follow the career of their choice while living a Christian life. The learning of the classical period would have been lost when the Roman Empire fell were it not for the monks and monasteries.

One of the earliest organizations for men in nursing, the Parabolani brotherhood, was established at this time. Responding to the needs created by the Black Plague, this group reportedly organized a hospital and traveled throughout Rome caring for the sick.

At the same time, monastic nurses such as the famous St. Brigid (an abbess in Ireland known for her healing of the lepers), St. Scholastica (a twin sister of St. Benedict), and St. Hilda, founded schools, tended to the sick, and gave to the poor (Donahue, 1996).

During this period (approximately 50 A.D. to 800 A.D.), the first hospitals were established, usually as a part of a nearby monastery that included grain fields, gardens, orchards, farm buildings, and eventually schools, in addition to the church. Many of these hospitals are still standing. There were more than 700 hospitals in England by the middle of the 16th century. The Hôtel Dieu in Lyons was established in 542 and the Hôtel Dieu in Paris around 652. The Hôtel Dieu in Paris was staffed by the first order specifically devoted to nursing, the Augustinian Sisters (Kalisch & Kalisch, 1995). The Santo Spirito Hospital in Rome, the largest medieval hospital, was established by papal order in 717 (Donahue, 1999).

The Crusades, which swept from northern Europe to the Mideast in response to the advance of the Ottoman Empire into Spain, France, and Eastern Europe, lasted for almost 200 years (1096–1291). Military nursing orders, such as the Knights Hospitallers of St. John, evolved as a result of the Crusades. The Knights was organized to staff two hospitals located in Jerusalem, and had as its grand master a monk named Gerard. He drew up codes and introduced the black robe with a white Maltese cross that became the uniform for the brethren (Kalisch & Kalisch, 1995). The same cross was later used on a badge designed for the Nightingale School; this badge was the forerunner of the nursing pin as we know it today. (The symbolism of the pin is discussed later in this chapter.) The Knights, organized as a nursing order, soon became famous for their hospitality and care and their numbers, possessions, and wealth increased. At times they were required to defend the hospital and its patients. In Germany, a women's order called "consorores" was founded specifically to perform hospital work. Although they took vows, the women were not granted the same status as the Knights, and they lived outside the monastic precincts.

Two other monastic orders were founded during this period: the Knights Templars in 1118 and the Knights of the Teutonic Order in 1190. The Hospitallers and the Templars played significant roles during the Crusades. Secular orders of nurses also came into existence at this time. Operating much like the monastic orders, members of these groups could terminate their vocations at any time and were not bound to the vows of monastic life. Examples of the secular orders include the Order of Antonines (1095); the Beguines of Flanders, Belgium (1184); the Misericordia (1244); and the Alexian Brothers, founded during the bubonic plague epidemic of 1348. The only nursing education offered to these dedicated people was in the form of an apprenticeship during which a newcomer would be assigned to a more experienced person for instruction.

The inquiring student is encouraged to seek greater depth of knowledge about the nursing orders, their purposes and goals, and the lives of those who devoted their energies to the care of the sick and the poor by consulting the nursing references given at the end of this chapter.

MUSLIM CULTURE

Far from Greece and Rome where western civilization had developed, the Islamic society was developed in the Mideast. In an area known today as Saudi Arabia, nomadic people, living primarily in tribes, struggled for existence on the arid desert of Arabia, while oasis settlements relied on agriculture. Large numbers of people traveled to Mecca (Makkah) to visit the *Ka'abah,* the House of God built by the Prophet Abraham, which, at that time, housed numerous idols belonging to the inhabitants of the city and to tribes. About 400 A.D., Mecca became a trading center (Peck, 2002). The Prophet Muhammad was born in Makkah in 570 A.D. At about age 40, he began to preach a religion that would later be identified by the name "Islam." His preachings were not well received by the people of Mecca; Muhammad and his small group of followers endured persecution and in the year 622 A.D., were forced to emigrate to the city of Madinah (once known as Yathrib), located 260 miles to the north. This migration (Hijrah) marked the beginning of a new era and also the beginning of the Muslim calendar. The city had abundant water supplies, which nourished dates and vegetables, and became a reprovisioning point for caravans traveling from the southern part of the Arabian Peninsula along the Red Sea to Syria and Egypt. As the religion grew, mosques were built for worshipers. The first was established at Quba; another adjacent to Muhammad's house soon became the social and economic center of the city. Muhammad spent 8 years strengthening the Islamic community and warding off aggressors. At the end of this time, he and his followers were able to enter Mecca without bloodshed, remove all idols from the Kaaba, and convert inhabitants of Mecca to Islam ("Al-Madinah Al-Munawwarah," 1998).

Both civil and religious life were given direction through the writings of Muhammad. Thirty years after his death in 632, these writings were incorporated into a book titled the *Koran (Qu'ran).* Muhammad formulated rules for good living that excluded gambling, lying, wine drinking, uncleanness, and eating unclean food. He advocated kindliness, honesty, hospitality, forgiveness, almsgiving, cleanliness, and eating only prescribed foods. (Jamieson & Sewall, 1944).

As the Islamic culture grew, the writings of Hippocrates and Galen were translated into Arabic. Although Muslim beliefs regarding uncleanness forbade dissection, an extensive materia medica developed. Hospitals were built.

Little has been written in nursing history books about the role of nursing in early Muslim cultures. Recently, attention has been drawn to an 11th-century Muslim "Nightingale" named Rufaida Al-Asalmiya, who was a nurse during the time of the Prophet Muhammad. Rufaido Al-Asalmiya's father was a healer. While assisting her father, Rufaido developed many nursing skills. With the permission of the Prophet Muhammad, she began to train women and young girls in the art of nursing. She is said to have developed the first code of nursing conduct and ethics, long before it was introduced in the Western world. When the holy war began, she is reported to have provided care to the Muslim army in battle, enjoining her Muslim nurses to assist her. She continued this care after the battle ended, setting up tents near the mosque of Nabvi, where she provided care and health education. A building at the Aga Khan University School of Nursing has been named in her honor (Jan, 1996).

The Servant Image of the Nurse

The Renaissance and the Reformation (occurring from the 14th through the 16th centuries) followed the Middle Ages. During the Renaissance, also known as the Age of Discovery, a new impetus was given to education, and, to some extent, to medical education. For example, Ambroïse Paré (1510–1590), a French surgeon, revived the method of tying blood vessels to stop hemorrhaging, believing that procedures based on acute observation were better than those based on ancient doctrines. Andreas Vesalium (1514–1564) published a treatise of surgery and anatomy that refuted the teachings of Galen, who up to that point had been the undisputed authority on medicine. Nursing education, however, was all but nonexistent during this period.

The **Reformation**, a religious movement inspired by the work of Martin Luther, began in Germany in 1517. It resulted in a revolt against the supremacy of the Pope and the formation of Protestant churches across Europe. Monasteries were closed, religious orders were dissolved, and the work of women in these orders became almost extinct.

The Reformation brought about a change in the role of women. The Protestant Church, which stood for freedom of religion and thought, did not grant much freedom to women. During the Reformation, women were deemed subordinate to men and were no longer venerated by their churches, but encouraged toward charitable activities. Their role was defined within the confines of the home; their duties were those of bearing children and caring for the home. Work in hospitals no longer appealed to women of high birth. Hospital care was relegated to **uncommon women**, a group comprising prisoners, prostitutes, and drunks (Fig. 4-2).

Women faced with earning their own living were forced to work as domestic servants; although nursing was considered a domestic service, it was not a desirable one. The nurse was regarded as the most menial of servants. Pay was poor, the hours were long, and the work was strenuous. Nursing care was not subject to inspection and was not governed by standards. The same bed linen might be used for several patients, even though suppurating wounds were common. Thus began what may be called the **"Dark Ages" of nursing**.

Charles Dickens (1936) described the image of nurses and nursing during this time through the characters of Sairey Gamp and Betsy Prig in his book *Martin Chuzzlewit*, which

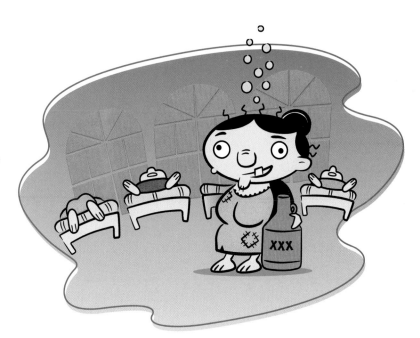

FIGURE 4-2   From the Middle Ages to the 19th century, nursing was often left to "uncommon women."

was written in 1843:

> She was a fat old woman, this Mrs. Gamp, with a husky voice and a moist eye, which she had a remarkable power of turning up, and only showing the white of it. Having very little neck, it cost her some trouble to look over herself, if one may say so, at those to whom she talked. She wore a very rusty black gown, rather the worse for snuff, and a shawl and bonnet to correspond.... The face of Mrs. Gamp—the nose in particular—was somewhat red and swollen, and it was difficult to enjoy her society without becoming conscious of a smell of spirits. Like most persons who have attained to great eminence in their profession, she took to hers very kindly; insomuch, that setting aside her natural predilections as a woman, she went to a lying-in or a lying-out with equal zest and relish (p. 318).
>
>   Mrs. Prig was of the Gamp build, but not so fat; and her voice was deeper and more like a man's. She had also a beard (p. 417).

The 16th and 17th centuries found Europe devastated by famine, plague, filth, and horror. In England, for example, King Henry VIII effectively had eliminated organized monastic relief provided to orphans and other displaced persons. Throughout Europe, vagrancy and begging abounded; those caught begging were often severely punished by being branded, beaten, or chained in galleys where they served as oarsmen. Knowledge of hygiene was insufficient; the poor suffered the most.

This servant image remains in modern day health care, as some individuals treat nurses as maids and others are unwilling to enter nursing because of the image. In the first World War, the International Red Cross tried to combat this image and produced a recruiting poster with the image of a Red Cross nurse on the battlefield and the statement, "Neither a nanny, nor a maid; A professional nurse" written in three languages.

The Beginning of Change

In the 17th century, social reform was inevitable. Several nursing groups were organized. These groups gave money, time, and service to the sick and the poor, visiting them in their homes and ministering to their needs. Such groups included the Order of the Visitation of Mary, St. Vincent de Paul, and in 1633, the Sisters of Charity. The last group became an outstanding secular nursing order. They developed an educational program for the intelligent young women they recruited that included experience in a hospital as well as visits to the home. Receiving help, counsel, and encouragement from St. Vincent de Paul, the Sisters of Charity expanded their services to include caring for abandoned children. In 1640, St. Vincent established the Hospital for Foundlings in Paris. Later, in 1809, the Sisters of Charity established a nursing order in the United States, under the direction of Elizabeth Bayley Seton. Other branches of this order were to follow, variously called the "Gray Sisters," the "Daughters of Charity," or the "Sisters of St. Vincent de Paul."

Those countries in Europe that remained Roman Catholic escaped some of the disorganization caused by the Reformation. During the 1500s, the Spanish and the Portuguese began traveling to the Americas. In 1521, Cortés conquered the capital of the Aztec civilization in Mexico and renamed it Mexico City. Early colonists to the area included members of Catholic religious orders, who became the doctors, nurses, and teachers of the new land. In 1524, the first hospital on the American continent, the Hospital of Immaculate Conception (Hospital de Nuestra Senora O Limpia Concepçion), was built in Mexico City. Mission colleges were founded. The first medical school in America was founded in 1578 at the University of Mexico, the second at the University of Lima before 1600.

Farther north, Jacques Cartier sailed up the St. Lawrence River in 1535 and established French settlements in Nova Scotia. Franciscan friars, Jesuits, Dominicans, and other settlers and explorers followed. In 1639, three Augustinian nuns arrived in Quebec to staff the Hôtel Dieu at Quebec, a hospital that opened that year. The Ursuline Sisters, an order of teaching nuns who accompanied the Augustinians from France, are credited with attempting to organize the first training for nurses on this continent. They taught the Indian women of the area to care for their sick during a smallpox epidemic. Jeanne Mance, who had been educated at an Ursuline convent, came to Montreal from France in 1642. She is considered to be the founder of the Hôtel Dieu of Montreal as well as the cofounder of Montreal itself. She returned to France in 1657 to gather financial support and staff, and returned with three French hospital nuns from the Society of St. Joseph de la Fleche to staff the Hôtel Dieu (Donahue, 1996).

In Europe, outstanding men of medicine made vital and valuable contributions to medical knowledge. Among lay persons influencing social change during this time was a young minister in Kaiserwerth, Germany, Theodore Fliedner (1800–1864). With the assistance of his first wife, Friederike, Fliedner revived the deaconess movement by establishing a training institute for deaconesses at Kaiserwerth in 1836. During a fund-raising tour through Holland and England, Pastor Fliedner met Elizabeth Fry of England, who had brought about reform at Newgate Prison in London. Greatly impressed with Mrs. Fry's accomplishments, the Fliedners followed her example and first worked with women prisoners in Kaiserwerth. Later they opened a small hospital for the sick, and Gertrude Reichardt, the daughter of a physician, was recruited as their first deaconess. The endeavors at Kaiserwerth included care of the sick, visitations and parochial work, and teaching. A course in nursing was developed that included lectures by physicians.

Friederike, who played a large part in helping to bring Theodore's visionary plans to fruition, was herself deeply dedicated to the deaconess movement. While away from home promoting deaconess activities, she learned that one of her children had died. A second child died shortly after her return and she herself died in 1842 after the birth of a premature infant. His second wife, Caroline Bertheau, who had some nursing experience before her marriage, also assisted Pastor Fliedner in his work. In 1849, Pastor Fliedner traveled to the United States, where he helped to establish the first motherhouse of Kaiserwerth deaconesses in Pittsburgh, Pennsylvania. With the help of four deaconesses, the Motherhouse of Kaiserwerth Deaconesses assumed responsibility for the Pittsburgh Infirmary, which was the first Protestant hospital in the United States. The hospital is now called Passavant Hospital.

In England, at about the same time, Elizabeth Fry (1780–1845) organized the Institute of Nursing Sisters, a secular group often called the Fry Sisters. Two other groups followed shortly; the Sisters of Mercy, a Roman Catholic group formed by Catherine McAuley (1787–1841), and another Catholic group called the Irish Sisters of Charity, formed by Mary Aikenhead (1787–1858).

Critical Thinking Activity

Knowing what you do about the history and early image of nursing, how will you, as a nurse of the future, advance the image of nursing? What aspects of the role are most critical? Who are the people who most need to be influenced? How do you think they can best be encouraged to select nursing as a career?

THE NIGHTINGALE INFLUENCE

In the latter half of the 18th century, one woman dramatically changed the form and direction of nursing and succeeded in establishing it as a respected field of endeavor. This outstanding woman was **Florence Nightingale**.

Born on May 12, 1820, the second daughter of a wealthy family, she was named after the city in which she was born—Florence, Italy. Because of her family's high social and economic standing, she was cultured, well traveled, and educated. By the age of 17, as the result of tutorage from her father, she had mastered several languages and mathematics and was extremely well read. Through the influential people she met, she was expected to select a desirable mate, marry, and assume her place in society.

Florence Nightingale had other ideas, however. She wanted to become a nurse, but this aspiration was unthinkable to her family because of the conditions that surrounded nursing. She continued to travel with her family and their friends and, in the course of these travels, met Sidney Herbert and his wife, who were becoming interested in hospital reform. She began collecting information on public health and hospitals and soon became recognized as an important authority on the subject.

Through friends she learned about Pastor Fliedner's institute at Kaiserwerth and visited it in 1850. Because it was a religious institution under the auspices of the church, her parents would permit her to go there, although she could not go to English hospitals. In 1851, she spent 3 months studying at Kaiserwerth, never returning home to live.

In 1853, she began working with a committee that supervised an "Establishment for Gentlewomen During Illness." She eventually was appointed superintendent of the establishment, a position she held from August 1853 to October 1854. As her knowledge of hospitals and nursing reform grew, she was consulted by reformers and by physicians who were beginning to see the need for "trained" nurses.

After the Crimean War began in March, 1854, war correspondents wrote about the abominable manner in which the British Army cared for the sick and wounded soldiers. Florence Nightingale, by then a recognized authority on hospital care, wrote to her friend Sir Sidney Herbert, who was then Secretary of War, and offered to take a group of 38 nurses to the Crimea. (At the same time, he had written a letter proposing that she assume direction of all nursing operations at the war front. Their letters crossed in the mail.) Her tireless efforts resulted in greatly reduced mortality rates among the sick and wounded.

When the war ended in 1856, Florence Nightingale returned to England as a national heroine but with her health broken. Much has been written of her "illness," some suggesting that it was brucellosis; others stating that it was, to a large degree, a neurosis; and more recently some declaring that it was posttraumatic stress disorder. She retreated to her bedroom, and for the next 43 years conducted her business from her secluded apartment.

Throughout her lifetime, Florence Nightingale wrote extensively about hospitals, sanitation, health, and health statistics, and especially about nursing and nursing education. Among the most popular books is "Notes on Nursing," published in 1859. She crusaded for and brought about great reform in nursing education.

In 1860, she devoted her efforts to the creation of a school of nursing at St. Thomas' Hospital in London, financed by the Nightingale Fund. The basic principles on which Miss Nightingale established her school included the following:

- Nurses would be trained in teaching hospitals associated with medical schools and organized for that purpose.
- Nurses would be selected carefully and would reside in nurses' houses designed to encourage discipline and form character.
- The school matron would have final authority over the curriculum, living arrangements, and all other aspects of the school.
- The curriculum would include both theoretic material and practical experience.
- Teachers would be paid for their instruction.
- Records would be kept on the students, who would be required to attend lectures, take quizzes, write papers, and keep diaries.

In many other ways, Florence Nightingale advanced nursing as a profession. She believed that nurses should spend their time caring for patients, not cleaning; that nurses must continue learning throughout their lifetime and not become "stagnant"; that nurses should be intelligent and should use that intelligence to improve conditions for the patient; and that nursing leaders should have social standing. She had a vision of what nursing could and should be. For further discussion of Florence Nightingale's definition of nursing, refer to Chapter 5.

Florence Nightingale received many honors from foreign governments, and in 1907 she was recognized by the Queen of England, who awarded her the British Order of Merit. It was the first time it was given to a woman.

Florence Nightingale died in her sleep at the age of 90 on August 13, 1910. The week during which she was born is now honored as National Nurses Week. The enthusiastic student is encouraged to learn more about this fascinating woman in Cecil Woodham-Smith's book *Florence Nightingale,* or by pursuing the topic of Florence Nightingale through the Internet.

THE MILITARY INFLUENCE

Through her experience in the Crimean War, Florence Nightingale first brought attention to nursing as a career and profession and to needed changes in health care delivery. Similarly, other wars have brought advances in how care is provided. In the following section, we will highlight some of those areas of **military influence**; however, it is impossible, in the context of this book, to provide more than just an overview (Fig. 4-3).

The American Revolution

All of the English colonies scattered along the Atlantic Coast of the United States were involved in the American Revolution. The hastily organized army existed without the benefit of a medical corps or trained nurses. The nuns of the Catholic Church, who also cared for those who were ill with epidemic diseases, such as scarlet fever, dysentery, and smallpox, nursed wounded soldiers. On the battlefield, women who had followed their husbands to the

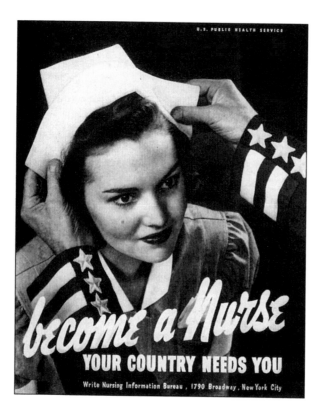

U.S. PUBLIC HEALTH SERVICE

become a Nurse

YOUR COUNTRY NEEDS YOU

Write Nursing Information Bureau , 1790 Broadway , New York City

FIGURE 4-3   Nurses were widely recruited for service in the military.

battlefield often nursed soldiers. Homes and barns near the battles were turned into hospitals. Other women contributed to the cause by making clothing and bandages or by helping to feed the soldiers from their own pantries.

When the war ended, the usual type of poverty existed, with invalids and cripples who needed care. However, the colonies were not sufficiently developed to have such services available. In response, a new type of institution evolved, which is perhaps the forerunner of today's clinic or hospital outpatient department. In 1786, the Philadelphia Dispensary was established and volunteer physicians treated those needing care at no charge. These dispensaries later became a major site for controlling disease. Vaccination against smallpox was one of the earliest preventive treatments offered.

The Influence of the Civil War

The Civil War broke out in the United States in 1861. Although social reform was on the rise, the nursing profession was still in an embryonic, unorganized stage. There was neither an army nurse corps nor an organized medical corps. There were no ambulance services or hospital units. Responding to the nursing needs created by the war, in which it is estimated that 618,000 men died (Donahue, 1996, p. 247), many men and women volunteered to help. After a brief training course, they performed nursing duties. The poet Walt Whitman is one of the better known individuals who became nurses during this time. Many religious orders also volunteered and provided service. A steamer, captured from the Confederates, was converted into a floating hospital and anchored near Vicksburg. Considered the first Navy hospital ship, the *Red Rover* was staffed through the volunteer efforts of the Catholic Sisters of Mercy, who became the first "Navy" nurses. An account of some of the contributions of nurses during the Civil War and afterward is found in Table 4-2. The serious need for trained nurses created by the Civil War was undoubtedly a significant factor in the development of nursing in the United States.

The Spanish-American War and the Boer War

These two conflicts occurred at about the same time in history. The United States entered the Spanish-American War in 1898, and the British went to war against the Boers of South Africa in late 1899. By this time, the Red Cross had organized and the United States, Canada, and Great Britain all had nursing schools to prepare young women for nursing roles.

In the early days of the Spanish-American War, little attention was given to the selection of nurses to care for the wounded. Volunteers, both men and women, included nurses with training, those partly trained, and the untrained. The entire system lacked organization; needed supplies were seriously deficient. These conditions attracted the attention of both the government and the people. Among groups addressing the concern was the Nurses' Associated Alumnae of the United States and Canada, who offered to develop a process through which better skilled nurses might be secured. When Mrs. Isabel Hampton Robb, the group's president, visited Washington for this purpose, she found the Department of Army Nursing already under the direction of Dr. Anita Newcomb McGee, a physician, who was setting up standards for selection. The management of the chosen nurses was given over to the Red Cross, which retained this role throughout the war.

Nursing occurred in the military camps. Anna C. Maxwell, on leave from the Presbyterian Hospital in New York, was Chief Nurse at one such camp. Among problems she encountered were inadequate water facilities, lack of laundry and laundry services, and inadequate medical supplies. In addition, many of her nurses became ill with typhoid fever.

When the war ended, nurse leaders exerted pressure to secure legislation to ensure an efficient army nursing service. A bill establishing the Army Nurse Corps was passed in 1901, and in 1908 the Navy Nurse Corps was established. Jane A. Delano was appointed Superintendent of the Army Nurse Corps. At about this time, the Red Cross began a complete reorganization, and William Howard Taft served as its president for 8 years. He also became president of the United States during this time.

In South Africa, the situation was much the same as in the United States—the need for more efficient and educationally prepared nurses was apparent. The British Army Nursing Service, organized in 1881 as a result of the Crimean experience, recruited Canadian volunteers who functioned under the direction of Georgina F. Pope. Canada was the first country to accord military rank to women. Britain soon learned that it needed a group of nurses who could be called upon in an emergency, and the Queen Alexandra's Imperial Military Nursing Service came into being.

History honors the contribution of a special nurse, Clara Maas, from the Spanish-American War; a commemorative stamp was issued in her honor. This 25-year-old nurse was so moved by the suffering of her patients with yellow fever that she volunteered to be bitten

TABLE 4-2.	NURSES OF THE CIVIL WAR AND THEIR CONTRIBUTIONS*
NURSE	**CONTRIBUTION**
Sojourner Truth (1797–1883)	Born into slavery and named Isabella, this African American was sold three times by the time she was 13, the last time for $300. She married an older slave and bore him 5 children, some of whom were also sold into slavery. In 1843 she changed her name to Sojourner Truth. She nursed Union soldiers, worked for improvement in sanitary facilities, and sought contributions of food and clothing for black volunteer regiments. She supported her travel from sales of her *Narrative of Sojourner Truth: A Northern Slave* (1850), dictated to Olive Gilbert because she was illiterate. She continued her work as a nurse/counselor for the Freedmen's Relief Association after the war (Whitman, 1985, pp. 814–816).
Dorothea Lynde Dix (1802–1881)	A Boston school teacher already known for her humanitarian efforts on behalf of the mentally ill, she was commissioned as Superintendent of Women Nurses for All Military Hospitals during the Civil War when she was over 60 years of age. Her authority was often challenged by the physicians.
Mary Ann Ball Bickerdyke (1817–1901)	Called "Mother" Bickerdyke by the troops, this Illinois woman challenged the work of lazy, corrupt medical officers. She served under fire in 19 battles. Her efforts were recognized by the government in the launching of the hospital ship, the *SS Mary A. Bickerdyke* in 1943.
Walt Whitman (1819–1892)	A well-respected poet, who worked as a volunteer in hospital wards after searching for a brother who had been wounded. Dressed wounds, wrote letters, read to soldiers, brought gifts and food. Later wrote about the war and suffering of soldiers.
Harriet Ross Tubman (1820–1913)	An abolitionist sometimes called "Conductor of the Underground Railroad" this black nurse was commended for caring for the sick and wounded without regard for color.
Mary Livermore (1820–1905)	Another untrained nurse of the Civil War, she later became a suffragist and advocated education for all women. Addressing the 6th annual convention of the Nurses' Associated Alumnae, she described the activities of the Civil War nurses.
Clara Barton (1821–1912)	Served as a Volunteer with the Sixth Massachusetts Regiment. Independently operated a large-scale relief operation. Was instrumental in founding the American Red Cross in 1882. Called "little lone lady in black silk" (Donahue 1996, p. 255).

TABLE 4-2.	NURSES OF THE CIVIL WAR AND THEIR CONTRIBUTIONS* *(Continued)*
NURSE	CONTRIBUTION
Kate Cummings (1828–1909)	A volunteer in the Southern army, her diaries chronicled the work of the "matrons" who served in the Confederate hospitals.
Louisa May Alcott (1832–1888)	Served as a volunteer nurse during the Civil War. From these experiences she wrote a small book entitled *Hospital Sketches,* which described the work of the volunteer nurses of the Civil War. The nurse character of the book was Miss Tribulation Periwinkle.
Jane Stuart Woolsey (1830–1891)	One of three sisters from a cultivated and elite northeastern family with colonial ancestry, Jane served the Union Army as supervisor of the nursing and cooking department. She provided much narrative to describe the conditions of the day, authoring a book entitled *Hospital Days.* Later she served as the directress of the Presbyterian Hospital in New York.
Abby Howland Woolsey (1828–1893)	A sister of Jane, she too served as a volunteer nurse for the Union Army and fought diligently for the abolition of slavery. Helped found the Bellevue Hospital Training School for Nurses and wrote one of the first books on the organization of nursing schools— *A Century of Nursing with Hints Toward the Organization of a Training School* (1876) (Whitman, 1985, pp. 904–906).
Georgeanna Muirson Woolsey (1833–1906)	Another Woolsey sister involved in war efforts, she benefited from a month-long nursing training experience in New York when selected by the Woman's Central Association of Relief as one of a group of a 100 for leadership potential. She wrote of her war experiences in a book entitled *Three Weeks at Gettysburg.* She later helped found the Connecticut Training School for Nursing in New Haven, enjoying the support of her husband, Dr. Francis Bacon (Whitman, 1985, pp. 903–906).
Susie King Taylor (1848–1901)	Born into slavery, as a young girl she secretly learned to read and write. While serving as a volunteer nurse for the Union Army, she also worked as a teacher.

*Much of the information contained in this table was gathered from the work of Kalisch & Kalisch, 1995, except as otherwise noted.

several times by the disease-carrying mosquito in an effort to determine how the disease was transmitted. Although she survived the first bite, she died of yellow fever from a subsequent exposure.

A memorial in Arlington National Cemetery honors the memory of the women who gave their lives as Army nurses in the Spanish-American War. It was erected by the Society of Spanish-American War Nurses.

World War I

In 1914, Austria declared war on Serbia, Germany invaded Belgium and France, and England became involved in the conflict. The United States joined them on April 6, 1917. Through Queen Alexandra's Imperial Military Nursing Service, England was prepared to meet the emergency needs for care. Navy and Air Force branches were added to that of the Army. As more nurses were required, the British Red Cross organized a Voluntary Aid Detachment composed of laypersons. These individuals were given short emergency courses to prepare them for service. When the United States joined the conflict, nurses from the Army and Navy Nurse Corps were ready to provide care to the wounded; other experienced nurses were recruited and enlisted. Despite continuous efforts to provide an adequate supply of nurses in both civilian and army hospitals, the lack of qualified nurses became more marked as time went on. The influenza epidemic of 1918 was of major proportions; pneumonia and typhus also claimed many lives, including those of doctors and nurses. It was at this time of great national need, that the Army Nursing Corps finally agreed to admit black nurses. By the time they actually entered the service, the war had ended.

Recognizing the demand for a long-term supply of military nurses, the Army School of Nursing was organized in 1918. Annie W. Goodrich served as its dean.

The experiences of the war also pointed to the serious need for uniformity in methods of nursing education. In response, England founded the Royal College of Nursing in 1916. Inspection and accreditation of schools became one of this group's major concerns.

Although there were many who made supreme efforts during World War I, Edith Cavell has been memorialized. An English nurse, Miss Cavell had organized the first school for nurses in Brussels, Belgium. During the battles that occurred in Brussels, the school and hospital offered care to the soldiers of all armies. As a result, Miss Cavell was arrested by the German soldiers and charged with helping Allied soldiers escape from occupied Belgium. She was sentenced to death and executed at dawn the next day, October 12, 1915.

In 1938, a statue sculpted by Francis Rich from Tennessee marble, titled "Spirit of Nursing," was erected at Arlington National Cemetery among the graves of nurses who had served their country. The only one of its kind to honor nurses in all the services, it was rededicated in 1971 (Klein, 1997).

World War II

In response to Germany's invasion of Austria and Poland, England declared war against Germany in September 1939. The United States entered the war after Japan attacked Pearl Harbor on December 7, 1941. Thus began a conflict that was to be known as a "total war" because it affected every nation in the world. In the United States, the National Nursing Council for War Service was organized in July 1940 to help meet the increasing need for individuals at all levels of preparation who could care for the sick and wounded. The U.S. Cadet Nurse Corps was established under the Bolton Act, which was authorized in June 1943. It provided funds for tuition, a monthly allowance, uniforms, and other expenses for women who would enter nursing and, upon completion of their education, serve in the military service. Volunteer nurse aides were given short, intensive training so that they might assist nurses in hospitals.

In World War II, nurses were given commissions as officers and had military rank, something that had not been true previously. This gave them a level of status and authority that supported their work. Nurses who were assigned to war zones, as opposed to working in military hospitals, often found themselves facing a serious dilemma. The Army had done nothing to prepare them for battlefield medicine or for life in the field. Wounded men were treated in field hospitals close to battle lines with supplies and equipment that might be inadequate, while bombs dropped around them. Although they were in the Army, the nurses considered themselves healers, not soldiers. Elizabeth Norman (1999) poignantly describes the situation in her book *We Band of Angels*:

> Then the shooting started, and they found themselves confronting as much danger and deprivation as any dogface in the field. The men who worked with them—doctors, medics, orderlies and attendants—were no longer "colleagues" and "staff," they were comrades in arms now, and "the girls," as so many referred to them, were no longer anomalies in the ranks, they were a military unit in the middle of battle. They were women at war (p. 39).

(Note: "dogface" was a slang term for the ordinary soldier.)

During this time, flight nursing came into existence as nurses were trained to assist with the air evacuation of sick and wounded soldiers and at ground medical installations. Nurses in these roles worked under extremely dangerous circumstances because the planes used to transport patients also were used to transport cargo. Because of this dual activity, the planes were not marked with the Geneva Red Cross or other insignia, and they remained fair game for enemy fighters.

Stateside, the country was involved in an industrial boom as defense plants mushroomed in response to military needs. Public health nurses moved into industry to carry out preventive health education and programs. Industrial nursing evolved on a national scale, with nurses employed in all types of manufacturing plants.

All of these activities left the country desperate for nurses. Serious shortages were felt in civilian hospitals and in military situations. Kalisch and Kalisch (1995) report that by the winter of 1944–1945, 65,000 nurses were enrolled in the Army and Navy and approximately 13,800 were employed in industry (p. 344). Nursing students began to carry much of the workload in hospitals that had nursing education programs.

The Korean and Vietnam Conflicts

On June 25, 1950, the Korean War broke out. Once again nurses were called into military service. Learning from the experiences of World War II, treatment centers located close to the front lines were established—the Mobile Army Surgical Hospital (MASH). Triage care evolved, made more effective by advances in antibiotics and medical technology. Flight nursing saw a significant resurgence, as the need for air evacuation of the wounded reached new heights.

The American commitment to Vietnam began about the same time as the Korean conflict. By 1963, approximately 15,000 military advisers were in South Vietnam and the first 13 nurses were placed on the staff at the Eighth Field Hospital in Nha Trang in March 1962 (Kalisch & Kalisch, 1995). Recruitment of nurses was once again a major activity; extraordinary incentives were offered because of widespread lack of support for the Vietnam conflict. Due to the guerrilla tactics of the Viet Cong, no military front existed. The country was partitioned into separate field zones and semipermanent, air-conditioned hospitals were constructed. Fixed installations were assigned to area-support missions, with ground evacuation of wounded almost impossible. Terrain and climate were tremendous obstacles. Advances in medical technology, however, permitted far better care than during any other combat situation. The contribution of nurses during this conflict was recognized publicly in a sculpture, designed by Glenna Goodacre, of three nurses and a wounded soldier erected near the Vietnam Memorial in Washington, D.C., in 1993.

On October 18, 1997, the Women in Military Service for America Memorial was dedicated at the Arlington National Cemetery. This marble, stone, and glass memorial is located at the gateway to the cemetery. The dedication included a special nurses' ceremony in which wreaths were placed at the "Spirit of Nursing" statue (Klein, 1997).

The Gulf War

The Iraqi Republican Guard invaded Kuwait on August 2, 1990 and seized control of that country. In an effort to deter any invasion of Saudi Arabia, Kuwait's oil-rich neighbor, the United States mounted Operation Desert Shield, the code name of the military action to eject the Iraqi army from Kuwait. When no withdrawal occurred, as mandated in a United Nations ultimatum, a U. S.-led coalition launched air and ground attacks against Iraqi targets, thus initiating the Gulf War, known by the code name Operation Desert Storm.

Again, nurses were deployed to the area of battle, setting up MASH units in conditions quite different from anything they previously had experienced. Often equipped with protective gas masks to combat any chemical warfare that might have been present, these nurses endured rocket attacks, the cold rains, hot winds, and dust and sand storms of the Arabian desert. Operating from tents, they mobilized triage areas, performed surgery, treated shrapnel wounds, and cared for the innocent Iraqi victims of war, many of whom were women and children, as well as wounded soldiers. As in other war situations, a major challenge was found in improvising equipment and techniques to handle emergency situations. If you are interested in learning more about nurses and the Gulf War, an extensive bibliography of articles related to the topic is available at *http://www.gulflink.osd.mil/gwv_bib/nursing.html*.

Critical Thinking Activity

Select a nursing leader of the past whom you would like to interview. Why did you choose that person? What would you like to ask that individual? How would you use the information that person shared with you? What would you tell that person if she or he asked you to describe nursing today?

EARLY SCHOOLS IN THE UNITED STATES

After the establishment of the Nightingale School in England, nursing programs flourished and the Nightingale system spread to other countries. In the United States, much of the push for nursing education occurred shortly after the Civil War, during which the lack of trained nurses presented a serious concern.

The Establishment of Early Schools

As with many other significant events that have evolved from a variety of influences, it is difficult to pinpoint the first nursing program in the United States. As early as 1798, a pioneer physician, Dr. Valentine Seaman, is said to have initiated the first system of instruction for nurses at New York Hospital (Donahue, 1996, p. 235). A society was formed in 1839 under Quaker influence, called the Nurse Society of Philadelphia, and a combined Home and School were opened. Historical records show that before 1850 some intermittent preparation was provided to individuals who cared for the sick. A plan of instruction also had been developed for women who would supply maternity service in the home, under the guidance of Dr. Joseph Warrington, who was obstetric physician to the Philadelphia Dispensary for the Medical Relief of the Poor.

In 1850, a commission of the Massachusetts Legislature recommended that institutions be formed to educate nurses. A plan for educating nurses was included in the formation of the New England Female Medical College, and a few nurses were educated through this institution. Other hospitals operated training programs, although the course of studies lasted only 6 months. The Woman's Hospital of Philadelphia, which operated under the direction of two female physicians, opened a training school in 1861, but it made little progress until endowed in 1872. Despite these efforts, the nursing services provided by most hospitals during the 1860s were disorganized and inadequate. In many cases, nursing care was provided by women who had been arrested for drunkenness or disorderly conduct and who were serving out 10-day sentences. The better hospitals benefited from the work of Catholic sisters or Protestant deaconesses, although most of them also were untrained.

In 1869, responding to the impetus given nursing during the Civil War, the American Medical Association established a committee to study the issue of **training for nurses**. The committee, chaired by Dr. Samuel D. Gross (1805–1884), was charged with identifying the best possible method to organize and manage institutions for training nurses. Their report concluded that every large hospital should have a nursing school; emphasized that the union between religious exercises and nursing would be conducive to the welfare of the sick; and recommended that schools be placed under the guardianship of county medical societies (Donahue, 1996, p. 265).

The efforts of several influential and socially prominent women of the time were significant in establishing structured training for nurses. An editorial written by Sarah J. Hale, editor of *The Godey's Lady's Book and Magazine,* entitled "Lady Nurses," advocated the elevation of nursing to the level of a profession. Ms. Hale further recommended providing an education "especially adapted for ladies who desire to qualify themselves for the profession of nurse" (Hale, 1871, pp. 188–189).

The New England Hospital for Women and Children is often credited with being the first hospital to establish a formal 1-year program to train nurses in 1872. It operated under the guidance of a female physician, Susan Dimock, who had received her medical education in Europe and had some knowledge of the work of Florence Nightingale. Five probationers started the program on September 1. It was from this school that Melinda Ann (Linda) Richards graduated in 1873, to become America's first trained nurse. This school was the alma mater for the first black nurse graduate, Mary Eliza Mahoney, in 1879.

By 1873, three additional schools had opened: the Bellevue Training School in New York City, the Connecticut Training School in New Haven, and the Boston Training School. Typically, these schools did not admit men. In 1888, the Mills School of Nursing at Bellevue Hospital opened to train male nurses for patient care. Separate schools to educate black nurses also opened; among them Spelman Seminary in Atlanta in 1886, Hampton Institute in Virginia and Providence Hospital in Chicago in 1891, and Tuskegee Institute in Alabama in 1892 (Kalisch & Kalisch, 1995). Table 4-3 identifies some of the early schools.

Similar movements to establish nursing schools were occurring in other countries. In 1868, a school was organized in Sydney Hospital, Australia. In Edinburgh, Scotland, a program was started at the Royal Infirmary. The Mack Training School in St. Catherines, Canada, was started in 1884.

Characteristics of the Early Schools

The life of the nursing student at the turn of the century was not an easy one. The strong militaristic and religious influences over nursing were embodied in the expectations held for nursing students. "Monastic and military traditions heavily influenced not only the actual workings of the schools of nursing but also the public's conception of them. The nurse in training was expected to yield to her superiors obedience characteristic of a good soldier and actions governed by the dedication to duty derived from religious devotion" (Kalisch & Kalisch, 1995, p. 111).

Typically, nursing students were about 21 years of age, single, and female. The first weeks or months of their education were spent as probationers, or "probies," and their duties, although helping with the operation of the hospital, did little to educate them as nurses. For example, they spent much of their time washing, scrubbing, polishing, folding, stacking, and the like. Rules of conduct were rigid and unforgiving; early superintendents saw it as their responsibility to "discipline" pupils, ensuring that they possessed good morals, and were honest, conscientious, obedient, respectful, loyal, passive, and devoted to duty. Nursing students were expected to be unselfish, thinking not of themselves but of the happiness and well-being of others (Fig. 4-4).

Initially, nursing education was largely an apprenticeship and resulted in students providing much of the workforce of hospitals. The workday was long and arduous, often starting at 5:30 in the morning and ending with nursing prayers very late at night, and consisted primarily of work on the hospital wards. The superintendent or her assistants provided instruction. There was no standardization of curriculum and no accreditation. The few lectures that were part of the program were usually given by physicians and scheduled at 8 or 9 PM after a

TABLE 4-3.	EARLY NORTH AMERICAN TRAINING SCHOOLS FOR NURSES*	
DATE	**NAME AND PLACE**	**COMMENTS**
1798	New York Hospital—New York	Dr. Valentine Seaman initiated a system of instruction for nurses. His lectures covered the topics of anatomy, physiology, maternal nursing, and care of children.
1839	Philadelphia Dispensary—Philadelphia	Dr. Joseph Warrington provided obstetric training to a group of women who would work with families who would otherwise not receive care. The Nurse Society of Philadelphia grew out of this training.
1861	Bellevue Hospital—New York	Dr. Elizabeth Blackwell converted Bellevue Hospital into a training center for nurses. About 100 women were trained to provide care during the Civil War in an intensive 4-week course.
1861–1862	Women's Hospital of Philadelphia—Philadelphia	Opened a training school, but it progressed slowly until 1872, when it became endowed—the first endowed school of nursing in America. Organized and conducted by two female physicians.
1862	New England Hospital for Women and Children—Boston	Dr. Marie Zakrzewska, a colleague of Dr. Blackwell's, offered a 6-month program to nurses.
1872	New England Training School—Boston	An expansion of the New England Hospital Program has been identified as the first formal school for nurses, under direction of Dr. Susan Dimock. The first graduate was Linda Ann Richards. Mary Mahoney, the first black nurse, also graduated here.
1873–May	Bellevue Training School—New York	First of a trio of schools modeled after the Nightingale model–Lavinia Dock was one of the early graduates.
1873–October	Connecticut Training School—New Haven	Second of the trio of schools started in 1873—introduced first textbook, *New Haven Manual of Nursing,* written by a committee of nurses and physicians.
1873–November	Boston Training School—Boston (attached to Massachusetts General)	Third of the trio—Linda Richards became superintendent of nurses in November 1894. Idea for school initiated by the Woman's Educational Association. Medical staff did not support initiation of the school.
1874	St. Catharine's General and Marine Hospital—Ontario, Canada—later called the Mack Training School	Patterned after the Nightingale schools, this program included instruction in the art of nursing, chemistry, sanitary science, physiology, and anatomy.

(*continued*)

TABLE 4-3	EARLY NORTH AMERICAN TRAINING SCHOOLS FOR NURSES* (Continued)	
DATE	NAME AND PLACE	COMMENTS
1877	Training School of the New York Hospital—New York	Offered an 18-month course to prepare graduates for nursing.
1878	Boston City Hospital Training School—Boston	Required graduates to complete a 2-year program of study.
1884	Toronto General Hospital—Toronto, Canada	Mary Agnes Snively became superintendent of this school, which had early beginnings in 1877.
1884–1885	Farrand Training School for Nurses—Harper Hospital, Detroit	Considered one of the better schools, students had two annual series of lectures, approximately 20 hours total.
1886	Spelman Seminary—Atlanta, GA	The first separate school to educate black nurses, who were often denied admission to other schools.
1888	Mills School of Nursing at Bellevue Hospital—New York	First school established for male nurses. Prepared them to give general patient care.
1889	Johns Hopkins School of Nursing—Baltimore	Program opened under direction of Isabel Hampton Robb. Mary Adelaide Nutting graduated in 1891.
1890	Montreal General—Montreal, Canada	Although wanting a nursing program as early as 1835, hospital conditions would not allow. Nora Gertrude Livingstone established school in 1890.

*Information for this table was gathered primarily from Donahue, 1996 and Kalisch & Kalisch, 1995.

long day of work. A 7-day workweek was the standard, and the help needed on the hospital units took precedence over the education of the young women. Lectures would be canceled if students were needed to care for patients.

As schools developed, facilities to house nursing students became necessary. Although some of the early programs provided sleeping quarters in the hospital, nursing students usually were housed in a building next to the hospital, often referred to as the "nurses' dormitory." A "housemother" often controlled the nurses' residence. In religious affiliations, a deaconess or Sister served the same purpose. Housemothers assured that codes of behavior were adhered to and that curfews were enforced. Violations usually resulted in expulsion from the program or the loss of a part of the uniform, such as the bib section of an apron. This signified to all that some infraction had occurred. Young women, who were attracted to nursing because of the imagined glamour of wearing a long crisp white apron and ministering to sick (though handsome) young men, often became discouraged with the severe duties and routine. The attrition rate was high in the early schools.

Although there were some changes in the curriculum—work hours were decreased, the length of study was increased, and the theory component was organized into specific areas of care such as medical, surgical, and obstetric nursing—hospital-based programs remained

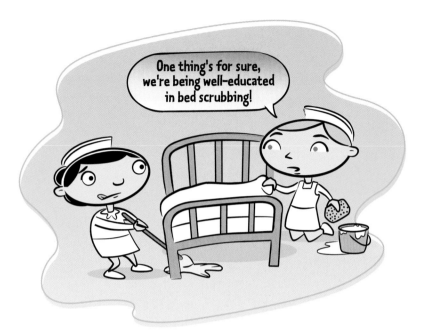

FIGURE 4-4   The duties assigned to probationers may have helped operate the hospital but did little to educate the nurse.

largely unchanged through the 1940s and 1950s. The following is a quote from a special publication developed on the occasion of the closing of a diploma school:

> In 1921, a nurse was discharged for "cigarette habit." Skirts of nurses' uniforms were getting shorter but there was periodic measurement to be sure some were not too short.
>
> The year 1924 would see Deaconess' first student protest. Student nurses were required to wear their hair long in those days. A number of them though made arrangements with a barber in the Victoria Hotel to stay open late one evening and they all went down and had their hair bobbed in the latest style. They were deprived of their caps for several weeks and ordered to wear switches and what-nots, their punishment comparatively slight, since "banks and other business regularly dismissed employees for social offense" (Deaconess Hospital School of Nursing 1980, p. 10).

Schools proliferated as even small hospitals established nursing programs, recognizing the valuable commodity available in students who provided the majority of care given. As early as 1905, early pioneers and advocates for nursing, concerned about the proliferation of schools, championed programs that offered a sound educational foundation and reasonable working hours. During the time Isabel Hampton was "Principal" of the Johns Hopkins Training School (a position she accepted in 1889 and continued until her marriage to Dr. Robb in 1894), she arranged for a regular period of 2 hours of free time during a day that was limited to 12 hours. She would have liked to limit the workday to 8 hours, however. Time was allowed for recreation and for meals (Jamieson & Sewall, 1944, p. 432).

Early Textbooks and Journals

There were few textbooks prior to 1900, a factor that complicated the learning process. Many of the lectures presented by physicians were given from notes they had taken while medical

TABLE 4-4.	EARLY NURSING TEXTBOOKS*	
YEAR	**AUTHOR**	**TITLE**
1878	A committee of physicians and nurses	*Hand-book for Family and General Use*
1885	Clara Weeks Shaw	*A Textbook of Nursing for the Use of Training Schools, Families and Private Students*
1890	Lavinia Dock	*The Textbook on Materia Medica for Nurses*
1893	Diana Kimber	*The first anatomy book for nurses, Anatomy and Physiology*
1889 (about)	Isabel Hampton	*Nursing: Its Principles and Practices for Hospital and Private Use*
1894 (about)	Isabel Hampton Robb	*Nursing Ethics*

*Information for the table was gathered primarily from Donahue, 1996 and Kalisch & Kalisch, 1995.

students. The first nursing textbook was reportedly the *Hand-book of Nursing for Family and General Use*, written by a committee composed of physicians and nurses associated with the Connecticut Training School at New Haven Hospital. Other books followed over the next 2 years. Table 4-4 describes some of the early textbooks.

Nursing journals also appeared toward the end of the 19th century. Five different journals for nurses were published before 1901. The first appeared in 1886 and was entitled *The Nightingale*. In 1889, under the direction of Mary E.P. Davis, a company was formed with 550 cash subscriptions, and a new journal called the *American Journal of Nursing* made its debut in October 1890 (Kalisch & Kalisch, 1995, pp. 115–116). The journal continues to be published today.

Critical Thinking Activity

Imagine that you are an instructor in an early nursing program. There are no textbooks. There are no nursing journals from which you can assign reading. How would you go about teaching the students for whom you are responsible? What would you see as the major concerns? How would the classes differ from those you are in today?

THE BEGINNING OF NURSING ORGANIZATIONS

By the end of the 19th century, changes were accomplished most effectively through organizations. Nursing pioneers saw this as an opportunity to bring about transformation in nursing practice and nursing education and began forming **nursing organizations**.

Nursing Organizations in England

In England, the establishment of an organization for nursing was driven by the energies of Mrs. Bedford Fenwick (Ethel Gordon Manson), a prominent leader who, in 1887, campaigned for nurse registration. She believed that standards were necessary to improve nursing. Although her ideas for nurse registration were not well accepted, she founded the British Nurses' Association in 1888. It grew rapidly to 1000 members by the end of the first year. It later became the Royal British Nurses' Association.

The American Society of Superintendents of Training Schools for Nurses

In 1893, the World's Fair and Columbian Exposition was held in Chicago to celebrate the 400th anniversary of Columbus' arrival in the United States. The Fair provided the meeting place for many professions and artisans. The first nurses' meeting was held in the Hall of Columbus from June 15–17, 1893, as part of the International Congress of Charities, Corrections, and Philanthropy. The nursing meeting was chaired by Isabel Hampton and was attended by American and Canadian nurses. Attendees included such individuals as Lavinia Dock—suffragist, nurse activist, historian, and educator—who spoke on the relation of training schools to hospitals. An address sent by Florence Nightingale was presented to the group. The papers presented were later compiled in a publication, *Nursing the Sick, 1893*. The day after the meeting, Isabel Hampton arranged a meeting of a small group of leaders to discuss the possibility of starting a nursing organization. This meeting resulted in the formation in 1896 of the American Society of Superintendents of Training Schools for Nurses, so named because most of the attendees were directors of nursing schools; the membership was restricted to those nurses associated with nurse training. Concern for the standards of nursing education was primary, and a committee to study nursing education was quickly appointed. In 1907, the Canadian members formed their own organization, the Canadian Society of Superintendents of Training Schools. The American organization changed its name in 1912 to the National League for Nursing Education (Donahue, 1996, p. 326).

In 1952, the National League for Nursing Education became the National League for Nursing when six organizations merged into one. The organizations involved in the merger were the National Organization for Public Health Nursing (est. 1912), the Association of Collegiate Schools of Nursing (est. 1933), the Joint Committee on Practical Nurses and Auxiliary Workers in Nursing Services (est. 1945), the Joint Committee on Careers in Nursing (est. 1946), the National Committee for the Improvement of Nursing Services (est. 1949), and the National Nursing Accrediting Service (est. 1949).

Nurses' Associated Alumnae of the United States and Canada

As the number of nurses increased throughout the United States and as hospitals formed individual alumnae groups, the need arose for an organization of trained nurses. At the third meeting of the American Society of Superintendents of Training Schools in 1896, a committee prepared a constitution and bylaws for such an organization with the delegates representing the various alumnae associations. The constitution was accepted a year later, and the Nurses' Associated Alumnae of the United States and Canada was formed. The first president was Isabel Hampton Robb. The purposes of the group were:

1. To establish and maintain a code of ethics
2. To elevate the standards of nursing education
3. To promote the usefulness and honor, the financial and other interests of the nursing profession. (American Nurses Association, 1941, p. 2)

When it was discovered that New York law would not permit foreign membership in an incorporated association, the words "and Canada" were dropped from the title in 1901 and Canadian participation was prohibited. In 1911, the name of the organization in the United States became the American Nurses Association (ANA).

In 1908, the Provisional Organization of the Canadian National Association of Trained Nurses was formed, which was renamed the Canadian Nurses Association in 1924. This group also had as its primary concerns the education of nursing students, the improvement of nursing care, the amelioration of conditions for nurses, and state registration of nurses to protect the public.

The International Council of Nurses

The International Council of Nurses, the oldest of all international nursing organizations, was formed in 1899. Founded by Mrs. Bedford Fenwick, it held its first meeting in Buffalo, New York, at the World Exposition in 1901. Mrs. Fenwick was the first president of the organization. The membership originally was composed of self-governing national nurses' associations rather than individual members, although, until 1904, individual members could belong because few countries had organized nursing associations. Its purpose was to encourage communication among nurses of all nations and to provide opportunities for nurses from all over the world to meet and discuss concerns about the profession and about patient care. At the present time, the International Council of Nurses meets once every 4 years.

Lists of nursing organizations can be found on the World Wide Web at the following sites: *http://dir.yahoo.com/health/nursing/organizations/* or *http://nursingworld.org/rnindex/* and click on links to nursing organizations. The links provided at those Web sites can help you to research individual organizations that may be of interest to you. As you review that list, you can understand why some critics suggest that nursing has too many organizations working in too many different directions.

Critical Thinking Activity

Research a particular nursing specialty organization. Why did you choose that organization? Who are the members of the organization and what is its purpose? Compare and contrast the philosophy of that organization with your own.

THE DEVELOPMENT OF HOSPITALS AND NURSING HOMES IN THE UNITED STATES

The history of hospitals in the United States can be traced back to the mid-1700s, when most cities built **almshouses**, also called poorhouses, at the time. Almshouses provided food and shelter for the homeless poor, and served as homes for the aged, the disabled, the mentally ill, and the orphaned. **Pesthouses** also were built at this time to isolate people with contagious diseases, especially those diseases contracted aboard ship. These facilities housed people suffering from cholera, smallpox, typhus, and yellow fever, and the more common communicable diseases such as scarlet fever. Pesthouses would open and close as needed.

Neither almshouses nor pesthouses were institutions from which most individuals would want to seek or receive care. They were crowded and unsanitary, with insufficient heat and ventilation. Cross-infection was common and mortality was high. Those with the financial means were cared for in their homes.

The first **hospital**, founded in what was to become the United States, was started in Philadelphia in 1751, at the urging of Benjamin Franklin. Franklin believed that the public had a duty to provide care to the poor, friendless, sick, and insane. A bill passed that year authorized the establishment of the Pennsylvania Hospital (Kalisch & Kalisch, 1995). The New York Hospital in New York City was established in 1773, primarily to prevent the spread of infectious diseases brought by sailors and immigrants. Massachusetts General Hospital in Boston opened its doors in 1816 and New Haven Hospital in Connecticut in 1826.

The early hospitals cared for people with acute illnesses and injuries but did not admit the mentally ill. Several separate hospitals were established for this purpose. The first such facility was established as a department of the Pennsylvania Hospital in 1752. The second was founded in Williamsburg, Virginia, in 1773; the third, known as Friends Hospital, was located near Philadelphia in 1817. By 1840, eight hospitals to treat the mentally ill had been established (Kalisch & Kalisch, 1995). The cruel and inhumane treatment of patients in the early mental hospitals is legendary. Dorothea Dix, mentioned in Table 4-1, campaigned vigorously for and brought about much reform in the area of mental health treatment. Although never educated as a nurse (she was a schoolteacher), Dix volunteered as a nurse during the Civil War and is included in the Nursing Hall of Fame because of her significant contributions to the profession.

The earliest hospitals left much to be desired. Most were housed in large buildings that had been converted into temporary quarters. Often they were dirty, rank with infection, and poorly ventilated. Linen was used for several patients before it was laundered, even though draining, suppurating wounds were common. The stench was overwhelming, and it is said that nurses used snuff to make working conditions more tolerable (Kalisch & Kalisch, 1995). Hospitals constructed during the early 19th century often followed a block plan in their design, and the buildings resembled large barns. In the 1850s, Massachusetts General Hospital constructed a facility divided into wards or pavilions, each one a separate building with high ceilings and good ventilation. The buildings were built of wood because it was believed they would need to be replaced after 20 years because of contamination (Kalisch & Kalisch, 1995, p. 22).

Factors Affecting the Development of Hospitals

Six major forces can be cited as influencing the growth of hospitals throughout the United States. Each played a unique role in the continued development of hospitals and patient care.

ADVANCES IN MEDICAL SCIENCE

By the end of the colonial period, two medical schools had been established in the United States. Before that time, physicians learned their skills through an apprenticeship with a practicing physician. As medicine became more of a science, advances occurred. One of the most significant was the discovery of anesthesia and the rapid progress in surgery that followed. The germ theory also did much to improve the practice of medicine because it inspired the development of agents or techniques that would sterilize or serve as antiseptics. The growth of hospitals in the United States was a direct result of such progress, which made hospitals safer and more desirable. The discovery of sulfa in the mid-1930s and antibiotics in the mid-1940s heralded even greater changes.

THE DEVELOPMENT OF MEDICAL TECHNOLOGY

The development of specialized medical technology was a natural successor to the advances in medical science. The first hospital laboratory was opened in 1889, and x-rays were used in diagnosis in 1896. The electrocardiogram (ECG) was invented in 1903 and the electroencephalogram (EEG) in 1929 (Haglund & Dowling, 1993).

CHANGES IN MEDICAL EDUCATION

Advances in medical education also had a significant impact on the development of health care in the United States. The Flexner Report (see Chapter 5) was completed in 1910, and it led to changes in the structure and content of curricula in medical schools. It also expanded the role of hospitals to include education and research and resulted in internships and residencies for medical students.

GROWTH OF THE HEALTH INSURANCE INDUSTRY

The growth of the health insurance industry is another factor responsible for the development of hospitals. Although there were some antecedents, most sources indicate that the first hospital insurance plan was initiated at Baylor University Hospital in 1929 to serve the needs of schoolteachers in Dallas, Texas (Raffel & Raffel, 1989). The approach used there was to form the model for Blue Cross plans around the country.

Today, figures vary as to what percentage of the population is protected against the costs of medical care by some type of insurance. A report based on the findings from *The Commonwealth Fund 1999 National Survey of Workers' Health Insurance* found that lack of insurance is a significant and growing problem. The study found that nearly one of five (19%) working-age adults lacked health insurance, and that two of five (41%) with incomes less than $20,000 lacked insurance ("Millions of working. . .", 1999). There is great concern for the millions of individuals who have no protection.

GREATER INVOLVEMENT OF THE GOVERNMENT

In early times, the government was involved in health care delivery primarily at a local level, building almshouses and facilities for the insane. By 1935, the government was providing

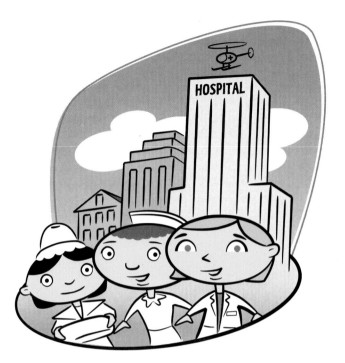

FIGURE 4-5   The growth of hospitals was significantly influenced by the emergence of modern nursing.

grants-in-aid to assist in the establishment of public health and other programs to furnish health assistance to citizens. The Hospital Survey and Construction Act of 1946 (also called the Hill-Burton Act) resulted in the construction of many hospitals and other health facilities. The initiation of Medicare and Medicaid in 1965 made another significant impact on the health care industry, because the legislation encouraged capital construction and the development of hospitals through the manner in which the system of reimbursement was structured.

THE EMERGENCE OF PROFESSIONAL NURSING

Another force that significantly influenced the growth of hospitals was the development of professional nursing. Haglund and Dowling (1993, p. 139) cite two ways in which advances in nursing contributed to the growth of hospitals (Fig. 4-5). First, they "increased the efficiency of treatment, cleanliness, nutritious diets, and formal treatment routines" that resulted in patient recovery. Second, they resulted in considerate, skilled patient care that made hospitals acceptable to all people, not just the poor. The role of the nurse and nursing influences the health care delivery system more today than ever before.

History of the Nursing Home

Like our acute care facilities, the nursing home had a rather harsh beginning. In the 19th century, the government constructed almshouses, or poorhouses, to shelter the destitute elderly. These facilities attracted a strange mixture of residents, including those who needed asylum and detention, as well as the poor, the chronically disabled, and the mentally ill. According to the moral perspective that prevailed at the time, poverty and disability were viewed as indications of an undisciplined, improvident, and even profligate life. A person who was housed in a "county poorhouse" often had no financial resources and no family to provide care and assistance, and endured a certain social stigma. In time, these almshouses became the community "dumping grounds" for all of society's cast-offs. The early facilities for the country's dependent elderly offered the same grim surroundings as the early hospitals. They were unsanitary, overcrowded, and poorly ventilated. Residents were expected to work to assist with their keep if they were able. Individuals who provided care sought employment there usually as a last resort. Appropriations to manage these facilities were meager because most citizens did not identify with the institutions that housed the poor and the transient, who probably had no history of contributing to the community.

As the United States grew as a society, various groups became concerned about the conditions that existed in the poorhouses. Eventually, patients were separated according to their condition and the mentally and chronically ill were reassigned to different hospitals. An increasing number of churches and fraternal organizations started homes to care for their elderly members. As a result of the Social Security Act of 1935, private (for-profit or proprietary) nursing homes emerged during that decade. Raffel and Raffel (1989, p. 205) state, "The original exclusion of benefits for patients in public institutions (since repealed) apparently stemmed from congressional concern about conditions in county poorhouses and a desire to get them closed."

In the postwar period, the Hill-Burton Act of 1946, which supported hospital construction, was expanded to include voluntary (nonprofit) nursing homes, and some states also developed grant programs. Since 1950, government funding for nursing home care has increased steadily and culminated in the 1965 Medicaid program, which by 1991 covered 40% of all nursing home costs (Collopy et al, 1991). Governmental regulation of nursing homes has become increasingly involved and complex.

As changes in funding occurred and as short-term acute care hospitals became increasingly specialized, the role of the nursing home changed. In the 1950s and 1960s, the deinstitutionalization movement, which saw large numbers of the elderly population discharged from mental hospitals, also affected nursing homes. Nursing homes began to assume the role of providing specialized care for the elderly. By the 1960s, this role was well established, but the nursing home industry was plagued by constant reports of substandard and negligent care and, in some instances, charges of absolute abuse of patients and misuse or embezzlement of their funds. This resulted in even greater scrutiny and regulation by the government.

Today, **nursing home** is a broad term that encompasses a wide spectrum of facilities ranging from special units in acute community hospitals to those that are a part of the campus of care retirement centers. Only about 6% have 200 beds or more. The facilities are licensed by the state in which they operate, and each state has its own definitions and requirements. Approximately 75% are certified by Medicare as "skilled nursing facilities," a necessary qualification if Medicare funds are to pay for the care. An even greater percentage are certified to care for Medicaid patients. All facilities receiving federal funds must meet federal as well as state standards. The major reason for admission to a nursing home is functional dependency rather than medical diagnosis. The use of nursing homes will continue to grow in the future as the population grows older.

The American Hospital Association

The American Hospital Association was founded in 1899 as the Association of Hospital Super-intendents, with a membership of nine. Its purpose was to establish and maintain high standards of hospital service, care of the sick, and control and prevention of disease. Nurses who held positions as hospital administrators were instrumental in the early development of this organization, although their roles might have been somewhat passive. It has been suggested that "this passivity cast a negative influence over nurse training standards" (Kalisch & Kalisch, 1995, p. 132). Today's American Hospital Association is an extensive organization with many activities.

Critical Thinking Activity

If you had the power to change one single event in the history of nursing, what would it be? Why would you make that change? How do you think it would have affected nursing today?

KEY CONCEPTS

- Nursing has its roots in all endeavors to care for the sick and injured; therefore, it is difficult to pinpoint a particular period in history when nursing first began.
- Nursing's history has influenced the way the profession is recognized by the public. There were three significant images of the nurse in the past: the folk image, the religious image, and the servant image.
- The "Dark Ages of Nursing" occurred during the Reformation, when only those individuals who could not find other employment cared for the ill.
- Florence Nightingale had a significant impact on the form and direction of nursing and established it as a respected field of endeavor. Many of her precepts are still a part of nursing.
- During times when the United States was at war, the serious need for trained nurses to care for the sick and wounded became a public concern.
- Early nursing schools were developed in the United States for the purpose of nursing service as much as for educating young women. The programs were rigorous; often a 7-day workweek consisted of 14-hour workdays.
- Nursing organizations, the forerunners of today's associations, began to emerge toward the end of the 19th century as the pioneers of early nursing saw the need for change in nursing education and nursing practice.
- Acute care hospitals have a history reaching back into the ancient past. Advances in medical science, the development of medical technology, changes in medical education, the growth of the health insurance industry, government involvement, and the emergence of professional nursing all affected the development of modern hospitals.
- Long-term care facilities have histories similar to that of acute care hospitals; both often started as facilities to house the poor and indigent. Today's nursing homes provide specialized care to the elderly or disabled and rehabilitation services to others.

RELEVANT WEB SITES

American Association for the History of Nursing (AAHN):
http:www.aahn.org/resource.html
American Association for the History of Medicine (AAHM): *http://www.histmed.org*
American Nurses Association Centennial Exhibit: Voices from the Past, Visions of the
Future: *http://www.ana.org/centenn/index.htm*
American Nurses Association Hall of Fame: *http://www.ana.org/hof/index.htm*
Archives of Nursing Leadership: *http://www.nursing.uconn.edu/ARCHIVE.HTML*
Black Nurses in History: *http://www4.umdnj.edu/camlbweb/blacknurses.html*
Boston University Nursing Archives: *http://www.bu.edu/speccol/nursing.htm*
British Columbia History of Nursing Group: *http://www.bcnursinghistory.ca*
Canadian Association for the History of Nursing:
http://www.ualberta.ca/~jhibberd/CAHN_ACHN
Center for Nursing Historical Inquiry:
http://www.nursing.virginia.edu/centers/cnhi/index.html
Center for the Study of the History of Nursing: *http://www.nursing.upenn.edu/history/*
Margaret M. Allemang Center for the History of Nursing: *http://www.allemang.on.ca/*
index.html
Men in American Nursing History: *http://www.geocities.com/Athens/Forum/6011*
National Information Center for Health Services Administration: *http://www.nichsa.org*
National League for Nursing: *http://www.nln.org*
Nursing Organizations Web site lists:
http://dir.yahoo.com/health/nursing/organizations/ or
http://nursingworld.org/rnindex/ and click on link to nursing organizations
References regarding Florence Nightingale:
http://www.nightingales.com
http://www.florence-nightingale-avenging-angel.co.uk/
Clendening History of Medicine Library—Florence Nightingale Resources:
http://clendening.kumc.edu/dc/fn
Florence Nightingale Museum Web site:
http://www.florence-nightingale.co.uk
http://www.countryjoe.com/nightingale

REFERENCES

Al-Madinah Al-Munawwarah: The City of the Prophet. (Spring, 1998, Vol. 15) Saudi Arabia, [On-line.]
Available at: *http://www.saudiembassy.net/publications/magazine-spring-98/madinah.htm*, (Accessed,
April 11, 2002).
American Nurses Association. (1941). ANA and you. New York: Author.
Collopy, B., Boyle, P., & Jennings, B.(1991). New directions in nursing home ethics (A Hastings Cen-
ter Report Special Supplement, March-April). *Hastings Center Report 21*(2):1–16.
Deaconess Hospital School of Nursing. (1980). *Eighty-one years of nursing: 1899-1980.* Spokane, WA:
Deaconess Hospital.

Dickens, C. (1936). Martin Chuzzlewit. In *The Works of Charles Dickens*, Vol. II. New York: Books Inc.

Donahue, M.P. (1996). *Nursing: The finest art*, (2nd ed.). St. Louis: CV Mosby.

Gunn, J.C. (1885). *Gunn's Newest family physician: or home-book of health: An approved household guide*. Chicago: Wm. H. Moore & Co.

Haglund, C.L., & Dowling, W.L. (1993). The hospital. In S.J.Williams & P.R. Torrens: *Introduction to health service* (4th ed., pp. 135–176). New York: Delmar Publishers, Inc.

Hale, S. (1871). Lady nurses. *Godey's Lady's Book and Magazine* 82:188.

Jamieson, E.M. & Sewall, M. (1944). *Trends in nursing history* (2nd ed.). Philadelphia: W.B. Saunders Co.

Jan, R. (1996) Rufaida Al-Asalmiya, the first Muslim nurse. *Image: Journal of Nursing Scholarship*. 28(3):267–268.

Kalisch, P.A. & Kalisch, B.J. (1995). *The advance of American nursing* (3rd ed.) Philadelphia: J.B. Lippincott Co.

Klein, J.A. (1997). Honoring female military nurses. *BRAVO Veterans Outlook*, August-September. [On-line.] Available at: *http://www.nursingnetwork.com/veterans.htm*. Accessed January 14, 2000.

Lake-Thom, B. (1997). *Spirits of the earth*. New York: Plume, published by Penguin Books USA Inc.

"Millions of working Americans can't afford to get sick." (Fall, 1999). *The Commonwealth Fund Quarterly*, [On-line.] Available at: *http://www.cmwf.org/publist/quarterly/index.asp*. Accessed January 9, 2000.

Norman, E.M. (1999). *We band of angels*. New York: Random House.

Nutting, M. A. & Dock, L. L. (1935). *A history of nursing*. New York: GP Putnam's Sons.

Peck, M.C. (2002). "Mecca." *World Book Online Americas Edition,* [On-line.] Available at: *http://www.aolsvc.worldbook.aol.com,* Accessed April 11, 2002

Raffel, M. W. & Raffel, N. K. (1989). *The U.S. health system: Origins and functions* (3rd ed.). New York: John Wiley & Sons.

Uprichard, M. (1973). Ferment in nursing. In E. Auld & L.H. Birum: *The challenge of nursing.* (pp. 24–31). St. Louis: CV Mosby.

Whitman, A. (1985). *American reformers*. New York: H.W. Wilson Co.

5

The Development of Nursing as a Profession

LEARNING OUTCOMES

After completing this chapter, you should be able to:

1. Analyze why the profession has had difficulty defining nursing.
2. Discuss the ways in which nursing differs from medicine.
3. Formulate a personal definition of nursing and identify a theorist who defines nursing similarly.
4. Identify the seven characteristics against which social scientists have evaluated professions and examine the ways they can be applied to nursing.
5. Compare and contrast the terms "profession" and "professional."
6. Explain how the image others hold of nursing affects the profession and the role of nurses.
7. Analyze areas of nursing about which studies have been conducted and discuss why each is important.
8. Discuss the concept of a universal language for nursing and describe how nursing classifications provide this.
9. Describe some of the traditions in nursing and explain why they were adopted.

KEY TERMS

Body of specialized knowledge

Characteristics of a profession

Classification systems

Code of ethics

Definition of nursing

Formal characteristics

Image

Institutions of higher education

Lifetime commitment

Medicine

North American Nursing Diagnosis Association (NANDA)

Nursing Interventions Classification (NIC)

Nursing nomenclatures

Nursing Outcomes Classification (NOC)

Nursing shortage

Occupation

Omaha System

Profession

Professional

Professional activity

Professional policy

Scientific method

Service to the public

Studies about nursing

Taxonomy

Traditions

What is nursing? Is nursing an art or a science? If it is both, which category should receive the primary emphasis? How can "hunches," "gut feelings," and "intuition" be useful in a world of practicality surrounded by scientific rationale, steeped in protocol, and immersed in critical thinking and clinical pathways? Should nursing be considered a profession or an occupation? What factors are affecting the emergence of nursing as a profession? Does nursing possess a unique body of knowledge? Is the nurse a professional? If so, what educational background qualifies the nurse for professional standing? Should the educational preparation for nursing occur in a variety of settings that award different degrees? How will the skills of graduates from various programs be differentiated in practice? Do different levels of competence exist in the practice of clinical nursing? What is the status of the nurse in relation to other members of the health care team? What is the language of nursing? Is a single language adequate? What is the role of the nurse in preventive care? What role belongs exclusively to the nurse? What forces have played a part in the development of that role? What is the future of the nurses' role? What should we remember from our past that can assist in the development of nursing in the future?

These are but a few of the questions being asked by nurses today. Not all the questions have clear or obvious answers. Some of the answers result in debate and dialogue among nurses, health care providers, and health care consumers. As a novice joining the ranks of those who have preceded you, you will benefit from a good understanding of the issues that have challenged, and in some instances plagued, nurses over the years. Most novice nurses develop an appreciation of nursing's heritage by learning about some of the nurses who helped to shape the profession. As a nurse in the 21st century, you may have many opportunities to directly influence the answers to these questions.

NURSING DEFINED

When you entered the nursing program in which you are now enrolled, what was your perception of nursing as a profession? Has that perception of nursing been changed by the experiences you have had as a nursing student? Some might ask, "So why spend so much time and effort trying to define nursing?" Chitty (1997, p. 143) helps answer that question. She states, "They [ie, definitions] are a good place to begin in attempting to understand any complex enterprise such as nursing." Over the years, the profession has worked at establishing a **definition of nursing**.

Defining nursing can be difficult. Nurses themselves cannot agree on a single definition, partly because of the history of nursing. Little is known about the work of the nurse in prehistory; however, Donahue (1996, p. 2) writes, "From the dawn of civilization, evidence prevails to support the premise that *nurturing* has been essential to the preservation of life. Survival of the human race, therefore, is inextricably intertwined with the development of nursing."

A major factor that has made it difficult to define nursing is that it is taught as encompassing both theoretic and practical aspects, but it is pursued (and continues to be defined) primarily through practice, a little-studied area. Benner (1984) states, "Nurses have not been careful record keepers of their own clinical learning. . . . This failure to chart our practices and clinical observations has deprived nursing theory of the uniqueness and richness of the knowledge embedded in expert clinical practice." She further discusses the differences between "knowing that" and "knowing how." When attempting to define nursing, we often stumble over these two concepts and how to combine the distinct and unique aspects of both.

Early Definitions of Nursing

A nurse is a person who nourishes, fosters, and protects—a person who is prepared to care for the sick, injured, and aged. In this sense, "nurse" is used as a noun and is derived from the Latin *nutrix,* which means "nursing mother." The word "nurse" also has referred to a woman who suckled a child (usually not her own)—a wet nurse. Dictionary definitions of nurse include such descriptions as "suckles or nourishes," "to take care of a child or children," "to bring up; rear." In this way, "nurse" is used as a verb, deriving from the Latin *nutrire*, which means "to suckle and nourish." With such an origin, it is understandable that people generally have associated nursing with women.

References to "the nurse" can be found in the Talmud and in the Old Testament, although the role of the nurse in these references is not clearly defined. The nurse in these texts was probably more similar to the wet nurse than to someone who cared for the sick.

> And Deborah, Rebekah's nurse died, and she was buried under an oak below Beth-el: so the name of it was called Allon-bacuth. (Gen. 35:6–8, Revised Standard Version of the Bible)

Over the centuries, the word "nurse" has evolved to refer to a person who tends to the needs of the sick. Florence Nightingale, in her *Notes on Nursing: What It Is and What It Is*

Not, described the nurse's role as one that would "put the patient in the best condition for nature to act upon him" (Nightingale, 1954, p. 133), a definition that often is quoted today.

In the past, nurses undoubtedly were more concerned about carrying out their responsibilities than about defining the role of the nurse. Through the years, we have seen the concept of the nurse grow and evolve from the nurse as mother, nourishing and nurturing children, to the nurse, without specific reference to gender, with responsibilities encompassing ever-expanding and challenging services to people needing health care.

Not surprisingly, the development of nursing as a profession, the defining of its role and language for society, and the placing of it among other attractive careers has been inextricably tied to the role of women in society at various times in history, and to the forces that have had an impact on society. If we are frustrated at what appears to be the slow development of nursing as a profession, we need to remember that it was 1916 when Margaret Sanger opened the first birth control clinic in the United States. And not until 1919, after 40 years of campaigning, were women in the United States granted the right to vote, through the 19th Amendment to the Constitution.

Distinguishing Nursing From Medicine

The formulation of clear and concise definitions of nursing also has been hampered by the lack of an obvious distinction between nursing and medicine. For example, it is not unusual to hear a prospective nursing student say, "I've always been interested in the medical field, so I decided to go into nursing." Something of an interdependence exists between medicine and nursing, and they have somewhat paralleled one another in historical development. However, anyone who has been involved in the profession of nursing for any period of time will be quick to assure you that distinct differences exist.

The primary differences between nursing and **medicine** are the purpose and goal of each profession, and the education needed to fulfill each role. Although the situation is much changed today, we must acknowledge that historically medicine has been perceived as a profession for men and nursing as a profession for women.

We can dismiss these stereotypes today, but they had an influence on the development of both professions. Finally, the subservient role of the nurse in relationship to the physician in the past—often referred to as the handmaiden of the physician—has been significant in shaping the definition of nursing.

In general, medicine is concerned with the diagnosis and treatment (and cure, when possible) of disease. Nursing is concerned with caring for the person in a variety of health-related situations. The caring aspects of nursing are well documented in nursing literature (Benner & Wrubel, 1989; Bevis & Watson, 1989; Carper, 1979; Watson, 1979). We think of medicine as being involved with the cure of a patient and nursing with the care of that patient. The role of the nurse in patient care (today we often refer to this as client care) also involves teaching about health and the prevention of illness, and caring for the ill individual. It also may encompass case management and is increasingly being practiced outside the walls of acute care facilities. Nursing takes place in the community and the home, in hospice centers, ambulatory care environments, schools and day care centers, and rehabilitation facilities. In all environments, nurses play a key role in promoting higher standards of health.

With advancing technology in the health care fields, the diverse areas of specialization, the different routes to educational preparation, and the distinct practice settings and roles occupied by the nurse, it is critical that nurses provide clear information for themselves and for the public. To state that you are a registered nurse (RN) says little about what you do. It conveys nothing about where you are employed or your educational background. For example, as an RN, you might be employed in a community hospital or in a long-term care facility; you might have a significant role in a critical care unit; you might have earned additional credentials and be working in advanced practice; or you might be a nurse educator.

Thus, you can see that the words "nurse" and "nursing" have been applied to a wide variety of health care activities, in many different settings, performed by people with a variety of different educational backgrounds. The old adage "A nurse, is a nurse, is a nurse" is out of place in a highly technical health care delivery system that struggles to keep "high touch" and "high tech" compatible.

The Effect of Technology on the Definition of Nursing

Technologic advances have significantly affected the definition of nursing and the role of the nurse; the methods by which care is delivered have been reshaped significantly. The acute care hospital provides care to patients who are much more acutely ill and who are diagnosed with conditions from which they would not have survived 25 years ago. Today, recovery is anticipated after careful evaluation and treatment that can require diagnostic procedures (eg, angiography, sonography, or tomography), delicate medical procedures, and specialized critical care nursing that requires a host of variously prepared health care providers. Critical thinking skills are essential to the successful performance of the diverse tasks expected of a nurse. Nurses in many positions have been required to assume ever-greater levels of responsibility. Only recently are nurses beginning to receive the official authority, autonomy, and recognition that should accompany those responsibilities.

Definitions of Nursing Theorists

Many would expect that any definition of nursing must indicate that it is both an art and a science. It is an art in the sense that it is composed of skills that require expertise, adeptness, and proficiency for their competent execution. It is a science in the sense that it requires systematized knowledge derived from observation, critical thinking, study, and research. As nursing has grown into a profession, many nursing theorists developed definitions of nursing consistent with their conceptual frameworks. Table 5-1 presents the definitions of some of the theorists.

In 1958, Virginia Henderson, a nurse educator, author, and researcher, was asked by the nursing service committee of the International Council of Nurses to describe her concept of basic nursing. Hers is still one of the most widely accepted definitions of nursing:

> The unique function of the nurse is to assist the individual, sick or well, in the performance of those activities contributing to health or its recovery (or to peaceful death) that he would perform unaided if he had the necessary strength, will or knowledge. And to do this in such a way as to help him gain independence as rapidly as possible. (Henderson, 1966, p. 15).

TABLE 5-1.	DEFINITIONS OF NURSING BY MAJOR THEORISTS	
THEORIST	**MAJOR THEME**	**DEFINITION**
Florence Nightingale (1859)	Environment/Sanitation	The goal of nursing is to put the patient in the best condition for nature to act upon him, primarily by altering the environment.
Hildegard Peplau (1952)	Interpersonal process	Nursing is viewed as an interpersonal process involving interaction between two or more individuals, which has as its common goal assisting the individual who is sick or in need of health care.
Faye Abdellah (1960)	Nursing problems	Nursing is a service to individuals, families, and society based on an art and science that molds the attitudes, intellectual competencies, and technical skills of the individual nurse into the desire and ability to help people cope with their health care needs, and is focused around 21 nursing problems.
Ernestine Wiedenbach (1964)	Nursing problems model	Nursing is a helping, nurturing, and caring service rendered with compassion, skill, and understanding, in which sensitivity is key to assisting the nurse in identifying problems.
Virginia Henderson (1966)	Development/Needs	Nursing's role is to assist the individual (sick or well) to carry out those activities . . . he would perform unaided if he had the necessary strength, will, or knowledge.
Myra Levine (1969)	Conservation and adaptation	Nursing means the nurse interposes her/his skill and knowledge into the course of events that affect the patient. When influencing adaptation favorably, the nurse is acting in a therapeutic sense. When the nursing intervention cannot alter the course of adaptation, the nurse is acting in a supportive sense.
Ida Orlando Pelletier (1972)	Interpersonal process	Nursing's unique and independent role concerns itself with an individual's need for help in an immediate situation for the purpose of avoiding, relieving, diminishing, or curing that individual's sense of helplessness.
Jean Watson (1979–1988)	Caring	The essence and central unifying focus for nursing practice is caring, a transpersonal value. Nurse behaviors are defined as 10 carative factors. Focuses on the spiritual subjective aspects of both nurse and patient and the "caring moment" relating to the time when nurse and patient first come together (LeMaire, 2002).
Dorothy Orem (1980)	Self-care	Nursing is concerned with the individual's need for self-care action, which is the practice of activities that individuals initiate and perform on their own behalf in maintaining health and well-being.

(continued)

TABLE 5-1.	DEFINITIONS OF NURSING BY MAJOR THEORISTS (*Continued*)	
THEORIST	**MAJOR THEME**	**DEFINITION**
Dorothy E. Johnson (1980)	Systems approach	Nursing is an external regulatory force that acts to preserve the organization and integration of the patient's behavior at an optimal level, under those conditions in which the behavior constitutes a threat to physical or social health, or in which illness is found.
Imogene M. King (1981)	Open systems approach	The focus of nursing is the care of human beings resulting in the health of individuals and health care for groups, who are viewed as open systems in constant interaction with their environments.
Rosemarie Rizzo Parse (1981)	Man-Living-Health	Nursing is rooted in the human sciences and focuses on man as a living unity and as qualitatively participating in health experiences. Health is viewed as a process.
Betty Neuman (1982)	Systems approach	Nursing responds to individuals, groups, and communities, who are in constant interaction with environmental stressors that create disequilibrium. A critical element is the client's ability to react to stress and factors that assist with reconstituion or adaptation.
Sister Callista Roy (1984)	Adaptation	The goal of nursing is the promotion of adaptive responses (those things that positively influence health) that are affected by the person's ability to respond to stimuli. Nursing involves manipulating stimuli to promote adaptive responses.
Martha E. Rogers (1984)	Science of unitary man	Nursing is an art and science that is humanistic and humanitarian, directed toward the unitary human, and concerned with the nature and direction of human development.
Katharine Y. Kolcaba (1992)	Holistic theory of comfort	The immediate desirable outcome of nursing care is enhanced comfort. This comfort positively correlates with desirable health seeking behaviors.

Nursing as Defined by Organizations

Both the American Nurses Association (ANA) and the National Council of State Boards of Nursing have established definitions of nursing.

AMERICAN NURSES ASSOCIATION DEFINITIONS OF NURSING

In 1965, the ANA published the "First Paper on Education for Nursing," which identified significant aspects of nursing. It stated that "essential components of professional nursing practice include care, cure, and coordination" (ANA, 1965, p. 107). ANA incorporated yet another definition into its Social Policy Statement published in 1980, which stated: "Nursing is the diagnosis and treatment of human responses to actual or potential health problems" (ANA, 1980, p. 9). That definition had a widespread effect, and we see its application in the language used in nursing diagnoses today.

NURSING AS DEFINED BY THE NATIONAL COUNCIL OF STATE BOARDS OF NURSING

In 1994, the National Council of State Boards of Nursing (NCSBN) again revised the Model Nurse Practice Act that was first developed in 1982 and revised in 1988. Although early publications of the Model Nurse Practice Act reflected the difficulty the committee experienced in arriving at a precise and succinct definition, the 1994 revision was clear. It stated, "The 'Practice of Nursing' means assisting individuals or groups to maintain or attain optimal health, implementing a strategy of care to accomplish defined goals, and evaluating responses to care and treatment" (NCSBN, 1994).

Legal Definitions of Nursing

The single most important part of any nurse practice act is the legal definition of nursing practice (see Chapter 7). This legal definition is critical because it provides the foundation and guidelines for education, licensure, scope of practice, and, when necessary, the basis for corrective actions against people who violate the practice act.

No state adopts the exact wording of any recommended definition, but most states include references to performing services for compensation, the necessity for a specialized knowledge base, the use of the nursing process (although steps may be named differently), and components of nursing practice. Several states include some reference to treating human responses to actual or potential health problems; this was first addressed in New York State's license law and was later incorporated in the ANA's "Nursing: A Social Policy Statement" (1980). Most states refer to the execution of the medical regimen, and many include a general statement about additional acts that recognize that nursing practice is evolving and that the nurse's area of responsibility can be expected to broaden.

Defining Nursing for the Future

As the profession grows and responsibilities change, undoubtedly we will continue to redefine and refine the definition of nursing. By being responsive to changes, nursing has become more closely aligned with professions such as law, theology, and education, in which changing practices have required greater precision and refinement of definitions of the profession.

Critical Thinking Activity

Analyze the definitions of the major nursing theorists. What concepts found in those definitions are most closely aligned with your perception of nursing? Develop your own definition of nursing and compare it to those of the theorists and to those of your classmates.

CHARACTERISTICS OF A PROFESSION

The meaning of professionalism has been a subject of debate for many years. The *Flexner Report*, issued in 1910, was one of a series of papers issued by the Carnegie Foundation about professional schools. The Flexner Report, which focused on medicine, provided the incentive for many future efforts to define and discuss the **characteristics of a profession** (Table 5-2). When nursing and nursing education were evolving in the United States, no one questioned whether nursing qualified as a **profession** or whether it was more

TABLE 5-2. CRITERIA FOR A PROFESSION		
FLEXNER (1915)	**BIXLER & BIXLER (1959)**	**PAVALKO (1971)**
• Activities must be intellectual (as opposed to physical) • Activities, because they are based on knowledge, can be learned • Activities must be practical rather than academic • Profession must have teachable techniques • Must have a strong internal organization of members • Practitioners must be motivated by altruism (a desire to help others)	• Uses a specialized body of knowledge • Enlarges the body of knowledge it uses and improves its techniques of education and service by the use of the scientific method • Entrusts the education of its practitioners to institutions of higher education • Applies its body of knowledge in practical services that are vital to human and social welfare • Functions autonomously in the formulation of professional policy and in the control of professional activity • Attracts individuals of intellectual and personal qualities who exalt service above personal gain and who recognize their chosen occupation as a lifework • Strives to compensate its practitioners by providing freedom of action, opportunity for continuous professional growth, and economic security	• Work is based on a systematic body of theory and abstract knowledge • Work has recognized social value • Requires a special amount of education to attain specialization • Provides service to the public • Group has freedom to regulate and control its own work behavior (autonomy) • Members are committed toward work as a lifetime or long-term pursuit rather than a stepping stone to another profession • Members share a common identity and possess a distinctive subculture • There exists a code of ethics

occupational in nature. As a matter of fact, evidence suggests that from an early date the word "profession" was associated with nursing. Strauss (1966) gives as an example a magazine article entitled "A New Profession for Women" that appeared in 1882. The article described nursing reform, and carried with it a picture of Isabel Hampton. Strauss (1966) also refers to the writings of Lizabeth Price, published in 1892, in which nursing was discussed as a profession.

From approximately the 1950s through the 1970s or mid-1980s, nursing periodically was reviewed against the characteristics of a profession that had been established in the sociologic literature. The activities for which nurses were responsible, their autonomy, the legal ramifications of practice, and particularly the education of future nurses were subjected to the scrutiny of sociologists and nursing leaders, who found it challenging to examine nursing against **formal characteristics** of a profession.

Some critics believe that nursing falls short of meeting these criteria. Some of nursing's leaders also would claim that nursing falls short of fulfilling a professional role (Newman, 1990; Schlotfeldt, 1987). Amid these challenges, other nurses are working to advance the standing of nursing through the development of a code of ethics, standards of practice, and peer review. In light of all this discussion and work, it might be helpful to explore how those major theoretic criteria could be applied to nursing (Fig. 5-1).

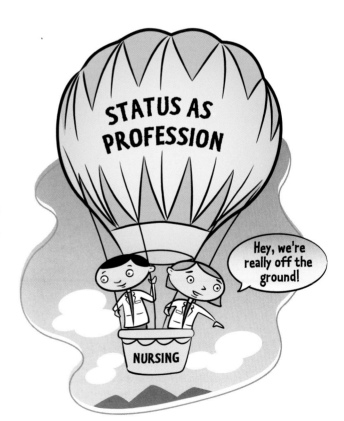

FIGURE 5-1   Some continue to question whether nursing truly can support the title of "profession."

A Body of Specialized Knowledge

A primary criticism leveled at nursing is that it has no **body of specialized knowledge** that belongs exclusively to nursing. Critics state that nursing borrows from biologic sciences, social sciences, and medical science, and then combines the various skills and concepts and calls it "nursing." Nursing leaders and theorists disagree whether nursing is a unique profession or one borrowed from other disciplines. In fact, this amalgamation and synthesis of some areas with application to another may be one of nursing's distinctive qualities. Nursing researchers also are working to develop an organized body of knowledge that is unique to nursing. Nursing theorists are challenging one another to identify and describe the general principles that govern nursing practice. (See Chapter 6 for more information on nursing theories.)

Similarly, nursing leaders are developing a language of nursing, which is discussed later in this chapter. As a result of these efforts, nursing is emerging as a profession with an established body of knowledge.

Use of the Scientific Method to Enlarge the Body of Knowledge

Critical to any profession is its ability to grow and change as the world changes. Equally important is the method by which those changes occur. Changes cannot take place in a haphazard, random, or hit-or-miss fashion; they must be well thought out. Data must be systematically gathered and carefully analyzed, the problem(s) must be correctly identified, alternative solutions must be sought, the best approach selected and implemented, and the results thoroughly evaluated. This is thought of as the **scientific method.** As a nursing student, you already recognize that this has been applied to nursing practice through the nursing process and through critical thinking. Tangible proof of this growth is the quick turnover in nursing textbooks. In a quality program, one seldom finds a clinical text in use that has not been published within the past 4 years. Accreditation criteria established for nursing programs by the national accrediting agencies require that libraries have up-to-date references and periodicals available to students either in print or through electronic reference resources. Nursing knowledge also increases because of nursing research and nursing practice. The number of nurses involved in nursing research is increasing. Journals focusing on clinical practice and the profession as a whole increasingly include news briefs or full articles reporting results of recent research affecting the practice of nursing. All of this reflects the continued growth of the body of knowledge in nursing through the use of the scientific method.

Education Within Institutions of Higher Education

Perhaps no issue in nursing has been more controversial than the education of its practitioners. Nursing's heritage, like that of medicine, was founded in apprenticeship. Students were assigned to experienced practitioners who taught the skills with which they were familiar. Once those skills were acquired, the student moved into the world of employment. Our earliest programs of education were located in hospitals rather than colleges or universities. (See Chapter 4 for more information on the history of nursing education.)

Over time, the settings in which nurses are educated have changed. Today, most nursing programs preparing RNs are located in **institutions of higher education** or collegiate settings (at either community colleges or senior colleges or universities). Controversy over the length of nursing education programs (associate degree versus baccalaureate degree) and the "technical" aspects of patient care continues (see Chapter 6). Additionally, not all nurses today are educated in colleges and universities. Particularly in the eastern part of the United States, hospital-based programs still provide an avenue to nursing education for prospective nursing students.

Control of Professional Policy, Professional Activity, and Autonomy

Most critics reviewing professions against professional standards emphasize the ability of any group to develop its own **professional policy** and to function autonomously. Some would suggest that this is an area in which nursing always has been weak, although current health care reform may assist the profession in achieving the full autonomy it has been seeking. Historically, the nurse worked under the direction of the patient's physician, often in a hospital setting. The physician wrote the orders for medical care to be implemented by the nurse; the agency or hospital set the policies under which that care was delivered. Only in the last 50 years has nursing made significant inroads in defining the unique role of the nurse in "care" as opposed to "cure" of the patient.

Today, we see much more **professional activity** than in years past. Nurses are responsible for planning and implementing the nursing care patients receive, and nurses are also accountable for the care provided. Nursing committees establish policies and protocols. Nursing diagnosis, once challenged as an inappropriate responsibility for nurses, has become a standard of good nursing care. In some practice settings, nurses are eligible for third-party payment; that is, insurance companies reimburse them for the care they have provided. One can anticipate that this situation will continue to improve with health care reform. Although nurses still carry out the medical regimen outlined by physicians, a more collaborative relationship is beginning to occur, and the contribution of the nurse is receiving more recognition. The practice acts of an increasing number of states provide prescriptive authority to advanced practice nurses who have completed the necessary educational preparation. The number of nurses seeking preparation and working in advanced nursing practice roles is increasing.

All health care professions are changing in response to public demand. Consumers are represented on licensing and accreditation boards, protocols exist for managing conditions and situations, and fees may be established by outside groups. Society is no longer willing to give any profession total autonomy.

A Code of Ethics

A critical standard established for professions is that there exists a **code of ethics**. The general standard for the professional behavior of nurses in the United States is the ANA Code for Nurses. This document was developed by the ANA and periodically is revised to address current issues in practice, the most recent revision occurring in 2001. Similarly, the International Council of Nurses, housed in Geneva, Switzerland, has developed a code for nurses that also addresses many of the issues outlined in the ANA code. The international code sets the standards for ethical practice by nurses throughout the world. Information on both codes and more discussion regarding the ethical conduct of nurses are found in Chapter 9.

Nursing as a Lifetime Commitment

Bixler and Bixler (1945) emphasized in their list of criteria for professions that a profession should attract people of certain intellectual and personal qualities, who exalt service above personal gain and who consider their chosen **occupation** to be their life work. Pavalko (1971) also identified as a significant criterion the **lifetime commitment** members have toward work, or at least a long-term pursuit rather than a stepping stone to another profession. Studies indicate that most people who prepare for a career in nursing remain in the profession. However, the "burnout" that occurs from stress (see Chapter 11) has become an increasing concern as nurses work long hours in understaffed situations and with team members who have less educational preparation.

Most individuals who have been nurses continue to identify themselves as nurses long after they retire. Today, there is a greater likelihood that individuals who enter the profession of nursing at one educational level will continue to advance in practice and education by pursuing additional degrees (and experience). The concept of "articulation" between variously positioned degree-granting institutions is in the forefront of nursing today, with the requirement that schools work together to develop such options sometimes legislated by the state governments. Articulation is the process of advancing from one level of nursing education to the next and receiving credit for previous learning; more discussion of articulation in nursing education is found in Chapter 6.

Service to the Public

Many theorists list altruism, **service to the public**, and dedication among criteria for professions. Some suggest that altruism, or the desire to provide for the good of society, must be the worker's motivating force. Nurses have long struggled with the ambiguity that can result from this concept. Possessing a history with a strong religious heritage, the giving of oneself at all costs helped frame the image of nursing and nurses. As nursing has come of age as a profession, we have recognized that "giving away" one's services should not be considered professional. Professions such as law, medicine, dentistry, and engineering have long required ample financial compensation for services provided. Because nurses expect appropriate remuneration for services rendered does not suggest that they are less than dedicated to the patients for whom they are caring. Providing service to the public should not mean sacrificing one's financial security. Collective bargaining, once viewed as antithetical to professionalism, is becoming an acceptable method of negotiating work-related issues and for assuring economic security for a wide variety of professions, including engineers, university professors, and even physicians who work for large organizations. Greater discussion of nurses and collective bargaining is included in Chapter 12.

Critical Thinking Activity

Select one of the characteristics of a profession that you believe nursing has difficulty meeting. Describe the actions that you believe should occur in the profession that would result in the profession fully meeting that criterion. How would you go about implementing those actions?

DIFFERENTIATING BETWEEN THE TERMS "PROFESSION" AND "PROFESSIONAL"

Nursing involves activities that may be performed by many different caregivers. These people include nursing assistants, practical (vocational) nurses, and RNs prepared for entry into nursing through any of several educational avenues (see Chapter 6). Each of these caregivers contributes to nursing as a profession. To meet the nursing needs of the public, it is essential that caregivers function at various levels of practice. This has led to confusion about the use of the terms **profession** and **professional.** Is there a difference between looking at the practice of nursing in its totality and the "professional" practice of nursing?

Legislated Definitions

In at least one instance, federal legislation has helped to establish a list of the characteristics of a professional. Public Law 93-360 (Labor Management Relations Act, 1947 [amended, 1959, 1974]), which governs collective bargaining activities, defines the professional employee as follows:

> (a) any employee engaged in work (i) predominantly intellectual and varied in character as opposed to routine mental, manual, mechanical, or physical work; (ii) involving the consistent exercise of discretion and judgment in its performance; (iii) of such a character that the output produced or the result accomplished cannot be standardized in relation to a given period of time; (iv) requiring knowledge of an advanced type in a field of science or learning customarily acquired by a prolonged course of specialized intellectual instruction and study in an institution of higher learning or a hospital, as distinguished from a general academic education or from an apprenticeship or from training in the performance of routine mental, manual, or physical processes; or
> (b) any employee, who (i) has completed the courses of specialized intellectual instruction and study described in clause (iv) of paragraph (a), and (ii) is performing related work under the supervision of a professional person to qualify himself to become a professional employee as defined in paragraph (a).

Based on this definition, all RNs are considered professionals.

Popular Views of a Professional

A popular view of a professional involves the approach a person has to the role that is required. Most professionals approach their activities earnestly, strive for excellence in performance, and demonstrate a sense of ethics and responsibility in relationship to their careers. Such people consider their work a lifelong endeavor rather than a stepping stone to another field of employment. They place a positive value on being termed professional, and perceive being termed nonprofessional or technical as an adverse reflection on their status, position, and motivation. Using this definition, we again find that it would apply to all RNs.

Certain people suggest that professionalism has a great deal to do with attitude, dress, conduct, and deportment. The attributes that are considered professional vary according to the personal values and stereotypes of the person doing the evaluating. For example, an early concept of the "truly professional" nurse was that of a person dressed in a starched white uniform and cap, whose hair was off her collar, and whose shoes were freshly polished. Some individuals would continue to support this concept of the "professional nurse." Others might perceive the "professional nurse" as one who consistently maintains appropriate boundaries with clients, who focuses on the needs of others, and who is tactful and skillful in interview techniques.

Other Definitions

The sociologic and legal definitions are much more restrictive than the popular concept associated with the term "professional." A communication block can result from people's using the term in different ways. When one person is using a restrictive, sociologic definition and the other person responds from a standpoint of personal belief and feeling, agreement is almost impossible. Styles offers a refreshing approach. She has used the word *professionhood* rather than professionalism and suggests that nurses would be better served by a set of internal beliefs about nursing (that force us to pay attention to our own image as the dominant figure) than by a set of external criteria about professions (Styles, 1982).

THE IMAGE OF NURSING TODAY

During the late 1970s and early 1980s, much time and energy were invested in studying the **image** of nursing, with much of this work done by Beatrice and Philip Kalisch, who have written prolifically about the topic. Their writing focuses on segments of an overall study of the image of the nurse in various forms of mass media, including radio, movies, television, newspapers, magazines, and novels. They believe that popular attitudes and assumptions about nurses and what nurses contribute to a patient's welfare can greatly influence the future of nursing. It is their contention that since the 1970s, the popular image of the nurse not only has failed to reflect changing professional conditions, but has been based on derogatory stereotypes that have undermined public confidence in and respect for the professional nurse. Nurses should be concerned about negative or incorrect images because such images can influence the attitudes of patients, policy-makers, and politicians (Fig. 5-2). Negative attitudes about nursing also may discourage many capable prospective nurses, who will choose another career that offers greater appeal in stature, status, and salary. This issue is of great concern today as the shortage of nurses promises to become severe (see discussion of the nursing shortage later).

Television and Motion Pictures

An important source of information in this country is television and motion pictures. From studying nurses on television, Kalisch and Kalisch found that nurses often had no substantive role in the television stories they investigated, with nursing being a part of the hospital background in programs that focused on physician characters. The role of the physician was viewed as more important and physicians scored high on such attributes as ambition, intelligence, rationality, aggression, self-confidence, and altruism. When a nurse was the focus of a program, the story line involved the nurse's personal problems, rather than her role as a nurse. The nurse often was portrayed as the "handmaiden" to the physician, and scored high on such attributes as obedience, permissiveness, conformity, flexibility, and serenity. It is interesting to note that nurses ranked lower than physicians on such items as humanism, self-sacrifice, duty, and family concern, all of which are values traditionally ascribed to nurses (Kalisch & Kalisch, 1982a). This may be changing as a result of programs introduced in the 1990s such as "ER" and "Chicago Hope," which depict nurses as responsible decision-makers.

Kalisch and Kalisch found a rise and fall in the image of nurses in motion pictures, with the high point occurring during the war years of the 1940s and the low point occurring in the 1970s, when the nursing profession was denigrated and satirized in many films. Because the largest proportions of moviegoers each year are adolescents, the image of nurses in movies will have an impact on the attitudes of students who are prospective nurses. The earlier, positive images of nurses usually came from films that were biographies of outstanding nurses, such as Sister Kenny, who worked with polio patients, or Edith Cavell, a World War I heroine (who was discussed in Chapter 4). For a time, the nurse-detective was a popular character in films; such nurses were portrayed as intelligent, perceptive, confident, sophisticated, composed, tough, and assertive. During the 1970s, however, nurses often were portrayed as malevolent and sadistic (eg, the roles of Nurse Ratched in *One Flew Over the Cuckoo's Nest* and Nurse Diesel in *High Anxiety*). This was the lowest point for the image of

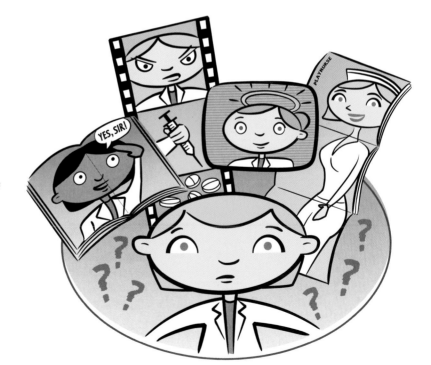

FIGURE 5-2   Nurses should be concerned about negative or incorrect images because these are sure to influence the attitudes of patients, policy makers, and politicians.

nurses in the history of film; nurses in film were lacking in such values as duty, self-sacrifice, achievement, integrity, virtue, intelligence, rationality, and kindness. Few films centered on the individual achievement or personal autonomy of the nurse. When compared with the physician's role, the nurse's role was portrayed as less important (Kalisch & Kalisch, 1982b). There is hope that this trend is reversing. The film *The English Patient*, which received the Oscar as Best Picture of the Year in 1997, added credibility to the role of the nurse by portraying the nurse character as caring, thinking, and involved.

The Image of the Nurse in Print

To study the image of nursing in novels, Kalisch and Kalisch analyzed 207 books. As with film and television, they found that the nurse in the novel was almost always female, single, childless, white, and younger than the age of 35. (The actual average age of nurses in the U.S. is 44.)

Because nurses almost always were depicted in novels as women, traditional female roles (ie, wife, mistress, mother) were emphasized. Three nurse stereotypes have resulted: the nurse as man's companion, the nurse as man's destroyer, and the nurse as man's mother or the mother of his children. The man in the novel is often a physician. Novelists of the 1970s and 1980s often maligned their nurse characters, ignoring the nurses' professional motivations and health care perspectives (Kalisch & Kalisch, 1982c).

Muff (1988) analyzed feminine myths and stereotypes and has elaborated on nursing stereotypes. After reading books about nurses written for school-aged children (eg, Cherry Ames, Sue Barton, Kathy Martin, and Penny Scott), she drew the following conclusions:

* Nursing is described as glamorous.
* Medicine and nursing are imbued with a sense of mystery and elitism.
* Nursing is simplistic.
* Nurses move from job to job.
* Nurses are subservient and deferential, following orders, and running errands.

All of the nurses in these books were educated in hospital-based diploma programs, earning the "RN" only after hours of hospital service, even though the Martin and Scott series were both written in the 1960s.

Muff (1988) also examined the role of the nurse as it is captured in the romance novel. In many instances, appearances (eg, the color and condition of the nurse's hair) were most important, and the nurse was portrayed as a "pure" girl, dressed in white, whose main aim was to get a man, usually a doctor. Women who were not looking for husbands were in nursing for altruistic reasons, and duty and self-sacrifice were glamorized. Muff also found that the image of the nurse in the novel usually could be placed into one of the following categories: ministering angels, handmaidens, battle-axes, fools, and whores. She stated that the stereotypes of nursing presented in television and film also usually fit one of these categories. When reviewing the nurse image on get-well cards, she had to add a new category, that of "token torturer."

Only newspapers and newsmagazines tended toward realism rather than fantasy. News articles examined the shortage of nurses, discussing reasons for it (such as working conditions, salaries, benefits, and hardships). Special feature articles also provided information about new or unique nursing roles, such as those of nurses in Vietnam. With the outbreak of war in the Middle East in 1991, nurses received positive recognition by the media. Nurses serving in reserve status with branches of the military were among the first called up when the conflict began. As our society recognizes the need to honor women as well as men for their contributions, nurses are often singled out for special recognition—especially during wartime. (See Chapter 4 for discussion of recognition honoring nurses.) Nurses also received recognition for their efforts to assist the wounded during the September 11, 2001 attack on the twin towers of New York's World Trade Center.

As we moved into the 1990s, it was hoped that the image of nursing would improve; to some extent that has been true. Suzanne Gordon, a journalist who is not a nurse became interested in the profession and has written about nurses and nursing. In *Life Support: Three Nurses on the Front Lines*, she realistically captures the challenges to the profession and addresses concerns about the undermining of nursing and of patients' healing through a health care system that is replacing caring with profit margins. However, the books have received more attention from nurses than from the people who most need to read them. In 1999, *Wit*, a play written by first-time playwright Margaret Edson after leaving a unit clerk job in a cancer research hospital, opened on Broadway. In this play, the nurse is the hero (Gordon, 1999).

In 1997, the University of Rochester conducted a study of nurses in the media, titled the *Woodhull Study on Nursing and the Media: Health Care's Invisible Partner*. It was named for Nancy Woodhull, the founding editor of *USA Today*, who became concerned about the lack of media coverage of nurses when she received care for lung cancer, which claimed her life in 1997. Commissioned by Sigma Theta Tau International, the study analyzed health care media coverage occurring in a single month. It examined more than 20,000 articles for content, of which 2,500 health care-related articles were studied in depth. The study found that nurses are "virtually invisible in media coverage of health care." It further found that "The few references to nurses or nursing were mostly in passing, with no in-depth coverage" (Sieber et al, 1998).

Although some might argue that nurses have better things to do than to worry about how the nurse is portrayed in the media, a consistently misrepresented image can negatively affect how the public views nurses. Therefore, nurses have responded to television advertisements or programs that portray nurses and nursing in a negative light with letters and telephone calls. Boycotts on the purchase of products that present nurses poorly in advertisements have proved to be an effective way to bring about change. In addition, various nursing organizations have waged campaigns to enhance the image of nursing by emphasizing nursing as a prestigious, desirable, and respected career.

Following the Woodhull Study, the ANA initiated a program titled "RN = Real News," which was a media outreach program to showcase nurses as experts in the area of health care. This initiative included a media speaker program and a media-training tool to help nurses gain the basic skills and confidence necessary for dealing effectively with the media (Stewart, 1999).

NURSING'S IMAGE AND THE NURSING SHORTAGE

Currently we are experiencing a serious **nursing shortage** that promises to become much worse before it gets better. For example, in a survey of 715 hospitals conducted in spring 2001 by the American Hospital Association, there were as many as 126,000 unfilled registered nursing positions nationwide (Trossman, 2002). The shortage is expected to reach serious proportions by 2010, when the gap will widen between the supply of and the requirement for registered nurses (Geolot, 2000). Authorities believe that the current shortage is not like previous shortages and that extraordinary means will need to be taken to reverse it.

A number of factors are suggested as contributing to the shortfall of registered nurses. First of all, nurses are getting older. In the United States, the average age of a nurse is 44, with many anticipating retirement within the next decade (Meade, 2002).

Another concern centers around the fact that members of the baby boom generation are beginning to enter their senior years, thus increasing the need for nurses in the health care system.

However, a factor that demands serious consideration relates to the fact that nursing has always been a female-dominated profession. Women today have more educational and occupational alternatives. Many other careers may seem more attractive than nursing in terms of the salary commanded, the working conditions, and the prestige given to the role. This has been realized by an overall dropping enrollment in nursing programs throughout the United States during the 1990s.

The shortage is of such import that various groups that command respect for their work have decided to study the issue or take action to try to encourage more individuals to study nursing. The Robert Wood Johnson Foundation funded a study with findings released in 2002. They recommended that a National Forum to Advance Nursing be created that would draw together a wide range of individuals affected by the shortage. The Forum would focus on helping nursing achieve higher standing as a profession. The Foundation has suggested that the Forum would focus efforts in several strategic areas that include:

- Creating new nursing models to address the shortage, study nursing's contribution to health care outcomes and create new models of health care provision.
- Reinventing nursing education and work environments to address the needs and values of and appeal to a younger generation of nurses.
- Establishing a national nursing workforce measurement-and-data collection system.
- Creating a clearing house of effective strategies to facilitate cultural change within the profession (Robert Wood Johnson Foundation, 2002).

In February 2002, Johnson & Johnson launched its "Campaign for Nursing's Future." In this program, they planned to spend $20 million during a 2-year period to attract more individuals to nursing. The campaign included television advertisements, a Web site (*http://discovernursing.com*), recruitment brochures, and posters and videos directed toward high-school-age individuals.

Health care organizations in collaboration with state nurses associations have created similar projects in local television markets. The sponsors of all these efforts hope that this will result in increased enrollment in nursing programs. In 2001, Nurses for a Healthier Tomorrow, a coalition of health care and nursing organizations, launched a new recruitment campaign to bring people into nursing. Their activities included a 30-second public service announcement, establishment of a Web site, and the development of posters and recruitment materials.

Another factor affecting the nursing supply is the limited number of spaces in nursing programs. As recently as 1993, a Pew report identified an excess of nurses and recommended that some nursing programs be closed (O'Neill, 1993). Because nursing education is costly, most educational institutions have not increased the size of their programs in the past decade. As applications increase, further efforts will be needed to increase the number of individuals who can be admitted.

To provide advice and recommendations to the Secretary of Health and Human Services and Congress on policy matters relating to the nursing workforce, the National Advisory Council on Nurse Education and Practice (NACNEP) was established. In 2001, this group focused on the shortage of nurses in practice; at its spring 2002 meeting, NACNEP addressed the shortage of nursing faculty.

As all areas employing nurses feel the effect of the shortage, serious concern has been voiced by educational institutions and organizations supporting educational efforts, such as the National League for Nursing, regarding the supply of educationally prepared nursing faculty. Again, in conjunction with Johnson & Johnson, scholarships have been made available in some geographic areas to nurses who would consider faculty positions.

Another aspect of the nursing shortage is the retention of current nurses. Some states have identified that there are a large number of RNs not currently working in the profession. Many experts have pointed to working conditions such as mandatory overtime, heavy workloads, and lack of respect in the workplace as reasons for people leaving. The ANA is focusing on actions that will improve the work environment and thus increase retention as means of addressing the nursing shortage.

How this will all play out is yet to be seen. Certainly, at no time in recent history has the need for nurses been more critical and the supply so limited.

Critical Thinking Activity

Interview five of your friends who are not nurses. What is their image of nursing? What do they understand of the role of the nurse? Do they view nursing positively? What recurrent information is mentioned?

STUDIES FOR AND ABOUT NURSING

Early in the 20th century, the quality of many nursing schools and their graduates was poor; many of Florence Nightingale's admonitions regarding nursing education had been forgotten. Nurses, doctors, friends, and critics of nursing became concerned that the preparation being offered was inadequate. Before the problem could be corrected, it was necessary to learn more about the programs and how nurses were being used in the employment market. To accomplish this, **studies about nursing** and nurses were initiated.

We recognize that many students in nursing are not excited by studies, especially not by those conducted years ago. However, we hope that when you have finished reading this section of the textbook, you will have gained an appreciation of the enduring effort made by nurses and interested colleagues to gain a greater understanding of the profession, with the goal of improving the profession and thus the care provided to the public. As you read you will, no doubt, recognize some recurring themes with which we continue to grapple today. Our discussion is limited to those studies that looked at the profession as a whole and does not include any of the myriad studies conducted each year, primarily clinical in focus, that form the basis for evidence-based practice and for the expansion of the body of nursing knowledge.

Although the first nursing studies were not begun until the early 1900s, the number of studies since the 1950s has been voluminous. It is impossible to look at any professional nursing publication and not find mention of some new study in progress. Efforts were made to classify and catalog references to these studies and to report them. One of the first was completed by Virginia Henderson, who prepared *A Nursing Studies Index*. In 1952, a group of nurses, under the sponsorship of the Association of Collegiate Schools of Nursing, launched a new journal called *Nursing Research*, which was designed to disseminate information about nursing research.

A single individual often conducted many of the early studies, with a particular purpose in mind. Through the years, studies often took the form of a "report" by a special group of individuals, often appointed by a governmental or professional agency. Although by no means inclusive of all studies and reports, Table 5-3 highlights some of the major significant studies of nursing that have provided benchmarks to the profession. Following is a discussion of some of the major studies and their impact on nursing.

Early Studies

One of the earliest nursing studies was carried out under the guidance of M. Adelaide Nutting in 1912. Published by the U.S. Bureau of Education, it was entitled *The Educational Status of Nursing*. The study investigated what and how nursing students were taught, and under what conditions students lived. Although it did not receive the attention it probably deserved, it began to establish nursing as a profession, suggesting that schools of nursing be independent from hospitals and leading the way to more studies.

The Winslow-Goldmark Report, sometimes called the Goldmark Report, followed in 1923. It was also referred to as *The Study of Nursing and Nursing Education in the United States* (Winslow-Goldmark Report, 1923) and was the work of a committee composed of physicians, nurses, and lay people. The report focused on the preparation of public health nurses, teachers, administrators, the clinical learning experiences of students, and on the financing of schools. Subsequently, the Yale University School of Nursing and the Vanderbilt University School of Nursing were established, funded by an endowment from the Rockefeller Foundation.

A three-part study, sponsored by the Committee on the Grading of Nursing Schools (a 21-member group of representatives from many nursing and medical professional organizations), was conducted between 1928 and 1934. The first part, which was socioeconomic in nature, was entitled *Nurses, Patients, and Pocketbooks*. It attempted to determine if there was a shortage of nurses in the United States. The second part, *An Activity Analysis of Nursing*, examined those nursing activities that could be used as a basis for improving the curricula in nursing schools. The third part, *Nursing Schools Today and Tomorrow*, described the schools of the period and made recommendations for professional schools.

In 1932, the National League for Nursing Education (later to become the National League for Nursing) conducted its first study, a comparative study of the bedside activities of graduate and student nurses. The study indicated that nursing care should be given by graduate nurses rather than students, and provided information about the number of tasks assigned to nursing students that had nothing to do with acquiring a nursing education.

TABLE 5-3.	MAJOR STUDIES ABOUT NURSING		
DATE	**NAME OF STUDY**	**PRIMARY INVESTIGATOR/SPONSOR**	**FOCUS AND RECOMMENDATION**
1912	*The Educational Status of Nursing*	M. Adelaide Nutting/U.S. Bureau of Education	What and how students were being taught and conditions under which they were living. Began to establish nursing as a profession.
1923	*Winslow-Goldmark Report on Nursing and Nursing Education in the United States*	Josephine Goldmark/ Rockefeller Foundation	The educational preparation of students including public health nurses, teachers, and supervisors. It pointed out fundamental faults in hospital training schools and resulted in the establishment of the Yale University School of Nursing.
	Committee on the Grading of Nursing Schools—a 3-part study	Francis Payne Bolton and contributions of thousands of nurses	
1928	*(1) Nurses, Patients, and Pocketbooks*	May Ayres Burgess/ statistician	An inquiry into the supply and demand for nurses. Demonstrated that there was an oversupply of nurses.
1934	*(2) An Activity Analysis of Nursing*	Ethel Johns and Blance Pfefferkorn	Looked at the activities that constitute nursing as a basis for improving curricula
1934	*(3) Nursing Schools Today & Tomorrow*	Ethel Johns	Described the nursing schools of the period and made recommendations about professional schools.
1937	*A Curriculum Guide for Schools of Nursing—* not truly a study of nursing, but often referred to as one because of its far reaching effects	National League for Nursing Education	A revision of a 1917 publication, it outlined the curricula for a 3-year course, emphasizing sound educational teaching procedures. Followed by many schools of the time.
1948	*Nursing for the Future*	Esther Lucille Brown/ Carnegie Foundation, the Russell Sage Foundation, and the National Nursing Council	Done to determine society's need for nursing. Described inadequacies in nursing schools. Resulted in recommendations that nursing education be placed in universities and colleges and encouraged recruitment of large numbers of men and members of minority groups into nursing schools.
1948	The Ginzberg Report or *A Program for the Nursing Profession—* a report of the discussions of the Committee on the Functions of Nursing	Eli Ginzberg/Columbia University	Reviewed problems centering around the shortage of nurses. Recommended that nursing teams consisting of variously educated nurses be developed.
1950	*Nursing Schools at the Mid-Century*	Margaret Bridgman/ National Committee for the Improvement of Nursing Services—Russell Sage Foundation	Studied the practices of more than 1000 nursing schools (including organization, costs, curriculum, clinical resources, and student health) and stimulated improvement in baccalaureate schools.

(continued)

TABLE 5-3.	MAJOR STUDIES ABOUT NURSING (*Continued*)		
DATE	**NAME OF STUDY**	**PRIMARY INVESTIGATOR/SPONSOR**	**FOCUS AND RECOMMENDATION**
1955	Patterns of Patient Care	Francis George and Ruth Perkins Kuehn/University of Pittsburgh	Assessed the amount of nursing service needed by a group of medical/surgical patients and determined how much of that care could be delegated to nursing aides and other nonprofessional people
1958	Twenty Thousand Nurses Tell Their Story	Everett C. Hughes/ANA and American Nurses Foundation	Looked at nurses, what they were doing, their attitudes toward their jobs, and job satisfaction. Formed basis for development of nursing functions, standards, and qualifications.
1959	Community College Education for Nursing	Mildred Montag/Institute of Research and Service in Nursing Education— Teachers College, Columbia University	Reported the findings of a 5-year study of eight 2-year nursing programs. Led to the establishment of more associate degree programs
1963	Toward Quality in Nursing: Needs and Goals	W. Allen Wallis— Consultant Group on Nursing—a panel of nurses in the health field/ U.S. Public Health Service	A report requested by the U.S. Surgeon General to determine funding priorities. Advised on the need for nurses, recruitment concerns, need for nursing research, and improvement of nursing education.
1970	An Abstract for Action (a report of the National Commission on Nursing and Nursing Education)	Jerome Lysaught/ANA, ANF, NLN, Mellon and Kellogg Foundations	Looked at current practices and patterns of nursing. Suggested joint practice committees, master planning for nursing education, funding for nursing education and research.
1979	The Study of Credentialing in Nursing	Inez Hinsvark/ANA	A review of credentialing—especially of nursing. Resulted in the appointment of a Task Force. Supported a freestanding credentialing center for nursing.
1983	National Institute of Medicine Study	Katherine Bauer/DHHS	Required by the Nursing Training Act of 1979, determined the need for continued outlay of federal money for nursing education. Resulted in 21 specific recommendations. Found that the shortage of nurses of the 1960s and 1970s no longer existed, that federal support of nursing education should focus on graduate study, and that the federal government should discontinue efforts to increase "generalist nurses."
1988	Secretary's Commission on Nursing	Lillian Gibbons/DHHS	Responded to serious nursing shortage. Validated the shortage. Recommended increased financial support of education and improved status and working conditions for nurses.
1990	Secretary's Commission on the National Nursing Shortage	Caroline Burnett/DHHS	Appointed for 1 year to advise on implementation of 1988 report. Had three main foci: recruitment and retention, restructuring of nursing service, and use of nursing personnel and information systems.

TABLE 5-3.	MAJOR STUDIES ABOUT NURSING (*Continued*)		
DATE	NAME OF STUDY	PRIMARY INVESTIGATOR/SPONSOR	FOCUS AND RECOMMENDATION
1991	*Report of the National Commission of Nursing Implementation Project (NCNIP)*	Vivian De Back/ANA, NLN, AACN, AONE, Kellogg Foundation	Looked at nursing education, practice, management and research, and developed recommendations for the future of nursing
1993	*Health Professions Education for the Future*	E.H. O'Neill/Pew Health Professions Commission— Pew Charitable Trusts	Reinforced the belief that the education of health professions was not adequate to meet the health needs of America. Identified competencies for 2005 and emphasized the need for nurse-midwives, nurse practitioners, and the role of nurses in health promotion.
1995	*Reforming Health Care Workforce Regulation*	Pew Health Professions Commission	Had as its mission assisting schools preparing health professionals to understand the changing nature of health care, the needs for the future, and how to design and implement the programs preparing these workers. Recommended reform of the licensing process, specifically elimination of exclusive scopes of practice.

The last of the early nursing studies that we mention was not really a study, but often is referred to as one because of its far-reaching impact. *A Curriculum Guide for Schools of Nursing*, published in 1937, was a revised version of a document published in 1917. It outlined the curricula for a 3-year course, emphasizing sound educational teaching procedures. It was read and followed by many schools that were operating programs at that time.

Midcentury Studies

By the 1950s, studies about nurses and nursing were numerous and dealt with many aspects of the profession. Only a few of the more significant studies are mentioned here.

Of particular significance was a study published in 1948 entitled *Nursing for the Future*. Conducted by Esther Lucille Brown, a social anthropologist, the study is also known as the Brown report. Funded by the Carnegie Foundation, the study was done to determine society's need for nursing and nurses, and recommended higher education for nurses. It prompted serious examination of professional education and pointed out weaknesses in the existing educational programs. The investigators recommended that basic schools of nursing be placed in universities and colleges, and encouraged the recruitment of large numbers of men and minorities into nursing schools. This report set the stage for studies of nursing education that followed in the 1950s and 1960s, and for recommendations that were to continue into the 21st century.

The Ginzberg report was published the same year. A report rather than a study, it reviewed problems centering on the current and prospective shortage of nurses. The conclusions and recommendations were published in the book entitled *A Program for the Nursing*

Profession. The report recommended that nursing teams consisting of 4-year professional nurses, 2-year registered nurses, and 1-year practical nurses be developed. This would ease the nursing shortage by enabling each member of the team to function in the role for which he or she was educationally prepared. Today we continue to struggle with the utilization of graduates according to their educational preparation.

In 1958, a study entitled *Twenty Thousand Nurses Tell Their Story* was published. It was part of a 5-year research project that was conceived by the ANA and financially supported by nurses throughout the country. The study looked at nurses, what they were doing, their attitudes toward their jobs, and their job satisfaction. As a result, nurses learned a great deal about themselves.

Another significant study was initiated by Mildred Montag and was published in 1959. This study on *Community College Education for Nursing* resulted in the establishment of associate degree nursing education (see Chapter 6).

Significant Studies of the 1960s and 1970s

In 1961, the Surgeon General of the U.S. Public Health Service appointed a 25-member panel called the Consultant Group of Nursing. This group was to advise him on nursing needs and identify the role of the federal government in assessing nursing services to the nation. In 1963, this group presented a report entitled *Toward Quality in Nursing*, which recommended a national investigation of nursing education that would place emphasis on the criteria for high-quality patient care.

After publication of *Toward Quality in Nursing*, the ANA and the NLN appropriated funds and established a joint committee to study ways to conduct and finance a national inquiry of nursing education. Later, the study was expanded to reflect on probable requirements in professional nursing that would occur over several decades to come, and to examine changing practices and educational patterns of the present time. Financing was obtained from the American Nurses Foundation, the Kellogg Foundation, the Avalon Foundation, and an anonymous benefactor. To conduct the study, the National Commission for the Study of Nursing and Nursing Education was set up as an independent agency and functioned as a self-directing group. The 12 commissioners were chosen for their broad knowledge of nursing, for their skills in related disciplines, or for their competencies in relevant fields, with no commissioner representing a particular interest group or position.

The study focused on the supply and demand for nurses, nursing roles and functions, nursing education, and nursing as a career. The commission found it necessary not only to examine these key concerns but also to relate these issues to the social system that provides care to the public.

The final report of the commission, *An Abstract for Action*, was published in 1970. It included 58 specific recommendations and concluded with four central recommendations. It also listed three basic priorities: (1) increased research on both the practice and education of nurses; (2) enhanced educational systems and curricula based on research; and (3) increased financial support for nurses and for nursing (National Commission, 1970).

In 1973, a progress report from the National Commission for the Study of Nursing and Nursing Education concerning the implementation of the recommendations of the original report was published under the title *From Abstract into Action*. The commission believed that it was imperative that nursing achieve the goals established in the recommendations so that nursing could emerge as a full profession and could assist in providing optimal health care for this country.

Studies of the 1980s

One of the major studies of nursing conducted in the 1980s was that of the National Commission on Nursing. This group was composed of 30 commissioners from disciplines such as nursing, hospital management, business, government, education, and medicine—all of whom were concerned about the current nursing-related problems in the health care system, especially the apparent shortage of nurses. The American Hospital Association, Hospital Research and Educational Trust, and the American Hospital Supply Corporation sponsored the commission. The group began its work in September 1980 and focused on areas that dealt primarily with the environments in which nurses worked, the relationship between nursing education and nursing practice, nursing issues, and the status of nursing as a profession (National Commission on Nursing, 1981). After systematically examining and evaluating data from a wide variety of sources and holding open forums to gain input, the final recommendations were published in 1983. Although the findings and recommendations are too lengthy to be included in this chapter in their entirety, it is important to mention the five major categories of issues identified by the study (National Commission on Nursing, 1981, p. 5):

1. The status and image of nursing, which includes changes in the nursing role
2. The interface of nursing education and practice, including models of education for preparing to practice
3. The effective management of the nursing resource, including such factors as job satisfaction, recruitment, and retention
4. The relationship among nursing, medical staff, and hospital administration, including nursing's participation in decision-making
5. The maturing of nursing as a self-determining profession, including defining and determining the nature and scope of practice, the role of nursing leadership, increasing decision making in nursing practice, and the need for unity in the nursing profession.

Many of the commission's findings were not surprising to people who were involved with nursing. Included were findings indicating that physicians and health care administrators often did not understand the role of nurses in patient care, and that traditional and outdated images of nurses (including Victorian stereotypes and traditional male–female relationships) impeded acceptance of current roles. Some physicians and administrators thought that nurses were overeducated and did not support an increase in the nurse's authority to make decisions concerning health care.

The findings that individuals and nursing groups are not unified in defining fundamental, professional goals for nursing, and that nursing, as a profession, lacks cohesiveness and a clear understanding of its role and direction, were not a revelation to many seasoned nurses. These same nurses also were not astonished to learn of the numerous and diverse associations that represent nursing but lack a way to determine common goals for nursing education, practice, and credentialing. The disagreement and confusion about educational preparation for nurses, and the controversy about entry into practice, were identified as further obstacles to the advancement of the profession (see Chapter 6). Clearly, there is a need for a system of nursing education that promotes realistic expectations, provides appropriate support for practice and advancement, and includes educational mobility in nursing. As we begin the 21st century, nursing continues to grapple with many of these issues. A number of the issues are ones with which nursing has struggled for years; most of them will not be completely resolved in the next decade. As a new graduate, you will have the opportunity to influence their outcome.

Following in the footsteps of the National Commission of Nursing was the National Commission on Nursing Implementation Project, which began in 1985. Funded for 3 years by the W. K. Kellogg Foundation, the project was cosponsored by the NLN, the ANA, the American Organization of Nurse Executives, and the American Association of Colleges of Nursing. Administered by the American Nurses' Foundation, its purpose was to provide leadership in seeking consensus about the appropriate education and credentialing for basic nursing practice, effective models for the delivery of nursing care, and the means for developing and testing nursing knowledge. The aim of this project was to lay the groundwork and take action wherever possible to support effective, high-quality nursing care delivery in the immediate and long-range future.

The results of another nursing study were released in January 1983. This 2-year study, mandated under the 1979 Nurse Training Amendments, was conducted by the Institute of Medicine Committee on Nursing and Nursing Education and was funded by the Department of Health and Human Services at a cost of $1.6 million. Basically, the study was to provide advice regarding federal support of nursing eduction, gain information about nurses and their employment, and make recommendations regarding measures to improve the supply and use of nurses. The study made 21 specific recommendations to Congress. Because the study found that the shortage of nurses in the 1960s and 1970s had largely disappeared, it was recommended that the federal government discontinue efforts to increase the supply of "generalist nurses." ("I.O.M. study . . . ", 1983).

The fallacies in these findings soon became apparent. Across the nation, nursing enrollments plummeted in the late 1980s. This drop in enrollment occurred at a time when nurses were assuming expanded roles and more nurses than ever were needed for the delivery of health care throughout the nation. The result was a serious national shortage of nurses, especially in certain settings and in specific areas of care, such as long-term care.

Studies of the 1990s

Responding to the need for more nurses, many studies of the early 1990s focused on the roles of nurses in the delivery of health care, on educational patterns that would encourage capable individuals to choose nursing as a career, and on programs that would facilitate educational mobility. Issues related to the nurse's image and the nursing shortage merged. A new Commission on the National Nursing Shortage replaced the Federal Commission on Nursing, and $275,000 was budgeted to assist in its function. This commission developed strategies to decrease the nursing shortage, which focused on recruitment, retention, restructuring of nursing services for the most effective use of nursing personnel, and gathering data about nursing and the information systems used in nursing.

Another group whose work has significantly affected nursing is that of the Pew Health Professions Commission (see Chapter 1). Although issued in the form of reports rather than a study, per se, the recommendations that have come from the Commission caused many nursing organizations to take a serious look at themselves and their activities. The reports of the Commission addressed issues related to nursing education, to credentialing, and to the supply of health care professionals. The recommendations in the first report regarding nursing education included the following:

* Recognizing the value of the multiple entry points to professional practice
* Consolidating professional nomenclature so that there is a single title for each level of nursing preparation and service
* Determining the practice responsibilities associated with different levels of nursing education
* Reducing the size and number of nursing education programs (with the suggestion that the reductions occur in associate degree and diploma programs)
* Expanding the number of masters-level nurse practitioner programs.

The second report dealt with credentialing issues and recommended that scopes of practice be eliminated and that unlicensed personnel be employed in health care (see Chapter 7 for more detail). It also addressed the need to ensure competence among today's licensed health care practitioners.

Studies of the 21st Century

As the nursing profession entered into the 21st century, it found itself perplexed with many of the concerns related to the impending nurse shortage. Various groups became involved in studying work force issues, with the primary research occurring on the state level, with individual states examining their current and potential workforce and establishing strategic plans to address the identified issues. An exception to the state studies is the one mentioned earlier in this chapter that was conducted by the Robert Wood Johnson Foundation and addressed the nursing shortage.

Critical Thinking Activity

Identify at least three areas in nursing that you believe need further study, and describe how you would begin to conduct those studies. Whom would you involve?

DEFINING A LANGUAGE FOR NURSING

For many, the development of a special language for nursing is a fairly new development. It began as an effort to develop a language that would describe the clinical judgments made by nurses that are not in medical language systems. However, as early as 1909, nurses with a strong eye to the future and professionalism recognized that nursing would someday need a language of its own. Ninety years ago, Isabel Hampton Robb wrote the following after attending a meeting of the newly formed International Council of Nurses.

> While attending a special meeting of the ICN in Paris, I was naturally at once struck by the fact that the methods and the ways of regarding nursing problems were . . . as foreign to the various delegations as were the actual languages, and the thought occurred to me that . . . sooner or later we must put ourselves upon a common basis and work out what may be termed a "nursing esperanto" which would in the course of time give us a universal nursing language (Hampton-Robb, 1909).

Defining a language for nursing primarily involves the development and refinement of **nursing nomenclatures** and **classification systems** that communicate information and guide data collection about nursing activities. The term "nursing nomenclature" refers to the words by which we name or describe phenomena in nursing. A "classification" is the systematic arrangement or a structural framework of these phenomena. As we move toward an international network of health care, the development of a language unique to nursing is viewed as critical to communication and decision making. Proponents of a specialized language for nursing emphasize the need for objective, science-based information to use in decision making. These data also provide the basis for accountability and the documentation supporting processes and outcomes of care. The data can be used further to answer research questions about nursing and nursing actions. In the age of information technology, uniform, accurate, and automated patient care data are required to conduct analyses that will result in improving the quality of care and costing out that care (Display 5-1). At present, the language of nursing primarily addresses nursing diagnoses, implementation activities, and nursing outcomes. Some would suggest that the existing systems are not adequate to reflect the entire scope of nursing practice and urge further development. We discuss the four systems that are currently most popular and summarize others that have gained attention (Table 5-4).

North American Nursing Diagnosis Association

The first steps toward a common language for nursing started in 1973 when Kristine Gebbie and Mary Ann Lavin of St. Louis University called the First National Conference on Classification of Nursing Diagnosis. National Conferences have been held regularly since then. The National

---

Display 5-1   **RATIONALE FOR THE DEVELOPMENT OF A CLASSIFICATION FOR NURSING**

- Permits recognition and communication with others by giving a name to the things nurses do
- Provides a uniform legal record of care
- Supports clinical decision making
- Lays the groundwork for nursing research
- Captures the cost of nursing services for billing and accounting purposes
- Generates a structured retrieval data base for quality assurance

TABLE 5-4.	MAJOR CLASSIFICATIONS FOR NURSING CARE RECOGNIZED BY THE AMERICAN NURSES ASSOCIATION	
TITLE	**WHAT IT IS**	**CHARACTERISTICS**
North American Nursing Diagnosis Association (NANDA)	A clinical judgment about an individual, family, or community response to actual or potential health problems that provides a basis for selecting a nursing intervention	Currently contains 71 conceptual areas and 143 terms
Nursing Intervention Classification (NIC)	A comprehensive standardized language, describing treatments that nurses perform in all settings and in all specialties	Includes 433 interventions, each with a definition and a detailed set of activities, organized in 27 classes and 6 domains
Nursing Outcomes Classification (NOC)	A variable concept that represents a patient or family caregiver state, behavior, or perception that is measurable along a continuum and responsive to nursing interventions	Contains 218 outcomes, each of which has a list of indicators in the evaluation of patient status, a measurement scale, and a short list of references
Home Health Care Classification	Adapted, revised, and expanded NANDA to include additional home health care nursing diagnostic conditions	Consists of 145 home health care nursing diagnoses, 50 of which were major nursing diagnostic categories and 95 subcategories. Designed for use in the home health care setting.
The Omaha System	A system of client problems, interventions, and client outcomes, referred to as the Problem Classification Scheme, the Intervention Scheme, and the Problem Rating Scale for Outcomes	Includes domains, problems, modifiers, and signs/symptoms; intervention categories, targets, and client-specific information; and outcome rating scales for knowledge, behavior, and status
Nursing Management Minimum Data Set	Establishes a standardized language to identify and collect those factors needed to manage nursing care across care settings	Defines 17 management variables that enable economic analyses and comparisons. Focuses on unit level data aggregation (Delaney & Huber, 1996)
Patient Care Data Set (PCDS)	Codifies patient problems and actions delivered by all caregivers during a hospital stay	Information gathered from hundreds of terms in patient records
Perioperative Nursing Data Set	Standardized language for documenting and evaluating perioperative nursing care	Designed for use in the perioperative nursing area
Systematized Nomenclature of Medicine (SNOMED)	Comprehensive system for indexing the entire medical record, including signs and symptoms, diagnoses and procedures	Allows full integration of all medical information in electronic medical record into a single data source

Group for the Classification of Nursing Diagnosis became a formal organization after the fifth conference and was renamed the **North American Nursing Diagnosis Association (NANDA)** in 1982. The Association has two main purposes: to develop a diagnostic classification system (also known as a **taxonomy**) and to identify and approve nursing diagnoses. The list of nursing diagnoses (concepts that are given word labels) continues to grow as nurses encounter diagnoses in clinical practice that have not been included and submit these to NANDA for consideration. As a student, you have some familiarity with nursing diagnoses from the nursing care plans you develop for patient care and in the case studies you discuss in your classes.

McCormick and Jones (1998) point out that a taxonomy refers to a hierarchical system that includes vocabulary and terms. After the first meeting of the 100 participants, 29 conceptual areas were identified, with approximately 100 terms. The current classification system contains 71 conceptual areas and 143 terms (Gordon, 1998).

The following is the definition of a nursing diagnosis accepted by NANDA:

> Nursing diagnosis is a clinical judgment about individual, family, or community response to actual or potential health problems/life processes. Nursing diagnoses provide the basis for selection of nursing interventions to achieve outcomes for which the nurse is accountable (North American Nursing Diagnosis Association, 1997).

Nursing Interventions Classifications

In 1996, work done at the University of Iowa on the classification of nursing interventions received attention. The **Nursing Interventions Classification (NIC)** is a comprehensive, standardized language describing actions that nurses perform in all settings and in all specialties, and includes both physiologic and psychosocial interventions. The interventions are numbered to facilitate computerization. There are 433 interventions, each of which contains a definition and a set of detailed activities that describe what a nurse does. The interventions are organized into 27 classes and 6 domains. They have been linked with NANDA and are in the process of being linked with the Nursing Outcomes Classification (University of Iowa, 1999a).

Nursing Outcomes Classification

Also developed at the University of Iowa, the **Nursing Outcomes Classification (NOC)** was published in 1997. Listed in alphabetical order, the classification includes 218 outcomes, 27 of which were developed after publication of the book. An outcome is defined as a variable concept representing a patient or family caregiver state, behavior, or perception that is measurable along a continuum and responsive to nursing interventions. Project developers believed that stating the outcomes as variable concepts rather than goals would allow the identification of positive or negative changes (or no changes at all) in the patient's status. Each outcome has a definition and a list of indicators that assist in evaluation of patient status. Outcomes thus far developed are at the individual patient or family caregiver level; outcomes for families and communities are beginning to be developed.

The outcomes are organized into 24 categories, called classes. Classes are grouped in six domains. The domains are Functional Health, Physiologic Health, Psychosocial Health, Health Knowledge and Behavior, Perceived Health, and Family. Because the work on outcomes is relatively new, you can anticipate that it will experience additions, refinements, and revisions (University of Iowa, 1999b).

The Omaha System

The **Omaha System**, another example of early classification efforts, is based on federally funded research conducted by the Visiting Nurse Association of Omaha from 1975 to 1993 (Martin & Scheet, 1992). It was designed as a three-part, comprehensive yet brief approach to documentation and information management for multidisciplinary health care professionals who practice in community settings. It offers terms and codes to classify the client's health-related concerns or problems, the interventions that nurses and other health care professionals use, and the client's outcomes (Zielstorff, 1998). Client problems can be identified for individuals, families, and groups. The interventions describe both plans and interventions for specific client concerns. The outcome scales evaluate a client's health-related changes through the use of problem-specific knowledge, behavior, and status ratings. The Omaha System is recognized by the ANA and has been translated into numerous languages. Automation and technology advances and health care delivery changes have markedly expanded its use nationally and internationally (Martin, 1999).

Other Classification Systems

Several other classification systems have emerged. In some instances, they were developed for a particular specialty.

THE NURSING MINIMUM DATA SET

In 1988, a Nursing Minimum Data Set (NMDS) was developed by Werley and Lang. It identified the four nursing elements of nursing diagnosis, nursing interventions, nursing outcomes, and nursing intensity (Clark, 1998). These elements have set the stage for classification activities by many other groups.

THE PATIENT CARE DATA SET

The Patient Care Data Set was developed at the University of Virginia in 1994 in work done by Ozbolt, Fruchtnicht, and Hayden. They gathered hundreds of terms from patient's records, from which they developed the Patient Care Data Set. It codifies patient problems and the actions of all caregivers during a patient's hospital stay (Zielstorff, 1998).

THE HOME HEALTH CARE CLASSIFICATION OF NURSING DIAGNOSES AND INTERVENTIONS

The Home Health Care Classification (HHCC) of Nursing Diagnoses and Interventions evolved from the work of Virginia K. Saba and associates at Georgetown University School of Nursing. It was developed to provide a structure for coding and categorizing home health care nursing services. It identifies 20 Home Health Care Nursing Components to classify. Working with NANDA Nursing Diagnoses, a list of 104 diagnoses were adapted, revised, and expanded to include additional home health care nursing diagnostic conditions. In its final format, it includes 145 diagnoses—50 major nursing diagnostic categories and 95 subcategories. The diagnosis statements also collected the actual outcome for each nursing diagnosis, which were used to measure the outcome of home health care (Saba, 1996).

THE PERIOPERATIVE NURSING DATA SET

Another recently developed nursing classification is the Perioperative Nursing Data Set (PNDS). It was developed by the Association of Operating Room Nurses to provide perioperative nurses with standardized language they could use for documenting and evaluating the care they provide. It was their intent to develop a unified language that would allow nursing care to be systematically quantified, coded, and captured in a computerized format in the perioperative setting. It consists of nursing diagnoses, nursing interventions, and patient outcomes related to delivery of nursing care in the perioperative setting (AORN Online, 1999).

THE SYSTEMATIZED NOMENCLATURE OF MEDICINE-REFERENCE TERMINOLOGY

The Systematized Nomenclature of Medicine-Reference Terminology (SNOMED-RT) represents an additional classification of terms. Although SNOMED-RT was developed in 1998, its development started as early as 1965 with the development of a Systematized Nomenclature of Pathology (SNOP). In 1976, the Systematized Nomenclature of Medicine (SNOMED) listed 44,587 terms, and in 1993, SNOMED International expanded to 130,580 terms (SNOMED, 1999). Although focusing primarily on medicine, SNOMED-RT is recognized by the ANA (SNOMED, 1999).

THE MINIMUM DATA SET FOR NURSING HOME RESIDENT ASSESSMENT AND CARE SCREENING

Although not referred to in terms of nursing language, the Minimum Data Set for Nursing Home Resident Assessment and Care Screening (MDS) bears some mention here. When the Omnibus Budget Reconciliation Act (OBRA) was passed in 1991, it required assessment of long-term care facility residents. This assessment, done on admission and every 3 months thereafter, must be standardized, comprehensive, accurate, and reproducible. It must be transmitted electronically to data centers in each state. Whenever problems are identified during the assessment, Resident Assessment Protocols (RAPs) must be instituted. The RAPs lists factors that might be associated with the problem, clarifying information to be considered in making a diagnosis, and describing the environment that will help reduce the symptoms. Complete documentation of the situation, including nature of the problem, complications, risk factors, referrals, and rationale for action is required of nurses (Eliopoulos, 1997). The MDS is used as the basis for determining payment to long-term care facilities. The implementation of the MDS nationwide has resulted in a significant collection of data that can be used as a basis for improving the care of the elderly.

The National Information and Data Set Evaluation Center

The National Information and Data Set Evaluation Center (NIDSEC) was established in 1995 by the ANA to review, evaluate against defined criteria, and recognize nursing information systems. Their mission is to "develop and disseminate standards pertaining to information systems that support the documentation of nursing practice, and evaluate voluntarily submitted information systems against these standards" (NIDSEC, 1999, p. 1). Within the framework of the NIDSEC, four dimensions of nursing data sets and systems are evaluated:

- Nomenclature (terms used)
- Clinical Content (the linkages among terms)
- Clinical Data Repository (how the data are stored and made accessible for retrieval)
- General System Characteristics (such as performance and attention to security and confidentiality)

Groups or vendors wishing to be recognized by ANA submit materials to a five-member review panel, who, after examining the application, submit a recommendation to the NIDSEC Committee. If accepted by the Committee, the recognition extends for 3 years, after which a new application must be submitted. At this writing, nine groups are recognized by NIDSEC.

The International Classification for Nursing Practice Project

The International Classification for Nursing Practice Project (ICNPP) is an effort of the International Council of Nurses (ICN). The goal of the Project is to provide "a unifying framework for existing systems and a system which can be used in countries which have none" (Clark, 1998). Now referred to as the ICNP, it is a classification of nursing phenomena, nursing actions, and nursing outcomes.

Although the United States has been involved in the development of classification and information systems for some time, the need for a unified language is now recognized internationally. Because cultural and language differences exist, many of the classification systems currently employed in the United States are not useful in other countries. For example, the concept of self-care reflects the cultural values and norms of American society but may be perceived quite differently in other cultures. In 1989, the ICN was asked to encourage member National Nurses Associations (NNA) to become involved in developing information and classification systems and nursing data sets that could be used by nurses in all countries to identify and describe nursing. The project began a year later. In 1996, an alpha version of the Classification of Nursing Phenomenon and Nursing Interventions was field tested, and a beta version was launched June 1999 at ICN's Centennial Conference. The objectives were reviewed and revised in 2000. The ICNP Programme has established formal evaluation and review process to advance the project and plans to release ICNP® Version 1 in 2005. The student wishing to learn more about this project is encouraged to research the topic by clicking on the ICNP link at *http://www.icn.ch*.

Critical Thinking Activity

Analyze the history of the development of a classification and nomenclature specific to nursing. Describe possible future developments, and provide a rationale for your answer. What do you see as major impediments and why? What do you believe will be the long-term benefits and why?

TRADITIONS IN NURSING

Because of its history, nursing has developed many **traditions**. Some of them are being questioned or eliminated, primarily because they are not practical in today's workplace (eg, the wearing of a nursing cap). It is worthwhile, however, to reflect just a little on the development of these traditions and to discuss their relationship to nursing. Earle P. Scarlett (1991, p. 6), a Canadian physician, writer, and medical historian, would support such discussion. He wrote:

> The truth of the matter is that any profession worthy of the name must forever be strengthening and re-creating its traditions. A profession is a sensitive organic growing thing, not a static order. And it is particularly important that we should remember this at the present time.

The Nursing Pin

The nursing pin may date back to the time of the Crusades, when Crusaders marched to Jerusalem to recover the Holy Land. Among the Crusaders were the Knights Hospitallers of St. John of Jerusalem. Their uniform, introduced by a man named Gerard, included a black robe with a white Maltese cross. The Maltese cross became a familiar sight on the battlefields of the Holy Land. Following the capture of Jerusalem in 1099, some of the Crusaders noted the excellent nursing care provided by the Hospital of St. John and decided to join the nursing group. The Maltese cross is an eight-pointed cross formed by four arrowheads joining at their points. The eight points of the cross signified the eight beatitudes that knights were expected to exemplify in their works of charity. When the Knights Templars and the Knights of the Teutonic Order were formed in 1118 and 1190, respectively, this symbol was carried forward. The Maltese cross later became a symbol of many groups who cared for the sick, including the United States Cadet Nurse Corps.

The actual symbolism of the pin relates to customs established in the 16th century, when the privilege of wearing a coat of arms was limited to noblemen who served their kings with distinction. As centuries passed, the privilege was extended to schools and to craft guilds, and the symbols of wisdom, strength, courage, and faith appeared on buttons, badges, and shields. It was probably this spirit that Florence Nightingale attempted to capture when she chose the Maltese cross as a symbol for the badge worn by the graduates of her first nursing school.

As nursing developed as a profession, each school chose a unique pin, awarded on completion of the program, as a public symbol of work well done. Many of the early schools, particularly those associated with hospitals supported by religious groups, incorporated the cross into their pin. The first Nightingale School of Nursing in the United States was at Bellevue Hospital and is credited with developing the first school badge or pin, which was presented to the class of 1880 (Kalisch & Kalisch, 1995, p. 82). A crane in the center symbolized the nurse's vigilance, an inner circle of blue suggested constancy, and an outer circle of poppy capsules symbolized mercy and the relief of suffering. The nursing journal *RN* has collected nursing pins from across the United States and has occasionally created a cover display of pins from that collection.

The Nursing Cap

The history of the nursing cap is less certain. Several explanations of the origin of the cap have been suggested. It probably evolved during the period of time when nursing was greatly influenced by religion. It may have originated in the habit worn by the Sisters of Charity of St. Vincent de Paul, who established the first modern school of nursing in Paris in 1864. Another opinion suggests that the cap was influenced by the Institute of Protestant Deaconesses, founded by Pastor Theodore Fleidner at Kaiserwerth in Germany, and the institution where Florence Nightingale studied. The white cap of the deaconesses of the early Christian era and the nun's veil of the Middle Ages have been said to be the forerunners of the nursing cap as we know it today (Mangum, 1994). The veil was modified to become a cap and was associated with service to others. We need to remember, also, that in Florence Nightingale's day, every lady wore a cap indoors. If you look at pictures of Queen Victoria, you notice the cap of plain white stiffened muslin framing her face. It was considered proper for women to keep their heads covered; thus, the cap would be viewed as the proper dress for a young woman of the day. The cap worn by students at Kaiserwerth when Florence Nightingale was a student was hood shaped, had a ruffle around the face, and tied under the chin. A final conjecture is that the cap originally was designed to cover and help to control the long hair that was fashionable in the late 19th century, when short haircuts were not acceptable for women.

In the United States and Canada, the head covering became smaller and lost its scarf or veil as women's hair styles changed and hair was worn shorter. (The hair-covering aspect remained a part of the cap in many areas of Europe.) As nursing education programs developed in hospitals, they each created their own cap and nursing pin as a symbol of that particular hospital and nursing school. Some of these were rather "frilly" and were fashioned after the cloth cone through which ether was dropped. Again, as hairstyles changed, the size of the cap also changed, until it became one of individual taste or preference. A "capping" ceremony was part of the ritual of the nursing student and is discussed later.

As the role of nurses changed and as high technology became a significant part of the hospital work environment, nurses found that caps were bothersome as they tried to carry out their duties. They were knocked askew by curtains, equipment, and tubing. By the 1980s, many hospitals no longer required the cap as a part of the uniform. Nursing programs responded by dropping the cap as a required article of dress. If students wished to have a cap, it was purchased from a local uniform store and had no particular identification with the program (Fig. 5-3).

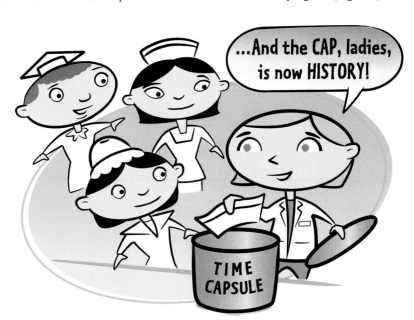

FIGURE 5-3   By the 1980s, many nurses were no longer wearing the cap as part of the nursing uniform.

The Nursing Uniform

Like the nursing cap, which is actually a part of the early nursing uniform, the requirement for special dress came from the religious and military history of nursing and has always been significant in nursing. This is due to the fact that dress provides a strong nonverbal message about one's image. The nurse attired in a white uniform, at least in the 1950s and 1960s, communicated an impression of confidence, competence, professionalism, authority, role identity, and accountability. As nurses have adopted more casual dress, some of this identity has been lost, and hospital committees, nursing programs, and nurses have spent considerable time discussing appropriate attire.

Early uniforms were long, usually stiffly starched, and had detachable collars and cuffs. A full uniform often included a long cape that would cover the uniform. Kalisch and Kalisch (1995, pp. 80–81) credit the New York Training School for Nurses at Bellevue Hospital with being the first school to adopt a standard uniform for student nurses, in 1876. The uniform consisted of a gingham apron worn in the morning and a white apron worn in the afternoon over a dark woolen dress. A well-bred young woman, Euphemia Van Rensselaer, is credited with updating the basic uniform, which students were opposed to wearing. Given 2 days' leave of absence to have a uniform made for herself, she created a tailored uniform consisting of a long gray dress for winter and a calico version for summer, both worn with a white apron and cap. The attractiveness of her appearance resulted in other students accepting the uniform as standard dress. Later, a more easily laundered dress that could be worn throughout the year replaced the gray dress for winter.

A regulation uniform became a distinguishing mark of each nursing school by the end of the 19th century. Typically, the uniform consisted of a bodice and skirt of white material, adjustable white cuffs, a stiff white collar, and a white cap. To maintain the feminine hourglass image popular at the time, a tightly laced corset was worn beneath the uniform and ankles were hidden from view. Some suggest that the adoption of a distinctive and attractive uniform played a significant role in developing a professional image for nursing, giving it status, respect, and authority.

By the 1900s, the uniform became more functional and the hemline was raised. By the mid-1960s, pantsuits became accepted and nurses in certain settings, particularly psychiatric and pediatric units, were challenging the appropriateness of uniforms, especially white uniforms. By 1970, significant changes were occurring in uniforms, with the acceptance of styles that were designed to "make the nurse more approachable." In psychiatric settings, "no uniform" became the standard of the day. Today, athletic shoes are acceptable in many institutions, and "scrubs" have become so accepted that they are featured in pamphlets advertising uniforms. In 1987, the Springhouse Corporation conducted a survey of nurses throughout the United States and found that most nurses prefer scrubs or lab coats worn over street clothes. The result of this change has been that nurses today are no longer identifiable by uniform. The stethoscope worn around the neck gives the consumer some clue to a person's position (ie, that the person is a health care worker rather than a maintenance person), and hospital identification badges provide further information, but sometimes do not include the person's full name.

There is still controversy over the appropriate attire for nurses. Mangum, Garrison, Lind, Thackeray and Wyatt (1991) recommended that nurses wear clothing that clearly distinguishes them as professional nurses. Although they did not suggest that nurses wear a cap, they advocated the more traditional white dress or pantsuit. Others have argued that what nurses wear matters less than what they know.

Ceremonies Associated With Nursing Programs

Long-standing traditions embraced by nursing include the ceremonies that mark various points along the educational paths of nursing students. Primary among these are the "capping" and the "pinning" ceremonies.

Capping ceremonies are not as common today as pinnings, probably because most nurses and nursing students no longer wear caps. Traditionally, the cap was awarded to students after they completed a certain part of the program. In hospital schools, it was awarded on completion of the probationary period, but more often it was given after the completion of the first year. Often held in a nearby church, a special ceremony was planned, to which students invited family and others who were interested in their progress. The director of the school, assisted by other school dignitaries and faculty, solemnly placed the cap on the head of each student. Students proudly wore the cap throughout the remainder of the program. Often a stripe was added to one corner of the cap to signify completion of the second year of study, and a black band was added at the time of graduation. Many colleges included these ceremonies when nursing education moved into those settings.

The second traditional ceremony in nursing, the pinning, was of even greater significance, and is continued by many schools today. The pinning heralded the completion of the program. Amid much pomp and circumstance, family and friends gathered to watch as the nursing director ceremoniously pinned the school pin on each new graduate. Graduates often recited, in unison, the Nightingale Pledge (Display 5-2), written in 1893 by Lystra E. Gretter, superintendent of Harper Hospital School in Detroit (Calhoun, 1993). This tradition is often repeated in nursing schools today, although the original pledge in some cases is modified. Some schools include additional tradition through the "passing of the lamp." A representative of the graduating class hands a lamp (symbolizing the lamp carried by Florence Nightingale) to a representative of the next graduating class, thus reinforcing the concept of the continual caring represented in nursing.

Display 5-2   **THE NIGHTINGALE PLEDGE**

I solemnly pledge myself before God and in the presence of this assembly:

To pass my life in purity and to practice my profession faithfully;

I will abstain from whatever is deleterious and mischievous and will not take or knowingly administer any harmful drug; I will do all in my power to maintain and elevate the standard of the profession, and will hold in confidence all personal matters committed to my keeping and all family affairs coming to my knowledge in the practice of my calling;

With loyalty will I endeavor to aid the physician in his work, and devote myself to the welfare of those committed to my care.

Gretter, 1893

As nursing education moved into institutions of higher education, some of the traditional ceremonies were discontinued. Some argue that the ceremony recognizing program completion in the collegiate environment is the college commencement, and that "special" celebrations for students of particular areas of study are not appropriate. However, in many large universities, the various disciplines now have separate ceremonies or an additional ceremony for their members. In other cases, the tradition is continued, although there is some tendency for graduates not to purchase a pin.

Critical Thinking Activity

Review the traditions established in nursing. Which is the most meaningful to you, and why? Which is the least meaningful to you, and why? Do you believe traditions should be continued in nursing? Provide a rationale for your answer.

KEY CONCEPTS

- In its development as a profession, nursing has struggled with its definition, its image, and its role in the health care delivery system. This is due in part to its history and the fact it has both theoretic and practical aspects. The role of the nurse in the health care delivery system has probably never been more important than it is today.
- Nursing is distinct from medicine. Medicine deals with diagnosis and treatment of disease and nursing is concerned with caring for the person.
- The position nursing occupies as a profession is often judged against sociologically developed characteristics of a profession. Not everyone agrees that nursing meets those standards.
- The standards of a profession typically include seven requirements: (1) possess a well-defined and well-organized body of knowledge; (2) enlarge a systematic body of knowledge and improve education; (3) educate its practitioners in institutions of higher learning; (4) function autonomously in the formulation of policy; (5) develop a code of ethics; (6) attract professionals who will be committed to the profession for a lifetime; and (7) compensate practitioners by providing autonomy, continuous professional development, and economic security.
- Nursing also has struggled with the terms "profession" and "professional." At times, the characteristics of the "professional" become confused with the formal concept of a profession.
- Nursing has struggled with its image. Various groups have waged campaigns to improve the image of nursing and thus make it a more attractive profession. A number of groups have launched campaigns to address this issue.
- The image of nursing today is viewed as a critical issue because of the nurse shortage. A positive image is needed to attract qualified individuals into the profession.
- Since the beginning of the 20th century, nursing has been a much-studied profession. Early studies dealt with nursing education; later studies dealt with the image of nursing, nurses themselves, and with nursing's role in health care delivery.

- As nursing has developed as a profession, more attention has been directed to establishing a unique classification and nomenclature for nursing. Efforts are being made to do this on an international basis.
- Nursing as a profession has many traditions, some of which are being challenged today. Among the traditions are the pin, the cap, the uniform, and nursing ceremonies.

RELEVANT WEB SITES

International Council of Nurses: *http://www.icn.ch/*
Nursing Classifications: *http://www.nursingworld.org* and type "Nursing Classifications" into the Search box
Nursing Shortage:
    American Organization of Nurse Executives: *http://www.aone.org*
    American Association of Colleges of Nursing: *http://www.aacn.nche.edu*
    Bureau of Labor Statistics: *http://www.bls.gov*
    Johnson & Johnson Nursing Campaign: *http://www.discovernursing.com*
    Nurses for a Healthier Tomorrow: *http://www.nursesource.org*
    The Forum on Health Care Leadership: *http://www.healthcareforum.org*
Nursing Theory Page: *http://www.ualberta.ca/~jrnorris/nt/theory.html*

REFERENCES

Abdellah, F. G. (1960). *Patient-centered approaches to nursing*. New York: Macmillan.

American Nurses Association. (1980). *Nursing: A social policy statement*. Kansas City, MO: American Journal of Nursing Co.

American Nurses Association. First Position on Education for Nursing. (1965). *American Journal of Nursing, 65*(12):106–111.

AORN Online: Research. Perioperative Nursing Data Set. (1999). [On-line.] Available at: *http://aorn.org/research/ pnds.htm*. Accessed November 1, 1999.

Benner, P. & Wrubel, J. (1989). *The primacy of caring*. Menlo Park, CA: Addison-Wesley.

Benner, P. (1984). *From novice to expert*. Menlo Park, CA: Addison-Wesley.

Bevis, E. O. & Watson, J. (1989). *Toward a caring curriculum: A new pedagogy for nursing*. New York: National League for Nursing.

Bixler, G. K. & Bixler, R. W. (1945). The professional status of nursing. *American Journal of Nursing 45*(9):730.

Calhoun, J. (1993). The Nightingale Pledge: A commitment that survives the passage of time. *Nursing & Health Care 14*(3):130–136.

Carper, B. A. (1979). The Ethics of Caring. *Advances in Nursing Science 3*:11–19, March.

Chitty, K. K. (1997). *Professional nursing concepts and challenges* (2nd ed.). Philadelphia: W. B. Saunders.

Clark, J. (1998 [Sept. 30]). The International Classification for Nursing Practice Project. 1998 Online Journal of Issues in Nursing. [On-line.] Available: *http://www.nursingworld.org/ojin/tpc7tpc7_3.htm*. Accessed October 31, 1999.

Delaney, C. & Huber, D. (1996). A Nursing Management Minimum Data Set (NMMDS): A report of an invitational conference. Chicago, IL: American Organization of Nurse Executives.

Donahue, M. P. (1996). *Nursing: The finest art* (2nd ed.). St. Louis: CV Mosby.

Eliopoulos, C. (1997). *Gerontological nursing* (4th ed.). Philadelphia: Lippincott-Raven.

Flexner, A. (1981). In Bernard, L. A. & Walsh, M.: *Leadership: The key to professionalism of nursing.* New York: John Wiley & Sons.

Geolot, D. (2000). *Resources and funding.* Paper presented at the Nurse Staffing summit (May, 2000) of the American Nurses Association, Washington, D.C.

Gordon, M. (1998 [Sept. 30]). *Nursing nomenclature and classification system development.* Online Journal of Issues in Nursing. [On-line.] Available: *http://www.nursingworld.org/ojin/tpc7/tpc7_1.htm.* Accessed October 4, 1999.

Gordon, S. (1999). Viewpoint: Nursing and wit. *American Journal of Nursing 99*(5):9.

Hampton-Robb, I. (1909). *Report of the third regular meeting of the International Council of Nurses.* Geneva: ICN.

Henderson, V. (1966). *The nature of a science of nursing.* New York: Macmillan.

"I.O.M. study sees need for funds in graduate, specialty areas." (1983). *American Journal of Nursing 83*(3):343, 344, 454.

Johnson, D. (1980). The behavioral system model for nursing. In Riehl, J.P. & Roy, C: *Conceptual models for nursing practice* (2nd ed., pp. 207–216) East Norwalk, CT: Appleton-Century-Crofts.

Kalisch, P. A., & Kalisch, B. J. (1995). *The advance of American nursing.* Philadelphia: J. B. Lippincott Co.

Kalisch, P. A. & Kalisch, B. J. (1982a). Nurses on prime-time television. *American Journal of Nursing 82*(2):264.

Kalisch, P. A. & Kalisch, B. J. (1982b). The image of the nurse in motion pictures. *American Journal of Nursing, 82*(4):605.

Kalisch, P. A. & Kalisch, B. J. (1982c). The image of nurses in novels. *American Journal of Nursing, 82*(8):1220.

King, I. M. (1981). *A theory for nursing: Systems, concepts, process.* New York: John Wiley & Sons.

Kolcaba, K. Y. (1992). Holistic comfort: Operationalizing the construct as a nurse-sensitive outcome. *Advances in Nursing Science, 1*, 1–10.

Labor Management Relations Act (1947) as amended by Public Laws 86-257 (1959) and 93-360 (1974), Section 2. [On-line]. Available: *http://www.nlrb.gov/publications/nlrb4.pdf*

LeMaire, B. (2002). Jean Watson, on her theory of caring. *Nurse Week (Mountain West Edition)* (3)40; 7.

Levine, M. E. (1969). *Introduction to clinical nursing.* Philadelphia: F.A. Davis.

Mangum, S. (1994). Uniforms and caps: Do we need them? In Strickland, O.L. & Fishman, D. J. *Nursing issues in the 1990s* (pp. 46–66) Albany, NY: Delmar Publishers.

Mangum, S., Garrison, C., Lind, C., Thackeray, R., & Wyatt, M. (1991). Perception of nurses' uniforms. *Image: The Journal of Nursing Scholarship* 23:127–130.

Martin, K. S. (1999). The Omaha System: Past, present and future. On-line Journal of Nursing Informatics, Volume 3(1). [Online] Available: *http://cac.psu.edu/~dxm12/art1v3n1art.html.* Accessed November 22, 1999.

Martin, K. S. & Scheet, N. J. (1992). *The Omaha system: Application for community health nursing.* Philadelphia: W. B. Saunders.

McCormick, K. A. & Jones, C. B. (Sept. 30, 1998). Is one taxonomy needed for health care vocabularies and classifications? Online Journal of Issues in Nursing. [Online] Available: *http://www.nursingworld.org/ojin/tpc7/tpc7_2.htm.* Accessed October 4, 1999.

Meade, J. (2002). *Health care's human crisis: The American nursing shortage.* Retrieved May 21, 2002 from the World Wide Web: *http://www.rwjf.org/newsEvents/nursing.jhtml*

Muff, J. (1988). Handmaiden, battle ax, whore. In Muff, J.: *Socialization, sexism and stereotyping.* (pp. 113–156) Prospect Heights, IL: Waveland Press, Inc.

National Commission for the Study of Nursing and Nursing Education: Summary, Report and Recommendations. (1970). *American Journal of Nursing, 70*(2):279.

National Commission on Nursing. (1981). *Initial report and preliminary recommendations.* Chicago: Hospital Research and Educational Trust.

National Council of State Boards of Nursing, Inc. (1994). *Model Practice Act.* Chicago, Il: The Council.

National Information and Data Set Evaluation Center. (1999). NIDSEC 3-year recognition. [On-line.] Available: *http://www.nursingworld.org/nidsec/index.htm.* Accessed November 1, 1999.

Neuman, B. (1982). *The Neuman System Model: Application to nursing education and practice.* East Norwalk, CT: Appleton-Century-Crofts.

Newman, M. A. (1990). Professionalism: Myth or reality. In Chaska, N.L.: *The Nursing profession: Turning points* (pp. 49–52). St. Louis: C.V. Mosby.

Nightingale, F. (1954). *Notes on nursing: What it is, and what it is not.* (An unabridged republication of the first American edition, as published by D. Appleton and Company in 1860.) New York: Dover Publications.

North American Nursing Diagnosis Association. (1997). *1997–1998. NANDA nursing diagnoses: Definitions and classification.* Philadelphia: Author.

Nursing World NIDSEC: home page. [On-line.] Available: *http://www.nursingworld.org/nidsec/index.htm.* Accessed November 1, 1999.

O'Neil, E. H. (1993). *Health professions education for the future: Schools in service to the nation.* San Francisco: Pew Health Professions Commission.

Orem, D. (1980). *Nursing: Concepts of Practice* (2nd ed.). New York: McGraw-Hill.

Orlando, I. J. (1972). *The discipline and teaching of nursing process.* New York: G.P. Putnam's Sons.

Parse, R. R. (1981). *Man-living-health: A theory of nursing.* New York: Wiley.

Pavalko, R. M. (1971). *Sociology of occupations and professions.* Itasca, IL: Peacock Publishers.

Peplau, H. E. (1952). *Interpersonal relations in nursing.* New York: G.P. Putnam's Sons.

Robert Wood Johnson Foundation. (2002). *The American nursing shortage: Strategies and recommendations for action.* Retrieved May 21, 2002, from the World Wide Web *http://www.rwjf.org/news Events/nursingStrategies.jhtml.*

Rogers, M. E. (1984 [May]). *Science of Unitary Human Beings: A Paradigm for Nursing.* Paper presented before the International Nurse Theorist Conference, Edmonton, Alberta.

Roy, C. (1984). *Introduction to nursing: An adaptation model* (2nd ed.). Englewood Cliffs, NJ: Prentice-Hall.

Saba, V. (1996). 4 Home Health Care Classification (HHCC): Nursing Diagnoses and Nursing Interventions. [On-line.] Available: *http://www.dml.georgetown,edu/research/hhcc.* Accessed October 31, 1999.

Scarlett, E. P. (1991). In M.M. Styles & P. Moccia. (Editors and Authors) *On nursing: A literary celebration.* (pp. 6–7) New York: National League for Nursing, Publication No. 14-2513.

Schlotfeldt, R. M. (1987). Resolution of issues: An imperative for creating nursing's future. *Journal of Professional Nursing*, 3:136–142.

Sieber, J. R., Powers, C. A., Baggs, J. R., Knapp, J. M., & Sileo, C. M. (1998). Missing in action: Nursing in the media. *American Journal of Nursing, 98*(12):55–56.

SNOMED. (1999). The History of SNOMED. Available: *http://www.snomed.org/what/sld005.htm.* Accessed November 1, 1999.

Stewart, M. (1999). Issues update: ANA puts nursing in media spotlight. *American Journal of Nursing, 99*(5):56–59.

Strauss, A. (1966). The structure and ideology of American nursing: An interpretation. In Davis, J.: *The Nursing Profession* (pp. 60–108) New York: John Wiley & Sons.

Styles, M. (1982). *On nursing: Toward a new endowment.* St. Louis: CV Mosby.

Trossman, S. (2002). The global reach of the nursing shortage. *American Journal of Nursing,* *102(3)*:85,87,89.

University of Iowa. (1999a). Nursing Interventions Classification (NIC): Overview. [On-line.] Available: *http://www.nursing.uiowa.edu/nic/overview.htm.* Accessed October 21, 1999.

University of Iowa. (1999b). Nursing Outcomes Classification (NOC): Overview. [On-line.] Available: *http://www.nursing.uiowa.edu/noc/overview.htm.* Accessed October 21, 1999.

Watson, J. (1979). *Nursing the philosophy and science of caring.* Boston: Little, Brown.

Wiedenbach, E. (1964). *Clinical nursing: A helping art.* New York: Springer Publishing Co.

Winslow-Goldmark Report. (1923). *The study of nursing and nursing education in the United States.* New York: Macmillan, 1923.

Zielstorff, R. D. (1998 [Sept. 30]). Characteristics of a good nursing nomenclature from an informatics perspective. *Online Journal of Issues in Nursing.* [On-line.] Available at: *http://www.nursingworld.* *org/ojin/tpc7/tpc7_4.htm.* Accessed October 4, 1999.

Educational Preparation for Nursing

After completing this chapter, you should be able to:

1. Compare the educational preparation of the nursing assistant, the licensed practical (vocational) nurse, the graduate of a hospital-based program, the associate degree graduate, and the baccalaureate degree graduate.

2. Explain the purposes of other forms of nursing education, including external degree programs, registered nurse baccalaureate programs, master's preparation, doctoral studies, nondegree programs, and articulated programs.

3. Identify factors that have prompted changes in nursing education, including studies and sociopolitical events, and analyze the effect of each.

4. Analyze the effects the American Nurses Association (ANA) Position Paper on Nursing Education would have had on nursing licensure if adopted nationwide.

5. Discuss the concept of differentiated practice and provide a rationale for its development.

6. Discuss the impact of technology on nursing education.

7. Identify factors that have influenced changes in nursing education and analyze the effect of each.

8. Analyze the ways in which nursing theories serve to advance the profession.

9. Define the continuing education unit, critique the major points supporting both mandatory and voluntary continuing education, and explain the mechanisms for documenting and recording continuing education.

KEY TERMS

Accreditation	Diploma programs	Position Paper
Advanced nursing practice	Educational mobility	Postsecondary education
Articulation	Entry into practice	Practical (vocational) nurse
Associate degree education	External degree	
Baccalaureate degree education	Generic program	Registered nurse baccalaureate program
Career ladder	Grandfather clause	Scope of practice
Community-based practice	Home health aide	Theorist/theory
	Hospital-based program	Titling
Competencies	Internships and residencies	Virtual university
Continuing education unit (CEU)	Interstate endorsement	Voluntary continuing education
	Mandatory continuing education	
Differentiated nursing practice	Nursing assistant	

Most professions provide a single route for the educational preparation of its practitioners. However, the development of nursing as a profession has resulted in three major educational routes that prepare graduates to write the National Council Licensure Examination (NCLEX) for registered nursing. These circumstances have resulted in alternatives and opportunities for prospective students. The benefits of these options for students and the public resulted in the Pew Commission identifying in their 1995 report the multiple-entry points to professional nursing practice as a strength of nursing (Pew Commission, 1995).

Despite this acknowledged strength, the existence of multiple-entry points has resulted in confusion for both consumers and employers. Health care consumers often find it difficult to understand the various nursing credentials—and probably have little interest in credentials as long as they receive satisfactory care. Employers have difficulty differentiating among the three major types of registered nurse (RN) graduates who, at least initially, enter the work environment performing similar activities. This confusion led to another recommendation from the Pew Commission: that nursing distinguish between the practice responsibilities of the graduates educated in each of the different educational environments. (Pew Commission, 1995), a task that has proven difficult at best.

An educator is charged with the responsibility of graduating a "safe" practitioner, but may not have a clear understanding of how the professional preparation provided by the various educational routes ought to differ in purpose, structure, and outcome. You will find that nursing leaders often vigorously debate aspects of the educational preparation of nurses, such as where it should take place, what content should be included in which programs and to what depth, which tests should measure the various competencies, and which credentials should be awarded.

The three traditional educational avenues that prepare men and women for registered nursing are hospital-based diploma programs, 2-year associate degree programs (primarily found at junior and community colleges), and baccalaureate programs (offered at 4-year colleges and universities). It is also possible for students to begin their nursing education in programs that culminate in a master's degree, and several programs now exist in which a student can earn a doctorate before being eligible to write the state licensing examination for registered nursing.

At least two other groups of caregivers are identified with nursing: the nursing assistant, who is certified, and the practical (vocational) nurse, who is licensed through a separate and different examination from that taken by the RN.

THE NURSING ASSISTANT

For years, individuals called nursing aides or assistants have provided care to patients in hospitals and long-term care facilities. In the past, these caregivers were hired without formal preparation for their responsibilities and were provided on-the-job training. The use of the nursing aides likely started during World War I, and certainly was reinforced during World War II when approximately 150,000 trained volunteer nursing aides served in wartime hospitals. Nursing aides or assistants have always provided the majority of care in nursing homes.

In 1987, Congress passed the Omnibus Budget Reconciliation Act (OBRA), which regulates agencies receiving federal funds, and includes an amendment regulating the education and certification of **nursing assistants** who work in nursing homes. The amendment stipulated that by October 1, 1990, all people working as nursing assistants in nursing homes (hospitals and assisted-living units were not included) would be required to complete a minimum of 75 hours of theory and practice and pass both a theory and practice examination to be certified. Certification falls under state jurisdiction, but is guided by federal regulations. In many states, the hours of preparation required exceed the 75 hours established by federal law. Following the federal legislation, the National Council of State Boards of Nursing Inc. developed the Nurse Aide Competency Evaluation Program (NACEP), which identifies the minimum skills a nursing assistant must attain and can be used to guide programs registering or certifying nursing assistants. The state agency responsible for certifying and maintaining the list of nursing assistants varies from state to state; most commonly, it is the board of nursing or the state department of health services.

The certified nursing assistant (CNA) functions under the direction of the RN or the licensed practical (vocational) nurse. Each state determines the skills that may be performed by the nursing assistant. Typically, these include basic nursing skills, such as changing bed linens; taking temperature, respiratory, and blood pressure readings for patients; bathing patients and helping with personal care; helping patients with eating, walking, and exercise programs; and supporting patients when they are allowed to get out of bed. The preparation of the CNA emphasizes the importance of a safe environment and includes instruction in the use of side rails and restraints, and patients' rights. A number of states also require a designated number of hours per year of continuing education.

Some nursing assistant programs also offer an additional period of training and education for roles as home health aides. The certification requirements for home health aides are similar to those of the nursing assistant. The **home health aide** is prepared to assist individuals with basic care in their home; thus the program of instruction includes content related to shopping for groceries, cooking, and doing laundry.

The training occurs in many settings, including high schools, long-term care facilities, hospitals, community colleges, regional occupational programs (ROPs), and privately operated programs. Some consider this preparation the first rung on the ladder of nursing education, and, in some states, the nursing assistant may be exempt from certain classes required in licensed practical (vocational) nursing programs. Some registered nursing programs establish certification as a nursing assistant as an admission requirement.

The criteria for hospital accreditation established by the Joint Commission on Accreditation of Healthcare Organizations now require that hospitals assure the competence of all employees, including nursing assistants. This led hospitals to the practice of hiring only those who were certified as nursing assistants in long-term care facilities and to the development of courses to prepare individuals as nursing assistants for acute care settings.

PRACTICAL NURSE EDUCATION

The **practical nurse** (titled **vocational nurse** in Texas and California) is no newcomer to the health care delivery system. In the past, the practical nurse was the family friend or community citizen who was called to the home in emergencies. This person, usually self-taught, learned by experience which procedures were effective and which were not. She would perform basic care procedures, such as bathing, and also would cook and perform light housekeeping duties for the family, much as the home health aide does today. Although controls on the licensing of practical nurses and the accreditation of their curricula were slower to evolve than those regulating professional nursing, states gradually enacted licensure laws governing practical nursing. By 1945, 19 states and one territory had licensure laws, but licensure of the practical nurse was mandatory in only one state (Kalisch & Kalisch, 1995). When more states began adopting mandatory licensure laws for practical nurses, many individuals who had been functioning in this capacity were granted a license by waiver, and were excused from any formal training (see Chapter 7 on credentialing). Most, if not all, of these people are now retired from nursing practice. By 1955 all states had licensure laws for practical nurses.

It is not clear when formal preparation for practical nursing began. Some suggest training programs were started in 1897 (Kalisch & Kalisch, 1995). A more popular belief is that the first programs were initiated through the YWCA in Brooklyn, New York, around 1892. The school established through the YWCA was known as the Ballard School, after Lucinda Ballard, who provided the funding to operate it. The course of study lasted approximately 3 months, and the students, called "attendants," were trained to care for invalids, the elderly, and children in a home setting. By 1930, there were only 11 schools of practical nursing, but between 1948 and 1954, 260 more were opened.

A YWCA may seem to many of us to be a strange place for a practical nursing program. In fact, however, YWCAs were an important source of inexpensive housing for many young women who, in the late 1890s and early 1900s, traveled from their homes to large cities in search of new careers and better lives. Because most of these women were untrained and had no marketable skills, the YWCA was a natural site for a school. Display 6-1 outlines some of the significant history in the development of practical nursing.

Display 6-1 HISTORY OF THE DEVELOPMENT OF PRACTICAL NURSING

1892 YWCA in Brooklyn, New York, establishes a program in practical nursing named after Lucinda Ballard, who provided the funding for it.

1907 Thompson School, is founded in Brattleboro, Vermont.

1908 The American Red Cross founds a practical nursing program.

1918 The Household Nursing Association School of Attendant Nursing begins in Boston.

1938 New York becomes the first state to require licensure for the practical nurse.

1941 The Association of Practical Nurse Schools (APNS) is founded.

1942 Membership in the APNS is opened to practical nurses and the name changed to the National Association of Practical Nurse Education and Service (NAPNES). The first planned curriculum for practical nursing is developed.

1945 NAPNES establishes and accredits service for schools of practical nursing; this program was discontinued in 1984.

1949 The National Federation of Licensed Practical Nurses (NFLPN) is organized.

1957 Working with the American Nurses Association, NFLPN seeks to clarify the role and function of the practical nurse. The National League for Nursing (NLN) establishes the Council on Practical Nursing.

1966 The Chicago Public School Program becomes the first practical nurse program to be accredited by the NLN.

1979 The NLN publishes a list of competencies of graduates of practical/vocational nursing programs.

1996 The National Council of State Boards of Nursing (NCSBN), working with NAPNES, offers a certification examination for licensed practical nurses in long-term care.

The general curriculum for practical nurses, which typically takes 1 year to complete, varies considerably from state to state and even from school to school. In many instances, the education is measured in clock hours instead of credit hours. Most of today's practical nursing educational programs stress clinical experience, primarily in structured care settings such as hospitals and long-term care facilities. Basic therapeutic knowledge and introductory content from biologic and behavioral sciences correlate with clinical practice; usually one third of the time is spent in the classroom and two thirds in clinical practice.

The educational preparation of the practical nurse takes place in a great variety of settings. High schools, trade or technical schools, hospitals, junior or community colleges, universities, or independent agencies may offer programs. If the rules and regulations of the state board(s) of nursing allow it, practical nursing and associate nursing degree programs can be incorporated in the community college, as part of a **career ladder** approach to nursing education. These programs sometimes are referred to as one-on-one programs; 1 year of preparation for practical nursing, followed by 1 more year qualifying the graduate to take the licensure examination for registered nursing. All nursing students in these colleges are grouped together for core courses during the first academic year. At the end of this time, a student has the option of stopping the educational program to seek licensure as a practical nurse, or continuing for an additional year to become an RN. Many students opt to do both. Graduates of these core programs in practical nursing usually have a broader and more in-depth understanding of the biologic sciences, and sometimes the social sciences (often also a part of the core curriculum), especially if these are college-level courses that are transferable to a 4-year institution. Because issues related to educational mobility and articulation between programs have received much attention (discussed later in this chapter), these combined programs have become popular.

Graduates of practical nursing programs take the NCLEX-PN; if they pass the exam, they use the title "licensed practical nurse" (LPN) or, in California and Texas, the title "licensed vocational nurse" (LVN). Their scope of practice focuses on meeting the health care needs of clients in hospitals, long-term care facilities, clinics, and the home. Typically, LPNs or LVNs care for clients whose conditions are considered stable, giving direct patient care; observing, recording, and reporting; administering treatments and medications; and assisting in rehabilitation procedures. An RN or a licensed physician directs their work.

As with the associate degree and hospital-based diploma programs for RNs, the educational preparation for practical nurses and the future of practical nursing have been topics of much discussion. Some advocate two levels of nurses: the practical nurse prepared with an associate degree and the RN prepared with a baccalaureate degree. Others would eliminate practical nursing altogether. In 1987, North Dakota became the first state (and to date the only state) to require all candidates taking the licensure examination for practical nursing to have completed an associate degree in practical nursing. With the "graying" of America, and the growing need for nurses in home health care and in long-term care facilities, practical nurses will continue to play a significant role in health care delivery.

DIPLOMA EDUCATION

The earliest type of nursing education in the United States took place in **diploma programs** administered by hospitals, and, therefore, also referred to as **hospital-based programs**. The first hospital with a nurse training school was the New England Hospital for Women, which accepted five probationers on September 1, 1872 (Kalisch & Kalisch, 1995). The characteristics of these early schools were discussed in detail in Chapter 4.

By the late 1940s and early 1950s, many hospital-based nursing schools had affiliated with nearby colleges and universities; these schools adopted general education requirements, such as anatomy, physiology, sociology, and psychology, as part of the curriculum. During this time, the National League of Nursing Education (later to become the NLN) assumed an active role in curriculum guidance and accreditation. Nursing programs gained a stronger educational foundation because they were required to align themselves more closely with other types of **postsecondary education,** that is, education occurring after the completion of high school.

Thus, diploma schools in operation today have sound educational programs that meet the criteria necessary for accreditation. They employ qualified faculty who have developed clinical learning experiences that meet the student's learning needs rather than the hospital's service needs (which often took priority in the past). These programs vary in length from 27 to

36 months. Many diploma schools are affiliated with a college or university so that postsecondary credit can be awarded formally. Graduates are provided with a foundation in the biologic and social sciences, and may have taken some courses in the humanities. There is a strong emphasis in diploma programs on client experiences. The course of study also includes experience in nursing management (for example, being in charge of a nursing unit). Graduates work in acute, long-term, and ambulatory health care facilities, fulfilling the responsibilities established by the scope of practice for RNs as defined by the state in which they are licensed.

During the mid-1960s, there was a significant decline in enrollment in diploma schools, a trend that has continued, so that today diploma programs comprise less than 10 percent of all basic RN education programs (American Association of Colleges of Nursing Education Center, 2002a). As more nursing education programs were moved to institutions of higher education, many hospital-based schools elected to discontinue their programs. Some merged with a local community college or university that assumed administrative responsibility for managing the nursing program, and awarded an associate or baccalaureate degree when graduation requirements were satisfied. The elimination of hospital-based programs has occurred most extensively in the western part of the United States.

Finances also played a role in this change. With increasing constraints on funding, many hospitals found that the costs associated with supporting a nursing program were too great. Many diploma programs existing today have strong endowments and private funding support.

ASSOCIATE DEGREE EDUCATION

The movement toward **associate degree education** began in 1952. Today, associate degree nursing programs prepare more graduates for licensure as RNs than do any of the other programs. Associate degree nursing (ADN) programs have the distinction of being the first (and, to date, the only) type of nursing education established on the basis of planned research and experimentation.

Four events undoubtedly influenced their beginning. First, these programs followed in the wake of the organization and growth of 2-year community colleges in the United States. Community colleges were organized specifically to offer the first 2 years of a traditional 4-year college program and bring many vocational and adult education programs to the community. The goal of the community college was to make some form of college education available to everyone. Second, the cadet nurse program, which was created during World War II, demonstrated that qualified students could be educated adequately in less than the traditional 3 years of the diploma program. Third, the development of associate degree education was influenced by the studies conducted on nursing education in the United States, as discussed in Chapter 5. The final factor influencing the development of associate degree education was the critical national nursing shortage of the 1950s, which occurred because nurses employed during World War II returned home to raise families. It was anticipated that the 2-year program would put graduates into the work market more quickly, thus helping reduce the shortage of nurses while, at the same time, helping to move nursing education into the overall system of higher education in America.

Associate degree programs have helped to solve the nursing shortage of the 1960s and the 1980s. These programs, which focused on preparing graduates skilled in bedside nursing, rapidly increased in number. Associate degree programs particularly appealed to men, minorities, and older students, who had not traditionally pursued educational preparation in nursing. Because most programs were located in community colleges, they tended to be more geographically accessible than the baccalaureate programs in 4-year colleges and universities, typically located in major urban areas.

Characteristics of Associate Degree Education

Associate degree education began with the Cooperative Research Project in Junior and Community College Education for Nursing at Teachers College, Columbia University. The original 5-year research project, which was directed by Mildred Montag, included seven junior and community colleges and one hospital school, located in six regions of the United States. This type of nursing education has expanded from these original programs in 1952 to more than 880 in 2003 (National Organization for Associate Degree Nursing, 2002).

The four basic characteristics of associate degree education originally included (NLN, 1973):

1. Encompassing the nursing program as an integral part of the college that controls and finances the program
2. Ensuring the members of the nursing faculty the same privileges and responsibilities granted to other faculty
3. Organizing a curriculum with a clearly stated philosophy, rationale, and conceptual framework, designed to be completed in 2 years
4. Ensuring that nursing students are treated the same as other community college students with regard to admission, progression, and graduation requirements. The programs are designed to award an associate degree on completion, and graduates are eligible to write the state licensing examination for registered nursing.

Today, these basic characteristics are still incorporated into the standards for accreditation of associate degree programs by the National League for Nursing Accreditation Commission (NLNAC).

In a typical program, approximately half of the credits needed for the associate degree must be fulfilled by general education courses such as English, anatomy, physiology, speech, psychology, and sociology; the other half must be fulfilled by nursing courses. Clinical learning experiences are carefully selected to correspond with the content delivered in classroom lectures; the pre- and postconferences help to reinforce the relationship between the two. Some modifications in this structure are occurring as associate degree educators strive to meet the expectations of employers and the community while remaining true to the concept of associate degree education.

The advent of associate degree education in nursing has brought greater diversity in the students who enroll in nursing programs (Fig. 6-1). Nursing students were traditionally a homogeneous group—typically single white women, ranging in age from 18 to 35, who graduated in the upper third of their high school classes. Associate degree programs (although they often impose selective admission policies on the "open door" philosophy of the community

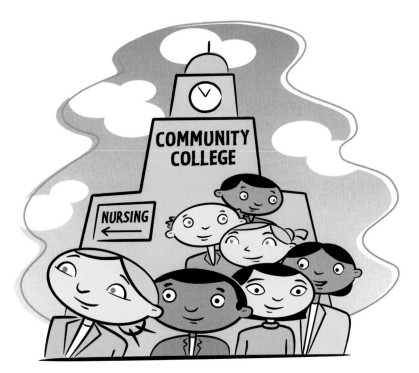

FIGURE 6-1   Associate degree programs attract older people, married women, minorities, men, and students with a wider range of educational experiences and intellectual capabilities.

colleges) attract older people, married women, minorities, men, and students with a wider range of educational experiences and intellectual abilities. People who already possess baccalaureate or higher degrees in other fields sometimes seek admission to an associate degree program, often because it can be completed in a shorter period of time than would be needed to earn another baccalaureate degree.

Concerns Facing Associate Degree Education

Associate degree education, like other educational programs, has experienced change. With these changes have come some concerns.

PRESSURE TO INCREASE CREDITS

As programs have developed, there has been a growing tendency to place more emphasis and time on nursing courses than on general education courses. Faculty members, prepared with master's degrees in nursing, and nursing advisory committee members from service settings have difficulty defining essential content. Faculty members often try to comply with requests from advisory committees for graduates who will need shorter orientation programs, and who will possess greater knowledge in certain specialty areas (eg, coronary care). The 1990 changes in the role of the graduate as defined by the Council of Associate Degree Programs of the National League for Nursing established the need for courses in the curriculum to include management principles and skills. Changes that some colleges have made in the basic requirements for all associate degrees have increased the number of non-nursing credits nursing students must complete; the concept of "core courses" that are taken by all students who graduate from a college has become popular. More content and a greater number of credit hours, selective admission criteria (that give preference to students who have completed general education course work), long waiting lists for entry, and students who cannot attend school on a full-time basis are all factors that have contributed to programs that can take as many as 3 to 5 years to complete, rather then the 2 years originally planned.

The recent shift to **community-based practice** also offers a challenge to associate degree educators. What part of the current curriculum should be cut to provide community experiences? How are community experiences to be supervised? What should be the balance between inpatient care and community experiences? Faculty members who have spent the greater part of their clinical nursing careers in acute care settings are often reluctant to divert even an hour from the time students spent on acute care hospital units.

According to the interpretive guidelines for NLNAC accreditation, the maximum number of credits for an associate degree in nursing is 108 quarter hours or 72 semester hours (NLNAC, 1999). Many schools have struggled to meet this criterion.

THE SELECTIVE ADMISSION PROCESS

Another concern with which educators struggle is the process used in selecting students for a nursing program. This challenge becomes more difficult to meet as the number of students seeking admission either increases dramatically or drops significantly, a phenomenon many programs have experienced during the last 15 to 20 years. As the demographics of students seeking admission become more diverse, the task of bringing to the program students who can realize success in their endeavors represents additional challenges to nursing faculty. In response to this problem, some programs have developed selective admission processes. Although this is common in 4-year schools and colleges, it is a departure from the open-door policy of most community colleges. Some nursing programs use a "waiting list," which honors the concept of "first come, first served." Other schools use systems similar to a lottery. Also popular are "factoring" or "point" systems that award numeric scores for courses completed, past work experience, cumulative grade-point average, or a combination of all of these, with the students acquiring the greatest number of points being selected for the next class. These factoring systems often require that a student spend at least a year in college to secure a position in the beginning nursing class.

MISUNDERSTANDINGS ABOUT ASSOCIATE DEGREE EDUCATION

For many years, associate degree education was poorly understood by employers, the public, and to some extent, nursing educators in baccalaureate and higher degree programs. Although this route to nursing education is now firmly established as credible preparation for a nursing career, it has continued to receive some opposition. The controversy regarding "entry into practice" and the preparation needed for "professional" nursing (which will be discussed later in this chapter) is renewed intermittently, although this issue has lost much of its original passion and dissension because of the nurse shortage that started in the late 1990s and became worse in the early 2000s. Thus, advocates for associate degree education continue to find themselves clarifying facts and emphasizing the contributions made by graduates of the programs.

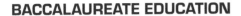

BACCALAUREATE EDUCATION

Baccalaureate degree education is that which occurs in a 4-year college or university. The first school of nursing to be established in a university setting was started at the University of Minnesota in 1909. The program existed as a quasi-autonomous branch of the university's school of medicine. The program was not very different from the 3-year hospital-based program; nothing was required in the way of higher general education, and graduates were prepared for the RN certificate only. Education took place predominantly through apprenticeship, and students provided service to hospitals in exchange for education. However, nursing education did become a part of an academic organization, with 16 colleges and universities having developed programs by 1916.

Many of the early programs offering a baccalaureate degree in nursing extended over a 5-year period. This allowed for 3 years of nursing school curriculum similar to that of the hospital-based programs, and for an additional 2 years of liberal arts. In 1924, the Yale School of Nursing became the first to be established as a separate department within a university; Annie W. Goodrich was its dean. However, the increase in the number of these schools was not rapid.

Although the development of baccalaureate education for nurses may not seem like a major step to young people today, you need to remember that it was not until 1920 that the 19th Amendment to the Constitution of the United States granted women the right to vote. Many people considered nursing to be a less than desirable occupation: vocational in its orientation; overshadowed by militaristic, religious, and technical characteristics; and confined to women. Liberal education, scholarship, and knowledge were thought to be incompatible with the female personality, and capable of interfering with marriage (for many years, nursing students were not allowed to be married). The nursing curriculum, with its emphasis on the performance of skills rather than on the philosophic and theoretic approaches used in the humanities, was not well accepted by universities. Opposition to collegiate education for nurses also came from physicians, who argued that nurses would be "overtrained." Physicians were not certain that a sound knowledge base was as important as the technical skills and manual dexterity that could be acquired with brief training at the bedside. Physicians also argued that a baccalaureate education would make nursing services too expensive.

Many nursing leaders have advocated for baccalaureate education as the minimum educational preparation for supervisory and administrative nursing roles. Baccalaureate education also provides the background needed for public health positions, including school nursing, and the educational base for entry into graduate education in nursing. In 1965, the ANA recommended baccalaureate preparation in nursing as the minimum educational preparation for entry into professional nursing practice, an issue discussed later in this chapter. The American Nurses' Credentialing Center now requires a baccalaureate degree for initial basic certification in a nursing specialty, and requires a master's degree for initial certification as a clinical specialist or nurse practitioner. Those certified before these new requirements took effect are permitted to maintain their certification. Although some of the other nursing specialty organizations that provide certification do not require a baccalaureate degree for certification, that situation also is changing in favor of more education.

Characteristics of Baccalaureate Education

Baccalaureate nursing programs are located in 4-year colleges and universities. A university nursing program is termed a basic or **generic program** when the program of studies includes an upper division (junior and senior years) nursing major that is built onto 2 years of liberal arts and science courses taken during the freshman and sophomore years.

Applicants to such programs must meet the entrance and graduation requirements established by the university, and those of the nursing school. The admission requirements usually specify academic preparation at the high school (or preadmission) level, including courses in foreign language and higher-level mathematics and science, and a high cumulative grade-point average. Relatively high scores on college admission tests also may be required.

During the freshman and sophomore years, students who pursue a nursing education take humanities, social, life, and physical science courses with college students who are preparing for other majors. In some schools, these courses may be completed on a part-time basis; however, this extends the overall course of study beyond 4 years. The number of required liberal arts and science courses may vary from program to program, but usually constitutes about one half the total number of credits specified for graduation—typically 120 semester credits or 180 quarter credits. Students usually begin their study of nursing content in their junior year, thus the term "upper-division major" in nursing. Nursing theory can be taught so that it builds on an understanding of the physical and biologic sciences and liberal arts studied the previous 2 years.

Until the 1980s, most schools offering the baccalaureate degree in nursing required sophomore level nursing courses. Curriculum restructuring and economic pressures gradually led many baccalaureate programs to eliminate sophomore level courses, with all nursing being taught in the last 2 years. More recently, some schools offering a baccalaureate degree in nursing have resumed introducing nursing content in the sophomore year of study. Nursing courses offered at this point often include an overview of the nursing profession and some of the fundamental nursing skills.

Students in baccalaureate nursing programs learn basic nursing skills. They also learn concepts of health maintenance and promotion, and disease prevention; supervisory and leadership techniques and practices are taught, along with an introduction to research. Clinical course work includes experience in public health nursing, community health settings, and leadership responsibility within the acute care hospital. Emphasis is placed on developing skills in critical decision-making, on exercising independent nursing judgments that call for broad background knowledge, and on working in complex nursing situations in which the outcomes are often not predictable. Acting as a client advocate, the graduate with a baccalaureate degree in nursing collaborates with other members of the health care team in structured and unstructured settings, and supervises those with lesser preparation. Baccalaureate graduates often work with groups as well as with individuals. Baccalaureate programs face some of the same pressures faced by associate degree programs with a demand for additional content to be added to an already full curriculum.

Changes in Baccalaureate Education

In recent years, the nature of baccalaureate education has changed. Some schools, seeking to add an advanced component, have included courses that permit a degree of specialization at the baccalaureate level (eg, supplemental courses in coronary or critical care nursing). Other schools are providing more grounding in research, either as preparation for graduate school or for a more varied role in nursing. There is another interesting variation in baccalaureate education in California. In that state, the rules and regulations for schools of nursing stipulate that all courses required by the Board of Nursing for licensure as an RN be offered within the first 36 months of full-time training, the first six academic semesters, or the first nine academic quarters, whichever is shortest (California Board of Registered Nursing, 1994). This means that all educational preparation required for application for licensure in California must be completed by the end of the junior year. The senior year is then open for specialty experience, preceptorships, or whatever a school might deem appropriate education. This variation in the licensure law has caused problems. Some students complete their junior year and successfully pass the licensing examination; these students may elect to drop out of school and work as RNs. Although they are licensed in the state of California in the category of "nongraduate" allowed by that state, these students have no educational credentials. This creates problems if they seek licensure in another state, because all other states (at the present time) require a degree or diploma for licensure. Table 6-1 provides a comparison of the major avenues to RN licensure.

MASTER'S AND DOCTORAL PROGRAMS THAT PREPARE FOR LICENSURE

Our discussion of the various educational programs for registered nursing would be incomplete without mention of the generic master's program. The concept of the master's degree in nursing developed at Yale and several other schools of nursing, where students admitted with a baccalaureate degree in another area were granted a master's degree in nursing after completing an established 2-year program of study that prepared them for RN licensure. Case Western Reserve University initiated the first program in which the student earns a doctorate in nursing (ND) before being eligible to write the licensing examination. Most of the graduates of these programs are engaged in teaching and research.

These programs reflect the thinking of some nursing leaders that the minimum preparation for professional nursing should be the master's degree. These programs also provide a higher degree to those people who possess basic baccalaureate preparation in another area of study and are making a career change. With increasing emphasis on the need for a baccalaureate degree for professional practice, this type of program provides a credible opportunity to those with baccalaureate degrees in another area of study. When programs of this type are not available, many students with degrees in other disciplines choose to pursue a 2-year associate degree in nursing. Even when other options are available, some people with degrees in other disciplines opt for the 2-year degree because it requires less time and expense.

A generic master's degree program or generic doctoral program is not without its problems for the graduate. Although the newly licensed individual is truly a novice in the field, the expectation of most employers is that the graduate degree represents an expert level of

TABLE 6-1.	EDUCATIONAL OPPORTUNITIES FOR REGISTERED NURSING: A COMPARISON		
	DIPLOMA	**ASSOCIATE DEGREE**	**BACCALAUREATE**
Location	Is usually conducted by and based in a hospital	Most often conducted in junior or community colleges, occasionally in senior colleges and universities	Located in senior colleges and universities
Length of study	Requires generally 24–30 months, but may require 3 academic years	Requires usually 2 academic or sometimes 2 calendar years	Requires 4 academic years
Requirements for admission	Requires graduation from high school or its equivalent, satisfactory general academic achievement, and successful completion of certain prerequisite courses	Requires that applicants meet entrance requirements of college as well as of program	Requires that applicants meet entrance requirements of the college or university as well as those of program
Program of learning	Includes courses in theory and practice of nursing and in biologic, physical, and behavioral sciences. May require that certain courses in the physical and social sciences be taken at a local college or university	Combines a balance of nursing courses and college courses in the basic natural and social sciences with courses in general education and the humanities	Frequently concentrates on courses in the theory and practice of nursing in the junior and senior years. Provides education in the theory and practice of nursing and courses in the liberal arts as well as the behavioral and physical sciences.
Clinical Component	Provides early and substantial clinical learning experiences in the hospital and a variety of community agencies; these focus on an understanding of the hospital environment and the interrelationship of other health disciplines	Requires as a significant part of the program supervised clinical instruction in hospitals and other community health agencies	Provides clinical laboratory courses in a variety of settings where health and nursing care are given
Opportunity for Educational Advancement	Little or no transferability of courses unless affiliated with a community college or university	Is structured so that some credits may be applied to baccalaureate degree	Provides the basic academic preparation for advancement to higher positions in nursing and to master's degree
Competency on graduation	Graduate is prepared to plan for the care of patients with other members of the health care team, to develop and carry out plans for the care of individuals or groups of patients, and to	Graduate is prepared to plan and give direct patient care in hospitals, nursing homes, or similar health care agencies, and to participate with other members of the health care team, such as	Graduate is prepared to plan and give direct care to individuals and families, whether sick or well, to assume responsibility for directing other members of the health care team, and to take on

TABLE 6-1.	EDUCATIONAL OPPORTUNITIES FOR REGISTERED NURSING: A COMPARISON (*Continued*)		
	DIPLOMA	**ASSOCIATE DEGREE**	**BACCALAUREATE**
	direct selected members of the nursing team. Has an understanding of the hospital climate and the community health resources necessary for the extended care of patients.	licensed practical nurses, nurses aides, physicians, and other registered nurses, in rendering care to patients.	beginning leadership positions. Practices in a variety of settings and emphasizes comprehensive health care, including preventive and rehabilitative services, health counseling and education, and care in acute and long-term illnesses. Has necessary education for graduate study toward a master's degree and may move rapidly to specialized leadership positions in nursing as teacher, administrator, clinical specialist, nurse practitioner, and nurse researcher.
Licensure	Must successfully complete state licensing examination	Must successfully complete state licensing examination	Must successfully complete state licensing examination

practice. Thus, the graduate must carefully discuss expectations with any employer and clarify his or her own preparation for the role.

SIMILARITIES AMONG ENTRY-LEVEL PROGRAMS

Currently there are as many similarities in the various avenues to nursing education as there are differences. These similarities may be grouped into several broad classifications, including academic standards, administrative concerns, and areas relating to students.

Academic Similarities

In the academic realm, several similarities stand out:

1. All graduates write the NCLEX for registered nursing in their state. All writers must meet the same minimum standardized score to pass the test and become licensed.
2. All schools preparing graduates for RN licensure must meet the criteria established for state board approval.
3. Most schools preparing for RN licensure (both associate degree and baccalaureate degree) have a similar number of credits of *basic* nursing education. Baccalaureate

degree programs add credits for research, community health nursing, and leadership components not taught or not taught in depth in associate degree programs.

4. All faculty are pushed to develop curricula responsive to the needs of today's health care delivery system, which demands greater efficiency, an ability to work in a highly technical environment, knowledge of new protocols, community experiences, and greater responsibility and accountability. A knowledge explosion and the emphasis on evidence-based practice challenges nurse educators to remain current of the newest developments and flexible when it comes to change.

5. All programs are placing a greater emphasis on critical-thinking skills, especially as related to decision making in the clinical area. Much energy is invested in finding the best method(s) to measure such thinking as an outcome of undergraduate education. These activities were accelerated by changing standards for accreditation developed by the National League for Nursing Accreditation Commission in the late 1990s.

6. The recruitment of faculty possessing master's and doctoral degrees is ongoing and critical. Salaries in education have lagged behind those in practice. The graduate with a master's degree can find interesting and challenging positions in hospitals, clinics, and even in private practice, that offer salaries far better than those offered in colleges and universities. More than one third of 4-year nursing schools cite faculty shortage as the primary reason for not accepting more students (NLN, 2002).

7. Members of the faculty are pushed to meet the increasing demands of education, clinical excellence, tenure, and possibly vocational certification or research. The workload and the time invested in performance of professional responsibilities often are greater than for instructors in other disciplines, even though they are considered colleagues in the educational setting.

Administrative Similarities

From an administrative perspective, four similarities are noted among entry-level programs:

1. Adequate financial support is a major concern. All nursing programs are relatively expensive to operate in comparison with other forms of education provided in colleges and universities. Federal and state agencies, as well as colleges and universities, are limiting funding and demanding greater accountability. In tough economic times, the nursing program—like the one at the University of California, Los Angeles (UCLA)—may be the one chosen to be phased out. Less financial assistance is available to students in the form of scholarships and loans than in the past. Tuition costs are rising. Lindeman (2000, p. 5) summarizes the situation ". . . nurse educators will work in a market driven, highly competitive, system of higher education preparing the next generations of nurses to work in a market driven, highly competitive, health care system."

2. Finding appropriate learning experiences is a challenge. Most programs find themselves competing with other schools for learning experiences in clinical agencies. To some extent, this competition is caused by changes in societal values and in the health care delivery system. Families are electing to have fewer children and, more recently in some areas, to deliver these children at home. The result has been fewer clients in the obstetric units of hospitals. Pediatric clients are managed on an

outpatient basis as much as possible, and hospitalization, when required, is kept to a minimum. The management of the client with psychiatric disturbances is moving from institutions to community mental health centers whenever feasible. The increase in the number and size of schools in urban areas creates a high demand for clinical facilities. Finally, there have been changes in the attitudes of the consumer and the agency toward having students provide care. The concept of the "teaching" hospital is not as viable as it once was. Consumers paying for the high cost of care want that care provided by qualified nurses rather than by students who are still learning.

3. Maintaining programs that prepare graduates for current practice. Health care has seen a myriad of changes in the last decade brought forth by technology, demographics, legislation, and other social and political factors. More clients live longer and receive care outside of the traditional acute care facility. Clients in those facilities are more critically ill, recovering from procedures unheard of even 10 years ago. Educators in all types of nursing programs struggle to construct and teach curricula that will prepare the graduate for entry into a profession that practices in a much larger arena, with much more technical equipment, and requiring greater critical thinking skills than ever before.

4. Decisions regarding national accreditation. Many schools wrestle with the decision of whether to seek recognition of their program through national accreditation. Historically, that recognition was granted through the National League for Nursing, which, through its autonomous arm, the NLNAC, still accredits all levels of nursing education programs. In the mid-1990s, the American Association of Colleges of Nursing (AACN) established the Commission on Collegiate Nursing Education (CCNE) as an autonomous arm of the AACN, and officially made its first accreditation visit to a baccalaureate degree program in the fall of 1998. Today, programs located in 4-year colleges and universities must choose from which of these two organizations they wish to seek recognition—a few choose to be accredited by both. At all levels, programs wrestle with the cost and additional work such recognition involves.

Similarities Relating to Students

Three similarities relating to students are noted:

1. Recruitment and selection of students is a major task. All schools must develop sound educational programs, while balancing student enrollments against recruitment and retention factors. In some years, the number of applications significantly exceeds the positions available in beginning classes; at other times, the number of applicants is lower than is desirable. At the same time, schools must be responsive to an increasingly diverse population that, at times, is not prepared for college-level studies. This has resulted in the development of selective admission policies that must be scrutinized carefully by school officials, and, in some areas, reviewed by the school's attorney for correct legal form and legal ramifications, before being accepted by the school's policy-making group. As nursing enrollments have declined, more time is involved in recruiting efforts.

2. Legal concerns are demanding more time and attention. Programs are caught up in more legal concerns than in the past, because applicants and students are seeking their "rights as individuals" and challenging admission, progression, and dismissal policies. The National Student Nursing Association Student Bill of Rights and Responsibilities is widely accepted by schools of nursing in the United States. It sets forth the students' basic rights and establishes grievance procedures if a student believes that these rights have been violated (see Chapter 3). Another legal concern relates to malpractice coverage for students. Some collegiate programs, now removed from the umbrella coverage of the hospital, ask that students purchase malpractice insurance as protection against any lawsuits that might arise as the result of errors committed in the learning process.

3. There is greater diversity in the student body. All programs are finding more diversity in the characteristics of applicants seeking admission. Programs are receiving more applications from men, minorities, older adults, and persons who possess degrees in other fields of study. Students with English as a second language present new challenges to nursing faculty in all types of programs. Special courses and other forms of assistance are being developed to enable students with academic challenges to succeed in nursing. One usually finds nursing educators united in their efforts to create quality programs that will graduate students who can function satisfactorily in a changing and challenging health care delivery system (see Table 6-1).

Critical Thinking Activity

Imagine that you could restructure nursing education for an ideal world. Where would you begin? How many levels of nursing education would you incorporate into your model? Would each level be terminal or articulated with others? Where would general education fit into your model? How would you see the graduate of each program functioning on the health care team? How would you see each level reimbursed for services?

OTHER FORMS OF NURSING EDUCATION

A number of factors have fostered the development of other forms of education for nurses. Most of these are seen in the expansion of higher educational offerings, due in part to the changing role of the nurse in health care delivery, and the need this creates for more adequate education to meet the requirements of that role. Another contributing aspect is the continuing push to make nursing truly professional. To increase nursing's professional component, there is a need for nurses who are interested and competent in research techniques and skills. A third significant reason for advancing nursing education relates to the need for leadership in nursing administration and education. Nurse educators, joining the ranks of other professionals in the academic environment, are required to possess equivalent educational backgrounds. Nurses who assume roles in nursing administration have found the need for a solid understanding of management and finance. Thus, RNs seek baccalaureate, master's, and doctoral degrees to support the complex roles into which they move.

Registered Nurse Baccalaureate Programs

During the last decade, there has been a constant increase in the number of nurses completing a baccalaureate degree through a **registered nurse baccalaureate** (RNB) **program.** These programs are designed for the RN, with either a diploma or an associate degree, who wishes to return to school to complete a baccalaureate degree in nursing. There are also master's degree programs that admit RNs with associate degrees who, after 3 years, graduate with a master's degree in nursing, receiving a baccalaureate degree partway through the program. Still other master's degree programs in nursing admit RNs with associate degrees in nursing and a baccalaureate degree in another field (see discussion below). Some schools also have added programs designed to admit the licensed practical (vocational) nurse, who will emerge with a baccalaureate degree in nursing. These programs carry different names in different parts of the country, including baccalaureate registered nurse (BRN) programs, two-on-two programs, and, in the Midwest, capstone programs.

There are many reasons for the increase in this form of nursing education, several of which were discussed above. In addition, many highly qualified young men and women enter associate degree programs because of cost and time factors and plan for more education several years after completing the original program. The nursing profession is endeavoring to increase the number of nurses prepared with baccalaureate and higher degrees.

The RNB programs vary greatly throughout the United States. In some instances, they exist in universities that already offer the generic baccalaureate program. The students may be completely integrated with generic baccalaureate students, partially separated from them, or in a totally separate program. Another form of RNB preparation is the two-on-two approach, in which RN students transfer into the college or university with junior standing and complete an additional 2 years of upper-division nursing classes. In some instances, this is the only nursing program offered by a college or university; that is, the college may not offer a basic program that prepares a graduate for licensure. Some schools offer nurse practitioner preparation in conjunction with the baccalaureate degree, although the current trend is to place this at the master's level.

Another general trend is to allow the transfer of credits in the natural and biologic sciences, and in basic courses such as psychology and sociology earned at junior and community colleges. Often, some transfer of credit is allowed for nursing courses (eg, 45 quarter credits or 30 semester credits), but the courses may be challenged by examination. Distribution requirements of the particular college or university must be satisfied, and upper-division nursing courses must be completed in such areas as physiologic nursing, community health, understanding nursing research, and supervision. A minimum of 2 years usually is required for completion of the program, although the time may be shorter or longer, depending on the number of requirements satisfied at the time of entry.

Some nurse educators criticized programs offering baccalaureate education to RNs when they were first launched; the ladder concept in nursing education was slow to develop. Three major issues were present.

1. Many nurse educators perceived associate degree education as technical in nature and therefore terminal (ending at the associate degree level), and did not accept it as a stepping stone to baccalaureate education.

2. There were problems associated with evaluating credits earned at lower-division level and equating them with upper-division course. How did nursing process taught at the Nursing 100 level correspond to similar content taught at the Nursing 300 level?

3. Decisions had to be made to determine whether additional courses designed specifically for the RN should be offered. What additional nursing courses were needed to form the upper-division major in nursing that would provide a foundation for graduate education? How was this student the same and how was this student different from the generic student?

Because the skills of the various graduates were not clearly delineated, it was difficult to develop a curriculum that would enable the RNB graduate to demonstrate specific outcome behaviors. When attempts were made to develop such programs, baccalaureate educators were confronted with another concern: they were working with adult students. This required them to rethink teaching and learning principles to provide effective education. Students were seeking a learning program that allowed for part-time study, provided more evening and weekend classes, and permitted part- or full-time employment—in other words, a program tailored to their life circumstances.

Today, RNB education and two-on-two educational programs flourish; schools with both generic and RNB programs may report more graduates from the RNB program than from the generic. At least four factors are responsible for the change in attitude toward RNB education. First, the ANA Commission on Nursing Education has provided a push to increase the availability of baccalaureate programs for RNs. Nursing educators are challenged to create and accept more innovative educational strategies.

The second factor comes from pressure within each state itself. Several states have enacted legislation, sometimes in response to the nursing shortage, that requires the development of a statewide plan for articulation between various types of nursing education programs. In most instances, the legislation establishes a date by which the plan will be implemented.

The third factor influencing the development of RNB programs has been a call for increased educational mobility from organizations in the health care arena. The American Medical Association (AMA) House of Delegates has suggested career mobility as one way to alleviate the nurse shortage. The Pew Commission recommended strengthening existing career ladder programs to make movement through these levels of nursing as easy as possible (de Tornyay, 1996). Some of the RNB programs currently in operation provide for part-time study or for studies completed through evening courses. The desirability of such approaches for nurses who must work to support their education is obvious. Other innovative RNB programs provide baccalaureate education to people living in areas geographically remote from colleges or universities. These programs use new technologies for distance learning, including the electronic transmission of information.

A final factor influencing the development of RNB programs relates to the allocation of federal dollars to assist students who are seeking to advance their preparation in nursing. Many of the scholarships and traineeships, once available to all students, have been directed largely to students who wish to continue their education in the area of advanced practice in nursing. Major nursing groups such as the ANA and the National League for Nursing (NLN) currently are lobbying Congress for additional funds directed toward nursing education including the creation of grants to provide scholarships to assist disadvantaged students and individuals entering or seeking advanced education in nursing.

The External Degree

The concept of an **external degree** is not new. Universities in Australia, the Soviet Union, and England have long recognized independent study validated by examination. The University of London has awarded college degrees earned in this fashion since 1836. The major difference between the external degree and the traditional educational experience is that students awarded an external degree are not required to attend classes or follow any prescribed methods of learning (however, they may choose to take some classes). Learning is assessed through highly standardized and validated examinations. This approach to education was not developed in the United States until about the mid-1950s, and then only in selected areas. New York's Empire State College and the University Without Walls consortium were the first schools in the United States to recognize the value of self-directed learning.

Now known as Excelsior University, the New York Regents External Degree (REX) Program of the University of the State of New York has become part of this movement. The New York Board of Regents established the College Proficiency Examination Program in 1961. Similar to the College-Level Examination Program tests developed by the Educational Testing Service, the examinations allow students to gain credit and meet the University's requirements without attending classes.

In 1971, the New York Board of Regents authorized an external associate degree program in nursing; the external baccalaureate degree in nursing was to follow in April 1976, with the first baccalaureate degrees awarded in 1979. The W. K. Kellogg Foundation provided funds to support the initiation of the program. The programs have grown in popularity.

The nursing program, like other external degree programs in arts, science, and business, uses an assessment approach and is primarily—although not exclusively—designed for those with some experience in nursing. It is philosophically based on principles of adult learning, which advocate flexible and learner-oriented education. Specifically, the responsibility for demonstrating that learning has occurred is placed on the student, and the responsibility for identifying the content to be learned and objectively assessing that this has occurred rests with the faculty. The nursing major is divided into cognitive and performance components. Cognitive learning is documented through nationally standardized and psychometrically valid written examinations. Clinical skills are evaluated through four criteria-referenced performance examinations at regional performance assessment centers throughout the country.

Despite objections, alternative and nontraditional avenues to nursing education appeal to the learner, and these programs continue to evolve. Nursing education, like nursing care, should be tailored to fit the consumer's needs. There are some limitations on the use of external degree programs. Some states do not accept New York Regents' degrees for initial licensure because their laws mandate that the educational process include supervised clinical practice. Some states will admit to the licensure examination for RNs only those external associate degree graduates who were LPNs and therefore have had supervised clinical practice in addition to clinical examinations.

NURSING EDUCATION AT THE GRADUATE LEVEL

The critical need for nurses with additional preparation to work in educational settings, in supervisory roles, as clinical specialists, and to fulfill the expanded role of the nurse has resulted in more programs at the graduate level.

Master's Preparation

There are a variety of models of master's preparation in nursing. Some less traditional approaches include outreach programs; summers-only programs; RN-to-MSN tracks (that provide a direct route to the master's degree for RNs who have graduated from diploma or associate degree programs); programs for students with special needs (such as RNs with non-nursing baccalaureate degrees); and programs that admit non-nurses and foreign graduates. Some schools offer off-campus classes, at times rotating sites, and some deliver core content by way of television or through other distance-learning technology. In at least one school, all classes are on Fridays. Several unique programs (eg, those at Yale University, Pace University, and the University of Tennessee at Knoxville) offer a master's degree in nursing after completion of a baccalaureate degree in another field. Such programs, called generic master's degree programs, were discussed earlier in the chapter.

Most programs require at least a full year for completion; many have been expanded to 2 years. Master's programs in nursing typically are found in senior colleges and universities that have baccalaureate programs in nursing. They have the option of seeking voluntary accreditation from the NLNAC or from the CCNE.

Doctoral Studies

The number of requests for admission to doctoral study in nursing has increased greatly since the early 1980s. The impetus for this movement stems from the need for advanced study for academic advancement or tenure in the educational setting, and reflects the need in nursing research for the advancement of the profession as a whole.

Before doctorates in nursing were offered, doctoral study in other fields allowed nurses to benefit from post-master's preparation. A doctorate outside the area of nursing was often the only doctorate available to persons seeking further education; doctorates in nursing are relatively new to the educational milieu, as opposed to such degrees in psychology, sociology, anthropology, or physiology. Certainly nursing can and has benefited from other disciplines.

Doctoral programs in nursing offer various degrees, such as the doctor of nursing science (DNSc), the doctor of science in nursing (DSN), the doctor of nursing education (DNEd), and the doctor of philosophy (PhD) in nursing. Other types of doctorates are available to nurses, such as the doctor of education (EdD) and the doctor of public health (DPH).

The difference in the preparation and function of graduates possessing the various degrees is confusing; typically, the nurse with a doctorate assumes a leadership role in education, often serving as a faculty member or the dean or director of a nursing program. These nurses also may choose to be involved in the research and development of a body of nursing knowledge.

Critical Thinking Activity

If nurse practitioners are to work in a collaborative way with physicians, and as primary care providers, what type and level of education do you believe they should complete? How would you ensure that this would occur? What standards regarding continuing education should be mandated for those involved in advance practice? Should it be more stringent than that required at the RN level? Defend your position.

ARTICULATED PROGRAMS

Today, as increasing numbers of graduates seek additional education beyond the associate degree or diploma, the "ladder" concept in nursing education is growing in popularity. This has resulted in more RN baccalaureate and "two-on-two" programs. Programs have been developed that provide direct **articulation** between lower-level and higher-level programs. As mentioned earlier, in some states legislation has been passed strongly encouraging, and in some instances mandating, articulation plans.

The purpose of an articulated program is to facilitate opportunities for students to start nursing education, stop when some goal is achieved, or keep moving up the educational ladder. Statewide articulation plans exist in several states. Many of the plans allow most of the work completed at the lower level to meet the requirements of the baccalaureate degree. Some schools, such as the University of Washington, have formalized RN-to-master's pathways.

Similar plans exist for articulation between practical (vocational) nurse programs and associate degree programs and some programs allow credit for nurse assistant preparation or require it for admission. Again, the articulated program allows students to move up the career ladder from practical nurse to associate degree nurse, to the nurse with a baccalaureate degree. Students in an articulated licensed practical nurse/associate degree program spend a year preparing to be an LP(V)N, and another year completing the associate degree. If they want to continue after this 2-year period, they can earn a baccalaureate degree at another institution after 2 more years of study. Some schools have established LPN-to-Baccalaureate Degree programs. From that point, a student may continue to work toward a master's degree (Fig. 6-2).

The multiple-entry, multiple-exit programs are not without problems. Initially, they are difficult to develop because of the tremendous amount of joint planning required. Questions arose regarding granting upper-degree credit (course work with 300 and 400 numbers) for studies completed with 100 and 200 numbers in the community college. Understanding what has been taught and determining how to evaluate current knowledge is important. This is particularly relevant to articulation between practical nurse programs and RN programs, where graduates of the practical program may know how to perform many of the nursing skills but may lack the theory base of RNs. Educators need to speak the same language and develop mutual respect.

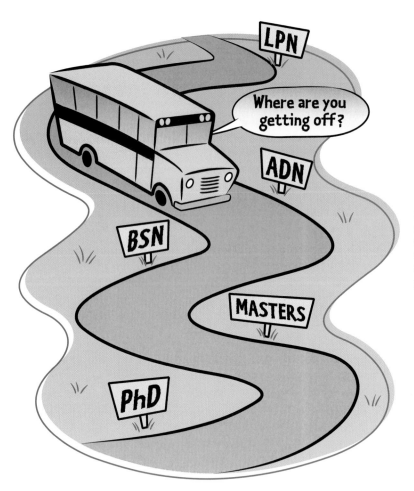

FIGURE 6-2 Among innovations occurring in nursing education over the past decade are programs that provide direct articulation between lower-level and higher-level programs.

NONDEGREE PROGRAMS

Specialized programs have been developed to help individuals prepare for roles of increased breadth and scope. Some programs are incorporated into the preparation leading to a particular degree; others exist as part of a school's continuing education program.

The RN anesthesia and midwifery programs both award a certificate after completion of a standardized and rigorous course of study, lasting from 18 months to 2 years. At one time, admission requirements stipulated licensure only; however, the trend is toward making a baccalaureate degree in nursing an admission requirement, and toward awarding a master's degree on completion of the program. Some states require a master's degree for the nurse anesthetist or nurse midwife.

More recent programs offer nurse practitioner and nursing specialist preparation in areas of nursing practice such as pediatrics, gerontology, family health, genetics, and women's health care. Recent health care reform has resulted in an increased emphasis on the role of **advanced nursing practice** in health care delivery, and more demand for educational programs to prepare these practitioners. The Pew Commission has encouraged the growing number of master's level nurse practitioner training programs (de Tornyay, 1996). Programs that prepare nurse practitioners concentrate study in specific areas during a period lasting from several months to a year or more. Requirements for admission vary tremendously. Most require licensure and a baccalaureate degree, and still others require that the education occur at the post-master's degree level. The American Nurses' Credentialing Center requires the master's degree for all those seeking initial nurse practitioner certification, and some states now require the master's degree for those seeking initial licensure as a nurse practitioner.

The proliferation of such programs has been so great that a complete listing is impossible. A student interested in pursuing such preparation is encouraged to write to the college or university of choice for information about available programs.

RESIDENCIES AND STRUCTURED ORIENTATION FOR THE NEW GRADUATE

When nursing education moved from hospital-based diploma programs into higher education, a new problem was created. Employers of the new graduates, who expected these graduates to function as experienced and qualified professionals on the day after graduation, complained that the graduates were not prepared to assume staff nurse positions within their institutions.

As nursing education moved into institutions of higher education, all clinical time was recognized in credit hours. If students worked on hospital units on weekends, they did so as hospital employees, not as a requirement of their education. As a result, students spent less time in the clinical area. Many graduates of diploma schools in the 1950s would have had as much as 4000 clock hours of clinical experience, albeit more as apprenticeship and service to the hospital than as a learning experience. Graduates of associate and baccalaureate degree programs, with integrated curricula and objective-based learning experiences, joined the work world with clinical learning time of 800 or fewer clock hours. Hospital-based programs also decreased their clinical hours as curricula were reorganized. Students in all programs now receive their clinical experience in a variety of settings as opposed to one primary health care facility where they become very familiar with policies, procedures and physical plant.

All of this has resulted in individuals graduating today needing orientation to the work facility and to their new role, and time to become efficient in using their newly learned skills. Although few would question the need for internships and residencies for new physicians, the need for similar experiences for new nursing graduates has not been readily accepted. The new graduates, unable to live up to expectations placed on them, often became frustrated and discouraged; some opted for less stressful situations, sometimes even outside nursing. Nursing educators, in defending the education provided, cited other professions, such as law and engineering, in which graduates needed time to adapt to the world of work.

As a result of efforts to address this concern, orientation programs, **internships, and residencies** for new graduates were instituted by hospitals. The programs were intended to ease the transition from the role of student to that of staff by providing the opportunity to increase clinical skills and knowledge, as well as self-confidence. These programs can last from several weeks to a year, and are designed for graduates of all nursing programs—associate degree, diploma, and baccalaureate. They often include rotations to various units in the hospital, including specialty areas, and they accommodate different shifts. Usually, some formal class work is associated with the experience, but the majority of the time is spent in direct patient care, often under the supervision of a preceptor.

Institutions receive some direct benefits from such programs in addition to securing a better-prepared employee, who remains in employment. Inadequacies in policy and procedure books have been uncovered and, as a result, these books have been rewritten. Performance evaluation tools that are more objective in format have emerged. Nursing practice throughout some agencies has become more standardized. Job satisfaction has increased. It is no longer unusual for hospitals to advertise planned orientation and internships as benefits offered to the new graduate seeking employment, a strong recruitment tool in times of nurse shortages.

The major disadvantage voiced by hospitals is the cost of operating such programs. When cost containment is crucial, hospitals are not anxious to deal with the additional costs of such programs. Another problem is that some employees who benefit from such programs may resign from their positions soon after completing an internship. This has resulted in hospitals stipulating a period of required employment following the orientation or internship.

FACTORS INFLUENCING NURSING EDUCATION

During the 20th century, society experienced tremendous change. Nursing, as a part of that society, has also experienced enormous change. A number of factors influenced nursing education.

The Brown Report

In 1948, Esther Lucille Brown, who was not a nurse (see Chapter 5), conducted one of the important early studies of nursing. She was concerned that young women were not choosing nursing as a profession, and believed, as a result of her study, that the majority of nursing schools failed to provide a professional education. In "Nursing for the Future," Brown (1948) recommended that nursing education move away from the system of apprenticeship that predominated at the time (see earlier discussion of hospital-based programs in Chapter 4), and move toward a planned program of education similar to that offered by other professions. She recommended that the schools be operated by universities or colleges, hospitals affiliated with institutions of higher learning, medical colleges, or independently. She also recommended that programs periodically be examined or reviewed, and that a list of accredited schools be published and distributed.

The Brown report attracted the attention of many nursing leaders, who shared her concerns about recruiting qualified women into nursing. The study took place shortly after World War II, and nurses who had been involved in the military had a new sense of autonomy and independence that they were not willing to leave behind. Committees were formed to respond to the suggestions put forth in the Brown study, particularly those related to the accreditation of programs. At the same time, the National League for Nursing Education (NLNE), later to become the National League for Nursing (NLN), recommended that hospital schools of nursing consider transferring control and administration of their programs to educational institutions. The NLNE also urged that federal grants be provided to nursing schools to allow for their improvement.

Development of the State Board Test Pool Examination

Along with the push for the improvement of nursing education, licensing authorities were pressured to establish a uniform licensing examination (see Chapter 7). The development of the State Board Test Pool Examination helped all schools to focus on common goals and laid the foundation for interstate endorsement of licenses.

National Accreditation of Nursing Programs

By 1952, the NLN had a temporary accreditation program in place, and was helping schools to find ways to improve their programs of instruction. The **accreditation** of programs had a noticeable effect on standards of nursing education. As a result of accreditation activities, schools were forced to look at the educational preparation of faculty, the workload of faculty and students, the structure of clinical teaching, withdrawal rates, and the state board examination scores. This system of program assessment enhanced the quality of education; graduation from a nationally accredited school meant added opportunities for advanced education or certain types of employment.

Changes in Nursing Service

While changes were occurring in the education of nurses, nurses in the workplace also experienced significant changes. With the advent of antibiotics and other major advances in medical protocols and medical technology during the mid 1900s, the public was receiving care in hospitals rather than treatment in the home. Births that previously took place at home now occurred in hospitals. Federal funds were allocated for the construction of hospitals. Increased hospitalization drove the need for qualified nurses to a new high. Hospitals were desperate to find nurses to fill needed positions, and nurses represented half of all hospital personnel.

The role of the nurse changed in response to changes in the workplace. Nursing staff began assuming responsibilities formerly associated with physicians. Unfortunately, they were also assuming responsibilities that could have been assumed by housekeeping, dietary, laboratory, and pharmacy departments. Nurses began spending more time managing personnel, delegating responsibilities, and carrying out other administrative duties. Nurses at higher levels in the organization needed higher levels of education (ie, baccalaureate and master's degrees).

The Report of the Surgeon General's Consultant Group

In 1961, the Surgeon General of the U.S. Public Health Service appointed a group to advise him of the federal government's role in providing adequate nursing services to the country. This group was known as the Surgeon General's Consultant Group on Nursing, and they published their report in 1963.

The report emphasized the need for more nurses, and identified the lack of adequate financial resources for nursing education as a major problem. Several other major concerns also were reported. Of critical importance were the reports that too few schools were providing adequate nursing education, that too few college-bound young people were being recruited into the profession, and that more nursing schools were needed in colleges and universities. (By now you are recognizing this as a recurrent theme regarding nursing.) Educational preparation at the baccalaureate degree level was recommended as the minimum preparation for nurses assuming leadership roles (U.S. Public Health Service, 1963).

The Surgeon General's Consultant Group on Nursing also recommended that federally funded low-cost loans and scholarships be made available to students in both professional and practical nursing programs. It advocated the use of federal funds to construct additional nursing school facilities and to expand educational programs. The Nurse Training Act of 1964 was an outgrowth of these recommendations.

THE AMERICAN NURSES ASSOCIATION POSITION PAPER

In the early 1960s, the educational preparation of nurses became a major concern of the ANA. The ANA believed that the improvement of nursing practice and the profession as a whole depended on the advancement of nursing education. After studying the issue for 3 years "A Position Paper on Educational Preparation for Nurse Practitioners and Assistants to Nurses" was published in December, 1965. It resulted in the **entry into practice** controversy.

The **Position Paper** took four major positions:

1. The education of all those who are licensed to practice nursing should take place in institutions of higher education.
2. Minimum preparation for beginning professional nursing practice at the present time should be baccalaureate degree education in nursing.
3. Minimum preparation for beginning technical nursing practice at the present time should be associate degree education in nursing.
4. Education for assistants in the health service occupations should be short, intensive pre-service programs in vocational education institutions, rather than on-the-job training programs (ANA, 1965, p. 107).

No other single action or position has affected nursing more or has there been any issue that has been more devisive than the ANA position paper. Gosnell (2002) states, "Overall, entry into practice has been one of the most contentious issues in all of nursing." For almost 40 years, the profession has been plagued with the issues it brought forth. A basic concern related to the fact that the roles, functions, and responsibilities (competencies) of programs offering three different routes to preparation for registered nursing were not clearly differentiated for graduates. All graduates took the same examination and performed similar activities when hired as new graduates in acute care facilities. That situation has not changed since the publication of the position paper.

Associate degree nursing programs in community colleges and hospital-based diploma programs took serious exception to the paper. To this group, not being considered "professional" was unacceptable and they were unwilling to compromise title or licensure. As a result, many individuals associated with these two groups dropped their membership in ANA because they could not support this position.

Because of the dissension the position paper created among nursing groups, little immediate action followed. However, groups slowly began to take action regarding the paper, with many nursing organizations supporting the position.

In an August 1986 meeting, representatives of the National Council of State Boards of Nursing (NCSBN) and the National Federation of Licensed Practical Nurses (NFLPN) voted without debate or opposition to take a "formal position of neutrality on changes in nursing education requirement for entry" (Hartung, 1986, p. 124). To date, the NCSBN has maintained that position; however, in August 1984, the membership of the NFLPN voted to support increasing the period of study in the practical nurse program to 18 months, and to support awarding an associate degree at the completion of the program of study. To date, only North Dakota has implemented these NFLPN recommendations.

Problems Associated With Changing Educational Requirements for Licensure

Several problems are associated with making any changes in educational requirements for licensure. Four major problems are related to titling, scope of practice, grandfathering, and interstate endorsement.

TITLING

One of the most controversial problems associated with changing requirements for licensure involves **titling,** or the use of titles. The RN title has a long history and is clearly recognizable to the public and to the health care community. Some states advocated using "RN" for the baccalaureate graduate and "LPN" for the 2-year associate degree graduate. Needless to say, this is unacceptable to associate degree graduates and students, who currently use the RN title if successful on state licensing examinations. It is also upsetting to graduates of current diploma schools, from which no degree is granted. They feel their contribution is being ignored. Others have suggested that the graduates of 2-year programs be titled "associate nurse" or "registered associate nurse." When a tertiary care hospital in South Dakota implemented differentiated nursing practice, the terms "associate nurse" for the associate degree graduate and "primary nurse" for the baccalaureate graduate were used. This approach again overlooks the diploma graduate. It is not likely that this issue can be resolved easily even as we make strong efforts to move toward differentiated practice (discussed later in this chapter).

SCOPE OF PRACTICE

Of equal concern is the description and delineation of the **scope of practice** for the two levels of caregivers. The scope of practice (discussed in Chapter 7) is that section of the Nurse Practice Act that outlines the activities a person with a particular license may legally perform. This would mean the separate testing of each level as currently exists between the RN and the practical nurse licensure examination. This problem might be of less concern if the nursing profession could agree on an approach to differentiated practice. As some states have moved toward plans for two levels of practice, the process of making nursing diagnoses and developing nursing care plans sometimes has been included in the scope of practice of the baccalaureate-prepared nurse only, a position totally unacceptable to associate degree advocates. Again, the diploma graduate is left out of the discussion.

THE GRANDFATHER CLAUSE

The application of the **grandfather clause** presents another challenge to nurses. Traditionally, when a state licensure law is enacted, or if a current law is repealed and a new law enacted, the grandfather clause has been a standard feature that allows persons to continue to practice their profession or occupation after new qualifications have been enacted into law. The legal basis for the process is found in the 14th Amendment to the U.S. Constitution, which says that no state may deprive any person of life, liberty, or property without due process of law. The Supreme Court has ruled that the license to practice is a property right. The grandfather clause has been used in nursing at various times in the past. For example, when psychiatric nursing became a requirement of all programs, nurses who graduated and were licensed without psychiatric nursing experiences were "grandfathered" into the new role. In other words, they continued to practice as RNs without taking a formal course in psychiatric nursing, and without being required to write a psychiatric examination to maintain their licenses. If nursing began to require a baccalaureate degree for individuals using the RN title, under the provisions of the grandfather clause, all associate graduates licensed before the implementation date for the change would continue to use the title "registered nurse." Those licensed after the change would use whatever new title was established. Although this serves to "protect" the title of currently licensed nurses, it does not prevent employers from writing job descriptions stipulating a baccalaureate degree as the minimum educational preparation acceptable for a particular position.

Complicating this matter is the fact that some nurses believe the grandfather clause should be conditional. If it were conditional, nurses licensed before the changes in the licensure law would continue to use their current title for a stipulated period of time—for example, 10 years. At the end of that period, if they had not completed the education mandated in the changes (or any other conditions that might have been added), they would have to use the title stipulated in the new law for nurses with their educational preparation. Because of the complexity and the difficulties associated with implementation, it is unlikely that conditional "grandfathering" will ever become a reality.

INTERSTATE ENDORSEMENT

A fourth concern is that of **interstate endorsement**. Nursing is one of the few professions to have developed a process whereby national examinations with standardized scores are administered in each state or jurisdiction, thus allowing a nurse who has passed the licensing examination in one state to move to another state and seek licensure without the need to retake and pass another examination. (However, with few exceptions, they do need to secure licensure in each state in which they practice.) Because nurses have been highly mobile, this has been a great advantage. As the profession examines multistate licensure, this issue takes on new dimensions. Issues related to interstate endorsement are discussed in greater detail in Chapter 7.

The Position Paper and Nursing Today

Because the initial thinking and work on the Position Paper occurred 40 years ago, nursing leaders are raising questions about its relevancy today. Gosnell (2002) points to differences in practice demographics, stating that in the early 60s, 75% of all nurses were educated in diploma schools of nursing, that 16% came from baccalaureate programs, and that associate degree nursing was in its infancy. By the year 2000, diploma programs had dramatically declined to just 6%, baccalaureate programs had doubled to 30%, and associate degree programs had risen to produce nearly 60% of all new graduates. Certainly the goal to place nursing in institutions of higher education was being realized but two thirds of the graduates possess less than a baccalaureate education, resulting in nurses being the least educated of all health professionals. Nelson (2002, p. 5) emphasizes that nursing exists in a climate in which "strong cooperative relationships and interdisciplinary teamwork are becoming increasingly important in delivering health care," and that a baccalaureate is essential if nurses are to maintain equal status with other health care professionals. Supporting the baccalaureate for entry, Nelson (2002, pp. 5–6) would "end licensure at the associate degree and diploma levels."

A different position has now been taken by the American Association of Colleges of Nursing (an organization of baccalaureate and higher degree nursing programs). Their Web site (*http://www.aacn.nche.edu/*) clearly states that they do not advocate changing licensure for associate degree nurses. They recognize the valuable role of associate degree nurses in health care and encourage articulation and continued education. They do support the baccalaureate degree as entry into "for what the organization holds to be professional-level nursing practice."

Donley and Flaherty (2002, p 8) observe that, "Under-educated members of the health team rarely sit at policy tables or are invited to participate as members of governing boards. Consequently, there is little opportunity for the majority of practicing nurses to engage in clinical or health care policy." They advocate a second position on education for nurses "that is grounded in the human, clinical, and professional realities of the twenty-first century."

Recognizing that any progress toward educational standardization or upgrading could jeopardize a substantial workforce for the health care industry, Joel (2002, pp. 4–5) points to the changed scope of nursing practice, the intellectual growth of the discipline, and the increased demands of the service environment and recommends "a longer and more demanding education than the baccalaureate degree."

At the Spring 2000 meeting, the ANA Board of Directors reaffirmed the long-standing position that baccalaureate education should be the standard for entry into professional nursing practice. Just prior to that decision, the American Nurses Credentialing Center (ANCC) decided to offer a new certification examination for nurses who hold a bachelor's of science in nursing and to offer the current exams to nurses with diplomas or associate degrees ("ANA Reaffirms . . .", 2000).

As some nursing groups set 2010 as the target year for requiring the baccalaureate in nursing as the educational preparation for entry into practice as an RN (Barter & McFarland, 2001), it becomes clear that this contentious issue is not one of the past but, rather, is one with which the nurses of tomorrow will continue to grapple.

Critical Thinking Activity

Take a stand on the ANA Position on Nursing Education. Provide a rationale for the position you have taken. What do you see as the outcome of the position paper? How would your position be implemented in the future? What implications might it have for nursing practice? Do you believe the salaries of nurses educated at different levels and practicing at differentiated levels should differ? Why or why not? If so, how?

DIFFERENTIATED PRACTICE

In the beginning of the 1990s, some nursing leaders began to reassess the entry-into-practice issue. Although the nursing shortage of the late 1980s and the push toward cost cutting in the 1990s may have encouraged its reevaluation, the review also may reflect a new thinking regarding the role of nurses and nursing and the role of all education in the United States. Many nursing leaders encouraged recognition of the need for different types of practitioners, prepared with different types of education, or differentiated practice. **Differentiated nursing practice** can be defined as "the practice of structuring nursing roles on the basis of education, experience, and competence" (Boston, 1990, p. 2).

Today, many groups support the concept of differentiated practice. The report of the Pew Commission (1995) advised that nursing distinguish between the different levels of nursing. The Commission recommended associate degree preparation for the entry-level hospital set-ting and nursing home practice, baccalaureate degree preparation for hospital-based care management and community-based practice, and master's degree preparation for specialty practice in the hospital and independent practice as a primary provider. The National Com-mission Nursing Implementation Project (NCNIP) also strongly supported differentiated practice.

The American Association of Colleges of Nursing and the American Organization of Nurse Executives established a Task Force on Differentiated Competencies for Nursing Practice funded by the Robert Wood Johnson Foundation. This group was later expanded to include representatives from The National Organization for Associate Degree Nursing. A joint publication of these three organizations, titled *A Model for Differentiated Nursing Practice*, is available at *www.aacn.nche.edu* (click on publications). It recognizes that nurses with differing educational preparation bring different capabilities to the patient care system.

Competency Expectations and Differentiated Practice

The task of describing and differentiating the **competencies** and the scope of practice of nurses graduating from various types of programs is one of the major challenges facing nurs-ing today. As stated earlier, graduates of baccalaureate nursing programs, associate degree programs, and hospital-based programs all write the same licensing examination, designed to assure minimum safe practice. This approach fails to recognize the broad range of functions in nursing, and the potential for improving the quality of care given, if different roles and responsibilities were identified. In the work environment of acute and long-term care facili-ties, little differentiation exists in beginning staff nurse positions.

If developed and implemented, realistic statements about competencies of each level or category of nursing education will facilitate the effective and efficient use of each category of graduate within the health care delivery system. Validated competencies also will provide a basis for the development of curriculum patterns to ensure adequate preparation of each cate-gory of caregiver, without running the risk of overeducating or undereducating at any one level.

The competencies also can serve as a foundation for educational mobility patterns in the profession, job descriptions in the health care system, and responsive reimbursement packages.

The Work of Organizations in Defining Competencies

Some work has been done toward describing the competencies of graduates of different programs in nursing. The Council of Associate Degree Programs revised a 1990 publication of the NLN titled "Educational Outcomes of Associate Degree Nursing Programs: Roles and Competencies," which was a revision of an earlier 1978 statement. The revision condensed what were previously five roles into three: Role as Provider of Care, Role as Manager of Care, and Role as Member within the Discipline of Nursing (NLN, 1990). The "Characteristics of Baccalaureate Education in Nursing," revised by the Council of Baccalaureate and Higher Degrees of NLN in 1994, accomplishes a similar purpose for baccalaureate education. Similarly, the Council of Diploma Programs and the Council of Practical Programs of NLN have developed competencies for graduates. (Since 1999 all the educational councils of NLN have been merged into one group.)

Since 1986, and every 3 years following that, the National Council of State Boards of Nursing has conducted several studies aimed at role delineation and job analysis of entry-level RNs. The purpose of these studies is to validate the NCLEX-RN. During 1997, the National Council developed a protocol for conducting a study to identify similarities and differences in the practice of all levels of licensed nurses within and across employment settings; they conducted the study in 1998 (National Council, 1998). In 1999 they published the *Role Delineation Study,* which describes the similarities and differences in the roles of nurse aides, licensed practical/vocational nurses, RNs, and advanced practice nurses.

Some of the most recent work related to defining competencies has come from the Pew Health Professions Commission's Final Report. The fourth report, which continued the theme of reforming health professions, addressed skills needed to function in health care in the 21st century. Twenty-one competencies were identified as critical to practice (Display 6-2) (Bellack & O'Neil, 2000).

Special Projects to Differentiate Practice

Several projects have been conducted throughout the United States in an effort to achieve a regional consensus among nursing service persons and educators on differentiated statements of scope of practice for each level of graduate. Some of the early projects included the Midwest Alliance in Nursing Projects, the first project funded by the W. K Kellogg Foundation and the second project by a grant from the Division of Nursing of the Department of Health and Human Services (Primm, 1987); the Healing Web Project, composed of representatives of nursing education and practice from six midwestern and western states; and the Sioux Falls Experience, a detailed project implemented to differentiate educational design.

Other states have developed sets of recommendations to enable differentiated practice. For example, in the Colorado Experiment, they first asked for a statewide plan to facilitate articulation of nursing education programs, allowing nurses to move from one educational credential to another without unnecessary replication of learning or curricular experience. The second recommendation called for a differentiated model for nursing practice that would

Display 6-2   **COMPETENCIES DEFINED BY THE PEW HEALTH PROFESSIONS COMMISSION**

1. Embrace a personal ethic of social responsibility and service.
2. Exhibit ethical behavior in all professional activities.
3. Provide evidence-based clinically competent care.
4. Incorporate the multiple determinants of health in clinical care.
5. Apply knowledge of the new sciences.
6. Demonstrate critical thinking, reflection, and problem-solving skills.
7. Understand the role of primary care.
8. Rigorously practice preventive health care.
9. Integrate population-based care and services into practice.
10. Improve access to health care for those with unmet health needs.
11. Contribute to continuous improvement of the health care system.
12. Advocate for public policy that promotes and protects the health of the public.
13. Continue to learn and help others learn.
14. Practice relationship-centered care with individuals and families.
15. Provide culturally sensitive care to a diverse society.
16. Partner with communities in health care decisions.
17. Use communication and information technology effectively and appropriately.
18. Work in interdisciplinary teams.
19. Ensure care that balances individual, professional, system, and societal needs.
20. Practice leadership.
21. Take responsibility for quality of care and health outcomes at all levels.

facilitate appropriate use of nurses with varying educational credentials and degrees of experience. This would be accompanied by a differentiated pay scale, to allow appropriate compensation of nursing personnel as career advancement or growth occurred. Movement from one role to another required completion of the appropriate additional degrees, although growth within each role was possible without acquiring formal education. Wide-scale implementation of this model has not yet occurred.

As heightened interest in differentiating practice occurs in various nursing settings, a number of states or groups within states have established groups to work on the issue. In some instances, the work has evolved from efforts to build systems of work-force development with the capacity to adapt to the rapid and continual changes in the nation's health care system. In some instances, one group may be focusing on program articulation, another on differentiated practice, and still another on work-force projection. Collectively, the efforts have taken on broad perspectives and goals that include gathering data about the current work force and making projections regarding future needs, standardizing the degree taxonomy of the state, adopting common nursing course content, sequencing and numbering systems, developing (sometimes mandating) stronger programs of articulation between graduates of various levels of nursing education, modeling differentiation in limited settings, and working at defining competencies and identifying roles.

Critical Thinking Activity

Given the situation we have today, with three routes to preparation for registered nursing, how would you suggest that the skills of the graduate of each program be differentiated? How should that influence nursing practice? How would you implement differentiated practice on the unit on which you currently are working? Do you believe there should be a difference in salary? What is the rationale for your answer?

FORCES FOR CHANGE IN NURSING EDUCATION

As the nursing profession advances, and as education remains responsive to the changes that occur, it is imperative that nursing education undergo modifications. A discussion of some of the most significant challenges follows.

Incorporating Computer Technology in Nursing Education

It is safe to say that in the last 10 years, nursing education has experienced no transformation more dramatic than the incorporation of computer technology into all aspects of teaching, learning, and health care. These changes encompass activities covering everything from entire degrees that can be earned in on-line courses, to separate courses that are taught on-line, to the incorporation of computer technology in the classroom and learning laboratory. In the health care setting, computers are used for patient records, business functions, and increasingly as a support to effective decision making.

COMPUTER TECHNOLOGY IN THE CLASSROOM

The computer plays a major role in nursing education and is as essential to the operation of colleges and universities as it is to the operation of hospitals. Additionally, it is an important instructional tool. The computer offers a variety of approaches to instruction that are appealing and helpful to a diverse student population. Classroom lectures and presentations are augmented by computer-assisted instruction (CAI) in the form of interactive and linear video programs, patient simulations, drill and practice routines, problem-solving programs, and tutorials, to name a few examples. Faculty use computers for word processing, literature review, and the development and scoring of tests. Some faculty use computers in the classroom to augment their lectures and discussions through Power Point presentations and other computer technology. E-mail and the Internet are also a part of most teaching environments. Some instructional programs are delivered to sites far from the main campus through distance learning modalities using computer technology. At the end of their program of study, all students demonstrate their ability to practice safely on computerized licensing examinations in the form of computerized adaptive testing (CAT). In the nursing skills laboratory, mannequins that can blink their eyes, have pupils that dilate, breathe, and have a heart beat and a pulse assist students in the process of learning about heart attacks, diabetic shock, and other emergencies.

Computer literacy among students and faculty is no longer an issue—it is the current state of the art. Nursing educators express concern about the initial cost of the equipment and programs needed for this instruction, as well as the increasing cost of keeping both equipment and programs current. For example, the mannequin mentioned above carries a price tag of $215,000. At a time when the budgets of educational institutions are experiencing severe cuts, people responsible for purchasing supplies and equipment increasingly must find creative ways to acquire needed items. Another challenge to faculty is finding time to evaluate the existing software and integrate it into the approved curriculum.

COMPUTERS IN THE HOSPITAL ENVIRONMENT

Today's health care settings could not operate without computers and computerized equipment. Computers are used for business operations, medical records, and collection of clinical data, such as vital signs and hemodynamic values. Computers may be voice activated for charting at the bedside, for use with nursing care plans, for communication from the physicians' office to nursing stations, for regulating the administration of medications, and for many other facets of operation and patient care. Most of the equipment used in today's modern hospital is computerized. New graduates move into a highly technical world when they seek their first nursing positions. The education they receive to prepare them for these positions also must include the skills necessary to work in this highly computerized environment.

DISTANCE LEARNING OPTIONS

Many students who are geographically bound and unable to relocate to a community offering baccalaureate or master's education in nursing have found distance learning to offer convenience and flexibility. It also appeals to the nurse who cannot quit work to attend school. Essentially, distance learning refers to a teaching/learning situation in which the student and the teacher are not present in the classroom. Distance education may be accomplished through on-line courses, through courses broadcast to distant sites, and through courses taught in areas distant from the campus. A wide variety of approaches are used.

For on-line courses, sometimes referred to as a **virtual university**, students register for a class and are given passwords and access to the system. They work with an instructor and other class members, discussing issues, sharing ideas, and testing theories without the need to commute to another area. These on-line programs use the power of the Internet to deliver learning that is independent of time and location. Often individuals in the group share a mailbox, which serves as an "electronic classroom" facilitating a group forum among students. Research material is available through an electronic library. Students usually concentrate on one subject at a time, with courses being sequenced but offered outside the constraints of established times. Students may sign on at any hour, day or night. The instructor may have posted a short lecture and provided discussion questions. Students complete reading and written assignments as in traditional learning situations, except that the written assignments are sent to the instructor, graded, and returned on-line. Computer conferencing allows the students to participate in class discussion, ask questions, and receive feedback. After completing one course, the students move to the next until degree requirements are met.

Although these programs offer much flexibility to students, they also demand a great deal of discipline on their part. A single course may require as much as 15 to 20 hours of study time per week. A student attempting such a program needs to be an independent learner.

Sufficient faculty time also must be provided for students to receive effective feedback regarding their efforts. Library resources are always a concern for distant learners, and colleges need to provide access to appropriate learning resources for distance learners. Mechanisms for evaluating the learning must be developed thoughtfully to ensure the integrity of resulting credentials.

Establishing Programs That Provide for Educational Mobility

The concept of educational mobility in nursing has been discussed earlier in this chapter in the section dealing with articulation. In current times, it certainly must be included as one of the forces for change in nursing education.

Increasing Community-Based Practice Experiences

Another significant change in nursing practice is the trend toward community-based practice. Most nursing programs, especially hospital-based and associate degree programs, have a history of being strongly oriented toward the hospital as the primary clinical teaching environment. "Community," as it was used in nursing education, was associated with public health nursing and was to be found in baccalaureate education only.

Earlier hospital discharge to the home and an increasing emphasis on prevention has created new demands on nursing. Nurses are expected to provide care in clients' homes, the workplace, schools, nursing homes, community health agencies, clinics, shelters, and community gathering places. As the arena in which nursing is practiced begins to shift, nursing educators are challenged to define what part of the nursing curriculum should be taught in a community setting. Often this requires different clinical teaching strategies and approaches. Some faculty are reticent to shorten any time in acute care facilities; many are uncertain how a community experience should be provided and evaluated. Others worry about the legal ramifications associated with having students in many different environments and in less-controlled situations. Tremendous strides have been taken in developing innovative approaches to community-based nursing; more will follow.

Increasing Emphasis on Nursing Theories and Research

As the nursing profession continues to grow, one of the areas receiving more emphasis is nursing theory and research. This emphasis will undoubtedly continue. As nursing education keeps pace with the advancement of nursing knowledge, there is a push to develop curricular patterns that respond to the work of nursing theorists. Most approval bodies, state and national, now stipulate that a nursing program must have a coherent organizing or conceptual framework around which the program of learning is developed. Some programs have chosen to select the approach of a particular nursing **theorist**, and structure the program of learning around that theorist's work. The program in which you are enrolled may reflect this trend. Perhaps one of the hospitals to which you are assigned for clinical experience also uses the principles of a nursing theory to structure the delivery of care, although this is less common than using a theory in curriculum development.

A **theory** is a "scientifically acceptable general principle which governs practice or is proposed to explain observed facts" (Riehl & Roy, 1974, p. 3). Because nursing as a developing profession is seriously involved in research, to build a sound body of nursing knowledge, theories are valuable to us. They provide the bases for hypotheses about nursing practice. They make it possible for us to derive a sound rationale for the actions we take. If the theories are testable, they then allow us to build our knowledge base and to guide and improve nursing practice

Today, there are many published nursing theories. In an attempt to structure and organize those theories, various authors have categorized or classified them. Not all are classified similarly. Included are general classifications such as the art and science of humanistic nursing, interpersonal relationships, systems, and energy fields. Other categories include growth and development theories, systems theories, stress adaptation theories, and rhythm theories.

Examples of growth and development theories with which you are probably familiar are those of Maslow, Erikson, Kohlberg, Piaget, and Freud. Most basic nursing texts incorporate a discussion of the concepts developed by these theorists. The theories are so named because they focus on the developing person. They have the common characteristic of arranging this development in stages through which a person must pass to reach a particular level of development. They allow nurses to monitor progress through the stages and evaluate the appropriateness of that progress. You will recognize Maslow for his approach to self-actualization, Erikson for his psychosocial development, Kohlberg for his theories of moral reasoning, Piaget for his approach to cognitive development, and Freud for psychosexual theories on which medicine later based the school of psychoanalysis. These theories are not truly theories of nursing, however, because they were not developed for the purpose of explaining, testing, and changing the practice of nursing. They represent some of the "borrowed" knowledge around which we build our profession.

Most nursing theories are developed around a combination of concepts. Among these concepts, four approaches usually include those directed to the human person, to health and illness, to the environment (or society), and to nursing.

Nursing theories usually are classified according to the structure or approach around which they are developed. Theories that speak to the art and science of humanistic nursing were among the earliest pure nursing theories developed. Some authors have looked back at the contributions of Florence Nightingale and have included her work in that grouping. Among others are Virginia Henderson and her *Definition of Nursing*, Faye Abdellah and the *Twenty-one Nursing Problems* (which is often cited as one of the early attempts at classification of nursing behaviors), Lydia Hall and her *Core, Care, and Cure* model, and Madeleine Leininger's *Transcultural Care Theory*.

Interpersonal process theories deal with interactions between and among people. Many of these theories were developed during the 1960s. Included in this grouping could be Hildegard Peplau's *Psychodynamic Nursing*, Joyce Travelbee's *Human to Human Relationship*, Ernestine Wiedenbach's *The Helping Art of Clinical Nursing*, and Imogene King's *Dynamic Interacting Systems* model, although the last also could be classified as a systems theory.

Systems theories are so named because they are concerned with the interactions between and among all the factors in a situation. A system usually is viewed as complex and in a state of constant change. It is defined as a whole with interrelated parts and may be a subsystem of a larger system as well as a suprasystem. For example, a person may be viewed as a system composed of cells, tissue, and organs. The person is a subsystem of a family, which in turn is a subsystem of a community. In a systems approach, the person usually is considered as a "total" being, or from a "whole" being viewpoint. Systems theories also provide for "input" into the system and "feedback" within the system. The systems approach became popular during the 1970s. Included in this group of theorists are Dorothy Johnson, Sister Calista Roy, and Betty Neuman.

Stress adaptation models are based on concepts that view the person as adjusting or changing (adapting) to avoid situations (stressors) that would result in the disturbance of balance or equilibrium. The adaptation theory helps to explain how balance is maintained and therefore directs nursing actions. One often finds Sister Calista Roy's adaptation model and Betty Neuman's work included in this group, but both also may be considered systems models, as mentioned above.

One of the most recent classifications of theories is by energy fields. These theories, although developed earlier, received growing recognition during the 1980s. Included in this group are the works of Myra Levine, Joyce Fitzpatrick, Margaret Newman, and Martha Rogers.

Humanistic Models are also fairly recent. These focus on man's humanness and needs for love, caring, personal meaning, and living in concert with the environment. Theorists noted for developing these theories include Jean Watson, Rosemarie Rizzo Parse, and Margaret Newman.

It is not our purpose to discuss and critique the many approaches to nursing theory. The student who wants to pursue nursing theorists further is encouraged to consult the section on further reading at the end of the chapter or follow links provided on the Web available at *http://www.enursescribe.com/nurse_theorists.htm*. Table 6-2 outlines the approaches of several recognized nursing theorists.

Critical Thinking Activity

Select one nursing theorist. Describe what you find interesting and attractive about her nursing theory. Give a rationale for your decision, and describe how using her theory might affect your practice of nursing.

CONTINUING EDUCATION

Continuing education in nursing is defined as "planned learning experiences beyond a basic nursing educational program. The learning experiences are designed to promote the development of knowledge, skills, and attitudes for the enhancement of nursing practice, thus improving health care to the public" (ANA, 1974). Continuing education programs are widely publicized in today's nursing literature. They often are presented just before and during major nursing conventions. Some professional meetings carry continuing education credit. Other continuing education programs exist as extensions of nursing programs at colleges and universities.

TABLE 6-2.	NURSING THEORIES AND THEORISTS
THEORIST	**THEORY OR MODEL**
Lydia Hall	Viewed illness and rehabilitation as learning experiences in which the nurse's role was to guide and teach the patient through personal caregiving. Role involves therapeutic use of self (core), the treatment regimen of the health care team (cure), and nurturing and intimate bodily care (care).
Dorothy Johnson	A behavioral systems approach that focuses on health viewed as a state of equilibrium that the nurse assists in maintaining or balancing.
Imogene King	A model in which three open systems interact with the environment: personal, individual, and social. Nurse's role is to assist individual to perform daily activities and includes health promotion and maintenance. Involves goal attainment.
Madeleine Leininger	Focused on a caring model that must be practiced interpersonally. Emphasized a transcultural approach.
Myra Levine	Developed around the four concepts of conservation of energy, structural integrity, personal integrity, and social integrity. Supports a holistic approach to nursing based on recognition of the total response of the person to the interaction between the internal and external environment.
Betty Neuman	A systems model influenced by Gestalt theory, stress, and level of prevention. Employs lines of resistance and lines of defense in creating a healthy being. Nurses are to identify the stressors and assist the individual to respond. Involves primary, secondary, and tertiary prevention.
Dorothea Orem	Recognized as a self-care theory of nursing, supports the concept that each person has a need for the provision and management of self-care actions to achieve "constancy." When the individual is unable to provide these, a self-care deficit exists. The role of the nursing system is to help eliminate the self-care deficit through wholly compensatory, partially compensatory, or supportive-educative actions.
Martha Rogers	Includes complicated approaches to health that involve helicy, resonancy, and complementarity. The holistic individual moves through time and space as part of an expanding universe with potential states of maximum well-being. Nurses act to promote symphonic interaction between man and environment by repatterning the human and environmental fields.
Sister Calista Roy	Identified as an adaptation model that conceives of the individual as being in constant interaction with a changing environment, thus requiring adaptation. Four adaptive modes, or ways in which a person adapts, are identified through: (1) physiologic needs, (2) self-concept, (3) role function, and (4) interdependence relations. The nurse's role is to assess a patient's adaptive behaviors and the stimuli that may be affecting the person to manipulate the stimuli in such a way as to allow the patient to cope or adapt.

Like so many other areas of nursing, continuing education is not new. In an article entitled "Nursing the Sick," written around 1882, Florence Nightingale wrote:

Nursing is, above all, a progressive calling. Year by year nurses have to learn new and improved methods, as medicine and surgery and hygiene improve. Year by year nurses are called upon to do more and better than they have done. It is felt to be impossible to have a public register of nurses that is not a delusion (Nightingale, as cited in Seymer, 1954, p. 349).

The first continuing education courses for nurses probably would be considered postgraduate instruction today. In 1899, Teachers College at Columbia University instituted a course for qualified graduate nurses in hospital economics. Nursing institutes and conferences were first offered to nurses in the 1920s; often these were given to make up for deficiencies in basic nursing curricula. Hospital in-service or staff development programs also were beginning to be discussed in nursing literature around this time. Today most hospitals employ someone who is responsible for the staff education program. By 1959, federal funds became available for short-term courses, giving much thrust to continuing education. In 1967, the ANA published "Avenues for Continued Learning," its first definitive statement on continuing education; and in 1973, the ANA Council on Continuing Education was established. The Council, which is responsible to the ANA Commission on Education, is concerned about standards of continuing education, accreditation of the programs, transferability of credit from state to state, and development of guidelines for recognition systems within states. In 1974, "Standards for Continuing Education in Nursing" was published by the ANA, and the federal government altered the Nurse Traineeship Act of 1972 to include an option that would provide continuing education as an alternative to placing more students into programs receiving federal capitation dollars.

By the 1970s, most nursing publications had something to say about continuing education for nurses. Practically all states were organizing or planning to organize some method by which the nurse could receive recognition for continued education. These systems were called continuing education approval and recognition programs, or continuing education recognition programs, and most state systems followed the guidelines and criteria prepared by the ANA.

The **continuing education unit (CEU)** became a rather uniform system of measuring, recording, reporting, accumulating, transferring, and recognizing participation in nonacademic credit offerings. The National Task Force on the Continuing Education Unit, which represented 34 educational groups, developed the definition of a CEU. Although nursing was not one of the groups, the profession has accepted the definition. Ten hours of participation in an organized continuing education experience under responsible sponsorship, with capable direction and qualified instruction, is equal to one CEU. Many states and organizations, however, simply report clock hours of instruction (Fig. 6-3). Following a system for accreditation and approval of continuing education in nursing that was developed and implemented by the ANA in 1975, programs or individuals offering courses for continuing education now receive authority to do so from a recognized body, thereby assuring quality programs and standardization in their approach.

Today, colleges, universities, hospitals, voluntary agencies, and private proprietary groups all offer continuing education courses to RNs. The cost of this education varies tremendously. Nurses can earn continuing education credits for merely attending meetings and conferences. Little attempt is made to assess whether learning has occurred. Professional journals include sections of programmed instruction that can be completed in the comfort of one's living room. These have an evaluation mechanism. Telecourses are offered by television. Workshops, institutes, conferences, short courses, and evening courses abound. Courses are available on the Internet. Yet some nurses do not feel the need to keep up with these current offerings.

An issue today is whether continuing education should be mandatory or voluntary. **Mandatory continuing education** affects licensure; that means that any nurse renewing a license in a state requiring (mandating) continuing education will have to satisfy that requirement. **Voluntary continuing education** is not related to relicensure. Government agencies and state legislatures are exerting pressure on nurses, as they have on physicians, attorneys, dietitians, dentists, pharmacists, and other professionals, to provide evidence of updated knowledge before license renewal.

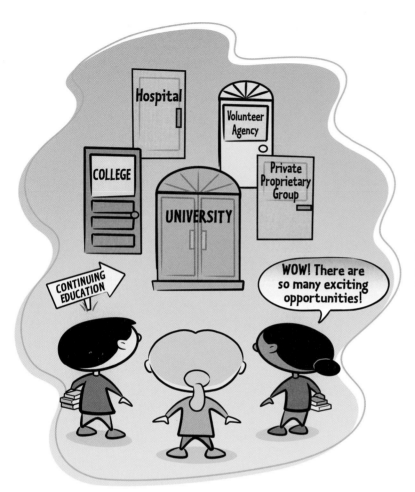

FIGURE 6-3   Today, colleges, universities, hospitals, voluntary agencies, and private proprietary groups are all offering continuing education courses to nurses.

A position supporting mandatory continuing education raises some questions. How should the learning be measured? Who should accredit the programs? How can quality be ensured? By whom and where should records be retained? Who should bear the cost? What should be the time frame for continuing education? How many hours, courses, and credits should be required?

You can contact the state board of nursing for information on specific requirements for that state.

Critical Thinking Activity

Do you believe continuing education should be a mandatory requirement for the renewal of one's license? Why or why not? If your answer is no, how would you ensure competence? If you believe it should be mandatory, what kind of record-keeping would you require? Who do you believe should keep the records?

KEY CONCEPTS

- Three major avenues to preparation for licensure as a registered nurse exist in the United States: the hospital-based diploma, the university-based baccalaureate degree, and the associate degree (usually offered in community colleges). Many similarities exist among these programs. In addition, various nontraditional approaches to nursing education have evolved.
- Educational programs prepare nursing assistants and licensed practical (vocational) nurses for roles in the health care delivery system. As these programs have grown, greater oversight of the programs by approval bodies has occurred.
- The nursing shortage of the 1990s coupled with recommendations or mandates from important groups has resulted in greater creativity and collaboration in educational approaches.
- Master's and doctoral programs that prepare nurses for leadership positions in the profession continue to grow, with more emphasis on the master's degree for advanced practice. The actual degree awarded at the end of doctoral studies varies.
- One of the most rapidly growing areas is that of advanced practice; this growth was accelerated by health care reform. Recommendations from major commissions have urged continued expansion of advanced practice programs.
- Many changes are occurring in nursing education. These include more emphasis on articulation and career ladder programs and a shift in educational settings from acute care facilities to community-based experiences.
- No change has affected nursing education as greatly as has the computer age. Entire programs can be completed on-line. Computer technology has changed the structure of the typical nursing classroom, and instructors prepare graduates who will be able to function in a health care environment that makes heavy use of computerized services.
- Nursing education has been influenced by the ANA Position on Nursing Education that advocated the baccalaureate degree as the minimum educational preparation for professional practice. Many nursing educators, particularly those in diploma and associate degree programs, disagreed with this position. This issue may take on new life in the 21st century.
- Models for differentiated practice are being encouraged; these models recognize and use graduates according to the competencies inherent in the program from which they graduated.
- Nursing theories continue to influence nursing and nursing education. Nursing theories assist us in building a body of nursing knowledge and describing and defining nursing practice.
- Continuing education, whether further education that results in a higher degree, or whether in the form of classes, seminars, or workshops that update and increase expertise, is being encouraged by more and more organizations. Staying current in practice is critical to safe client care.

RELEVANT WEB SITES

American Association of Colleges of Nursing: *www.aacn.nche.edu*
Commission on Collegiate Nursing Education: *www.aacn.nche.edu/Accreditation*
National Council of State Boards of Nursing: *www.ncsbn.org*

National League for Nursing: *www.nln.org*
National League for Nursing Accreditation Commission: *www.nlnac.org*
National Organization for Associate Degree Nursing: *www.noadn.org*
Nursing Theorists: *www.enursescribe.com/nurse_theorists.htm*

REFERENCES

American Association of Colleges of Nursing. (2002a). Your Nursing Career: A look at the facts. [On-line] Available: *http://www.aacn.nche.edu/education/Career.htm.*

American Association of Colleges of Nursing. (2002b). Associate Degree in Nursing Programs and AACN's Support for Articulation. [On-line]. Available: *http://www.aacn.nche.edu/Media/Backgrounders/ADNFacts.htm.*

American Nurses Association's first position on nursing education. (1965). *American Journal of Nursing, 65*(12):106–111.

American Nurses Association. Standards for Continuing Education for Nursing. (1974). Kansas City, MO: American Nurses Association.

ANA reaffirms commitment to BSN for entry into practice—supports new certification program to be offered by ANCC. (2000). [On-line]. Available: *http://www.nursingworld.org/pressrel/2000/pr0225b.htm.*

Barter, M. & McFarland, P. L. (2001). BSN by 2010: A California initiative. *Journal of Nursing Administration, 31*(3) 141–144.

Bellack, J. P. & O'Neil, E. H. (2000). Recreating nursing practice for a new century. *Nursing and Health Care Perspectives 21*(1):14–21.

Boston, C. (1990). Differentiated practice: An introduction. In C. Boston: *Current issues and perspectives on differentiated practice* (pp. 1–3). Chicago, IL: American Organization of Nurse Executives.

Brown, E. L. (1948). *Nursing for the future.* New York: Russell Sage Foundation.

California Board of Registered Nursing. (1994). *Laws relating to nursing education licensure: Practice with rules and regulations.* Sacramento: California Board of Registered Nursing.

de Tornyay, R. (1996). Critical challenges for nurse educators. *Journal of Nursing Education 35*(4):146–147.

Donley, R. & Flaherty, M. J. (2002, May 31). Revisiting the American Nurses Association's first position on education for nurses. *Online Journal of Issues in Nursing* [On-line]. Available: *http:nursingworld.org/ojin/topic18/tpc18_1.htm.*

Gosnell, D. J. (2002 [May 31]). Overview and summary: The 1965 entry into practice Proposal–Is it relevant today? *Online Journal of Issues in Nursing.* [On-line]. Available: *http:nursingworld.org/ojin/topic 18/tpc18ntr.htm.*

Hartung, D. (1986). Organizational positions on titling and entry into practice: A chronology. In *Looking beyond the entry Issue: Implications for education and service,* NLN Publication No. 41-2173. New York: National League for Nursing.

Joel, L. A. (2002, May 31). Education for entry into nursing practice: Revisited for the 21st Century. [On-line]. *Online Journal of Issues in Nursing* Available: *http://nursingworld.org/ojin/topic18/tpc18_4.htm.*

Kalisch, P. A. & Kalisch, B. J. (1995). *The advance of American nursing* (3rd ed.). Philadelphia: J. B. Lippincott.

Lindeman, C. A. (2000). The future of nursing education. *Journal of Nursing Education, 39*(1):5–12.

National Council of State Boards of Nursing. (1998). National Council Update. *Issues 19*(4):10–11, Chicago: Author.

National League for Nursing Accreditation Commission. (1999). Interpretive guidelines for standards and criteria 1999: Associate degree programs in nursing. New York: Author.

National League for Nursing. (2002). Public policy agenda 2002. New York: Author.

National League for Nursing. (1990). Educational outcomes of associate degree nursing programs: Roles and competencies. Publication No. 23-2348, Council of Associate Degree Programs. New York: National League for Nursing.

National League for Nursing. (1973). Characteristics of associate degree education in nursing. Publication No. 23-1500, Council of Associate Degree Programs. New York: National League for Nursing.

National Organization for Associate Degree Nursing. (2002). Associate degree nursing (ADN) facts [On-line]. Available: *http://wwwnoadn.org/and_facts.htm.*

Nelson, M. A. (2002 [May 31]). Education for professional nursing practice: Looking backward into the future. [On-line]. *Online Journal of Issues in Nursing.* Available: *http://nursingworld.org/ojin/topic18/tpc18_3.htm.*

Pew Health Professions Commission. (1995). Critical challenges: Revitalizing the health professions for the twenty-first century. San Francisco, CA: UCSF Center for the Health Professions.

Primm, P. L. (1987). Differentiated practice for ADN- and BSN-prepared nurses. *Journal of Professional Nursing, 3*(4):218–225.

Riehl, J. P. & Roy S. C. (1974). *Conceptual models for nursing practice.* New York: Appleton-Century-Crofts.

Seymer, L. R. (1954). *Selected writings of Florence Nightingale.* New York:Macmillan.

U. S. Public Health Service. (1963). Toward quality in nursing: Needs and goals. Report of the Surgeon Generals' Consultant Group on Nursing. Washington, D.C.: U.S. Government Printing Office.

Legal and Ethical Responsibility and Accountability for Practice

A well-grounded understanding of the legal and ethical dimensions of practice provides the foundation for professional nursing. This unit begins by exploring the issue of credentials for health care providers. It discusses the basic concerns related to credentialing, provides a rationale for credentials, and emphasizes the responsibility of health care providers (especially nurses) to the public.

The unit continues with a discussion of the legal ramifications of practice. Concrete examples provide help in understanding specific legal issues of importance to consumers and health care providers. The role of the nurse as a witness concludes this chapter.

Ethical and bioethical issues associated with health care constantly challenge us as professionals and as members of society. Each new technologic advance brings additional questions and concerns to our attention. The unit concludes with a discussion of these major questions and provides an understanding of the basis of ethical decision making and the factors that significantly affect it. Some of the specific problems are explored in the hope that considering them before you become directly involved will help you to address the issues more comfortably as you move into a professional role.

7

Credentials for Health Care Providers

LEARNING OUTCOMES

After completing this chapter, you should be able to:

1. Define and discuss the concept of credentialing in the health professions.
2. Describe how each of the following types of credentials differ: diploma, certificate, license.
3. Outline the purposes of accreditation.
4. Identify and analyze the major elements addressed by nursing practice acts.
5. Outline the role of the State Board of Nursing or other state regulatory authority.
6. Differentiate between licensure by examination and licensure by endorsement.
7. Discuss personal strategies to avoid violating the provisions of the Nurse Practice Act and encountering the disciplinary process.
8. Discuss issues in licensure, including assuring continued competence, multistate licensure, and licensure for graduates of foreign nursing schools.
9. Explain the various uses of certification in nursing.
10. Discuss current trends in credentialing within the health care workforce.

KEY TERMS

Accreditation	Enacted (statutory) law	Party state
Advanced practice nurse (APN)	Frequency	Permissive licensure
	Grandfathering	Reciprocity
Certificate of completion	Home state	Remote state
Certificate	Injunctive relief	Revocation
Certification	License	Rules and regulations
Computerized adaptive testing (CAT)	Licensure by endorsement	Site-based certification
	Licensure by examination	Site-based examination
Credentials	Mandatory licensure	State Board of Nursing
Criticality	Multistate licensure	Sunset laws
Degree	NCLEX-PN	Telenursing
Diploma	NCLEX-RN	
Disciplinary action	Nurse practice act	

 Credentials are written documents that communicate to others the nature of one's competence and provide evidence of one's preparation to perform in a specific occupation. The basic rationale for legal credentials in health care occupations is that providing a standard mechanism for judging competence protects the safety of the public. Further, those who are engaged in careers in health occupations want to be assured that the standards of practice in their discipline remain high. They do not want to be replaced by people with less educational preparation and skill who are willing to work for lower wages (Fig. 7-1). Credentials also are used by organizations or institutions to demonstrate the quality of their care to the public.

TYPES OF CREDENTIALS IN HEALTH CARE

There are many types of health care credentials; examples include diplomas, certificates, degrees, accreditation, and licenses. Each of these serves a different purpose. Not all are available for each different health occupation.

Diplomas, Degrees, and Certificates of Completion

A school or business offering instruction awards a **diploma** or **certificate** to those who complete a designated program of study. An example is the diploma awarded on graduation from high school or college. A business that provides instruction in using computer programs might present certificates to those who complete the course. Licensed practical nursing programs offer a **certificate of completion**. Hospital-based programs preparing registered nurses (RNs) offer a diploma. College-based nursing programs offer academic **degrees**, such as the associate, baccalaureate,

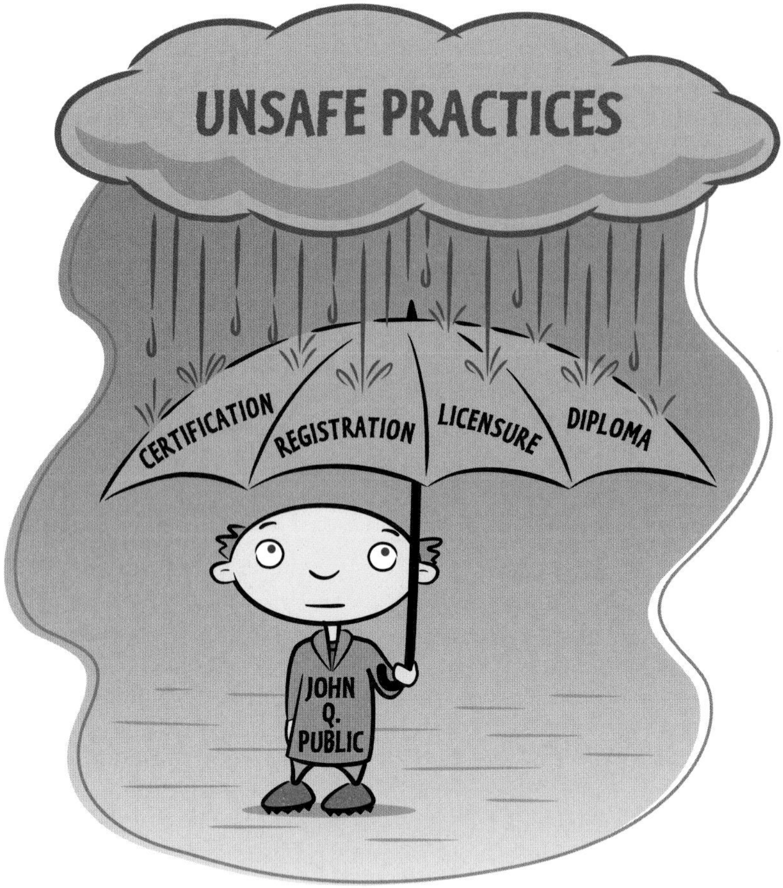

FIGURE 7-1 Various forms of credentialing ensure the public of qualified caregivers.

or master's degree, which require the fulfillment of certain general education courses and course work that prepares you for a particular career, such as nursing. When only a diploma or educational certificate is available, it is necessary to know about the educational institution and the specific educational program to evaluate the person's abilities. That is the purpose of accreditation.

Accreditation

Accreditation is a process whereby educational institutions or programs are surveyed and evaluated against previously determined standards. Some accreditation recognizes the entire educational institution, such as the accreditation offered by regional bodies for colleges and universities. If an institution's programs meet published standards, it is awarded accreditation. The standards include agreed-upon criteria that are designed to measure quality, value, and amount. An associate, baccalaureate, or master's degree awarded by this accredited institution would reflect a standard of postsecondary education approved by the accrediting organization. Although a nonaccredited institution might award a degree, there is no guarantee that the school meets educational standards; therefore, the degree might not be accepted as adequate evidence of qualifications. Many educational credentials are acknowledged only if offered by an accredited educational institution. Similarly, only course work completed at an accredited institution may be accepted for transfer. You may have experienced the need for this type of accreditation if you transferred academic credits from one college to another. A regionally accredited college or university usually limits direct transfer of coursework to that which was completed at an accredited institution.

Some academic accreditation is "specialized," meaning that it applies only to a particular program in an institution, or to a particular type of professional–technical education. This accreditation requires that the specific program meet professional standards for excellence established by a specialized accrediting agency. An educational institution might have general accreditation for its degrees but still not have specialized accreditation. Sometimes this is because of the cost of the accreditation process, or because of a philosophic stance that additional accreditation is not needed if the institution has general accreditation. Certain educational organizations are not degree-granting institutions, and therefore are not eligible for general accreditation, but they are still eligible for specialized accreditation. This is true of hospital-based diploma schools of nursing.

The national accreditation of nursing programs is a specialized accreditation. The National League for Nursing Accrediting Commission (NLNAC), a subsidiary organization related to the National League for Nursing, accredits nursing programs at all levels: practical nursing, hospital diploma nursing education, associate degree nursing education, and baccalaureate and higher-degree educational programs. The Commission on Collegiate Nursing Education (CCNE), a subsidiary organization of the American Association of Colleges of Nursing, also began accrediting baccalaureate and higher-degree nursing programs in 1999. Advanced practice nursing organizations such as the American Association of Nurse Anesthetists provide specialized accreditation for institutions offering advanced practice/nurse practitioner programs.

Licensure

A **license** is a legal credential conferred by an individual state that grants permission to that individual to practice a given profession. The individual seeking licensure must have demonstrated an essential degree of competency necessary to perform a unique scope of practice prior to receiving the license (National Council of State Boards of Nursing, 2002d). A wide variety of health professionals are licensed in different states. Most states require licensing only of those who have more direct contact with clients. Physicians, dentists, pharmacists, and nurses are licensed in all states. The licensing of other health care workers varies. An individual state or province determines eligibility for licensure and the type of testing required based on the practice act for that profession within that state. Each state develops and enforces its own practice act, which includes the scope of practice for the profession the license represents. (We will discuss practice acts later in this chapter.)

Permissive licensure is a voluntary system whereby an individual may choose to become licensed to provide evidence of competence, but a license is not required to practice. **Mandatory licensure** is a requirement that all individuals must obtain a license in a particular jurisdiction to practice. Mandatory licensure is instituted when there is a compelling public interest in licensure to protect the public. All states and Canadian provinces have mandatory licensure for nurses. Most licensing laws specify completion of a state-approved educational program and require successful completion of a written examination prescribed by the state. Some professions, such as dentistry, require candidates to pass both a practical examination and a written examination. Nursing is unique in having a standard licensure process in every state and territory in the United States. This was developed through the cooperative action of the state boards of nursing. A national examination may exist for other professions, but its application may vary. For example, there is a national licensing examination for pharmacy, but California prepares and administers its own examination and does not use the national pharmacy examination. There are national medical board examinations, but some states administer independent medical examinations. Even when the same examination is used for licensure, as in pharmacy, some states require that a person new to the state retake the licensing examination when applying for a license in that state.

Some states require completion of continuing education to renew a health care license. Pharmacists were one of the first groups required to pursue continuing education to remain licensed. Continuing education is required for licensure renewal of nurses and physicians in many states. The cost of monitoring continuing education has been a barrier to its adoption in some states (see Chapter 6).

Certification

For some groups, a standard credential is available in the form of **certification** provided by a nongovernmental authority, usually a professional organization. Workers with this credential are referred to as "certified" or sometimes as "registered." This type of credential should not be confused with a legal license. Certification usually is granted on completion of an educational program and the passing of a standardized examination, both of which are prescribed by a professional organization or group. Certification does not include a legal scope of practice.

Some organizations provide certification for several related occupational groups. One such organization is the National Accrediting Association for Clinical Laboratory Sciences (NAACLS). Members of the various professional groups involved in laboratory science cooperated in setting up this association. The purpose of this organization is to make the laboratory science credentialing system more independent and as objective as possible. This organization awards the title medical laboratory technician (MLT) and medical technologist (MT) to those who have met the educational standards and passed the certification examination for each of those credentials. All groups in the field of laboratory science recognize these as professional credentials. Some states have made certification by this body the required criterion for practice in clinical laboratory sciences.

While some professional organizations conduct their own certification, in most instances they have established an independent national entity with the sole purpose of credentialing to assure objectivity and enhance confidence of others in the process.

One of the concerns regarding certification is the potential for confusion that exists because regulatory agencies (such as State Boards of Nursing) and professional associations may use the term "certification" differently and in different contexts (NCSBN, 2001). In nursing, certification is used for identifying licensed RNs who have specialized or advanced competence in a specific area of nursing. Certification in nursing will be discussed in more detail later in this chapter, after the discussion of basic licensure.

Critical Thinking Activity

Choose an allied health occupation found in a health care facility in which you have clinical practice. Investigate the credentials needed for that occupation and how they would be obtained in your state. Analyze a way in which you could work collaboratively with an individual in this health occupation.

NURSING LICENSURE IN THE UNITED STATES

Through a regulatory process set up in each state, only individuals who meet predetermined qualifications are permitted to practice nursing. The government agency that has the legal authority to regulate nursing is the Board of Nursing. They enforce the Nurse Practice Act enacted by the legislature of each state.

The History of Credentialing in Nursing

Nursing leaders historically have maintained an ethical position that accountability to the public for quality nursing care is essential. The public, however, often has no method for evaluating the competence of an individual nurse. Therefore, in the United States, the nursing profession has tried to ensure that nurses have credentials that can be recognized by everyone.

Recognizable credentials were not always available for nurses. Before the Nightingale schools became prevalent in England, and nursing schools were established in the United States, little training was available to those who wanted to provide nursing care. Nurses with some training and those without typically worked side by side. After schools of nursing became common, a rudimentary means of identifying the qualifications of a caregiver was the certificate of completion issued by the nursing school. This was the first true nursing credential.

However, because the quality of education offered in the nursing schools varied greatly—programs varied in length from 6 weeks to 3 years—it became apparent that a completion certificate was not an adequate guarantee of competence. Nursing leaders were concerned about this situation; they believed that clients had no way to judge a particular nurse's competence, or whether they might suffer from the care administered by a poorly prepared nurse.

In 1896, the Nurses' Associated Alumnae of the United States and Canada was created. This organization later evolved into the American Nurses Association (ANA). One of the major concerns of the association was the establishment of legal licensure for nurses. The route toward legal licensing for credentialing was long and difficult. Nurses, legislators, and the public had to be educated about the value of licensure for the profession and encouraged to support it. Display 7-1 presents a chronology of nursing licensure. An interesting historic note is that Florence Nightingale was opposed to nursing licensure although she initiated a registry for nurses. She believed that only continuing education and practice could assure competence and that a license approved at one time could not.

Display 7-1 THE HISTORY OF NURSING LICENSURE

1867	Dr. Henry Wentworth Acland first suggested licensure for nurses in England.
1892	American Society of Superintendents of Training Schools for Nurses organized and supported licensure in the United States.
1901	First nursing licensure in the world: New Zealand
1903	First nursing licensure in the United States: North Carolina, New Jersey, New York, and Virginia (in that order)
1915	ANA drafted its first model nurse practice act.
1919	First nursing licensure in England
1923	All 48 states had enacted nursing licensure laws.
1935	First mandatory licensure act in the United States: New York (effective 1947)
1946	Ten states had definitions of nursing in the licensing act.
1950	First year the same examination used in all jurisdictions of the United States and its territories: State Board Test Pool Examination
1965	Twenty-one states had definitions of nursing in the licensing act.
1971	First state to recognize expanded practice in the nursing practice act: Idaho
1976	First mandatory continuing education for relicensure: California
1982	Change to nursing process format examination: National Council Licensure Examination for Registered Nurses (NCLEX-RN)
1986	Only state to require baccalaureate degree for initial RN licensure and associate degree for licensed practical nurse licensure: North Dakota (effective 1987)
1994	Computer-adapted testing initiated nationwide
1998	Mutual Recognition Nurse Licensure Compact finalized. Utah is the first state to become part of the Compact.

The ANA campaigned vigorously for the adoption of state licensing laws. These early laws provided for permissive licensure. The requirements for permissive licensure included graduating from a school that satisfied certain standards established in the practice act for that state and passing a comprehensive examination. Only those who had met these standards could use the title "registered nurse;" others used the title "nurse." An employer or a member of the public then could differentiate between an RN and an individual who used the title "nurse," but had not met the standards required to be registered. Under this system, no one was required to have a license to practice nursing and there was much variability in standards from one state to another.

The community benefited from these standards because an established credential attested to an RN's level of competence. The individual licensed as an RN profited by better job availability and salary when employers differentiated between those with licenses and those without licenses.

The set of laws regulating the practice of nursing is termed the **Nurse Practice Act**. North Carolina passed the first law providing for permissive licensure in 1903. By 1923, all the existing 48 states had permissive licensure laws. Alaska and Hawaii passed licensure laws while they were still territories, and continued to recognize these laws when they became states.

After permissive licensure laws came into being, nurses' activity regarding licensure became less intense because most individuals graduating from nursing schools sought and received licenses to practice. However, there was still concern that some persons were practicing nursing without having demonstrated skill and knowledge. The majority of those functioning without licenses were nursing school graduates who had failed the licensing examinations; they were referred to as graduate nurses, rather than RNs. Other nurses who practiced without licenses included individuals who had been educated as nurses in foreign countries.

To end this situation and provide greater protection to the public, many nurses began to call for mandatory licensure. Mandatory nursing licensure requires that all persons who wish to practice nursing meet established standards for education, pass standardized examinations, and secure a license to practice in the state, province, or territory in which they wish to work.

The first mandatory licensure law took effect in New York in 1947. Today, mandatory licensure is the standard in the United States and Canada, and in most other countries. Therefore, if you wish to work as a nurse in any state, territory, province, or other country, you must obtain a license that is valid in that jurisdiction before you begin working. Even though you are licensed to practice in one place, that does not allow you to practice elsewhere without seeking a new license in that jurisdiction.

Although the terms "registered nurse" and "licensed practical nurse" (or licensed vocational nurse, as used in Texas and California) were protected in law, the more general term "nurse" has not been protected traditionally. Many individuals describe themselves as nurses, when their roles in health care are assistive. Their employers also may refer to them as "nurses" to support their status. Some states have made "nurse" a protected term. In these states, only RNs or practical (vocational) nurses may use the title "nurse." Others, such as certified nurses' aides/assistants and medical assistants, may use only their specific title.

Current Nursing Licensure Laws

The authority for establishing a licensure law lies with the legislature of each jurisdiction. The group initiating the action may spend months preparing and planning the content of the bill and gaining the support of legislators for its ideas.

A proposed change in the law enters the legislative process through an elected member of the legislature who has been persuaded that the change is in the best interest of the public. That individual introduces a bill. (See Chapter 3 for an overview of how a bill becomes a law.)

During the legislative process, individuals and organizations may affect the content of the proposed legislation by influencing the legislators to amend the bill. Amendments to a bill may change the content dramatically and cause the originators of the bill to reconsider their support. Once the appropriate legislative body passes a bill, it becomes the **enacted or statutory law**. This law cannot be changed without another vote of the legislative body.

Rules and Regulations

Each state has its own set of administrative **rules and regulations** to carry out the provisions of laws regulating nursing. These rules and regulations are established by an administrative body, usually the **State Board of Nursing**, that is given responsibility for administering the Nurse Practice Act. This responsibility is authorized in the Nurse Practice Act itself. (See the section later in this chapter on the Role of the Board of Nursing.) Most states require that public hearings be held regarding proposed rules and regulations, but the board has the authority to make the final decision. The rules and regulations must be within the scope outlined by the legislation that was passed. Those that are accepted by the appropriate board have the force of law unless they are challenged in court and are found not to be in accord with the legislature's intent. These rules are termed the administrative law.

In some states, the Nurse Practice Act is detailed and specifies most of the critical provisions regarding licensure and practice. In other states, the practice act is broad, and the administrative body is given a great deal of power to make decisions through rules and regulations. Both the Nurse Practice Act and state rules and regulations govern nursing in every state.

Nursing Licensure Law Content

In the early 1900s, the ANA, assuming its leadership role in nursing licensure, formulated a model nurse practice act to be used by state associations when planning legislation. The most recent ANA revision of this model was in 1990 by the ANA Congress for Nursing Practice (ANA, 1990). When the responsibility for overseeing the licensure process shifted to the National Council of State Boards of Nursing (NCSBN) that group also developed a model nurse practice act. In addition, the NCSBN has written the Model Nursing Administrative Rules. The NCSBN continues to update its model act and model rules and regulations as part of its role in supporting the state boards of nursing, with the most recent update in 2002. (NCSBN, 2002a and 2002b).

We recommended that you carefully read the Nurse Practice Act for the state in which you will practice. A copy of the act may be obtained from the State Board of Nursing (check the NCSBN web site [*http://www.ncsbn.org*]). Many states make these documents available on-line. In some states, one act includes both practical nursing and registered nursing; other states have two separate but similar acts. Historically, the role of the nursing assistant was not outlined in nursing laws. As federal legislation mandating classes and certification for nursing assistants in long-term care took effect, some states modified laws and rules and regulations to address the role of the nursing assistant. In other states, regulations governing nursing assistants rest within a different department of the state government.

The following general topics usually are covered in state licensure laws for nursing.

PURPOSE

The purpose of regulating the practice of nursing is twofold: regulations protect the public, and they make individual practitioners accountable for their actions. Note that the protection of the status of the licensed individual is not the reason for licensure. With this in mind, you can better understand the inclusion of some other topics in the act.

DEFINITIONS

All of the significant terms in the act are defined for the purpose of carrying out the law. This is where the legal definition of nursing and the scope of practice are spelled out.

The NCSBN has given the following definition: "the 'practice of nursing' means assisting individuals or groups to maintain or attain optimal health, implementing a strategy of care to accomplish defined goals, and evaluating responses to care and treatment. This practice includes, but is not limited to, initiating and maintaining comfort measures, promoting and supporting human functions and responses, establishing an environment conducive to well-being, providing health counseling and teaching, and collaborating on certain aspects of the health regimen. This practice is based on understanding the human condition across the lifespan and the relationship of the individual within the environment" (NCSBN, 2002a, p. 3). The National Council document then proceeds to distinguish between RN practice and licensed practical/vocational nurse practice.

No state adopts the exact wording of any recommended definition, but most states include references to performing services for compensation, the necessity for a specialized knowledge base, the use of the nursing process (although steps may be named differently), and components of nursing practice. Several states include some reference to treating human responses to actual or potential health problems; this was first addressed in New York State's license law and was later incorporated in the ANA's "Nursing: A Social Policy Statement" (1980). Most states refer to the execution of the medical regimen, and many include a general statement about additional acts that recognize that nursing practice is evolving and that the nurse's area of responsibility can be expected to broaden.

Definitions of practical (vocational) nursing are more restrictive, and usually state that the individual must function under the direction of an RN or physician, in areas demanding less judgment and knowledge than is required of the RN. In the NCSBN model act, this is referred to as "a directed scope of nursing practice" (NCSBN, 2002a , p. 4). Practical nurse standards usually focus on data collection rather than comprehensive assessment, and specify that the practical nurse contributes to the plan of care and the evaluation of care rather than being accountable for them.

A variety of nursing assistants are employed in health care facilities; they may have titles such as mental health technician, nursing assistant, or medication technician. The preparation of and scope of practice for these individuals is a matter of serious concern to the public. Laws regarding educational requirements and legal definitions of scope of practice have been adopted for nursing assistant practice. Through the OBRA 1987 regulations for long-term care facilities, a nationwide standard was established for the training and certification of nursing assistants employed in these facilities. Each state administers the regulations and is free to raise the standards but may not lower them.

QUALIFICATIONS FOR LICENSURE APPLICANTS

The most common basic requirements for licensure are graduation from an approved educational program and proficiency in the English language. Some states make the educational requirements more specific—requiring, for example, high school graduation and either an associate or baccalaureate degree, or a diploma in nursing, for the RN applicant.

All states require a passing score on a comprehensive examination, but do not specify in the law which examination; the current licensing examinations are discussed later in this chapter. Many states require that an applicant be of "good moral character." There is usually a requirement for disclosure of criminal convictions, some of which are a barrier to licensure. Some require "good physical and mental health," but more commonly there is a requirement for disclosure of any illness or medication use that might affect practice.

TITLING

This section of the law specifies the titles to be used for those who have met the licensure requirements. In some states, only the titles registered nurse and licensed practical nurse are regulated. Many states also regulate the use of titles for advanced practice, such as nurse practitioner and nurse midwife. Titles used in these expanded roles vary from state to state. Some current titles are advanced nurse practitioner (ANP), advanced practice registered nurse (APRN), nurse practitioner (NP), and advanced registered nurse practitioner (ARNP). In some states, the specialized nurse uses the title of a specific certification, such as certified registered nurse anesthetist (CRNA), certified nurse midwife (CNM), family nurse practitioner (FNP) and pediatric nurse practitioner (PNP)(ANA, 2000).

GRANDFATHERING

Whenever a new law is written, it usually contains a statement specifying that anyone currently holding a license may continue to hold that license if and when requirements for the license change. This is termed **grandfathering**. Without this provision, the enactment of a new law would require individuals who are currently licensed to reapply and to show that they meet the new standards.

However, not all changes in the law are grandfathered. When new requirements are instituted that the legislature believes are important for the safety of the public, all currently licensed individuals may be required to meet the new standards within a given time period. For additional discussion of grandfathering, please refer to Chapter 6.

LICENSE RENEWAL AND CONTINUING EDUCATION REQUIREMENTS

The length of time for which a license is valid and any requirements for its renewal are specified in the law. In some states, license renewal requires only the payment of a fee; other jurisdictions require evidence of continuing education for renewal. The documentation of continuing education may be the submission of records or it may be attested to by signing a form. For example, California requires that the person seeking to renew an RN license list all continuing education courses taken, along with the number of continuing education units earned and the provider number of the agency offering the courses. In many states where the applicant is not required to submit records at the time of renewal, a procedure for random checking ensures compliance with the law. Continuing education requirements vary greatly, with the most common requirement being an average of 15 hours per year (NCSBN, 2002d).

FINANCIAL CONCERNS

Although the Nurse Practice Act itself usually does not specify the fees to be charged for obtaining or renewing a license, general restrictions on the method of calculating fees and on how the fees may be used are often included in the act. The act may specify how the expenses of the Board of Nursing are to be met and who has legal authority to make decisions regarding the use of funds.

All states charge a fee for processing an application for licensure. At initial licensure, there is also a fee for taking a licensing examination (approximately $200), which is paid to the company that prepares and scores an examination. In addition, there is a fee each time a license is renewed. For specific information on current licensure fees, temporary permits, and continuing education requirements, contact the Board of Nursing in the state in which you will practice.

NURSING EDUCATION PROGRAMS

Some state laws describe the requirements of nursing education programs in only the most general terms, leaving the details up to the Board of Nursing; in other states, the laws are specific. The law may specify the number of years of education required, the courses or content that must be included, and the approval process for particular programs. If the law is general, then the board sets more specific standards. A nursing education program in a state must fulfill the requirements of the state law for graduates to be eligible for licensure.

GROUNDS FOR DISCIPLINARY ACTION

Disciplinary action refers to all penalties that may be imposed against an individual who has violated provisions of a licensing law. The Nurse Practice Act for a state identifies the bases for disciplinary action, and the Board is empowered to prosecute those who violate the law. Disciplinary actions may include fines, reprimands, restrictions on practice (such as working only under supervision), suspension of a license for a specified period, or **revocation** (removal) of a license. The board may be authorized to ask a court to halt a specific practice that it believes is contrary to the law until a full hearing can be held. This is called **injunctive relief.** This term refers to the court order called an injunction that requires an individual or organization to stop a particular activity. The Board may also immediately suspend a license pending investigation if the situation holds a serious threat to the public.

Disciplinary action can only be taken based on criteria stated in the law (Fig. 7-2). Most courts have supported revocation of a license only when the offense was related in some way

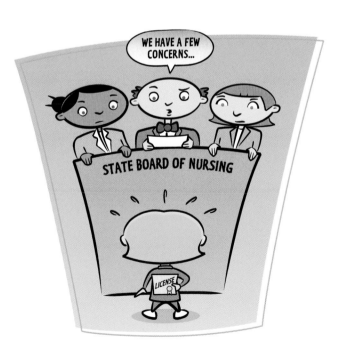

FIGURE 7-2   A nursing license may be revoked by the State Board of Nursing.

to practice issues that affected the public safety. Thus, most modern nurse practice or disciplinary acts contain specific concerns such as the following:

* Fraud in obtaining a license
* Conviction of a felony
* Practicing while chemically impaired
* Harming the public
* Practicing outside the scope of practice

Some states also have clauses that call for license revocation for individuals who default on government-sponsored educational loans or on agreements regarding service in return for scholarship aid (New Legislation, 1996).

EXCEPTIONS

Certain provisions may allow those who are not licensed to act as nurses in specific situations. Performing as a student while in an educational program is usually the primary exception. Those who are caring for family members or friends without pay are also exempted from license regulations. Those who are practicing nursing in a federal agency, such as a military hospital, are exempted from seeking a license in the state where they are stationed as long as they maintain a current license in another state. Some states are adopting exceptions for self-directed care by the disabled. In these situations, a paid care provider may perform certain care that is usually considered nursing when directed to do so by the mentally competent, physically disabled client. This includes administering medications in the home and carrying out specific care procedures, such as catheterization.

ADMINISTRATIVE PROVISIONS

Each law requires administrative specifications detailing when the law will become effective and when a previous act will no longer be in force. Such provisions are of particular interest to nurses when a law is first passed, because nurses want to know when changes affecting them will take place.

Advanced Practice Nurses

Advanced practice nurses include nurse practitioners, nurse anesthetists, and nurse midwives. Licensure requirements for advanced practice vary from state to state, although work is being done to develop uniform APRN licensure requirements. Many, but not all, require the master's degree in nursing. Gradually, states are moving toward the master's degree as the standard. None of the states administers a state licensing examination for advanced practice nursing.

Often the law requires that a person be certified for advanced practice by the ANCC or a nursing specialty organization (see section on certification later in the chapter) to receive a license as an advanced practice nurse. This certification includes testing. The requirements and methods for obtaining certification remain with the organization granting the certification, but the nurse receives a license from the state to practice in the expanded role. This is true of certified nurse anesthetists, who are all certified through the Council on Certification of Nurse Anesthetists, but who receive legal status to practice in anesthesia by the appropriate authority in their state. Some states do not specifically mention advanced practice nurses, but the Board of Nursing approves specialty practice based on the provisions in the basic act. In still other states, advanced practice nurses are governed under the medical practice act. Contact the Board of Nursing in the state in which you are interested for information about advanced practice.

The NCSBN has adopted the position that the testing and licensing of nurses in advanced practice is the responsibility of the legal jurisdiction. Therefore, the NCSBN is developing a testing program for advanced nursing practice. In 1996, the NCSBN began a study process that could lead to a state-run testing program. That process is continuing at the time of this writing. Another of the goals of this study is the standardization of other licensing requirements for advanced nursing practice across the country.

Those who now certify advanced practice nurses have voiced opposition to this plan ("Boards will weigh . . .", 1996). The ANA does not believe that regulating advanced practice through the law and state-administered testing is the best method of ensuring safety in expanded practice. Some of the laws regulating advanced practice have provided for physician review of nursing's scope of practice. The ANA is concerned that these laws will take autonomy away from nursing and allow medicine to control some aspects of the nursing profession. The ANA also is concerned about the rigidity of these laws, which may not allow for evolving nursing roles. The ANA holds the position that the licensure law should regulate minimum safe practice, and that the profession should regulate advanced practice. A parallel process is used in medicine, in which there is only basic licensure and a physician in specialty practice is regulated by specialty boards in the profession.

The Role of the Board of Nursing

The Board of Nursing (or its equivalent) is legally empowered to carry out the provisions of the law. The membership of the board, the procedures for appointment and removal, and the qualifications of board members are determined by the Nurse Practice Act. The board has the power to write the rules and regulations used in daily operations.

The governor of the state usually appoints the members of the State Board of Nursing. The law specifies the occupational background of the candidates; nominations may be made by nurses' organizations and other interested parties. North Carolina is the only state in which the RN members of the state board are elected by the RNs in the state.

Boards of nursing range in size from 7 to 17 members. Prerequisites for educational background of nurses who serve as board members vary from state to state. Some states require that the board include nurses from different occupational areas, such as education and nursing service. Most states have at least one public member of the board. A few have at least one physician on the nursing board.

Most states have a single board for RNs and LPNs. In some states, two separate boards exist. Each state board has a paid staff that usually is headed by an RN who is employed as the executive director of the State Board of Nursing. The executive director is responsible for administering the work of the board and seeing that rules and regulations are followed. Some duties related to professional licensure may be performed by a centralized state agency acting in that capacity for all licensed occupations. The responsibilities of these centralized agencies may range from administrative matters (such as collecting fees, managing routine license renewals, and providing secretarial services) to decision making, relegating individual boards like the Board of Nursing, to an advisory status.

Each state board must operate within the framework of its own state law regarding the practice of nursing, but all cooperate with one another through the NCSBN. For example, state boards acting together through the NCSBN contract with the company that prepares the licensing examinations for RNs and practical nurses that are used throughout the United States. They also cooperate with the ANA and the National League for Nursing (NLN) in some matters, but maintain the separation that is required of a governmental body.

The Board of Nursing typically must perform the following functions:

1. Establish standards for licensure
2. Examine and license applicants
3. Provide for interstate endorsement
4. Renew licenses, grant temporary licenses, and provide for inactive status for those already licensed who request it
5. Enforce disciplinary codes
6. Provide rules for revocation of license
7. Regulate specialty practice
8. Establish standards and curricula for nursing programs
9. Approve nursing education programs

OBTAINING A NURSING LICENSE

There are two different procedures for obtaining a nursing license; one is used for obtaining an initial license and the other for obtaining a license when the nurse is already licensed in another jurisdiction. The initial licensure process is called **licensure by examination.** Obtaining a license in a second jurisdiction is called **licensure by endorsement.** In both instances, the applicant for licensure must meet all provisions of the law (such as educational preparation, language proficiency, and legal residency status) in the state where he or she is seeking licensure. In the initial licensure process, the applicant must take and pass the standard licensing examination (NCLEX). When seeking licensure by endorsement, the applicant is not required to take another examination; the licensing examination results from the initial state are accepted as proof of minimum safe practice, but other requirements must be met. This process is discussed later in the chapter.

Licensure by Examination

The establishment of a licensing examination was an important part of early efforts to achieve a professional standard for the RN. When each state adopted a licensing law, it also established a mechanism for examining license applicants. A major achievement in the history of nursing licensure was the formation of the Bureau of State Boards of Nurse Examiners, which eventually led to the use of an identical examination in all states in 1950. The original examination, called the State Board Test Pool Examination, was prepared by the testing department of the NLN, under a contract with the state boards. Although each state initially determined its own passing score, most states agreed on an acceptable test score; eventually all states adopted a common passing score for the State Board Test Pool Examination. The current examination, called the **NCLEX-RN** for registered nursing and the **NCLEX-PN** for practical nursing, is used in all states and territories of the United States. Beginning in October 2002, a new testing company, Pearson Professional Testing of Minnesota, was granted the contract for preparing and administering all NCLEX examinations.

CONTENT OF THE EXAMINATION

Traditionally, the content of the nursing examination was divided into the categories of medical, surgical, obstetric, pediatric, and psychiatric nursing. Because nursing had changed in nature and these categories no longer adequately reflected nursing practice, the NCSBN adopted a different examination plan, which was implemented in July 1982. For this new examination, the National Council supported a research study, called the "RN Job Analysis," that identified nursing behaviors critical to maintaining a safe and effective standard of care. This research has been repeated periodically to ensure that the test plan remains relevant to current nursing practice.

In all of these studies, newly licensed, practicing RNs are studied to determine both the frequency and the criticality of various behaviors. **Frequency** refers to how often the behaviors are required of the newly practicing RN. **Criticality** refers to those actions that, if performed incorrectly or omitted, could cause serious harm to the client. These studies are reflected in the "Test Plan for the NCLEX Examination for Registered Nurses (2001)" (NCSBN, 2001).

The NCLEX-RN examination questions are organized into categories based on the interaction of client needs and the steps of the nursing process. The four client needs (safe effective care environment, health promotion and maintenance, psychosocial integrity, and physiologic integrity), with their subcategories, form the basis of the exam. The nursing process is divided into five steps: assessment, analysis, planning, implementation, and evaluation. These two sets of concepts form a matrix in which each question tests a step of the nursing process and one subcategory of client need. Another set of broad concepts (caring, communication and documentation, cultural awareness, and self-care) is integrated into the test. The multiple-choice questions in the examination typically are based on situations that require a nursing response. They are designed to test judgment and decision making, not simply knowledge of facts. Setting priorities, delegating, and communicating with the health team are aspects of that judgment. The entire test plan is explained in the test plan booklet distributed to those who are applying to take the examination. The test plan is also available for downloading without charge from the NCSBN (NCSBN, 2001; NCSBN, 2002c).

The NCLEX-PN has a similar construction pattern. A "PN Job Analysis" study is conducted, and then the test plan is developed. The most recent PN Job Analysis was completed in 2000; the newest test plan for the PN was approved in 2001 and implemented in April 2002. The practical nurse is expected to assume a more dependent role in assessment; therefore, the category is titled data collection. Analysis is not part of the test plan. Whereas the RN examination includes management of care, the PN examination focuses on coordinated care. Even when topics are the same, the level of judgment expected of the PN differs from that expected of the RN. The newest test recognizes that many LPNs are employed in long-term care settings, with clients older than 65 years of age, and, therefore, has a life-span focus that emphasizes the older population. (NCSBN, 2001; NCSBN, 2002c).

PREPARING AND ADMINISTERING THE EXAMINATION

Preparing questions for the examination is a complex process. Nursing educators and RNs who work with new graduates are brought together as item writers. Together they write questions based on the test plan. Content experts who are also nurses currently working with new graduates review all questions. Another panel of individuals reviews the questions for bias. Each question then is verified for accuracy by using current nursing references; test-construction experts also review the structure of all of the questions. The final versions of all questions are tested by inclusion in a nongraded part of the license examinations being given to new graduates; the questions are evaluated for their level of difficulty and appropriate use as part of a future scored examination.

In addition to assuming responsibility for test preparation, the testing service administers the computerized tests through contracted testing centers, scores the examinations, and reports scores to the state boards. The testing service is authorized to sell statistical information related to the examinations to the states and to individual schools.

COMPUTERIZED ADAPTIVE TESTING

All NCLEX examinations (both RN and PN) are now administered through **computerized adaptive testing (CAT).** The CAT consists of a bank of examination questions administered through a computerized system. CAT had its first field trials in 1990, was tested across the country in 1993, and was adopted for all testing beginning in April 1994.

In this computerized test, the multiple-choice questions are on a computer screen. The computer contains a large bank of questions; different individuals may be presented with different questions. The computer program evaluates each response, and then selects an appropriate question to present next, choosing a slightly harder question if the previous question was answered correctly, or an easier question if the response was incorrect. The computer program ensures that all essential aspects of the test matrix plan are part of every examination. The development of questions and the design of the computer program ensures that all tests are equivalent even when not identical. On the NCLEX-RN, the minimum number of questions that might be administered is 75 and the maximum is 265. The maximum length of time for the examination is 5 hours, but a candidate performing either especially well or very poorly might complete the exam in just 1 hour. One break is required after 2 hours of testing, and others may be taken at the discretion of the applicant. Testing ends when the scoring analysis (see "Scoring the Examination") clearly indicates a pass, clearly indicates a fail, the maximum number of questions have been answered, or the maximum time has been completed.

Each candidate for licensure makes an individual appointment at a testing site. Security at the center is tightly monitored using photo identification and thumb prints. The computers are located in a quiet room without distractions. No test study materials are allowed at the testing center and no food or drink is allowed in the test environment. An erasable noteboard is provided for notes or calculations. An optional on-screen calculator is provided.

Each question, along with its possible answers, is presented on a separate screen; if there is a brief situation, it appears on the same screen as the question and answers. Only two keys are used throughout the examination: the space bar moves between the alternative answers, and the "enter" key must be pressed twice to make a selection. A mouse is also available for movement and selection. A selection must be made to move to the next question. It is not possible to go back to a question previously answered. In April 2003, two new types of questions will be used. One involves keyboard entry of short answers, and the other allows the person to select several answers from the multiple options, other than only one correct answer. A tutorial on how to use the computer, including the on-screen calculator, along with some practice questions are provided to assure that the individual understands the process. When the individual has completed enough questions for the computer program to determine either a "pass" or a "fail," the testing session is ended.

SCORING THE EXAMINATION

The computer calculates the score as the applicant answers questions. Based on the computation made as the applicant progresses, additional questions are presented to clearly determine whether the applicant meets the standards for safe, effective practice in all areas of the test plan. The score used to determine a pass or a failure is not a raw score (ie, the number correct), but is derived from a complex statistical process that takes into consideration both the difficulty of a question and whether the response was correct. As soon as the statistical computation provides a clear prediction of "pass" or "fail," the test is terminated. If the computerized score has not provided a clear prediction of pass or fail by the end of the examination (either time is up or maximum questions are answered), the performance on the last 60 questions becomes key to determining pass or fail. The test was not designed for the purpose of differentiating levels of excellence, only for demonstrating basic safe practice, and this is what the pass or fail communicates.

Although the computer immediately determines a score (upon the completion of the examination), the individual is not notified of the result at that time. The scoring information is communicated to the Testing Service, which then notifies the appropriate board. The Board of Nursing then notifies the individual whether he or she received a "pass" or "fail."

Every 3 years, the National Council of State Boards considers the appropriateness of the passing standards for both the PN and RN examinations. In October 1997, the decision was made to increase the passing standard for the NCLEX-RN beginning in 1998, based on the increased expectations placed upon nurses in their work environments (NCSBN, 1997). In 1998, the NCSBN approved a change in the passing standard for the PN examination. This increased standard took place in April 1999, coincident with the implementation of the new NCLEX-PN Test Plan (NCSBN, 2002c). The passing standards for the PN exam have not been changed since that time.

PREPARING FOR THE NCLEX

Each individual must determine how best to prepare for the licensure examination. This is determined based on background and preferred study style. A review of the knowledge basic to nursing is important for most individuals. This may be done using course notes and texts. Those who become anxious in testing situations may want to focus on exercises to decrease anxiety during the examination. Those who find the process of test taking difficult can gain greater self-confidence by practicing test-taking techniques. This can be done through printed tests in books or computerized test preparation programs.

For both the NCLEX-RN and the NCLEX-PN, many commercial study aids are available. To prepare applicants to take the examination, the NCSBN has authorized the preparation of a study book that explains the examination, how it was written, and the scoring system, and that provides sample questions to familiarize applicants with the way the test is written. The NCSBN also provides an on-line NCLEX-RN study program available by subscription. Many companies also prepare NCLEX-RN and NCLEX-PN review books, sample examination questions, audiotapes, and computerized practice examinations that are used to prepare for the licensing examinations. Manuals that outline standard nursing practice relative to many different health care problems may be useful for reviewing nursing content. Live and videotaped review courses, both by individual schools of nursing and by commercial publishers, are available to those who want assistance with preparation.

Critical Thinking Activity

A student about to graduate from a registered nursing program in New York wishes to practice nursing in New Jersey. Investigate the steps she should take to ensure that she may legally practice nursing in New Jersey as soon after graduation as possible.

Licensure By Endorsement

The process of obtaining a nursing license in a new state (when already licensed in another state) is called licensure by endorsement. Sometimes people incorrectly assume **reciprocity** exists among all states for nursing licenses. Technically, reciprocity is the type of recognition provided for such items as a driver's license; you can drive in any state as long as your license from your state of residence is valid. A similar type of recognition for nursing licensure has been developed between some states (see Multistate Licensure, below), but is not the universal pattern.

In licensure by endorsement, each case is considered independently, based on the rules and regulations of the state. However, due to the uniformity of licensing laws throughout most of the United States and its territories, nurses have enjoyed easy mobility between geographic areas.

Because the same licensure examination and same passing standards are used nationwide, no state requires that the examination be retaken. Basic educational and legal requirements of the individual state where a license is sought must be met. Sometimes a nurse moving to a new state must meet the current criteria for new licensure. In other states, a nurse must fulfill only the requirements that were in effect at the time of the original licensure. A state may require a nurse to meet other criteria, such as those for continuing education, before granting licensure by endorsement. In all cases, appropriate paperwork must be completed, necessary fees paid, and a license obtained before a nurse may begin employment.

A temporary license, which allows the applicant for licensure by endorsement to be employed while credentials are being verified and processed, is available in some states. Other states require that a permanent license be obtained before any employment is legal in those jurisdictions.

If a nurse wishes to maintain licensure in more than one state, this may be done by paying the renewal fees and meeting other requirements for continued licensure, such as continuing education, in each state. Some nurses hold licenses in several different states to be able to work as a traveling nurse or to choose work in different locations. Nurses working close to state lines may need more than one license to be employed by an agency that operates in more than one state. This might be true of a nursing education program that has clinical sites in two adjacent cities or a home care agency with clients in two states.

At present, North Dakota does not offer straightforward licensure by endorsement to all nurses licensed in other states. In North Dakota, an associate degree is required for initial licensure as a practical nurse, and a baccalaureate degree is required for initial licensure as an RN. All nurses registered in North Dakota were grandfathered into their licenses when this change in licensure regulations occurred. An RN or LPN from another state who does not have the required degree and who seeks licensure by endorsement in North Dakota must meet specific conditions and standards identified by the North Dakota Board; the conditions may include enrollment in an educational program to obtain the required degree. Based on individual evaluation, a temporary license may be granted while the individual fulfills the conditions specified for a regular license. North Dakota recently joined the multistate recognition compact. This means that those nurses with a diploma or associate degree and an RN license in another compact state will be able to work in North Dakota without the requirement to obtain the baccalaureate degree.

Critical Thinking Activity

An RN who has been working in San Jose, California for 10 years decides to relocate to Orlando, Florida. What are the steps that the nurse should take to ensure that she is able to work as an RN in Florida? Where should she seek information about the needed steps?

MULTISTATE LICENSURE

Multistate licensure involves an individual receiving an RN license in one state and being legally permitted to practice in additional states without obtaining additional licenses for those states. The Multistate Licensure Compact is the agreed-upon standard for mutual recognition of registered nursing licensure that was adopted by the NCSBN. Those states that have entered into the NCSBN Multistate Licensure Compact have all passed legislation adopting the terms of the compact into their licensure laws (NCSBN, 1998). This law applies only to basic registered nursing licensure and does not apply to any form of advanced practice nursing.

All of the states that have signed the compact are referred to as **party states.** A person's **home state** is the state in which an individual resides and in which that individual has a registered nursing license. An individual maintains only one license, the license granted in the home state, but is legally permitted to practice in any party state. When renewing a license, the individual renews in the home state. The individual nurse cannot hold a license in two party states at the same time. When an individual changes residence to a new party state, he or she would apply for a new home state license based on residency. If an individual wished to practice in a nonparty state, that person would still need to apply for a license in the nonparty state before practicing nursing.

A **remote state** is a place other than the nurse's home state where the patient or recipient of nursing practice is located. For purposes of this law, nursing care is located where the patient is, not where the nurse is. The individual nurse must comply with the state laws regulating nursing practice in the state in which the client is located. Any party state where nursing care occurs (whether the home state or the remote state) may institute disciplinary action based on appropriate procedures. The home state is notified of the action being taken in the remote state through a coordinated information system. When a remote state institutes disciplinary action, they may revoke the privilege to practice in that state only. Only the home state may revoke the license itself. If an individual has been assigned to some type of alternative program (such as drug treatment and monitoring) as part of the disciplinary process by any party state, the conditions of the disciplinary process must prohibit the individual from practicing in other states in the compact until the problem is resolved.

A computerized data bank titled NURSYS was completed in 2000. This data bank contains disciplinary information from every state and is used in the Multistate Compact states to track disciplinary concerns (Ventura, 1999). Noncompact states may also submit disciplinary information through the Health Care Integrity and Protection Data Bank (HIPDB) maintained by the NCSBN.

As you can see, the RN who is licensed in a Multistate Licensure Compact state who chooses to work outside the home state, must follow the directives contained in the compact and become familiar with the nursing practice act in any state in which clients are located. The State Board of any state participating in the compact will provide complete information on the specific requirements to be met.

States Involved

At the time of this writing, 18 states have enacted the necessary legislation to participate in the multistate licensure compact (Arizona, Arkansas, Delaware, Idaho, Iowa, Indiana, Maine, Maryland, Mississippi, Nebraska, New Jersey, North Carolina, North Dakota, South Dakota, Tennessee, Texas, Utah, and Wisconsin). For the most current information on participating states visit the National Council of State Board of Nursing (*http://www.ncsbn.org*).

Reasons Nurses Seek Multistate Licensure

Under standard licensing laws, the nurse who practices in more than one state must hold multiple nursing licenses. This is both costly and complex. As the health care system grows more diverse, it is not uncommon for a health care-providing organization to operate across state boundaries.

Telenursing includes the use of telecommunications technology (eg, telephone, fax, computers, teleconferencing, interactive television, and video phone) to provide nursing services to individuals and groups. A telenurse may be in one state, with a client in a distant state, thus raising questions regarding licensure requirements for a nurse who serves clients in more than one state. Does the nurse who provides telephone monitoring and advice for the client in another state need to be licensed in that client's state? Another area of concern is the nurse who works for an agency that serves clients across state borders. This nurse needs to visit clients in more than one state. The nursing case manager may follow clients in several states. All of these create situations in which both health care agencies and individual nurses would like a simpler system for licensing for work in multiple states.

Concerns Regarding Multistate Licensure

Not all nurses have supported multistate licensure. The ANA has identified that nurses could be practicing side-by-side who have differing requirements for relicensure; for example, one home state requires continuing education and another does not. Some state attorneys general have given opinions that it would be unconstitutional in their state to allow another state to control the requirements for practice. Privacy concerns regarding the data stored in the NURSYS system are another area of concern. The multistate licensure system may save money for the nurse who practices in multiple states because only one license would be purchased. However, if fewer nurses are licensed in the state, but the same number practice in the state, one would expect that disciplinary costs would remain even. The cost of licenses for all nurses, therefore, would have to rise to assure adequate funds to support disciplinary costs (Ventura, 1999).

A major concern is the disciplinary process. Although the board of nursing can investigate nursing practice and enforce its own standards in the state, it cannot change the licensure status of the person whose licensure is in a different state; this fact is troubling to some boards of nursing. They are concerned that they would be unable to protect the public adequately. A person disciplined in a remote state still would possess what would appear to be a valid home state license, but perhaps would not legally be able to practice in the remote state. For the individual nurse, the differences in licensure regulations could result in the same behavior being the cause of disciplinary action in one state but not in others; however, if the license were removed, then it would be invalid in all states. Simpson (1999) suggests that technology can solve most of these concerns if it is applied effectively. The ANA has expressed concern that multistate licensure would facilitate bringing in out-of-state nurses for strike breaking and thus interfere with valid collective bargaining. (See Chapter 12 for a further discussion of collective bargaining.)

The future holds many exciting possibilities for nursing but also poses many potential pitfalls. This is a complex issue, because state licensing agencies are charged with protecting the public and have legitimate concerns regarding such areas as disciplinary action.

REVOCATION OR LIMITATION OF A LICENSE

A license to practice any occupation becomes a property right of the individual once the state has awarded it. As long as the individual renews a license by paying the appropriate fees and meeting any requirements, such as continuing education, a license cannot be revoked without cause. The possible reasons for revoking or limiting a license are spelled out in the law. (The common reasons were listed earlier, in the discussion of disciplinary provisions of the law.)

The procedure for revoking a license includes a fact-finding process and a hearing, which functions in many ways like a court proceeding. The state board or a specially designated hearing board is responsible for conducting the hearing and making a decision. The board may provide a license with conditions, suspend a license until certain conditions are met, or revoke a license completely. For example, a nurse faced with charges of chemical dependency might be directed to enter a treatment program, to refuse employment involving direct responsibility for clients or access to drugs, and to be monitored for compliance. If these conditions are met, the individual may be allowed to work in a restricted environment and then be reinstated to full rights and privileges of licensure when treatment is completed. The board's decision may be appealed in a court of law in most states. If a board of nursing finds that the individual's actions constitute a felony, the board is obligated to report that to the criminal authorities for prosecution.

The individual being investigated for any violation of the Nursing Practice Act, or who is in the hearing process, should have an attorney who is knowledgeable about professional disciplinary issues for legal counsel from the time of notification of the complaint. According to Malugani (2000), the majority of nurses facing disciplinary action fail to take this important step to protect themselves. The state nurses association or the local chapter of the National Association of Nurse Attorneys can often provide referrals of attorneys who are familiar with the disciplinary process. Although attorney costs are substantial, a license to practice nursing is extremely valuable to the individual nurse. Some malpractice insurance policies include payment for attorney fees in the case of disciplinary action. (see Chapter 8.)

As a licensed professional, you should be aware that you are responsible to your clients and to the state for your practice. You can act to protect your license through maintaining current knowledge and appropriate standards of practice. You should also understand and abide by the scope of practice as described in your individual nurse practice act. If you take a position in a new state, be sure to become informed about that state's Nurse Practice Act.

Critical Thinking Activity

A nurse in your state receives a notification from the Board of Nursing that a complaint has been lodged with the board regarding her practice. Find out what the process would be in your state for this nurse to respond to the complaint. What resources will this nurse need? What are the possible consequences if the complaint is sustained?

SUNSET LAWS

Most laws remain in effect until the legislature votes to rescind or replace them. Because this has resulted in archaic laws remaining in effect for many years, some states have passed what are known as "sunset laws." **Sunset laws** provide that any regulatory act, such as the Nurse Practice Act, will automatically be rescinded after a predetermined length of time if not reauthorized. In states with sunset laws, nurses cannot wait for an opportune time to support changes in the Nurse Practice Act. Instead, they must identify when sunsetting will occur and work in advance to sustain the current law or make changes. The advantage of sunset laws is that they guarantee that the legislature will review and evaluate agencies and programs.

LICENSURE OF GRADUATES OF FOREIGN NURSING SCHOOLS

Many nurses from other countries have immigrated to the United States and sought licensure to be able to work in their new home. Some nurses have come to the United States for additional education and need a license to engage in clinical practice associated with that education. Still others are attracted by the better salaries and living conditions for nurses in the United States. During the nursing shortage of the early 1980s, and again in the current nursing shortage, employers in the United States actively recruited foreign nurses, sometimes providing support for travel and relocation expenses.

All graduates of foreign nursing schools who want to practice nursing in the United States must provide verification that their nursing education meets state requirements, and they must take the appropriate NCLEX examination. In the past, institutions would sometimes hire foreign nurses into lower-paying positions until they obtained a license. When many did not pass the examination, they felt exploited by the system.

The U.S. Department of Labor, the Department of Health and Human Services, the Immigration and Naturalization Service, the ANA, and the NLN were different agencies and organizations concerned about the safety of the public and about the well-being of the foreign-educated nurse. To address these problems, these organizations and governmental agencies collaborated in the development of an independent organization called the Commission on Graduates of Foreign Nursing Schools (CGFNS). This organization reviews foreign educational credentials, assures English language proficiency by evaluating scores on the English language proficiency examinations, and administers a nursing proficiency examination to foreign-educated nurses. Based on these data, the CGFNS provides certification to Boards of Nursing, educational institutions, and the Immigration and Naturalization Service of the nursing education status of the individual seeking to go to school or work in the United States. Nurses may take the CGFNS examination in 40 sites around the world before undertaking expensive relocation. Up to 85% of foreign-educated nurses who have obtained CGFNS certification pass the licensing examination. This contrasts to the 5% to 10% who passed the licensing examination without CGFNS screening (CGFNS, 2002). Because many foreign-educated nurses still come to the United States without having taken the CGFNS examination, it also is offered in selected cities in the United States. Some states make CGFNS certification a requirement for graduates of foreign nursing schools who wish to take the NCLEX-RN.

During the nursing shortages, recruitment of foreign-educated nurses is prevalent. Special immigration regulations allow these nurses to obtain the special-preference visas from the U.S. Immigration and Naturalization Service, or a work permit from the U.S. Labor Department. The foreign-educated nurse must obtain CGFNS certification to get this visa.

Several concerns have been expressed regarding this process. In many of the countries from which nurses emigrate to the United States, there are also nursing shortages. Thus, the United States depletes other countries of an important health resource. In some instances, U.S. nurses have believed that overseas recruitment took the place of addressing the workplace problems that contribute to the shortage.

INTERNATIONAL NURSING LICENSURE

Nursing education and nursing licensure differ greatly throughout the world. Additionally, practice patterns and expectations of nursing behaviors may differ between countries. In Australia, nursing education has been moved into university settings, and future applicants for licensure in that country will be required to have a university education. In Italy, nursing education is now consolidated under broad, multisite programs administered by university nursing departments. The European Union is moving toward a system that allows freer movement of professionals between the nations of the E.U. The nations of Eastern Europe face many drastic changes in their health care systems as they change internally and form different relationships with the West. Nursing education was restricted during Soviet domination, and many nurses had limited nursing educational opportunities, with basic nursing education sometimes occurring at the high school level. These nurses are now seeking ways to broaden nursing education in their own countries and to interface with the international nursing community.

Because of these great differences, nursing credentials are not easily transferred internationally. The International Congress of Nurses (ICN) has supported the development of effective licensure legislation worldwide. In 1988, the ICN launched a project called "Nursing Regulation: Moving Ahead," which was funded by the W. K. Kellogg Foundation. This ongoing project involved nurses and officials from 77 countries in seminars and studies. To date, nursing licensure laws in the United States have not been affected by this study, but it has supported the development of licensure laws in some parts of the world.

Individuals who are interested in international nursing need to consider their language proficiency and educational backgrounds. Not all countries welcome nurses educated elsewhere. They may have a surplus of nurses and wish to avoid displacing local nurses. Others are concerned that nurses educated in affluent societies such as the United States and Canada may understand little about the health care needs and nursing practices in a developing country. Organizations actively working in the international health field, such as the World Health Organization and medical relief organizations, usually will provide information on opportunities and licensure requirements in various countries. The ICN in Geneva can provide addresses of appropriate governmental authorities to contact regarding licensure in certain countries.

CERTIFICATION IN NURSING

As mentioned earlier, **certification** in nursing is primarily a professional, and not a legal, credential and focuses on knowledge and skills related to a particular area of practice. The definition of certification adopted by the Interdivisional Council on Certification of the ANA (1978) states: "Certification is the documented validation of specific qualifications demonstrated by the individual registered nurse in the provision of professional nursing care in a

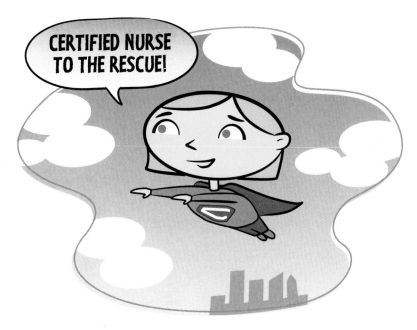

CERTIFIED NURSE TO THE RESCUE!

FIGURE 7-3 Certified nurses provide an expert level of practice and may serve as a resource to others.

defined area of practice." Certification is available from many professional nursing and health care organizations (Fig. 7-3).

ANCC Certification

In 1988, the ANA established a credentialing center called the American Nurses' Credentialing Center (ANCC), which assumed all of the ANA credentialing activities. The ANA invited all other organizations providing credentialing for nurses to join; some joined, but many retained their individual programs.

ANCC certification is a method of recognizing nurses who have special expertise. Applicants must demonstrate current practice and knowledge beyond that required for licensure as an RN. After submitting evidence of completing all requirements, a nurse may take the national examination for a specific certification. Certification is granted for a period of 5 years, after which a nurse may renew the certification by submitting new evidence of current practice and ability. Display 7-2 lists the various certification credentials available from the ANCC.

Effective in 1998, as approved by the House of Delegates in 1991, individuals seeking certification as generalists in all specialties were required to have a baccalaureate in nursing; those seeking certification as specialists or advanced practice nurses needed a master's degree in nursing. In 2000, responding to the voices of RNs, the ANCC revised its certification program. There are now two basic types of certification. Registered Nurse, Certified (RN, C.) is awarded to those with diplomas or associate degrees in nursing who meet the certification requirements. Registered Nursing Board Certified (RN, BC) is awarded to nurses with a baccalaureate or higher degree who meet differing certification requirements. The master's degree remains the requirement for certification as a clinical nurse specialist, a nurse practitioner, or other advanced practice roles.

Display 7-2 NURSING CERTIFICATION AVAILABLE THROUGH THE AMERICAN NURSES' CREDENTIALING CENTER

Generalists*
Cardiac Rehabilitation
CE/Staff Development
College Health
Community Health
General Nursing
Gerontological
Home Health
Medical-Surgical
Pediatric
Perinatal
Psychiatric and Mental Health
School Nurse

Nurse Practitioners (master's degree required)
Acute Care
Family
Pediatric
Adult
Gerontological
School

Clinical Specialists (master's degree required)
Community Health
Home Health
Gerontological
Medical-Surgical
Adult Psychiatric and Mental Health
Child/Adolescent Psychiatric and Mental
   Health

Nursing Administrators
Nursing Administration
Nursing Administration, Advanced
   (master's degree required)

**Modular (specialty certification or additional
   test required)**
Nursing Case Management
Ambulatory Care

A new plan that includes "board certified" for BSN preparation and "certified" for diploma and associate degree education was announced in 2000.

In addition to certifying individuals in specialty practice, the ANCC provides an accreditation mechanism for institutions or organizations desiring to be an "approver" or a "provider" of nursing continuing education programs. State nurses associations and specialty organizations often seek accreditation as approvers of programs. Accreditation as a provider assures the nurse consumer that the continuing education offering meets appropriate standards ("Consultation services . . .", 1999).

American Board of Nursing Specialties

In 1991, eight national nursing certification programs joined to establish the American Board of Nursing Specialties. These organizations were the American Nurses' Credentialing Center of the ANA, the American Board for Occupational Health Nursing, the American Board of Neuroscience Nursing, the Association of Rehabilitation Nurses, the Council on Certification of Nurse Anesthetists, the National Board of Nutritional Support Certification, the Nephrology Nursing Certification Board, and the Orthopaedic Nurses Certification Board. According to their report, in 1991 these eight organizations represented more than 65% of the total

| **Display 7-3** | **NURSING CERTIFICATION AVAILABLE THROUGH THE SPECIALTY NURSING ORGANIZATIONS*** |

Addictions Nursing	Neonatal Intensive Care Nurse
Childbirth Educator	Neonatal Nurse Practitioner
Critical Care Nursing	Nephrology Nursing
Diabetes Educator	Neuroscience Nursing
Emergency Nursing	Nurse Anesthetist
Gastroenterology	Nurse Midwife
Healthcare Quality	Occupational Health Nursing
Holistic Nursing	Oncology Nursing
Hospice Nurse	Ophthalmic Nursing
Inpatient Obstetric Nurse	Orthopedic Nursing
Intravenous Nursing	Pain Management
Lactation Consultant	Plastic and Reconstructive Surgical Nursing
Legal Nurse Consultant	School Nurse
Low-Risk Neonatal Nurse	Urology Nursing
Maternal Newborn Nurse	Women's Health Nursing

Educational requirements vary.

number of RNs certified in specialty practice ("Specialty certification . . .", 1991). The goals of this board are to ensure quality in specialty nursing, to improve the public's perception of specialty nurses, and to provide specialty nurses who bring a consistent standard of education and experience to their practice. This is a major breakthrough in the entire certification process for nursing. This Board has established a peer review process for certification organizations that provides evaluation and recognition of the certification granted (Display 7-3).

Other Certification Programs for Registered Nurses

Other specialty organizations in nursing also have certification programs. Most are administered by a separately titled and funded certification organization that is closely related to the specialty organization. This administrative structure is set up to protect the sponsoring organization from economic liability, to preserve tax-exempt status, and to provide a more objective approach to the credentialing process. Information on any of these specialty certification programs can be obtained by writing directly to the organization. Some of these organizations require a BSN for certification, but others certify based on the RN license, role-specific education and practice, and an examination. The Oncology Nurses Society adopted the BSN as a requirement, but in December 1999, announced the requirements were changing to admit any RN meeting other requirements. Their rationale for the change was that they were unable to demonstrate any practice differences between those prepared with various basic nursing credentials once they had the required specialty education and practice. This illustrates the constant changes that are occurring in the field of nursing.

The National Association of Pediatric Nurse Associates/Practitioners (NAPNAP) supports an independent certification for the pediatric nurse practitioner. This has resulted in certificates being awarded in the same area by two organizations. NAPNAP and the ANCC have had joint conferences regarding certification, with the hope of developing one jointly sponsored certification; however, fundamental differences still exist between the two organizations on how authority for determining standards should be established.

The Association for Women's Health, Obstetric and Neonatal Nursing (AWHONN), formerly called the Nurses' Association of the American College of Obstetricians and Gynecologists (NAACOG), sponsors certification for nurses working in women's health care, obstetrics, and neonatal nursing.

The American Association of Critical Care Nurses (AACCN) sponsors certification of nurses in the critical care arena. Their certification confers the title Critical Care Registered Nurse (CCRN). Although this certification is not required to work in critical care, it attests to ongoing practice in critical care, along with continuing education directly related to the critical care field and a passing score on a critical care examination.

The American College of Nurse Midwives sponsors a certification program for nurses specializing in nurse midwifery. Nurses graduating from approved midwifery programs apply for certification through this organization. Approved programs may be at a postbaccalaureate, nonmasters degree level or at a master's degree level.

Some organizations of health care workers offer credentialing to individuals in specific occupations that may include nurses. For example, the Society of Gastroenterostomal Assistants offers certification to individuals employed in gastroenterology laboratories. This certification is available to both RNs and LPNs. The Association for Practitioners in Infection Control certifies individuals who are professionals in infection control, including physicians, public health officers, and nurses.

Critical Thinking Activity

An RN with 5 years of general medical-surgical acute care experience is interested in working in the critical care unit of a hospital in your community. Seek information regarding how this nurse could obtain a critical care position in your community. Compare that process with what would be required of you as a new graduate to move into such a position.

Certification for Licensed Practical Nurses

Certification for LPNs (LVNs) is available for those practicing in long-term care. The National Association of Practical Nurse Education and Service (NAPNES) determined that many LPNs have responsible positions in long-term care and that recognition of their abilities through certification would be appropriate. They contracted with the National Council of State Boards of Nursing to develop and administer a certification examination. Those taking this examination use the title CLTC (Certified in Long-Term Care). This is the only nursing certification available to LPNs. LPNs may be eligible for certification programs that are not specifically nursing.

THE FUTURE OF CREDENTIALING IN HEALTH CARE

Because credentialing in nursing involves so many different aspects of education, licensure, and certification, it has confused the public, nurses, and other health care professionals. The ideal credential clearly communicates qualifications and competence; therefore, it is important for nursing to have a credentialing system that can be understood by others. Current changes are moving nursing closer to an effective credentialing system.

Institutional Control of Credentials

Many new health care occupations related to new procedures and processes in medical care are being developed as new technology develops. Those who believe the state should take positive action to protect the public continue to exert pressure to license additional health care providers. Those who oppose credentialing of additional individual groups of health care workers believe that modern-day employers are able to assess workers and to differentiate among them on the basis of competence. Some who oppose credentialing of individual health occupations believe that licensing the institution that hires the employees would be an adequate safeguard for the public.

Another approach to credentialing in health care is certifying specific competencies rather than an entire field of practice. Those advocating this approach believe that it would facilitate the development of individuals with a broad range of competencies suited to a particular setting. For example, in a rural area one individual might be certified as competent to perform certain basic x-ray examinations (such as for simple fractures), basic laboratory studies (such as complete blood count and urinalysis), and some basic client care procedures (such as bathing, toileting, feeding, and positioning). Because more complex procedures are sent to a larger center and there is no need for a full-time person in any of these positions, basic care would be made available in a convenient and low-cost manner. Certification of specific competencies by the employing agency is sometimes referred to as **site-based examination** and **site-based certification.** One concern about this method of certifying competencies is the focus on technical skills, without adequate recognition of the knowledge base needed for decision making and judgment. Other concerns are the complexity of keeping track of the many specific competencies, and the difficulty with job mobility when competencies are not standardized.

Pew Report

A comprehensive reform of all health care workforce regulation was proposed by the Center for the Health Professions (Finocchio et al, 1995). Based on a study supported by the Pew Charitable Trust, the report titled "Reforming Health Care Workforce Regulation" (commonly referred to as one of the "Pew Reports on Health Care Workforce Regulation"), made 10 recommendations for changes in regulations. These are found in Display 7-4. These recommendations are based on what is termed a SAFE focus: Standardized where appropriate, Accountable to the public, Flexible to support optimal access, and Effective and Efficient in

Display 7-4   **RECOMMENDATIONS FOR REFORMING HEALTH CARE WORKFORCE REGULATION**

1. Standardize regulatory terms.
2. Standardize entry-to-practice requirements.
3. Remove barriers to the full use of competent health professionals.
4. Redesign health professional board structures and functions.
5. Educate the public.
6. Collect data on the health professions.
7. Develop, implement, and evaluate continuing competency requirements.
8. Reform the professional disciplinary process.
9. Develop tools to evaluate regulatory effectiveness.
10. Understand the organizational context of health professions regulation; develop partnerships to streamline regulatory structures and processes.

The Center for the Health Professions. "What's the fuss?" Front & Center, San Francisco: University of California, Summer, 1996.

protecting and promoting the public's health, safety, and welfare. Many of the recommendations, such as educating the public about health professional regulation and collecting data on the health professions, are supported by almost everyone. Others, such as developing, implementing, and evaluating continuing competency requirements, raise many questions in the minds of both health professionals and regulatory boards.

The National Council of State Boards of Nursing provided leadership in a national meeting in December of 1995 to discuss the Center for Health Professions' recommendations and their implications for nursing regulation. The response of those in attendance was that nursing has supported the broad goals of the recommendations and has achieved goals in many areas. However, there was concern that the stated goals are unfocused and go beyond what can be accomplished through regulation alone. Although some of the policy suggestions in the report are controversial, there appeared to be a willingness to engage in constructive dialogue and encourage the participation of legislators, consumers, and health professionals in decision making. In August 1996, the NCSBN published a detailed response to the Pew Report as a special section in its Issues Newsletter. For each recommendation, a discussion and specific policy option were provided (Lund et al, 1996).

Continued Competency

Once an individual receives a license to practice as a health professional, a serious event (or series of serious events) must occur for that license to be removed. Even in states that require continuing education, the question has been asked "How can anyone be sure that an individual who was judged competent through an examination at one time is still competent years later?" The National Council of State Boards of Nursing has defined competence as "the application of knowledge and the interpersonal, decision-making, and psychomotor skills expected for the nurse's practice role, within the context of public health, welfare, and safety." The NCSBN has further indicated that the nurse should be expected to perform as necessary for the particular situation or restrict practice if the RN cannot safely perform (Green & Ogden, 1999).

In 1996, the Center for the Health Professions provided grants for the State Initiatives Program to Reform the Healthcare Workplace. Some states established specific programs to examine competency issues. Focusing on the concern regarding continued competency, state boards of nursing, nurses associations, and others have worked together. The states of Kentucky, Oklahoma, Texas, and Nebraska are addressing the issue of continued competence (Green & Ogden, 1999; Burback & Exstrom, 1999).

One concern that has emerged is the difference between identifying beginning competence as a generalist in all areas of nursing, and the expectation of higher-level competence in a special sphere of nursing that is needed by the experienced nurse. There are clear differences in roles of nurses between urban and rural settings, between acute care and long-term care, between ambulatory care and inpatient care. The role of the employer in assessing the nurse's competency is another area of discussion. The Joint Commission on the Accreditation of Healthcare Organizations requires that accredited organizations have a program in place to evaluate competency of all employees.

The expectation for personal self-assessment and growth also must have a place in the search for continued competence. What responsibility should nurses take in identifying their own learning needs, seeking appropriate professional development opportunities, and monitoring their own learning from those opportunities? Should nurses be required to establish professional goals? To keep portfolios documenting self-assessment and professional development? To take advanced examinations? Chapter 9 offers suggestions for a personal self-evaluation plan. Whatever the rules and regulations, nurses do have a professional, ethical obligation to maintain their own competence.

KEY CONCEPTS

- Credentials are written proof of qualifications and may include diplomas conferred by educational programs, certification, or registration by professional groups, and legal licenses conferred by governmental agencies.
- Permissive licensure allows for those meeting certain standards voluntarily to be licensed, whereas mandatory licensure requires that all individuals who wish to practice in the field be licensed to practice.
- Nursing leaders began efforts to obtain legal licensure in 1896. The first permissive licensure law was passed in 1903 by North Carolina, and the first mandatory licensure law was passed in New York in 1947.
- Legal rules governing nursing practice are found in the licensure law passed by a legislative body. Further provisions governing nursing are found in the rules and regulations established by the administrative agency in which the legislation vests authority.
- The nursing practice act usually contains a definition of nursing, and addresses qualifications for licensure applicants, use of titles, renewal and continuing education requirements, grandfathering, financial concerns, nursing education programs, disciplinary action, violations and penalties, administrative provisions, and expanded nursing roles.

- The Board of Nursing (or its equivalent) is the administrative agency with the authority to carry out the provisions of the Nurse Practice Act.
- A license to practice nursing must be obtained from the state or province in which you wish to work. An initial license is termed licensure by examination, and subsequent licenses may be obtained in other jurisdictions through licensure by endorsement.
- Advanced practice nurses are regulated by each state. Most require professional certification in an advanced practice nursing specialty to be licensed in that role.
- Multistate licensure involves a compact between certain states that allows nurses who are licensed in those states to work freely among all the compact states without the need for obtaining additional licenses.
- The NCLEX-RN examination is administered through a computerized plan that covers the five steps of the nursing process and four areas of client needs, and that identifies competence for entry-level safe nursing care.
- Graduates of foreign nursing schools must have their credentials reviewed and may be required to take the CGFNS examination, which reviews both nursing content and English language ability, before being admitted to take the NCLEX examination.
- A license may be revoked by the State Board of Nursing, a designated disciplinary board, or a court of law based on specific reasons stated in the Nurse Practice Act.
- Certification provides evidence of specialized clinical knowledge and ability beyond the basic level. Certification as a nurse practitioner may be used as a basis for legal approval to practice in an expanded role.
- Concerns about the future of health care worker credentialing include issues of public accountability and continued competence.

RELEVANT WEB SITES

Certification information:
American Nurses Association: *www.nursingworld.org*
Lippincott/AJN: *www.nursingcenter.com/prodev/ce_certification.asp*
Licensure information:
Commission on Graduates of Foreign Nursing Schools: *www.cgfns.org*
National Council of State Boards of Nursing: *www.ncsbn.org*

REFERENCES

American Nurses Association. (1991). *Nursing's agenda for healthcare reform*. Washington, DC: American Nurses Publishing Co.

American Nurses Association Congress for Nursing Practice. (1990). *Suggested state legislation: Nursing Practice Act, Disciplinary Diversion Act, Prescriptive Authority Act*. Kansas City, MO: American Nurses Association.

American Nurses Association. (1980). *Nursing: A social policy statement*. Kansas City, MO: American Nurses Association.

American Nurses Association. (2000). States recognizing advanced practice under independent acts, separate title of advance practice acts or regulations. Available on-line at *www.nursingworld.org/ gova/charts/titles.htm*, Accessed August 10, 2002.

Boards will weigh plan to test NPs. (1996). *American journal of Nursing, 96*(6):69, 73.

Burback, V. & Exstrom, S. (1999). Continued competency in Nebraska: Process and progress. *Issues 20*(2): 1, 5–11.

"Consultation services now available for ANCC magnet and accreditation programs." (1999). *American Nurse 31*(5):11.

Finocchio, L. J., Dower, C. M., McMahon, T., Gragnola, C. M., & the Taskforce of Health Care Workforce Regulation. (1995). *Reforming health care workforce regulation: Policy considerations for the 21st century*. San Francisco: Pew Health Professions Commission.

Green, A. & Ogden, B. S. (1999). Three state nursing boards examine continued competency. *American Nurse 31*(2). [On-line]. Available: *www.nursingworld.org/tan/99marapr/competen.htm*. Accessed August 6, 2002.

Lund, E., Bouchard, J., Graves, C., Osman, C., VanWingerden, C., Bosma, J., Creal, D., Hutcherson, C., & Sheets, V. (1996). National Council of State Boards of Nursing's response to the Pew Taskforce on Health Care Workforce Regulation. *Issues 17*(3): Special Section 1–6.

Malugani, M. (2000). Nurse, interrupted: A disciplinary action can put a wrinkle in your career and tie you up in knots. *Nurseweek* [On-line]. Available: *www.nurseweek.com/news/features/00-08/ discip.html*. Accessed August 10, 2002.

National Council of State Boards of Nursing. (1997). New test plan for RN approved. *Issues, 18*(4):1.

National Council of State Boards of Nursing (1998). Nurse licensure compact: Final version, November 6, 1998. [On-line]. Available: *www.ncsbn.org*. Accessed March 9, 2003.

National Council of State Boards of Nursing. (2002a). *Model Nursing Practice Act* (revision). Chicago: National Council of State Boards of Nursing.

National Council of State Boards of Nursing. (2002b). *Model Nursing Administrative Rules* (revision). Chicago: National Council of State Boards of Nursing.

National Council of State Boards of Nursing. (2002c). *Test Plan for the NCLEX for Practical Nurses.* Chicago: National Council of State Boards of Nursing. (also available at *www.ncsbn.org*).

National Council of State Boards of Nursing. (2002d). Nursing Regulation. [On-line]. Available: *www.ncsbn.org/*

National Council of State Boards of Nursing. (2001). *Test plan for the NCLEX for registered nurses.* Chicago: National Council of State Boards of Nursing. (also available at *www.ncsbn.org*).

Simpson, R. L. (1999). Tech talk on multistate licensure. *Nursing Management 30*(1):12–13.

"Specialty certification groups form organization." (1991). *American Nurse, 23*(4):20.

Ventura, M. J. (1999). The great multistate licensure debate. *RN 62*(5):58–63.

Washington State Department of Health. (1996). New legislation. *The Nursing Commission Newsletter, 2*(1):2. Olympia, WA: Author

8

Legal Responsibilities for Practice

LEARNING OUTCOMES

After completing this chapter, you should be able to:

1. Differentiate the two general sources of law and explain how they apply to nursing.
2. Explain the role of institutional policies and protocols in legal decision-making.
3. Describe situations in which inappropriate nursing actions may violate criminal law.
4. Discuss liability in relationship to nursing practice, including situations in which liability is shared by employers or supervisors.
5. Analyze the value to you as an individual nurse of purchasing professional liability insurance.
6. Explain the nurse's role in supporting patient rights through informed consent and advance directives.
7. Discuss the nurse's responsibility in the specific issues that can constitute malpractice.
8. Explain the most commonly recurring legal issues in nursing.
9. Identify factors that contribute to a suit being instituted against a health care professional, and explain how an individual nurse might prevent legal suits.
10. Explain the various aspects of a legal action.
11. Outline the role of the nurse when testifying for a legal proceeding.

KEY TERMS

Administrative ruling	Emancipated minors	Misdemeanor
Advance directive	Enacted law	Negligence
Assault	Ethics	Patient Self-Determination Act (PSDA)
Battery	Expert witness	Perjury
Civil law	False imprisonment	Plaintiff
Common law	Felony	Privileged communication
Consent	Fraud	Prudent professional
Constitutional law	Futile	Reckless endangerment
Crime	Guardian	Regulatory law (administrative)
Criminal law	Informed consent	Standard of care
Criminal negligence	Intentional tort	Standard of practice
Defendant	Judicial law (decisional or case law)	Statute
Deposition	Law	Statutory law
Directive to physicians	Lawsuit	Substitutionary decision-maker
Discovery	Liability	Testimony
Do not resuscitate (DNR) (No Code)	Living will	Tort
Durable power of attorney for health care	Malpractice	Witness to fact
	Mature minor	

Every newspaper contains reports of sensational cases being decided in our courts. Concerns about lawsuits and liability are voiced in every business. Health care remains at the forefront of professions where legal issues constitute a major area of concern. The wise nurse considers legal issues before a crisis arises and uses sound information to help guide action in situations where questions arise. This chapter provides basic information you will need in that process.

UNDERSTANDING THE SCOPE OF THE LAW

Legal issues are those that are decided by law. **Law** may be defined as "a rule of conduct or action prescribed or formally recognized as binding or enforced by a controlling authority" (Judson & Hicks, 1999, p. 4). They are put in place to assure that behavior that would threaten public safety is controlled. **Ethics** are the principles of conduct governing one's relationships with others—basic beliefs about right and wrong. Legal and ethical issues are often discussed together because they go hand in hand, with one supporting the other. Ethics also may address questions that are entirely different from those addressed by the law. Hall (1996, p. 49) stated, "Law is the minimum ethic, written down and enforced; behavior that is not merely desired but mandated." In this chapter, we focus on how the law affects nursing practice. Ethics are introduced here and are discussed in more detail in Chapter 9.

Examples and situations relating to legal issues discussed throughout this chapter are given to help you understand the application of the specific concepts. Many more factors would be considered in arriving at an actual legal decision than can be presented in a paragraph or two. It is the interaction of multiple factors that makes it impossible to provide absolute predictions regarding legal outcomes in specific situations; that is, data may be interpreted differently by judges and juries, resulting in different outcomes, although cases may appear similar.

If you have a question about a specific personal situation, you would be well advised to consult an attorney who is experienced in medicolegal matters. The facility where you are employed may have a legal counselor who is available to you. Another source of legal aid is your nurses association attorney. If you desire private counsel, suitable names may be recommended by the nurses association in your state or the local bar association. And, of course, you may·always identify and seek the services of an attorney in your community who works in the area of law about which you are concerned.

SOURCES OF LAW

If nurses know the source of law, then they know how it can be challenged and changed, and how powerful it can be. There are three general sources of law: *statutory law, regulatory (administrative) law,* and *common law*. All are relevant to nursing practice (Fig. 8-1).

Statutory Law

A **statute** is a rule or formal regulation established by governmental legislative authority, such as the Congress, the state legislature, or the city council, that appears in writing. A violation of a statute is legally punishable. Statutory law is published in codes. A key aspect of all statutory law is that it is written down as specific rules. In the United States, **statutory law** includes constitutional law and enacted law. All laws are in a hierarchy of authority, with constitutional law having the greatest authority and enacted law the next. Regulatory law, to be discussed below, is below statutory law in authority.

CONSTITUTIONAL LAW

Constitutional law is the law established by the federal government and based on the U. S. Constitution. The Constitution was developed and passed by the Continental Congress and then ratified by all the states. The Constitution establishes the general organization of the federal government, and specifies the federal power and limitations to that power. The powers not specifically given to the federal government in the Constitution are retained by the states. Amendments to the U. S. Constitution require similar passage and ratification by the states. The first amendments were contained in the Bill of Rights, which was passed a few years after the Constitution was established. The amendments have the same status as the original provisions. Each state has its own constitution that acts as the highest law for that individual state. Many other nations, such as Great Britain, do not have a constitution or equivalent document. In those countries, the enacted law is the highest level of law.

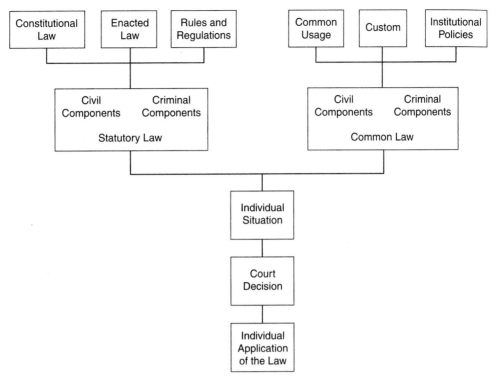

FIGURE 8-1   Civil law and criminal law both may affect a nursing situation.

ENACTED LAW

Enacted law includes all bills passed by legislative bodies, whether at the local, state or province, or national level. Enacted laws of the U. S. federal government all carry the designation "USC" in their official title. The federal Social Security Act (42 USC 401) is an example of federally enacted law. Enacted laws of states or other governing bodies carry a similar designation. Nurse practice acts in the various states are examples of enacted law at the state level.

Regulatory Law

Regulatory law (also referred to as executive or administrative law) includes the rules and regulations established by governmental agencies to carry out enacted law. These also appear as carefully written rules that apply to everyone. At the federal level, the Centers for Medicare and Medicaid Services (CMS) writes regulations governing the payment of Medicaid and Medicare funds that were authorized through legislation. At the state level, the State Board of Nursing is authorized through enacted laws to establish and enforce rules and regulations that govern the practice of nursing in that particular state. The rules and regulations they establish protect the safety of the public by defining standards for nursing education and practice (see Chapter 7). Rules and regulations of administrative bodies can be enforced in court.

Common Law

Common law derives from common usage, custom, and judicial law (judicial decisions or court rulings). It is based in the English common law. Because it is based on occurrences of events, common law is less clear and exact than statutory law; it is composed of many actions and documents that are not specific written rules that apply to everyone. Common law is fluid and changes over time. In general, statutory law and regulatory law carry more weight in court than does common law.

COMMON USAGE AND CUSTOM

As the term seems to imply, courts are empowered through the concept of common law to examine the common usage and custom in a community for patterns that reflect the community's standards for behavior. Common usage and custom are not usually written down and specific. However, written documents can be used to support common usage and custom in specific cases. For example, when examining standards of professional practice in a court case, the court may examine documents that specify standards of professional practice as reflecting common usage. These documents may be changed by the organization writing the standard and thus are not fixed.

The issue of abandonment of a patient illustrates how common usage applies to nursing. An individual state may not have a written law that dictates that a nurse cannot leave a seriously ill patient without ensuring that someone else will provide care, but common practice and custom (which could be supported through the testimony of nurses and other health care workers) require that nurses do not abandon their patients. Failure to meet this standard might be deemed a violation of common law even when no statute exists.

JUDICIAL LAW

Judicial law (also referred to as decisional, or case law) is derived from decrees or judgments from the courts. Judicial decisions or rulings in court cases apply statutory, regulatory, and common law to specific situations. These decisions then become precedents for interpretations of all types of law in other cases. Court rulings are binding within the jurisdiction of the particular court that determines them, but are used in a more general way (as guidelines) in other jurisdictions. In any specific situation, the final determination of the application of all types of law is the decision of the court in that case, although in most instances a decision may be appealed to higher courts.

OTHER FACTORS AFFECTING LEGAL DECISIONS

In addition to the sources of law discussed above, several other factors can affect how laws are interpreted and enforced. These factors also play an important role in our legal system.

Administrative Rulings

An **administrative ruling,** also referred to as an advisory opinion, made by a state board or by an attorney general provides a guideline based on an interpretation of the enacted and regulatory law relative to a specific situation, and is not a final legal decision. Different boards and attorneys general might vary in their opinions. The validity of an opinion stands until the issue is brought before a court, and the court rules on the situation and provides a final decision. The court decision may or may not support the advisory ruling.

Rights and Responsibilities in Health Care

Rights and responsibilities have both legal and ethical aspects. In the United States, basic rights are specified in the first 14 amendments to the Constitution and are part of statutory law. This section of the Constitution is called the Bill of Rights and is an example of one of the limitations placed on the federal government. These rights protect the individual from governmental interference in basic areas of life. From these primary rights, other rights are deduced. For example, although the right to privacy of medical records is not specifically discussed in the Bill of Rights, the right to be secure in one's own home against unreasonable search and seizure is guaranteed. This basic right has led to court decisions supporting the right to privacy regarding one's own affairs, including medical records.

In other countries, rights may be more limited, or may be part of the statutory law enacted by a legislative body. These laws may carry less weight than the U. S. Constitution. Some countries have no counterpart to the rights found in the United States.

Some of the rights of which we speak are not legally supported, but are based on ethical beliefs. For example, we often speak of a "right to health care." There is no legal basis for this right in the United States, but many people believe an ethical basis exists. In some countries, such as Canada and Great Britain, health care is a right supported by the law. In these countries, health care for all has been established through legislation and administrative rules and regulations.

In the United States, patient rights within the health care system are the matter of considerable debate. Currently Congress is considering the adoption of a patient's bill of rights that would create federal laws guiding actions in relationship to patient rights. At this writing, such a document has not yet been passed. For current information check Congress's Web site (*http://thomas.loc.gov*). Recent attention has been directed to the patient's right to pain management. While managing pain has always been a health care goal, most providers did not think of it in terms of the patient's right to pain relief. The Joint Commission on Accreditation of Healthcare Organizations (JCAHO) has added requirements to accreditation standards requiring that agencies have comprehensive plans for managing pain effectively and demonstrate that those plans are used. In at least one instance, a family successfully brought suit against a nursing home for the failure to manage terminal pain in their loved one (Furrow, 2001). Therefore, it behooves all health care providers to recognize this as a newly developing legal right.

Responsibilities often accompany rights. If a right is guaranteed, the government and designated others have legally mandated responsibilities to ensure that the right is upheld. In the matter of the right to privacy of medical records, for example, all health care workers have legally mandated responsibilities to ensure that privacy is upheld.

Institutional Policies and Protocols

Institutional policies provide guidance in the proper actions to be taken in specific situations, and identify the individuals responsible for taking action. Established agency policies may be considered the **standard of practice** for that agency and, therefore, common usage (common law) by the court, and may become important as a basis for legal decisions. Policies may protect the institution itself and the employees of an institution from legal difficulties if they are based on current practice and sound legal advice.

Members of the hospital staff who have expertise in the practice area under consideration usually develop the specific policy. An attorney also may be consulted to ensure that policies conform to legal requirements. Final approval of policies often rests with the board of trustees, directors, or commissioners, who have ultimate responsibility for the financial and legal management of the organization.

Institutional policies are changed in response to new situations and new expectations in society. Usually there is an established institutional route for the change or expansion of a hospital policy. Nurses may be in a position to recognize the need for such a change as they use a policy and compare it with the latest professional information.

A protocol or procedure provides specific guidelines on performing a task. The purpose of protocols and procedures is to ensure that there is consistent, sound practice in an institution. Just as policies must be updated, so should protocols and procedures (see Chapter 12).

CLASSIFICATION OF LAWS

Law is divided into civil and criminal components. Both statutory law and common law may be subdivided in this way.

Criminal Law

Criminal law addresses the general welfare of the public. A violation of criminal law is called a **crime** and is prosecuted by the government. On conviction, a crime may be punished by imprisonment, parole conditions, a loss of privilege (such as a license), a fine, or any combination of these. The punishment is intended to deter others from committing the crime and to punish the violator. A crime may be classified as either a **misdemeanor** or as a **felony**. A misdemeanor is a lesser infraction of the law and is punished by a fine or an imprisonment of less than a year. A felony represents a more serious violation of the law, and carries heavier fines and longer periods of imprisonment, perhaps even death (Guido, 2001).

Civil Law

Civil law regulates conduct between private individuals or businesses, and is enforced through the courts as damages or money compensation. A *tort* is a violation of a civil law in which another person is wronged. Private individuals or groups may bring a legal action (a **lawsuit**) to court for breach (or breaking) of civil law. The judgment of the court results in a plan to correct the wrong and may include a monetary payment to the wronged party. Nurses may find themselves involved with both civil and criminal laws, either separately or within the same situation.

CRIMINAL LAW AND NURSING

Because a violation of any law governing the practice of any licensed profession may be a crime, you must be aware of the extent of the Nurse Practice Act of the state in which you are practicing. Where the Nurse Practice Act requires that actions (such as administering drugs) be performed only under the direction of a physician, that explicit authorization must exist. Standing orders that refer to specific situations, as well as the usual orders written for an individual patient, may both be adequate authorization. However, custom or usual practice will not substitute for the specific authorization required by law. A violation of a professional practice act may be prosecuted as a crime even if no actual harm occurred to the patient.

It is costly to the state to undertake criminal prosecution; therefore, even when they are discovered, some violations of criminal law are not prosecuted in court. Knowing this, some nurses make the error of believing that "minor" violations are acceptable. Even when not prosecuted in court, criminal action could result in the loss of a job and in the loss of a license to practice nursing.

For example, the Nurse Practice Act does not give the nurse the authority to diagnose disease and prescribe medication, regardless of the situation. The Medical Practice Act and the Nurse Practice Act on Advanced Nursing Practice contain this authorization. To give a medication without an order is a violation of the law and is a crime, even though the client may not be harmed.

Violation of laws related to the care and distribution of controlled substances is also a crime. Altering or changing narcotic records is a crime even if no diversion of drugs occurred. While finding where the error in a narcotic record occurred may be a tedious and time-consuming process, as a nurse, you need to look beyond temporary convenience to the potential consequences of your action.

Nurses also have been charged by states with committing crimes while in the role of caregiver. These legal actions may be based upon such charges as **reckless endangerment** or **criminal negligence**. These are situations in which the actions of the professional fall outside the bounds of simple error and reflect a serious lack of concern or attention to the safety of the patient. Errors resulting in the serious injury or death of a patient are investigated and may be prosecuted and tried by the criminal courts. A license to practice nursing may be temporarily withdrawn while such charges are investigated and tried. If the individual is found innocent, the license then may be restored. If the individual is convicted of the crime, the nursing license may be revoked, in addition to sentencing and other penalties.

In the state of Colorado, criminal charges were brought against three nurses for negligent actions that resulted in the death of an infant. Through a series of actions by the nurses, the infant was given a 10-fold overdose of intravenous (IV) penicillin. This case clearly shows that the state has the power to prosecute as a crime professional conduct that results in serious harm or death (Fiesta, 1999). Many nurses are distressed by the actions of the prosecutor in the Colorado case because the facts as currently known do not seem to indicate a criminal level of negligence (Curtin, 1997).

Nurses who commit felonies such as theft, abuse, or deliberate harm to a patient are always charged under both criminal laws and the laws regulating nursing practice. Nurses who commit felonies outside of the care setting can be prosecuted under criminal law and under the law regulating nursing practice if the felony reflects on their fitness to practice nursing. For example, an individual who was prosecuted for selling narcotics usually would have action taken under the Nurse Practice Act as well.

CIVIL LAW AND NURSING

Civil law relates to legal disputes between private parties. Malpractice actions brought in health care situations involve civil law.

Torts

Torts are civil wrongs committed by one person against another person or a person's property (Guido, 2001). The wrong may be physical harm, psychological harm, harm to livelihood, or some other less tangible value, such as harm to reputation. The action that causes a civil wrong may be either intentional or unintentional. An **intentional tort** is one in which the outcome was planned, although the person involved may not have believed that the intended outcome would be harmful to the other person. For example, preventing a patient from leaving against medical advice may be based on concern for the patient, but it is illegal and to do so is an intentional tort.

An unintentional tort is a wrong committed against another person or property that was not intended to happen. The most common cause of an unintentional tort is negligence.

Negligence

Negligence is a general term that refers to conduct that does not show due care (Guido, 2001). If harm is caused by negligence, it is termed an unintentional tort and damages may be recovered. Negligence is a broad term that has many applications in society. All negligence has the following four essential characteristics (Fiesta, 1994):

1. Harm must have occurred to an individual.
2. The negligent person must have been in a situation where he or she had a duty toward the person harmed.
3. The person must be found to have failed to fulfill his or her duty. This is called "breach of duty." This might include either doing what should not have been done (commission of an inappropriate action) or failing to do what should have been done (omission of a necessary or appropriate action). This is also referred to as failing to act as a reasonably prudent person. A reasonably prudent person in this context means someone who demonstrates careful and thoughtful action. Some authorities emphasize that this includes the responsibility to foresee possible results of a situation and act appropriately (Guido, 2001).
4. The harm must be shown to have been caused by the breach of duty.

Display 8-1	ESSENTIAL ELEMENTS OF MALPRACTICE

- Harm to an individual
- Duty of a professional toward an individual
- Breach of duty by the professional
- Breach of duty as the cause of harm

Malpractice

Malpractice is a term used for a specific type of negligence. It refers to the negligence of a specially trained or educated person in the performance of his or her job. Therefore, malpractice is the term used to describe negligence by nurses in the performance of their duties.

Malpractice is professional negligence; liability resulting from improper practice based on standards of care required by that profession (Shinn, 2001). The professional person must have had a professional duty toward the person receiving the care. For example, the nurse was performing the professional activities of a nurse for the person needing the care (in either a paid or volunteer capacity). Additionally, the harm that occurred to this person or to the property must be based on a failure to act as a **prudent professional** and in accordance with professional standards in the situation (Fig. 8-2). This is a higher standard than is required of the general public; it demands appropriate professional judgment and action (Guido, 2001) (Display 8-1).

Just as all parts of the situation are clear in some general negligence situations and not in others, the professional duty is similarly clear in some instances and not in others. The nurse who is assigned to care for a patient in a hospital clearly has a duty to that patient. In some situations, duties overlap and more than one nurse might have a duty toward the same patient; whether a supervisor, another nurse on the unit, or a nurse visitor has a professional duty to a patient might be in dispute. Again, the court would decide whether a duty was present.

Critical Thinking Activity

You have taken a new position as a home health nurse. One of your patients is an elderly woman with a long history of diabetes who has a leg ulcer. Your role is to assess the patient in relationship to her diabetic management and wound care, and teach as needed. While you are in the home, her husband tells you that he has been having pain in his knee and asks if you would examine it and tell him whether it is all right to use a heating pad on it, and whether he should take ibuprofen or some Tylenol. Do you have a duty to help him? Why or why not? What will your response be? What legal issues are involved in this situation? If you advise him and your advice turns out to be incorrect, what legal action could he take?

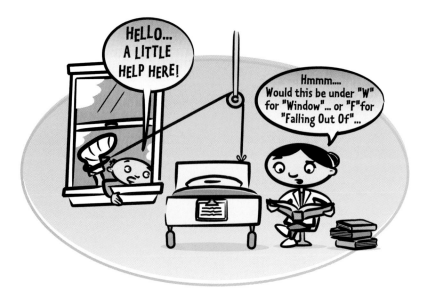

FIGURE 8-2   A reasonably prudent nurse uses common sense as well as nursing theory.

A breach of duty, as mentioned earlier, is a failure to act as a prudent professional, that is, according to the **standard of care** for the profession in a particular situation (Killion & Dempski, 2000). Standards of nursing care are determined in variety of ways. State boards of nursing set some standards; accrediting agencies such as the Joint Commission and professional nursing organizations set others. Federal administration codes may set standards such as nurse–patient ratio in federally funded institutions. Standards of care also appear in policies, protocols, and procedures of the institution. Current nursing references, educational material, and articles may contribute to an understanding of an appropriate and current standard of care. Still other standards of care are determined by seeking the input of an expert professional. To determine that a breach of duty was present in a particular case, a court will officially determine what constitutes a professional standard of care for that situation. This includes the application of both statutory law and common law, as previously discussed.

The final question becomes one of identifying the cause of the harm that occurred. Malpractice is present only if a breach of duty was the cause of the harm. The presence of harm is often clear. For example, if a person fractured a hip, no one would dispute that this was harm. However, the cause of a fractured hip might be the person's own responsibility, not the responsibility of someone else. When the harm is so clear and the responsibility for the harm so straightforward that it does not need to be proved in court, the legal term *res ipsa loquitur* is used. This is Latin for "the thing speaks for itself." In this case, the harm and responsibility do not need to be proved, because all would agree that harm occurred and who was responsible. This may be invoked in a case where a surgical instrument is left in an abdomen and causes harm. There is no way that the instrument could be in the abdomen if the surgical team had not placed it there and overlooked its removal. Everyone would agree that a surgical instrument in the abdomen that caused pain and failure to heal was harm to the person. Expert witnesses would not be needed to make this determination. Remember that, as discussed earlier in the chapter, a breach of duty may be either the omission of a correct action or the commission of an incorrect action.

LIABILITY

A **liability** is an obligation or debt that can be enforced by law. In the case of malpractice, a person found guilty of any tort (whether intentional or unintentional) is considered legally liable, or legally responsible, for the outcome. The person legally liable usually is required to pay for damages to the other person. These may include actual costs of care, legal services, loss of earnings (present and future), and compensation for emotional and physical stress suffered. Although liability is legally determined by a court, an individual who believes that he or she would be held legally liable if a court were consulted, may agree to pay damages (or that individual's insurance company may agree to pay) without actually going to court. This may be done even when the person denies true negligence or malpractice, but chooses to settle the issue because a court case would be more costly than the damages to be paid.

Personal Liability

As an educated professional, you are always legally responsible or liable for your actions (Bernzweig, 1996). Thus, if a physician or supervisor asks you to do something that is contrary to your best professional judgment and says, "I'll take responsibility," that person is acting unwisely. The physician or supervisor giving the directions may be liable also if harm results, but that would not remove your personal liability.

Personal Liability

SITUATION

The registered nurse (RN) giving medications on a large medical unit notes that an order for digoxin (a heart medication) is considerably larger than the usual dose. She looks up the medication in a reference book and finds that she is correct about the dosage. The ordered dose is several times the usual dose. The nurse then calls the supervisor and explains the situation.

The supervisor double-checks the order with the RN and then states: "Dr. Jones is an outstanding physician. I am sure he has a good reason for ordering this dose. Go ahead and give the medication as ordered. I'll take responsibility." The nurse then gives the medication, and the patient suffers a toxic reaction.

The RN could be held liable for giving the incorrect amount of medication. She had the knowledge and judgment to recognize that the dose was much larger than usual, and she failed to check with the physician. A statement by the supervisor does not remove the nurse's personal responsibility for her own actions. Because even a competent physician might make an error, the nurse had a responsibility to clarify the order. The supervisor and the physician could be held liable in addition to the nurse, but not instead of her.

Although each person is legally responsible for his or her own actions, the example above illustrates that there are also situations in which a person or organization may be held liable for actions taken by others.

Employer Liability

The most common situation in which a person or organization is held responsible for the actions of another is in the employer–employee relationship. In many instances, an employer can be held responsible for torts committed by an employee. This is called the doctrine of *respondeat superior* (a Latin term for "let the master respond"). The law holds the employer responsible for hiring qualified persons, for establishing an appropriate environment for correct functioning, maintaining correct policies and procedures, and for providing supervision or direction as needed to avoid errors or harm. Therefore, if a nurse, as an employee of a hospital, is guilty of malpractice, the hospital also may be named in the suit. The employer's liability may exist even if the employer appears to have taken precautions to prevent error.

It is important to understand that this doctrine does not remove any responsibility from the individual nurse, but it extends responsibility to the employer in addition to the nurse. If, for example, a hospital has a procedure that does not conform to good nursing practice as you know it, and you follow that procedure, you will still be liable for any resulting harm. You are expected to use your education and experience to make sound judgments regarding your work.

Employer Responsibility for a Staff Nurse

A nurse working in a long-term care facility is responsible for planning and coordinating the care of a severely debilitated resident. This elderly man is totally dependent for all activities of daily living due to a recent stroke. He is not eating and drinking adequately. He faints and is discovered to have very low blood pressure and a rapid weak pulse. He is sent to the local hospital, where he is admitted for dehydration secondary to inadequate fluid intake. Investigation reveals that no assessment of his fluid or nutritional status has been recorded, nor was there any plan to ensure that nutritional and fluid needs were met.

Both the nurse and the long-term care facility in this situation might be found liable for harm that resulted. The nurse had a personal, professional responsibility to accurately assess the resident and to institute care to meet his basic needs. The facility also had a responsibility to make sure that policies, procedures, and protocols were in place to ensure appropriate assessment and care, and that employees followed through on them.

Supervisory Liability

In the role of charge nurse, head nurse, supervisor, or any other role that involves delegation, supervision, or direction of other people, the nurse is potentially liable for the actions of others. The supervising nurse is responsible for exercising good judgment in a supervisory role, including making appropriate decisions about assignments and delegation of tasks. If an error occurs and the supervising nurse is shown to have exercised sound judgment in all decisions made in that capacity, the supervising nurse may not be held liable for the error of a subordinate. If poor judgment was used in assigning an inadequately prepared person to an important task or oversight was inadequate, the supervisory nurse might be liable for resulting harm. The extent of the subordinate's responsibility would depend on his or her level of education and training. People with limited education or training might not be liable for some errors; the more education subordinates have, the more likely they will be liable also. (See Chapter 14 for more discussion of delegation.)

Supervisory Responsibility for an Educated Staff Member

Two sudden admissions to the coronary care unit create a situation in which additional help is needed to care for the patients in the unit. A "float" nurse is sent to the CCU to assist. The charge nurse does not ask the temporary float nurse whether she has education or experience in coronary care, nor does the temporary float nurse volunteer this information. The temporary float nurse, however, has no background or experience in coronary care.

The temporary nurse is assigned by the charge nurse to the complete care of two patients. Because of the float nurse's inability to accurately interpret the monitors, a potentially life-threatening problem is not identified until the patient "arrests." Resuscitation efforts are successful, but the patient suffers some brain damage.

Both the charge nurse, who assigned the inadequately prepared nurse to total care, and the temporary nurse could be found liable: the charge nurse for incorrectly assigning the nurse, and the temporary nurse for not recognizing her own limitations. The educational preparation of the temporary nurse gave her the background to understand that she did not possess the expertise needed in this situation. If the situation were changed so that the temporary nurse was reviewed for expertise in coronary care and found to have that expertise, then the charge nurse might not be liable for the error of the temporary nurse. The supervisory function of ascertaining level of preparation and ability to meet the standards of the job would have been carried out.

Supervisory Responsibility for Staff Member With Limited Education

The RN is working on a unit that assigns a nursing assistant to work with each RN. One evening, the regular nursing assistant is absent due to illness. A new nursing assistant is assigned to work with the RN. During the evening, the RN asks the nursing assistant to monitor the new postoperative patient. The RN lists for the nursing assistant the items that are to be checked: vital signs, hourly urine output, pain, and condition of the dressing. Each hour, the RN stops the nursing assistant, asks if the patient is doing okay, and receives an affirmative reply. When the RN stops to chart, he reviews the last 4 hours of flow sheet information listed by the nursing assistant. He sees that the urine output has been only 15 mL/hr for the last 4 hours. When he questions the nursing assistant, he learns that the nursing assistant had no idea what information needed to be reported immediately. The RN completes an assessment and calls the physician. The patient is found to have developed renal failure.

The RN might be found negligent in this case for assigning the nursing assistant to monitor a critical postoperative patient without proper direction or supervision. The nursing assistant might not be found negligent because she had no basis for recognizing the seriousness of the situation or for recognizing her own lack of ability to meet the responsibilities involved in this assessment. She could carry out the tasks assigned and had done those correctly.

Limits on Patient's Claim to Negligence

Several situations may be viewed by the court as a valid defense to a patient's claim that negligence has occurred. Contributory negligence is based on the concept that the patient contributed to the injury by not acting prudently in that circumstance. For example, the patient may not have followed instructions, may have provided false information that led to improper treatment, or may not have followed warnings about the side effects of medications (Killion & Dempski, 2000).

Courts also may incorporate the use of comparative negligence. If this is used, the court would determine what percentage of the injury resulted from the patient's negligence and what part rested with the nurse, and reduce the damage award accordingly (Killion & Dempski, 2000).

LIABILITY INSURANCE

Liability insurance transfers the legal and any settlement costs related to a suit from the individual to a large group. The expectation is that most individuals will not be sued, and that the pool of premiums therefore will adequately cover the costs of those who are sued, the administrative costs of managing the policies, and the profit for the insurance company. Individuals benefit by transferring risk from themselves to the insurance company for the cost of the insurance policy.

A liability insurance crisis exists in the United States. The cost of liability insurance for primary health care providers (such as physicians and nurse practitioners) has escalated at an extraordinary rate. Some of the factors that have caused this are the large judgments that have been made, the number of suits that have been brought, the large fees that attorneys receive, and the high profits of insurance companies. Nurses in independent advanced practice have been especially affected by the increase in premiums, because their incomes have traditionally been moderate and they cannot charge fees sufficient to cover insurance costs that may equal those of physicians. Nurses who are employed in more traditional roles are able to obtain malpractice insurance for a modest cost.

The American Nurses Association (ANA) has initiated a data bank related to legal claims against nurses. The organization is asking all RNs to provide information to it regarding legal action in which they have been named as a defendant. The ANA's purpose is to have adequate records to support its contention that the low level of suits against nurses in all areas of practice should translate into low-cost liability insurance.

Some states have initiated legislation that allows for awards to cover actual losses and costs of care, while limiting awards for pain and suffering and other nontangible factors. Sometimes this legislation has been accompanied by restrictions on insurance company rates. Laws in some states are being amended to restrict the monetary liability of any party according to the percentage of responsibility. Liability laws continue to be a major concern for nurses, because nurses are being named in an increasing number of suits, although the total number is still low.

Institutional and Individual Insurance

Many hospitals and other institutional employers carry liability insurance that covers both the institution and its employees. Some hospitals may limit the coverage that their policies provide for individual employees in an effort to hold down costs. Kihm (1999) pointed out that when health care institutions merge, are bought out, or go bankrupt, liability insurance coverages might be called into question. Some institutions have chosen to self-insure part of their liability requirements. If such an institution goes bankrupt, there are no funds left to pay liability claims and pending claims may revert to individuals named in the suits.

In some states, nonprofit hospitals have charitable immunity. This means that the nonprofit hospital cannot be held legally liable for harm done to a patient by its employees. The employees of that nonprofit hospital are still legally liable for their own actions. When the institution does not bear any of the financial responsibility in a lawsuit, the individual employee is more exposed to financial risk. In Massachusetts, a nonprofit hospital that was protected by the state's charitable immunity laws was involved in a liability suit. Because the hospital was protected, the entire judgment fell on the individual nurse (Kihm, 1999). The trend in legislation is toward the repeal of laws providing for charitable immunity. Those active in the consumer movement have argued that no institution should be relieved of responsibility in such a blanket fashion. If you are employed by a nonprofit or governmental institution, you should learn whether the law in your state provides charitable immunity for the institution.

Even if an employer carries liability insurance, it is usually advisable for the individual professional to carry an independent policy. An independent policy will cover you in voluntary activities as well as on the job. It also will follow when you move from one employer to another. If a legal action is instituted against you, the individual liability insurance policy provides independent legal counsel. In a state where the institution has charitable immunity, it supports the individual nurse who may be sued when the institution is protected from a lawsuit. Many nursing liability policies also provide coverage for legal expenses incurred in defending your license in a disciplinary proceeding.

Keep in mind that insurance is not the only source of payment for a judgment. Judgments may be levied against most tangible assets, including houses, cars, and savings; judgments also may be levied against future earnings. Married nurses who reside in community property states should realize that one half of the assets of a family may be vulnerable to a judgment. Community property states at this time include Arizona, California, Idaho, Louisiana, Nevada, New Mexico, Texas, Washington and Wisconsin. These factors combine to support the need for the individual professional to carry liability insurance that will provide legal counsel and protection in the case of any judgment.

Analyzing Liability Insurance Coverage

Individual liability insurance for RNs is available from a variety of insurance companies (directly through their agents) and through professional organizations that offer coverage as a service to members. When investigating individual liability insurance, ask the agent or company the questions in Display 8-2.

Asking these questions can help you to compare policies from different insurance carriers. When coverage appears equal, you might ask how long a company has been in business and how long it has been providing nursing liability insurance. You want to be insured with a reliable, stable company.

The nurse employee should investigate just as carefully liability insurance coverage that is carried by the hospital. Questions 1 through 4 in Display 8-2 apply to institutional

Display 8-2   QUESTIONS TO ASK REGARDING INDIVIDUAL LIABILITY INSURANCE

1. In what situations would I, as an individual, be covered?
2. In what situations would I not be covered?
3. How is my coverage affected by my actions? For example, if I failed to follow hospital policy, would I still be covered?
4. What are the monetary limits of the policy?
5. Does the policy provide me with an attorney?
6. Is the policy renewable at my option? What factors affect renewability?
7. Does the insurance cover incidents that occurred while the policy was in force, regardless of when the claim is brought (claims-occurred insurance coverage), or does it cover incidents only if I am currently insured (claims-brought insurance coverage)?
8. What is the cost compared with other policies?

insurance policies as well as to individual insurance policies. In addition, you should ask the questions in Display 8-3 about any institutional policy.

Critical Thinking Activity

You are accepting a position in a clinic. When might you ask about professional liability insurance coverage? Formulate specific questions. Identify the person who would be the best source of this information. How will you proceed if this person does not have the information you seek? If the interviewer tells you that the clinic is well covered by liability insurance, will you purchase personal malpractice insurance? Why or why not?

Display 8-3   ADDITIONAL QUESTIONS REGARDING AN INSTITUTIONAL LIABILITY POLICY

1. Does the policy provide me with a personal attorney, or will the same attorney be working for the hospital?
2. At what point would the hospital no longer be responsible and would I become personally responsible?
3. How would my job be affected if a lawsuit were filed or payment awarded based on an action against me? (Check institutional policy as well as the insurance company policy).
4. Does the insurance company have the right to seek restitution from me if it pays a claim based on my actions?

(It is important that you have accurate answers to these questions so that you can make an informed decision regarding your need for an individual policy.)

NATIONAL DATA BANK

In the United States, the federal government maintains a "National Data Bank" on licensed health care providers. This is separate from and has a purpose different from the data collected by the ANA or the NCSBN. By law, the court or relevant board must report to this data bank all judgments, settlements paid, or convictions for malpractice, and all situations in which a health care provider's privileges to practice are curtailed or withdrawn. All institutions must consult this data bank for information before giving any health care provider privilege to practice in the institution. The purpose of the National Data Bank is to protect the public from incompetent professionals who could continue to practice by moving from one place to another.

LEGAL ISSUES COMMON IN NURSING

Some legal issues recur frequently in nursing practice. It is wise for the nurse to understand these particular issues as they relate to individual practice.

Duty to Report or Seek Medical Care for a Patient

A nurse who is caring for a patient has a legal duty to ensure that the patient receives safe and competent care. This duty requires that the nurse maintain an appropriate standard of care and that the nurse take action to obtain an appropriate standard of care from other professionals when that is necessary. For example, if a nurse identifies that a patient needs the attention of a physician and fails to make every effort to obtain that attention, the nurse has breached a duty to the patient. In a recent study, the "failure to rescue" individuals experiencing life-threatening complications was linked to a lower number of RNs (Needleman et al, 2002). This is a critical RN function.

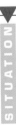

Failure to Seek Medical Care for a Patient

The RN is caring for a postoperative patient during the night. The patient's blood pressure begins to drop and the pulse begins to rise. The nurse's assessment indicates that the patient may be bleeding internally. The nurse institutes a plan for close nursing monitoring and calls the surgeon to describe the situation. The surgeon gives a telephone order to increase the IV fluid rate and states that he will see the patient in the morning. The patient's condition continues to deteriorate, but the nurse does nothing further to ensure that a physician examines the patient.

If the outcome is unfavorable, the nurse can be found to have breached a duty to the patient. The patient relies on the nurse to provide appropriate care and to identify when a physician is needed. The nurse could have made more telephone calls to the surgeon and failing the success of that, could have followed the facility's procedure for asking another physician (such as the emergency department physician) to see the patient.

The nurse has a duty to continue all efforts to obtain appropriate medical care for the patient. If the nurse had followed all procedures, sought another physician, and continued efforts when initial attempts were unsuccessful, the nurse would not have breached a duty. The nurse cannot guarantee a physician's care, but can guarantee that the patient will not be left without an advocate.

Additionally, the nurse has a responsibility to critically examine medical orders that are written for a patient. Although the nurse is not responsible for the medical order itself, the nurse's education provides a background to identify obvious discrepancies or problems. In one reported case (Anonymous, 1997), two doctors left conflicting orders, which the charge nurse then transcribed. The court ruled that the nurse had a duty to understand the patient's plan of care and to communicate with the doctors who had written the conflicting orders.

Confidentiality and Right to Privacy

Confidentiality and the right to privacy with respect to one's personal life are basic concerns in our society. All information regarding a patient belongs to that patient. This right has been inferred from interpretation of the federal constitution, but is explicitly stated in some state laws. The federally legislated Health Information Privacy and Protection Act (HIPPA) is demanding major efforts of all health care providers in regard to protecting patient privacy. In theory, the rights identified in HIPAA should protect a patient's privacy. Only information that the patient specifically releases may be shared with others. However, third-party payers (such as insurance companies and HMOs) will not reimburse for care if they do not receive the records they request. The result is that patients must often sign statements giving blanket approval for all information to be sent to the third-party payer. They may be unaware of exactly what information is sent or who may see it.

When computerized records are transmitted to insurance companies, they no longer contain only a brief statement of diagnosis and treatment; they may contain detailed accounts of interactions between a patient and a mental health professional, health information of a sensitive nature, and genetic information that could be used inappropriately. Because increased use of computerized records can result in easier retrieval and cross-referencing of records from many sources, the general public, health care providers, and government officials are becoming more concerned about potential invasions of privacy. Safeguards must be built into all computerized medical record systems that prevent unauthorized access and the tracking of those who do access the system.

A nurse who gives out information without authorization from the patient or from the legally responsible **guardian** can be held liable for harm that results. If you have any question about who the legally responsible guardian of a patient is, be sure to consult with your administrative authority. If there is not a court-appointed legal guardian, then specific state laws identify who becomes the responsible guardian when the person is unable to give personal consent. The hospital administration should be able to ascertain the correct guardian.

Only those professional persons involved in the patient's care who have a need to know about the patient can be allowed routine access to the record. A physician who is not involved in the patient's care or who does not have an administrative responsibility relative to that care is not allowed routine access. Persons not involved in care can be allowed access to the record only by specific written authorization or by court order. You should be cautious about what information you share verbally and with whom.

Medical records professionals state that it is not uncommon for attorneys, family members, media representatives, or law enforcement officials to request access to patient records or specific patient information without having express consent of the patient, or a legal court order to view the records or be given information. Those unfamiliar with laws regarding privacy sometimes reveal information inappropriately. If you are ever approached for patient information by someone who purports to have authority, your best course of action is to refer that individual to appropriate administrative personnel, who can determine the validity of the request.

Breach of Confidentiality

A nurse in a small community hospital discusses with a friend the admission of a woman community member for treatment of cancer. The nurse's friend then talks to others, who talk to still others, until there is widespread knowledge of the patient's cancer in the community. The woman's daughter hears about her mother's cancer diagnosis at school and is very upset.

The nurse could be held liable for revealing this information in a suit charging breach of privacy and confidentiality. The harm is the emotional distress to the woman and her family. If the breach of confidentiality could be traced to the nurse's conversation, the nurse's action would be considered the direct cause of harm.

A newer concern is that more health care agencies are using fax machines to send patient information to one another and even between departments within an institution. Faxes have a legitimate purpose in that continuity of care is enhanced when information is shared. When you send a document by fax machine, it is difficult to assure that confidentiality is maintained. Facilities are being mandated by HIPAA to keep fax machines in areas not accessible to the public. Some facilities have a policy requiring that you call ahead and designate a specific person to be present to receive the fax. The cover page often states that this is confidential material and should not be read by anyone other than the designated recipient. If your facility or agency has no policy regarding the safeguarding of faxed information, you would be wise to raise the concern.

Other new areas of concern are the Internet and e-mail. Through these avenues, a health care provider may consult with other professionals to provide the best diagnostic and treatment services to the patient. However, on-line computer communications are not private. Those with the necessary skill may intercept and read any e-mail or Internet message. Therefore, the identity of patients must be protected in any such communication.

Defamation of Character

Any time that shared information is detrimental to a person's reputation, the person sharing the information may be liable for defamation of character. Written defamation is called libel. Oral defamation is called slander. Defamation of character involves communication that is malicious and false. Sometimes such comments are made in the heat of anger. Occasionally, statements written in a patient's chart are libelous. Severely critical opinions may be stated as fact. An example of such a statement might be "The patient is lying," or "The patient is rude and domineering." Patients may charge that comments in the chart adversely affected their care by prejudicing other staff against them. Libel and slander may also be charged when written comments or verbal statements are made regarding another health care provider. Thoughtless or angry comments that impugn the abilities of a physician or that might cause a patient to lose trust in a physician can be slander.

The prudent nurse will chart only objective information regarding patients and give opinion in professional terms, well documented with fact. A chart might read: "The patient states . . . Observation reveals . . ."; this provides factual information for the reader without making potentially libelous accusations. In conversations, the prudent nurse avoids discussing patients and carefully considers any comments about other health care providers before making them.

Defamation of character also may be charged by a health care provider who believes that statements made by another professional are false, malicious, and have caused harm. There are accepted mechanisms for confidentially reporting inappropriate care or errors; these should be used, and critical statements to uninvolved third parties should not be made. In many states, licensed professionals are required to report poor practice or illegal acts on the part of other professionals. Criticism reported without malice and in good faith, through the appropriate channels, is protected from legal action for defamation.

Privileged Communication

Privileged communication refers to information shared by an individual with certain professionals that does not need to be revealed, even in a court of law. This individual is said to possess privilege—that is, has the privilege of not revealing information. All states consider certain types of communication (between client and attorney, between patient and doctor, or between an individual and a member of the clergy) privileged. Not all states recognize the nurse–patient relationship as one in which privileged communication takes place; even those states that recognize nurse–patient communication as potentially privileged do not consider *all* communication between patients and nurses privileged. It is important that you understand that privilege is a limited concept. Only a court can determine if privilege exists in any specific case. If a court does not determine information to be privileged, then you are legally obligated to testify about the communication.

Informed Consent

Every person has the right to either **consent** (agree) to or to refuse health care treatment. The law requires that a person give voluntary and **informed consent**. Voluntary means that no coercion exists. Informed means that a person clearly understands the choices being offered.

CONSENT FOR MEDICAL TREATMENT

Consent for medical treatment is the responsibility of the medical provider (eg, physician, dentist, nurse practitioner). Information to be shared with the client include a description of the procedure, any alternatives for treatment, the risks involved in the procedure, the probable results, including problems of recuperation, and anything else generally disclosed to patients (Shinn, 2001). This consent may be either verbal or written. Written consent usually is preferred in health care to ensure that a record of consent exists, although a signature alone does not prove that the consent was informed. A blanket consent for "any procedures deemed necessary" usually is not considered adequate consent for specific procedures. The form should state the specific proposed medical procedure or test.

The courts do not accept the patient's medical condition alone as a valid reason for withholding complete and accurate information when seeking consent. Currently, there are no clear guidelines as to what constitutes complete information. What constitutes adequate information about various alternative approaches to treatment is often unclear. Is it always necessary to discuss a treatment the physician does not believe is a good choice? Must all risks be discussed? Courts have generally supported the idea that commonly accepted alternatives and usual risks need to be disclosed, but that marginal or unusual treatments and rare or unexpected risks do not have to be discussed.

The law places the responsibility for obtaining consent for medical treatment on the physician. It is the physician's responsibility to provide appropriate information, and he or she is liable if the patient charges that appropriate information was not given. A nurse may present a form for a patient to sign, and the nurse may sign the form as a witness to the signature. This does not transfer the legal responsibility for informed consent for medical care to the nurse. If the patient does not seem well informed, the nurse should notify the physician so that further information can be provided to the patient. Although the nurse would not legally be liable for the lack of informed consent, the nurse has ethical obligations to assist the patient in exercising his or her rights and to assist the physician in providing appropriate care (see Chapter 9 for discussion of the ethical obligations regarding informed consent).

CONSENT FOR NURSING MEASURES

Nurses must obtain a patient's consent for nursing measures undertaken. This does not mean that exhaustive explanations need to be given in each situation, because courts have held that patients can be expected to have some understanding of usual care. Consent for nursing measures may be verbal or implied. The nurse may ask, "Are you ready to ambulate now?" The patient answers, "Certainly," providing verbal consent. Alternatively, the nurse may state, "I have the injection the doctor ordered for you. Will you please turn over?" If the patient turns over, this is implied consent.

The nurse should remember that the patient is free to refuse any aspect of care offered. Like the physician, the nurse is responsible for making sure that the patient is informed before making a decision. Good nursing care requires that you use all means at your disposal to help the patient comprehend the value of proposed care. For example, the postoperative patient needs to understand that getting into a chair is part of the plan of care, not a convenience for the nurse or simply a change to prevent boredom. Thus, a patient's refusal of care is accepted only after the patient has been given complete information. The nurse would then carefully document this situation.

COMPETENCE TO GIVE CONSENT

A person's ability to make judgments based on rational understanding is termed *competence*. Dementia, developmental disabilities, head injuries, strokes, and illnesses creating loss of consciousness are common causes of an inability to make judgments. Determining competence is a complex issue. The patient's illness, age, or condition alone do not determine competence. Legal competence is ultimately determined by the court. The general tendency of the courts has been to encourage whatever decision-making an individual is capable of and to restrict personal decision-making as little as possible.

When a person is determined legally to be incompetent, a legal guardian is appointed and consent is obtained from the legal guardian. A legal guardian is constrained from making some types of decisions. For example, if the health care action could be identified as injurious to the individual involved, a court may need to be consulted regarding consent for that specific action. An example would be the decision about discontinuation of dialysis for an incompetent individual. When such an individual leaves no clear indication regarding personal wishes, the health care providers might insist on getting a court decision before accepting the consent of the guardian to terminate the dialysis.

Health care providers often encounter those for whom no legal determination of competence has been made, but who do not seem able to make an informed decision; examples include the very confused elderly person, the inebriated person, and the unconscious person. The law in each state specifies who is allowed to give consent in such situations. Frequently, this is the spouse, the parent, the children, or the siblings. There are also guidelines to follow in determining that a person cannot give his or her own consent. Your facility policy should contain directions to guide you in obtaining legal consent; if it does not, you should consult an administrative person for a decision. In situations where there are several persons in the category, such as children of an elderly person, agreement regarding decisions is needed before proceeding. Determining who is able to give legal consent in such a situation is not a nurse's responsibility.

Competence may change from day to day, as a person's physical illness changes. The person who has had major surgery and is receiving large doses of narcotics for pain may not be able to reason clearly. Forty-eight hours later this same individual may be perfectly alert and capable of considering complex issues. An individual may be competent to make some decisions, such as "I don't like rice and I won't eat it!" but incompetent to make others; for example, decisions regarding financial matters. These differences in competence require care providers to adjust their own planning to incorporate patient self-determination whenever possible, even when the person is legally incompetent. If a person truly is not capable of making decisions, the nurse should attempt to present necessary nursing actions in a way that elicits cooperation and avoids confrontation over decisions.

WITHDRAWING CONSENT

Consent may be withdrawn after it is given. People have the right to change their minds. Therefore, if after one IV infusion a patient decides not to have a second one started, that is his or her right. As a nurse, you have an obligation to notify the physician if the patient refuses a medical procedure or treatment.

When individuals are participating in any type of research protocol for care, they are free to withdraw from the research study at any time. If you are caring for individuals who are part of a research process, you have obligations to protect the patient's right to make decisions even if they are contrary to the interests of the researcher.

CONSENT AND MINORS

The parent or legal guardian usually provides consent for care of a minor. You also should obtain the minor's consent when he or she is able to give it. Increasingly, courts are emphasizing that minors be allowed a voice when it concerns matters that they are capable of understanding. This is especially true for the adolescent, but this consideration should be given to any child who is 7 years of age or older. Often courts seek not *consent* from the minor but rather an indication that they understand the purpose of the care. For adolescents, the court may ask that negotiation with the minor occur. When a minor refuses care and the legal guardian has authorized that care, you should not proceed until legal clarification is given. Your nursing supervisor should be consulted.

Minors who live apart from their parents and are financially independent, or who are married, are termed **emancipated minors**. In most (but not all) states, an emancipated minor can give consent to his or her own treatment. Some states have specific laws relating to the **mature minor**, allowing a sexually active minor to give personal consent (without also obtaining parental consent) for treatment of sexually transmitted disease, or for obtaining birth control information and supplies (see Chapter 10). You should be sure of the law in your own state if you practice in an area where this is a concern. Most institutions have developed policies to guide employees in making correct decisions in this and other areas dealing with consent.

Advance Directives

Advance directives are legal documents stating the wishes of an individual regarding health care in situations in which he or she is no longer capable of giving personal informed consent. They are completed in "advance" of the situation in which they might be needed and "direct" the actions of others. There are several types of advance directives, such as a living will and a durable power of attorney for health care.

THE LIVING WILL

A **living will** or **directive to physicians** provides information on preferences regarding end-of-life issues such as types of care to provide and whether or not to use various resuscitation measures. The basis of a living will is an *if–then* plan. Most commonly, they declare that *if* "I am terminally ill and not expected to recover," *then* "I want this care given and do not want this care given." The *if* condition may also include that the person is in a persistent vegetative state and not expected to recover function and capacity. The condition stated as the *if* must be diagnosed by a physician. Many states require that two physicians must agree that the person is terminally ill or in a persistent vegetative state. Even when this is not the law, health care agencies often require this as a policy. The determination of the patient's condition must be recorded in the chart by the physician. Although living wills or directives were originally advisory for families and physicians as they made decisions, some states have now passed laws requiring that these documents be honored. If the physician does not agree with the decision of the patient, then the physician in that state is obligated to withdraw from care and refer the case to another physician.

If the living will requests that no resuscitation or limited resuscitation efforts be undertaken, the physician must write orders limiting resuscitation in the record. However, remember that living wills may also request that all possible resuscitation efforts be made.

Living wills or directives to the physician may address other aspects of care in addition to resuscitation efforts. For example, they may indicate whether the individual wants to be tube fed if he or she is in a persistent vegetative state, whether surgery should be used in certain instances, or whether IV fluids or ventilator support should be used. Some advance directives are many pages long as the person addresses many different possible concerns.

DURABLE POWER OF ATTORNEY FOR HEALTH CARE

A **durable power of attorney for health care** is a document that legally designates a **substitutionary decision-maker** should the person be incapacitated. This document may be combined with a living will that contains specific advance directives, such as those discussed above. Thus, the person identifies a preferred legal decision-maker if he or she is incapacitated and at the same time provides directions for that substitutionary decision-maker regarding the decisions.

If an individual has designated a substitutionary decision-maker for health care, this supercedes all general legal designations for decision-makers. In a society where there are many different family constellations and relationships, durable powers of attorney for health care are an important personal decision. For example, individuals who live in life partnerships other than marriage must have a durable power of attorney for health care to provide that life partner with decision-making ability for emergencies or critical situations. For the adult with no living parents or spouse and multiple siblings, the designation of one person as a decision-maker may diminish family conflict and facilitate the provision of the care the individual wishes.

DO NOT RESUSCITATE ORDERS

Limitations on resuscitation in the event of a cardiac arrest may take many forms. The most comprehensive is that the order reads **"Do not resuscitate" (DNR) or "No Code,"** meaning that no resuscitation efforts of any kind are to be made. There would be no CPR, no resuscitative drugs, and no ventilatory support. This is often the choice of the person who has a life-threatening disease and for whom resuscitation would only serve to prolong illness and discomfort. In some instances, the person may request a limited resuscitation effort, such as CPR and medications but no mechanical ventilation. Facilities may have a variety of ways to designate these limitations on resuscitative efforts and to communicate these directions to those providing care. An important understanding for nurses is that in the absence of a written order from a physician, other care providers are obligated to initiate resuscitation if an arrest occurs.

In many states, there are laws that designate under what circumstances a physician might write a DNR order in the absence of a living will. If the patient has not completed a living will and is not expected to recover, the physician may determine that resuscitation would be futile. **Futile** means that it would not add appreciably to life or have the potential for success. Laws or policies usually require the agreement of two physicians that resuscitation would be futile. After this medical determination, then the person who legally is the substitutionary decision-maker is consulted, provided information regarding the patient's condition, and asked to consent to a DNR order. This entire process must be documented in the patient's record.

All care providers must understand that a DNR order does not limit other types of care that will be provided. Treatment of wounds to promote healing, pain management, resolution of other physical problems such as nausea or constipation, antibiotic administration to control treatable infections, oxygen to ease breathing are all examples of care that will still be appropriate. In some instances, radiation therapy to reduce tumor growth would be administered.

In some instances, an additional order may be written that specifies "comfort care only." This order again occurs after consultation with the patient as able and family as appropriate. When this order is written, treatment of infections and other problems may not be undertaken. The focus becomes maximum comfort in the face of impending death. The patient for whom comfort care only is ordered should receive the same concerted focus on end-of-life care that would occur in a hospice setting.

Nurses sometimes find themselves in situations in which they believe that the patient's condition is futile and that a DNR or comfort-care-only order would be appropriate, but the physician has not made this determination or, having made this determination, has not consulted with the family regarding a DNR order. These become difficult situations for nurses because they have no decision-making authority, and yet they are the ones who legally must carry out the resuscitation. Much depends upon the nurse–physician working relationships and their ability to discuss difficult issues together. Some care facilities encourage care conferences where these matters can be raised for discussion.

PATIENT SELF-DETERMINATION ACT

In 1990, the U. S. Congress passed the **Patient Self-Determination Act** (PSDA).This Act took effect in 1992 and required that, on admission to any health care service (hospital, long-term-care center, or home care agency), patients be given an opportunity to determine what life-saving or life-prolonging actions they want to be carried out. Much of the impetus for this legislation was the belief that many individuals were having their lives prolonged in situations in which they would have preferred this not be done. The Act requires the agency to provide adequate information for the individual to make an informed decision regarding these important matters. As a result of this legislation, agencies reviewed and revised policies and protocols regarding consent. In many agencies, a nurse has the responsibility to provide the education and obtain a signature on a document indicating preferences.

Information regarding the results of the PSDA is being analyzed by several government agencies to determine whether there has been a change in practice. Some have suggested that the manner in which self-determination and the possible alternatives are explained greatly influences patient choices; one suggestion has been that these matters first be discussed in the health care provider's office, before admission. When this is possible, it allows for more time to consider alternatives and consult significant others. The final decision is then made away from the pressure of the health care environment. (See Chapter 10 for a further discussion of planning for end-of-life issues.)

Emergency Care

Care in emergencies has many legal repercussions; therefore, the judgment that an emergency exists is important. Certain actions may be legal in emergencies and not legal in nonemergency situations. In emergencies, the standard procedures for obtaining consent may be impossible to follow. Further, in emergencies, personnel must sometimes take on responsibilities that they would not undertake in a nonemergency situation. Critical thinking on the part of all health care professionals is essential when differentiating an emergency from a nonemergency.

Most facilities that provide emergency care have policies and procedures designed to ensure adequate support for claiming that an emergency exists. Thus, the policy will often state that at least two physicians in the emergency department must examine the patient and concur that the emergency requires immediate action, without waiting for consent. This ensures maximum legal protection for the physician and the institution.

CONSENT IN EMERGENCIES

If a true emergency exists, consent for care is considered to be implied. The law holds that if a reasonable person were aware that the situation was life threatening, he or she would give consent for care. An exception to this is made if the person has explicitly rejected such care in advance; an example is a Jehovah's Witness carrying a card stating his personal religion, and that he does not wish to receive blood or blood products. This is one reason emergency department nurses should check a patient's wallet for identification and information related to care. Checking a patient's wallet should be done with another person, and a careful inventory of contents made and signed by both. There should be little concern about liability in taking emergency action if this is completed.

STANDARDS OF PRACTICE AND EMERGENCIES

Standards of practice in emergencies also differ from those in nonemergency situations. In hospital emergencies, the nurse sometimes may be in the position of identifying an emergency and whether a needed action is one that only a physician usually performs. The hospital is expected to have a policy and procedure, which the nurse would follow, to verify and document the situation fully. This usually involves consultation with a supervisory nurse and verification of the emergency situation, as well as attempts to obtain medical assistance. Again, critical thinking by the nurse is essential to determine whether a true emergency exists.

When "life or limb" is truly in danger, the courts have held that a nurse can do those things immediately necessary, even if they usually are considered medical functions, provided the nurse has the essential expertise to perform the actions safely and correctly. The matter of having essential expertise is crucial; this is why all members of an emergency response team must learn all aspects of the "code" procedure. If, for any reason, the physician were unable to respond to the code, a nurse who was prepared with this essential expertise would assume the role of the leader.

Nursing Action in a Hospital Emergency

In an orthopedic unit, it is common to care for patients with new casts. A young man with a newly applied long-leg cast is admitted through the emergency department at 6 PM. The nurse assigned to this patient's care carefully makes all the appropriate observations throughout the evening and documents his findings. The nurse notes that the leg is beginning to swell and that the edges of the cast are beginning to cut into the skin. At that time, the nurse notifies the supervisor that a problem is developing, and that he thinks the physician should be notified. The supervisor agrees and the nurse begins trying to contact the physician. The nurse continues to make observations, noting increasing swelling, color changes in the exposed toes, and loss of sensation. The physician cannot be reached and no other physician is immediately available.

The nurse follows the hospital procedure for seeking medical attention and for determining when an emergency exists. After consultation with the supervisor, the nurse decides that an emergency exists and that the cast needs to be cut open to relieve the pressure. Deciding to cut a cast open and cutting the cast are considered medical responsibilities in this hospital.

The nurse has been taught how and when to use a cast cutter in emergency situations. Thus, the nurse possesses the essential expertise. The nurse, with the supervisor's approval, cuts open the cast and secures it in place with an elastic bandage. All observations made, consultations carried out, attempts to notify the physician, and the final action taken are documented carefully in the patient's record. Hospital policy was followed throughout the situation to ensure that all necessary steps had been taken.

Although this action went beyond usual nursing practice, it would not be considered a violation of either the nursing or the medical practice acts, because an emergency existed and the results of inaction would have been serious. Additionally, the nurse had the expertise and was prepared to carry out the necessary action safely. This emergency care usually is limited to specific technical procedures that the nurse has learned. It does not include diagnosing disease or prescribing medication, unless there are specific standing orders relative to the situation.

PROTOCOLS AND EMERGENCIES

Most health care agencies have established protocols for nursing action in a variety of emergency or even urgent situations. These provide directions for nursing action that would usually be a physician's order. For example, if the patient's blood pressure is dropping precipitously, the protocol might indicate that the nurse would start an IV infusion with a specified fluid to maintain circulating volume and to provide IV access for emergency drugs. The administration of oxygen to a person suffering acute respiratory distress is another situation frequently covered by a protocol. When emergencies occur, the nurse is protected from a charge of practicing outside the scope of the RN by following the protocol that was approved by the medical staff.

NONINSTITUTIONAL EMERGENCY CARE

Emergencies encountered outside the health care environment present other problems. Anyone rendering aid in an emergency is expected to behave as a reasonably prudent person would in such a situation. The nurse rendering aid in an emergency must behave as a reasonably prudent nurse in that situation. Thus, the standard is higher than for the nonprofessional person, although the nurse is not expected to perform as if he or she were operating in a health care setting. The physical situation and the psychological situation are both considered when determining what is a reasonably prudent nursing action.

All states and Canadian provinces have "Good Samaritan" statutes that excuse negligence on the part of rescuers in an emergency; the term refers to a person who voluntarily helps another in need (Killion & Dempski, 2000, p. 13). These laws are of interest to health care professionals, who are concerned about lawsuits. These statutes vary in content and comprehensiveness but relieve a professional of some liability when reasonable care is used. These laws often make people feel more secure when rendering aid.

Each nurse must make an individual decision about rendering emergency aid in a specific situation. The decision involves ethical as well as legal considerations. If the profession of nursing is a public trust and nurses are truly involved in the business of caring, then failure to aid an individual who is in serious danger is an ethical violation of that trust. To date, there has been no instance of a nurse being sued for coming to the aid of someone in an emergency situation (Bernzweig, 1996). Professional liability insurance does provide coverage when the nurse assists in this way, which may make you feel more comfortable about rendering emergency aid. Vermont was the first state to mandate that anyone encountering an emergency render assistance (Guido, 2001). You should check to see whether such a statute has been enacted in your state.

In many states, emergency personnel must render all possible aid, including all resuscitative measures, when they are called to an emergency situation. This has sometimes resulted in the resuscitation of a terminally ill person who had previously stated that resuscitation was not desired. As more individuals receive terminal care in their homes, this will become an increasing concern.

Legislation allowing for patient self-determination regarding emergency responders has now been passed in some states. The law usually stipulates the precise circumstances under which an individual may provide an advance directive regarding emergency procedures, and how that directive must be documented so that emergency personnel can honor it. For example, the individual may be required to wear a specific armband and the DNR order may be posted on the door of the refrigerator or other prominent position in the home. All emergency responders must be aware of their responsibilities regarding advance directives.

Fraud

Fraud is deliberate deception for the purpose of personal gain and is usually prosecuted as a crime. However, it may also serve as the basis of a civil suit. Situations of fraud in nursing are not common. One example would be trying to obtain a better position by giving incorrect information to a prospective employer. By deliberately stating (falsely) that you had completed a nurse practitioner program to obtain a position for which you would otherwise be ineligible, you are defrauding the employer. This may be prosecuted as a crime, because you are also placing members of the community in danger of receiving substandard care. You may also commit fraud by trying to cover up a nursing error to avoid legal action. Courts tend to be more harsh in decisions regarding fraud than in cases involving simple malpractice, because fraud represents a deliberate attempt to mislead others for your own gain and could result in harm to those assigned to your care.

Assault and Battery

Assault is saying or doing something to make a person genuinely afraid that he or she will be touched without consent. **Battery** involves touching a person when that individual has not consented to the action. Neither of these terms implies that harm was done; harm may or may not occur. For an assault to occur, the person must be afraid of what might happen because the individual appears to have the power to carry out the threat. "If you don't take this medication, I will have to put you in restraints" is an example of an assault. For battery to occur, the touching must occur without consent. Remember that consent may be implied rather than specifically stated. Therefore, if the patient extends an arm for an injection, he cannot later charge battery, saying that he was not asked. But if the patient agreed because of a threat (assault), the touching still would be considered battery because the consent was not freely given.

Assault and battery are crimes under the law. However, most of these cases in health care are instituted as civil suits by the injured party, rather than as criminal cases by the governmental authorities.

Assault and battery are most commonly treated as criminal cases when they involve suspected abuse of a patient. Most of us in health care are shocked and dismayed to learn of instances where care providers were abusive. Individuals who have difficulty with impulse control and anger may become frustrated with a patient and threaten, push, shove, or otherwise harm the individual. Most jurisdictions have laws requiring that anyone who knows of abuse to an individual, whether a child, a developmentally delayed adult, or an elderly person, report that abuse to the proper authorities. Within an institution, there should be policies and procedures for this type of reporting. Appropriate authorities must conduct a careful investigation to ensure protection of the rights of the person accused.

False Imprisonment

Making a person stay in a place against his wishes is **false imprisonment**. The person may be forced to stay either by physical or verbal means. It is easy to understand why restraining a patient or confining a patient to a locked room could constitute false imprisonment, if proper procedures were not first carried out. Again, false imprisonment is a crime, but when it occurs in health care it is most often the basis of a civil suit rather than a criminal case.

The law is less clear about keeping a patient confined by nonphysical means. If you remove a patient's clothes for the express purpose of preventing his leaving, you could be liable for false imprisonment. Threatening to keep a person confined with statements such as "If you don't stay in your bed, I'll sedate you" can also constitute false imprisonment. If a person needs to be confined for his or her own safety or well-being, it is best to help the person understand and agree to that course of action.

Any time a patient poses a danger to self or others, the law requires that the least restrictive means available be used to protect the patient and others. Health care providers are obligated to document the behavior of concern, problem-solve alternative actions, and then try those alternative actions before resorting to any type of restraint. Documentation of this entire process is essential. Nurses who determine the need for restraints must obtain a physician's order as soon as possible. Be sure to follow the policies of the facility.

In a conventional care setting, you cannot restrain or confine responsible adults against their wishes. All persons have the right to make decisions for themselves, regardless of the consequences. The patient with a severe heart condition who defies orders and walks to the bathroom has that right. You protect yourself by recording your efforts to teach the patient the need for restrictions and by reporting the patient's behavior to your supervisor and the physician.

In the same context, the patient cannot be forced to remain in a hospital. The patient has the right to leave a health care institution regardless of medical advice to the contrary. While this might not be in the best interests of the person's health, the patient has the right to decide to leave against medical advice (AMA). Again, you document your efforts in the record and follow applicable policies to protect the facility, the physician, and yourself from liability.

False imprisonment suits are a special concern in the care of the psychiatric patient. Particular laws relate to this situation. In the psychiatric setting, you may have patients who have voluntarily sought admission. The same restrictions on restraint or confinement that apply to patients in the general care setting apply to these patients. Other patients in the psychiatric setting may have been committed involuntarily according to the laws of the state. Specific measures may be used to confine the involuntarily committed patient. Laws in terms of situation, type of restraint allowed, and the length of time restraining may be used usually to define these measures. If you work in a psychiatric setting, you should review specific policies regarding restraint to protect patients, and to assist staff in functioning within the legal limits.

Medication Errors

Medication errors are one of the most common causes of adverse outcomes for hospitalized patients (IOM, 2000). The incidence of errors related to medications ranges from 4% to 17% of all people being admitted to a hospital (Bates et al, 1993, 1995; Lesar et al, 1990). In these studies, antibiotics, analgesics, and cardiovascular drugs most frequently were associated with errors. Errors had many different sources, including inappropriate medication for the condition being treated; incorrect dosage or frequency of administration of medication; wrong route of administration; failure to recognize drug interactions; lack of monitoring for drug side effects; and inadequate communication among members of the health care team and the patient.

Many different health care team members were responsible for the errors and many different team members can prevent errors. Although individuals must exercise extraordinary care and follow procedures carefully, systems for medication administration also need to be carefully scrutinized. Some errors result from drugs with similar names; look-alike medication containers contribute to other errors; still other errors are created by poor systems for communication, in which handwriting problems may contribute to lack of clarity. Verbal orders have such a potential for error that most systems are set up to avoid them as much as possible.

When medication errors do occur, the health care professionals involved should institute corrective action immediately and communicate with the patient and family. Fiesta (1998) points out that if health care professionals are not straightforward with patients and families, fraud or intentional concealment may be charged and may contribute to the awarding of punitive damages as well as ordinary damages. Most malpractice insurance will not cover punitive damages.

FACTORS THAT CONTRIBUTE TO MALPRACTICE CLAIMS

A suit usually does not always follow the poor results or harm that may on occasion occur in the course of nursing practice. An understanding of the factors that enter into whether a suit is instituted may be helpful to you.

Social Factors

Much is being written about changes in the public's attitudes toward health care personnel. Health care is big business, and patients complain increasingly of not being accepted and respected as individuals. Patients are more willing to bring suit against someone who is part of a large, impersonal system.

Health costs are high, and some people think hospitals and physicians have the ability to pay large settlements, whether directly or through insurance. If a patient's own income is lessened or disrupted by an illness, he or she might bring suit as a solution to economic difficulties. Increased public awareness of the size of monetary judgments that have been awarded may also be an economic incentive to initiating a suit.

Suit-Prone Patients

Some people are more likely to bring suit, for real or imagined errors. If these people are recognized as being suit-prone patients, it is possible for you to protect yourself through increased vigilance regarding care and thorough record-keeping. Although we would warn you to guard against stereotyping, the following general descriptions may help you to avoid problems. Suit-prone patients usually are identified by overt behavior in which they are persistent fault-finders and critics of personnel and of all aspects of care. They may be uncooperative in following a plan of care and sensitive to any perceived slight.

Persons who exhibit hostile attitudes may extend their hostile feelings to the nurses and other health care persons with whom they have contact. The nurse who becomes defensive when faced with hostility only widens the breach in the nurse–patient relationship. It is necessary to pay careful attention to those principles of care learned in psychosocial nursing that deal with how to help the hostile patient. Assisting patients in solving their own problems and offering support are the best forms of protection for the nurse.

Another type of patient who appears more suit-prone is the very dependent person who uses projection to deal with anxiety and fear. These individuals tend to ascribe fault or blame for all events to others and are unable to accept personal responsibility for their own welfare. Again, meeting these patients' needs with a carefully considered plan of care is the answer.

A common error is to withdraw and become defensive when confronting a suit-prone patient; this reaction occurs partly because a situation is unpleasant and partly because a staff member feels personally threatened by the patient's behavior. This reaction increases the likelihood of a suit if a poor result occurs.

Another incorrect nursing response to the suit-prone patient is to become more directive and authoritarian. This tends to increase the patient's feeling of separation and distance from the staff and again increases the likelihood of a suit.

When the staff is helped to view the patient as a troubled person who manifests his or her problems in this manner, sometimes they find it easier to be objective. The patient is in need of all the skill that the thoughtful nurse can bring to the emotional problems. The entire health team needs to develop a careful and consistent approach, which provides security and stability to the patient and family. The suit-prone patient does not always end up suing; much depends on the response of health care personnel.

Suit-Prone Nurses

Nurses may also be suit-prone. Nurses who are insensitive to the patient's complaints, who do not identify and meet the patient's emotional needs, or who fail to recognize and accept the limits of their own practice may contribute to suits instituted not only against the nurse but also against the employer and the physician. The nurse's self-awareness is critical in preventing suits (Fig. 8-3).

Staff members may contribute to a patient's distrust of care through complaining about working conditions, telling patients about problems occurring on the unit, and disparaging other health care providers. There is a distinction between informing a patient that you must meet someone else's needs, and therefore will not return for a specified period of time, and giving the patient the impression that you do not have time to attend to his or her needs.

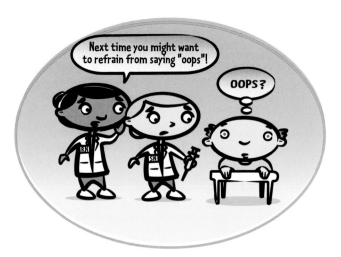

FIGURE 8-3   Certain things can be done to prevent malpractice suits.

PREVENTING MALPRACTICE CLAIMS

The most significant thing you can do to prevent malpractice claims is to maintain a high standard of care. To do this, you may work at improving your own nursing practice and also the general climate for nursing practice where you work. You can do this in many ways.

Self-Awareness

Identify your own strengths and weaknesses in practice. When you have identified a weakness, seek a means of growth. This may include education, directed experience, or discussion with colleagues. Be ready to acknowledge your limitations to supervisors, and do not accept responsibilities for which you are not prepared. For example, the nurse who has not worked in pediatrics for 10 years and accepts an assignment to a pediatric unit without orientation and education is setting the stage for an error to occur. The standard of care does not change for an inexperienced nurse (Killion & Dempsey, 2000). As a professional, you should not accept a position if you cannot meet the criterion of being a reasonably prudent nurse in that setting. In instances of true emergency (eg, disaster, flood), courts may be more lenient, but "we need you here today" is not an emergency.

Adapting Proposed Assignments

As discussed previously, nurses may find themselves assigned to units where they have little or no experience with the types of patient problems they will encounter. It is reasonable to be assigned to assist an overworked nurse in a special area if you can assume duties that are within your own competence, and allow the specialized nurse to assume the specialized duties. It is not reasonable or safe for you to be expected to assume the specialized duties.

Thus, if you were not prepared for coronary care, you might go to that unit, monitor the IV lines, take vital signs, and make observations to report to the experienced coronary care nurse; the experienced nurse then would be able to check the monitors, administer the specialized medications, and make decisions. Note that this does fragment the patient's care, and would not be appropriate as a permanent solution, but could alleviate a temporary problem in a safe manner.

Following Policies and Procedures

It is your responsibility to be aware of the policies and procedures of the institution that employs you. If they are sound, they can be an adequate defense against a claim, providing they were carefully followed.

For example, the medication procedure may involve checking all medications against a central medication Kardex®. If you do this and there is an error in the Kardex, you might not be liable for the resulting medication error because you followed all appropriate procedures and acted responsibly. The liability would rest with the person who made the error in transcribing the medication from the physician's orders to the Kardex. If, however, you had not followed procedure in checking, you might also be liable because you did not do your part in preventing error. As discussed previously, policies are often designed to provide legal direction.

Changing Policies and Procedures

As nursing evolves, changes are needed in policies, procedures, and protocols. Part of your responsibility as a professional is to work toward keeping these up to date. Are there written policies to deal with emergency situations? Statements such as, "Oh, we've always done it this way" are not adequate substitutes for clearly written, officially accepted policies. Often facilities that are reluctant to make changes based on the suggestions of individual nurses are much more receptive to new ideas when the legal implications of outmoded practice are noted. References such as the guidelines produced by the Agency for Health Care Policy and Research (AHCPR) and articles with research results may provide strong support for needed changes in practice.

Documentation

Nurses' records are unique in the health care setting. They cover the entire period of hospitalization, 24 hours a day, in a sequential pattern. Your record can be the crucial factor in avoiding litigation. Documentation in the record of observations made, decisions reached, actions taken, and the evaluation of the patient's response are considered much more solid evidence than verbal testimony, which depends on one's memory.

Because each case is determined by the facts as well as by the applicable law, clear documentation of all relevant data is important. For legal purposes, observations and actions that are not recorded may be assumed not to have occurred. Documentation needs to be factual, legible, and clearly understandable. Only approved abbreviations should be used. Narrative notes should have clear statements, and errors should be corrected according to the policy of the facility. Liquid erasing fluid, erasures, and heavy crossing out may be interpreted as attempted fraud in record keeping. You should avoid any statement that implies negligence on the part of any health care provider. Although primarily focusing on physician's records, Kightlinger provides examples of how poorly kept health care records actually may contribute to the likelihood of a successful suit (Kightlinger, 1999). Nurses should be aware that their notes protect not only themselves but often other members of the health care team and the facility.

Properly kept records also may protect you from becoming liable for the error of another, by demonstrating that you did everything in your power to prevent harm, including consulting with others. These records might include a complete log of telephone calls to a physician and consultation with any relevant supervisor. Documentation should support that you followed all relevant policies and procedures when an emergency occurred. Although it is easy to become impatient with the time required by "paper work," complete and clear documentation is often the basis of a successful defense against a claim of malpractice.

One concern about problem-oriented records and charting "by exception" is that these formats may provide less-detailed information and may be less helpful in defense against litigation. This does not have to be the case. You can use any system of charting and record keeping to create appropriate and adequate documentation of care. If you identify something that needs to be recorded and cannot find a provision within your system to make that recording, you can be sure that others have experienced the same difficulty. You might begin inquiries toward establishing a clear mechanism for the record keeping that concerns you. When nurses serve on committees to review and plan charting procedures, it is wise for them to seek consultation with the attorney for the facility. This helps to ensure that the plan for record keeping is legally sound as well as professionally useful.

ELEMENTS OF A LEGAL ACTION

Any legal action begins with the process of discovery, and then may be dropped, settled out-of-court, or go to trial for settlement.

Discovery

In a civil lawsuit (one between parties for the recovery of damages), a lengthy discovery process leads up to the trial. **Discovery** involves gathering information through documents (such as previous medical records and results of mental and physical examinations), interrogatories (written questions answered under oath), and depositions. **Testimony** refers to an individual's verbal or written account of a situation.

A **deposition** is a formal proceeding in which each attorney has an opportunity to question a witness outside of court, and a sworn verbatim record is made by a court reporter. On occasion, the deposition may be videotaped (Killion & Dempski, 2000). Depositions are often held in attorneys' offices or in a health care facility for the convenience of the health care providers. Sometimes depositions are taken to preserve the testimony of a witness for trial and are used in place of live testimony at trial. Most depositions in which you would participate, however, would be depositions for discovery purposes.

Settlement Out of Court

Often cases are settled before trial because of information obtained in the discovery process. The person bringing suit may be persuaded that no malpractice occurred or that it cannot be proved, and may drop the suit. On the other hand, the persons or institutions being sued (or their insurance companies) may determine that it is in their best interests to avoid a trial and agree to pay damages; this is often done without admitting that malpractice occurred. A settlement may require that no party to the settlement reveal its terms to others. Often the cost in time and money to defend a malpractice case exceeds the cost of a settlement. However, any settlement must be reported to the National Practitioner Data Bank. This has made many health care professionals reluctant to settle a legal action for reasons of finances and convenience.

Trials

A trial is a legal proceeding that takes place in a courtroom and is presided over by a judge. Some trials are settled before the judge (or panel of judges) alone, and others also have a jury present. In most instances, a trial is a public hearing and anyone can attend and listen to the proceedings. The various witnesses may appear in person or, when agreed to by both sides, a deposition may be accepted in place of in-person testimony. The judge has full authority over all that takes place in the courtroom.

The **plaintiff** is the individual bringing suit. The **defendants** are all those being named in the suit. Each side presents its witnesses who are examined (questioned) by the attorney. The attorney for the other side then is able to cross-examine (question) that witness about any of the information presented. The final decision is made by a vote of the jury meeting in private or by the judge, who considers all the information and makes a ruling. Monetary awards may be made at the time of the decision or may be established by further deliberation.

THE NURSE AS WITNESS

In the course of your practice as an RN, a time may come when you are asked to serve as a witness in a legal proceeding. Several kinds of cases may involve the nurse as a witness to fact or as an expert witness. When you become involved in any legal action, you should be sure that you understand both your rights and your obligations in regard to legal action.

As a witness, you will be required to swear (take an oath) or affirm to tell the entire truth. Failure to tell the entire truth is **perjury**, which is a crime. You are expected to answer the questions asked of you to the best of your ability; however, you do not have to provide an answer that would incriminate yourself, nor do you have to answer a question for which you do not remember or know the answer. It is perfectly permissible to state, "I do not remember" or "I do not know" if you do not.

It is helpful to use words and terms that can be understood by those who are not familiar with medical terminology, or to explain medical terminology when its use is essential. If hypothetical situations or cases are presented for your response, be sure to note the differences between the hypothetical case and the one currently under consideration before you respond.

Be brief and direct when answering questions. Answer the question asked of you. In clinical practice, nurses often use rephrasing techniques to gain information from clients. This should not be done when giving testimony (Shinn, 2001). Do not volunteer additional information that has not been asked for by the attorney. You may open up entire areas of inquiry that would not be considered without your comments. It is the attorney's job to ask the questions to bring out the facts to which he or she wants you to testify. The opposing attorney will have an opportunity during cross-examination to ask you additional questions that the attorney believes are necessary for the facts of the case. However, be cautious about simply answering "yes" or "no." In some instances, an explanation is essential; a simple answer may sound as if you did not perform appropriately (Guido, 2001).

A **witness to fact** is an individual who has firsthand knowledge of the specific situation that is the basis of the legal action. As a witness to fact, you will be testifying to the exact situation and circumstances of the event or events in question. You should always consult an attorney before talking to anyone about a matter in which you have been asked to testify, especially a malpractice action (Display 8-4).

For example, a nurse might be asked to testify as a witness to fact when a person has been injured (for example, in an automobile accident) and you or your organization were involved in the care of that person. Your testimony in such a case might be on behalf of the injured person, to help describe the injuries and the care received for those injuries. For example, you may be asked to testify regarding the care given in a burn center to a victim of an electrical accident, who received considerable nursing care during the recovery period.

Another situation involving the nurse as a witness to fact is one in which a patient brings a lawsuit against persons or organizations who have provided health care that the patient believes was below the standard of the community. Medical malpractice is alleged in such a situation. For example, the nurse may have to give evidence regarding medical record notes, or care given to the patient in the days before the alleged malpractice occurred. Sometimes a nurse is asked to provide information regarding the standards of care on a particular unit and the usual practices of the unit staff.

In both of these situations, the nurse's concern is with the specific factual details of a particular case. The nurse will be testifying only to what he or she has observed or done, not to

---

Display 8-4   **GUIDELINES FOR TESTIFYING**

- Answer only the questions asked.
- Do not volunteer additional information.
- Admit if you do not remember.
- Refer to your written documentation to support your answers.
- Be brief and direct.
- Do not use medical or technical terminology unless essential—then explain your terms.
- Explain when a simple yes or no would be misleading.
- Note differences between hypothetical cases presented and the one under considerations.

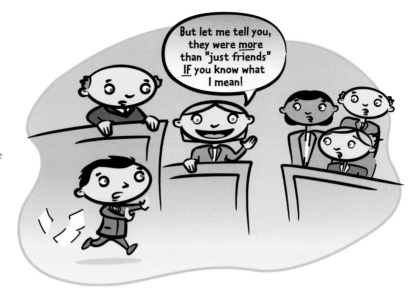

FIGURE 8-4 When testifying in court you should answer only the questions asked. Do not introduce other information.

hearsay. When nurses are asked to testify as to the facts of a situation, they sometimes believe that because they have done nothing wrong they do not need legal counsel. The law is complex, and you could jeopardize the position of an institution for which you work, or even jeopardize yourself and your professional future, with unwise statements. The person who is bringing suit may alter or amend the original complaint to involve new defendants, including you. If you have liability insurance, you should advise your insurance company of your role as a witness, and an attorney will be assigned to talk with you. If you are covered by an employer's policy, you should consult with the appropriate administrative representative immediately to obtain legal counsel. This attorney should assist you in understanding the questions in the case, your role, and how you can protect yourself in the situation (Fig. 8-4).

A nurse also may be involved in a lawsuit as an expert witness. An **expert witness**, under Rule 702 of the Federal Rules of Evidence, accepted in the federal courts and many state courts, is defined as "a witness qualified as an expert by knowledge, skill, experience, training, or education" who may testify in the form of an opinion or otherwise. The purpose of testimony as an expert witness is to provide information and opinion that can be used by the judge or jury to understand complex areas of care and make a decision. A nurse may provide a professional opinion, related to his or her area of expertise, on the appropriate care for a given situation. Nurses serving as expert witnesses usually have many years of experience, specialty education, and perhaps certification in their area of specialty.

KEY CONCEPTS

- Law includes those rules of conduct or action recognized as binding or enforced by government.

- Statutory law includes all written laws and governmental codes.
- Constitutional law, which has the greatest authority in any jurisdiction, is found in the U. S. Constitution and in state constitutions.
- Enacted law includes those laws passed by legislative bodies.
- Regulatory law, also referred to as administrative or executive law, includes those rules and regulations established by administrative bodies within the government.
- Common law includes judicial law, also referred to as case law, and common usage or custom.
- Civil law encompasses those laws regulating private conduct between individuals.
- Criminal law regulates actions having to do with the safety of the community as a whole.
- Violations of criminal law are considered crimes, whereas violations of civil law are considered torts.
- Legal rights are derived from constitutional guarantees and carry with them responsibilities. Other rights are ethically determined, and while not supportable by law, do govern the behavior of health care professionals.
- Malpractice actions brought against health care workers involve civil law. Nurses may be involved in cases related to intentional torts, negligence, or malpractice.
- The individual who is negligent or has committed malpractice is legally liable for the effects of that action. This means there is an obligation to the individual wronged.
- Liability may be focused on the individual, the supervisor, or the employer.
- Liability insurance may be purchased that transfers the cost of being sued and the cost of any settlement from the individual to a large group.
- A number of legal issues recur in nursing. Among these are the duty to report or seek medical care for a patient, protection of the patient's confidentiality and right to privacy, defamation of character, privileged information, issues related to informed consent, medication administration, and issues related to different types of emergency care.
- There are many legal issues surrounding consent by the patient or by a substitutionary decision-maker. These include the provision of advanced directives such as living wills (directives to the physician) and durable power of attorney for health care.
- Nurses also can be involved in criminal cases related to fraud, assault and battery, and false imprisonment. In some cases, however, a civil suit may be brought against a nurse, in which case, the nurse may not be prosecuted for criminal behavior.
- Many factors contribute to malpractice claims. These include social factors, characteristics of suit-prone patients, and characteristics of suit-prone nurses.
- A nurse can do many things to prevent malpractice claims. Being aware of your own practice, accepting only those assignments for which you are prepared, following policies and procedures, and properly documenting care are among the most important.
- A legal action may include a process of discovery, dropping the action, settlement out of court, or a trial.
- Nurses may be called as witnesses in trials because of their expertise in a particular area, or because of personal knowledge of the case. You must understand both your rights and your obligations regarding legal action before giving a deposition or testimony.

RELEVANT WEB SITES

Board of Nursing Web sites (see links from the National Council of State Boards of Nursing *www.ncsbn.org*) may contain the statutes relating to nursing and information on advisory opinions regarding nursing practice in that state.

Health Care Practice: *www.healthcarepractice.com*

St. Louis University and the American Society of Law, Medicine, and Ethics: *www.painandthelaw.org*

University of Texas Medical Branch, Center for Nursing Ethics, Law, and Policy: *www.son.utmb.edu/nursing/ethicslp/*

Note: Official state Web sites with statutes are available in some jurisdictions.

REFERENCES

Anonymous. (1997). Court case: A failure to communicate. *Nursing 97 27*(2): 32.

Bates, D. W., Cullen, D. J., Laird, N., et al. (1995). Incidence of adverse drug events and potential adverse drug events: Implications for prevention. *JAMA* 274: 29–34.

Bates, D. W., Leape, L. L., Petrycki, S. (1993). Incidence and preventability of adverse drug events in hospitalized adults. *Journal of General Internal Medicine* 8: 289–294.

Bernzweig, E. P. (1996). *The nurse's liability for malpractice* (6th ed.). St. Louis: Mosby–Year Book.

Curtin, L. (1997). When negligence becomes homicide. *Nursing Management 28*(7): 7–8.

Fiesta, J. (1999). Do no harm: When caregivers violate our golden rule, part 2. *Nursing Management 30*(9): 10.

Fiesta, J. (1998). Law for the nurse manager: Legal aspects of medication administration. *Nursing Management 29*(1): 22–23.

Fiesta, J. (1994). *The law and liability* (2nd ed.). New York: John Wiley & Sons.

Furrow, B. R. (2001). Pain and the law. *Journal of Law, Medicine, & Ethics 29*: 28–51, [On-line]. Available: *www.painandthelaw.or/aslme_content/29-1/furrow.pdf.* Accessed August 18, 2002.

Guido, G. W. (2001). *Legal and ethical issues in nursing.* Upper Saddle River, NJ: Prentice Hall.

Hall, J. K. (1996). *Nursing ethics and law.* Philadelphia: WB Saunders.

Judson, S. & Hicks, S. (1999). *Law and ethics for medical careers* (2nd ed.). Columbus: Glencoe.

Institute of Medicine (IOM). (2000). To err is human: Building a safe health care system. [On-line]. Available: *http://books.nap.edu/books/0309068371/html/index.html.* Accessed January 22, 2003.

Kightlinger, R. (1999). Sloppy records: The kiss of death for a malpractice defense. *Medical Economics 76*(8): 109–113.

Kihm, N. C. (1999). My hospital will cover me. *The Washington Nurse. 29*(4): 32–33.

Killion, S. W. & Dempski, K. M. (2000). *Legal and ethical issues.* Thorofare, NJ: Slack, Inc.

Lesar, T. S., Briceland, L. L., Delcoure, K., Parmalee, J. C., Masta-Gornic, V., & Pohl, H. (1990). Medication prescribing errors in a teaching hospital. *JAMA* 263: 2329–2334.

Needleman, J., Buerhaus, P., Mattke, S., Stewart, M., & Zelevinsky, K. (2002). Nurse staffing levels and the quality of care in hospitals. *New England Journal of Medicine 346*(22): 1715–1722.

Shinn, L. J. (2001). What to do if you are sued. In The ANA nursing risk management series I: An overview of risk management. (pp. 13–31) [On-line]. Available: *http://nursingworld.org/mods/mod310/cerm1ful.htm.*

Ethical Concerns in Nursing Practice

LEARNING OUTCOMES

After completing this chapter, you should be able to:

1. Discuss the concepts of ethics and morality and their application in the health care field.
2. Describe four ethical theories that may be used to guide ethical decision-making.
3. Explain how personal religious and philosophic viewpoints, the Codes for Nurses, and the Patient's Rights documents are used as bases for ethical decision-making.
4. Analyze ways in which sociocultural and occupational factors affect ethical decision-making for nurses.
5. Outline a framework for ethical decision-making.
6. Discuss how ethics relates to commitment to the patient, commitment to personal excellence, and commitment to nursing as a profession.
7. Analyze how ethics impact specific work situations, such as your obligations related to a chemically impaired nursing colleague or to boundary violations.

KEY TERMS

Autonomy	Ethical dilemma	Right
Beneficence	Ethics	Standard of best interest
Boundary violations	Fidelity	
Chemically impaired professional	Ideal observer theory	Theory of social justice
	Justice	Utilitarianism
Codes of ethics	Morality/Morals	Values
Cultural relativism	Natural law	Values clarification
Deontology	Nonmaleficence	Values conflict
Distributive justice	Paternalism	Veracity

Decisions that must be made regarding ethical and moral issues are primarily concerned with what is "right" or "good" for an individual. In nursing today, it is impossible to escape situations that call for judgments requiring serious consideration of what is right or best for our clients, their families, and the community. Although some of these decisions can be based on the clinical knowledge that you have been developing, many will require additional expertise in the realm of ethical and moral decision-making.

You have already had exposure to some of these decisions, such as the decision not to resuscitate a patient, or the decision to withdraw or withhold treatment. You already understand that these decisions are not made easily.

Fortunately, there are guiding principles to assist us in the process. And as you work at the process of applying critical thinking to your nursing decisions, you have learned to look seriously at the assumptions that have been made. Assumptions are often based on ethical and moral values. All of these are good reasons why, as nurses, we need knowledge of ethics, morality, and the process of ethical decision-making.

It is not possible in this text to explore the topic of ethics in depth; however, we provide an overview of the topic in this chapter. To assist you in understanding some of the terminology used in the discussion of ethics (and as a point of reference), we have provided a list of definitions in Table 9-1. Some of these terms are fully explained in the text of this chapter; others are not. We discuss some of the approaches to ethical decision-making and give examples of its application in health care. We also provide some direct application to your performance as a nurse and to personal decision-making. As you read about ethical issues and conflicts, and discuss them in your classroom or with a classmate, we urge you to respect others by listening carefully to them and honestly attempting to understand their positions and their accompanying values and beliefs. Only by considering all aspects of an issue can we seek and find understanding for ourselves.

UNDERSTANDING THE CONCEPT OF ETHICS

Since the time of Socrates and the Golden Age of Greece, philosophers have attempted to provide a logical approach to the questions of human conduct that arise in our lives. Why do we act the way we do? What constitutes good and evil, ethical and unethical? What are the factors that result in various cultures embracing different values? How are we to be guided in our decision-making? How will the ethics of care affect our professional performance? We continue to search for answers to these questions.

In the formal sense, **ethics** is a branch of philosophy (the study of beliefs and assumptions) referred to as moral philosophy. The word ethics is derived from the Greek term *ethos*, which means customs, habitual usage, conduct, and character.

Closely associated with the concept of ethics is that of **morals.** This word, derived from the Latin *mores*, means custom or habit. Morals are the basic standards for what we consider right and wrong. Morals or standards are often based on religious beliefs and, to some extent, social influence and group norms.

Together, the two words ethics and morals form constructs related to conduct, character, and motives for action. Thiroux (1998) suggests that ethics seems to pertain to an individual's character, whereas **morality** speaks to relationships between human beings. In either case, we

TABLE 9-1.	TERMINOLOGY RELATED TO ETHICS
TERM	**DEFINITION**
Absolutism	View that there is only one correct moral principle or code for which there are no exceptions
Altruism	Behavior motivated by concern for the well-being of others and that is intended to benefit others
Amoral	State or quality of being indifferent to morality
Categorical imperative	From Immanuel Kant's ethics, the view that for an act to be moral, it must be able to be applied to everyone
Cultural relativism	View that there is enormous variety in the mores and morals of people in different cultures and times, and no single cultural position is correct
Descriptive ethics	Focuses on what people actually do in given situations
Ethics	Specific area of study of morality that concentrates on human conduct and human values (from the Greek *ethos*, meaning character, habitual uses, customs)
Ethical/Moral egoism	When one considers only his or her own good or self-interest
Ethical/Moral nihilism	View that no universally valid or true moral principles exist
Ethical/Moral objectivism	View that universally valid and true moral principles exist
Ethical/Moral relativism	View that no universally valid or true moral principles exist but, rather, that all moral principles are valid relative to culture or individual choice
Ethical/Moral skepticism	View that we cannot know whether there are universally valid moral principles
Ethics of care	Focuses on those traits valued in intimate personal relationships, such as compassion, love, sympathy, and trust
Hedonism	View that good can be defined as that which is pleasurable
Meta-ethics	Deals with the extent to which moral judgments are reasonable or justifiable
Moral	Generally accepted as dealing with what is good and what is bad, what is right and what is wrong
Moral agent	Person capable of making distinctions between what is right and what is wrong
Moral philosophy	Branch of philosophy that examines beliefs and assumptions about the nature of certain human values
Moral thought	Individual cognitive evaluation of right and wrong, good and bad
Naturalism	View of moral judgment that regards ethics as dependent on human nature and psychology
Normative ethics	Examines individual rights and obligations as well as common good
Philosophy	Intense and critical examination of beliefs and assumptions (from the Greek words *philia*, meaning love or friendship, and *sophia*, meaning wisdom)
Practical ethics	Use of ethical theory and analysis to examine moral problems
Situational ethics	View that one's actions are governed entirely by the situation rather than by principles or rules
Subjectivism	View that moral principles are applicable to the agent alone, that what is right for one might not be right for another
Virtue ethics	Places emphasis on the agents or people who make choices and take actions

typically describe the behavior we observe as good, right, desirable, honorable, fitting, or proper; or, we might describe the behavior as bad, wrong, improper, irresponsible, or evil.

Quickly you will realize that such perceptions are based on **values**, and that each of us (and each society) has a differing set of values. Videbeck (2001) states, " . . . values are abstract standards that give a person a sense of what is right and wrong and establish a code of conduct for living." Some examples could include hard work, honesty, sincerity, genuineness, and being clean. Values are most commonly derived from societal norms, religion, and family orientation and provide the framework for making decisions about the actions we take every day. For example, if you were born in the United States, you may have been raised to believe it is unethical to restrict women's right to vote. Those in some other societies have been raised to believe that this is the ethical way to structure public life.

We all have been in a situation in which we experienced a **values conflict**. This occurs when we must choose between two things, both of which are important to us. For example, if you are a new mother, you probably would like to spend all of your time with your child; however, if you also must help provide support for the family, and that requires leaving the child to go to work, you have a values conflict.

Most of the time we don't think about our values—we just accept them. We are most likely to think about them when we have a difficult decision to make, when something goes wrong, or when we find ourselves in a conflict because of differing values. In nursing we work with a diverse patient population and therefore are exposed to a variety of values and ethical standards. The need to give conscientious care to all patients often forces us to examine our own values.

The process of becoming more conscious of and naming what one values or considers worthy is known as **values clarification** (Burkhardt & Nathaniel, 1998). We examine what we believe is good, bad, beautiful, worthy, meaningful, and so forth, and explore the process of determining our personal values. This increases our self-awareness or understanding of ourselves and assists us in making choices. It facilitates decision-making, because we have a better grasp of our own value systems.

Having a good understanding of yourself will be helpful when you are faced with an ethical dilemma. An **ethical dilemma** occurs when an individual must choose between two unfavorable alternatives. For example, assisted suicide provides an ethical dilemma for many. Although they certainly are opposed to seeing a loved one spend the last months of life in great pain and suffering, they equally are opposed to assisting with an earlier death. Ethical dilemmas usually have no perfect solution, and those making decisions may find themselves in the position of having to defend their decisions. Although there are times when a difference in values and decisions can be accepted, at other times differences put people into direct conflict. Should you experience such a situation, we urge you to be constructive (rather than destructive) in the methods you choose to work toward resolving the differences. Listen carefully without interrupting and be willing to hear what others have to say. Seek clarification using gentle questioning. Respect cultural differences and be attentive to body language. Explain the context of your point of view and try to picture the other person's perspective of what you are saying.

Critical Thinking Activity

Identify situations you might confront in nursing in which your personal religious or philosophic values would be involved. What would be the consequences of following the dictates of your value system? Do conflicts exist between your value system and actions required by the situation? If so, how will you recognize the differences and how will you deal with them? Are there any other alternatives? What might they be?

BASIC ETHICAL CONCEPTS

Various authors and theorists identify different concepts as basic to ethics. Those concepts that are most frequently addressed include rights, autonomy, beneficence, nonmaleficence, justice, fidelity, veracity, and the standard of best interest. Identifying how they apply to a particular situation and balancing their competing claims often present a challenge.

Rights

Typically, we think of a **right** as a just claim or entitlement, or as something that is owed to an individual on a legal, moral, or ethical basis. In common usage, this is often extended to include privileges, concessions, and freedoms. Rights form the basis of most professional codes and legal judgments. (See Chapter 8 for more discussion of rights as used in the legal sense.) The discussion of the other ethical concepts is founded on the belief that people are entitled to certain rights. We deal with the issue of "rights" any time we are talking about the right of a person to self-determination. If a patient is admitted to a hospital and refuses treatment, and there is a strong indication that the patient could recover, should the physicians and nurses respect the patient's right to self-determination? The problems that occur when one individual's rights come in conflict with the values of another provide us with many challenges and dilemmas.

SELF-DETERMINATION RIGHTS

Federal legislation has been passed to ensure that individual rights are respected. The Patient Self-Determination Act, also known as the Danforth amendment, is discussed in Chapters 8 and 10. This act was created because of our society's fundamental belief in the individual's right to decide. However, this act does little to recognize cultural diversity and sensibility to groups such as Chinese-Americans, who have a unique but different set of values and well-defined role relationships, in which the role of family in making health care decisions is strongly valued (Fung, 1994).

RIGHTS AND CULTURAL RELATIVISM

Although the concept of rights is almost taken for granted in our Western culture, there are some who suggest that there are no human rights and that we cannot talk about rights, the violation of rights, or moral judgments, because the validity of all moral judgments is culturally relative. In other words, all rights and judgments must be able to be applied to all cultures. This concept is known as **cultural relativism**. Carried to the fullest extent, the concept of cultural relativism would limit us to determining when rights are being violated in our culture (Buchanan, 1996). Cultural relativism embraces the notion that groups and individuals hold different sets of values that must be respected. If the same values are not held by all cultures, then they are not considered valid and should not be applied in any situation. This is an interesting concept to consider in relationship to health care practices with which we, in the Western culture, have great difficulty, such as female circumcision. Although it is appalling to us, in some non-Western cultures, concerns about virginity, ability to attract a husband, the husband's sexual pleasure, and religious beliefs dictate that female children be circumcised. Members of these cultures do not view this practice as mutilation; rather, it is thought to result in the improved appearance of female genitalia, and to be referred to as uncircumcised is a terrible insult (Lane & Rubinstein, 1996). Such beliefs challenge our tolerance of other's values.

RIGHTS OF THE UNBORN

There are many times when we grapple with whose rights should be respected. The most obvious example of this situation occurs when we consider the rights of the unborn to life versus the right of the mother to make choices regarding her own body. This issue is one that has continued to divide members of our society and is often an issue brought forth when candidates are running for election. The concern becomes even more contradictory, paradoxical, and convoluted when we consider that some states will permit a late-term abortion; however, in that same state, if an automobile accident occurs in which a pregnant woman is killed (thus also killing the fetus she is carrying), the offending driver can be charged with two cases of manslaughter—both the mother and the unborn child.

RIGHTS OF PRIVACY AND CONFIDENTIALITY

An area receiving much attention today is that of the rights of the patient to privacy and the confidentiality of medical information. This has surfaced as a major concern because sensitive health records are now computerized and can be e-mailed, telecommunicated, faxed, or copied to various individuals or groups who may have an interest in the information. In 1996, Congress passed legislation in the Health Insurance Portability and Accountability Act that required steps be taken or legislation be passed to ensure the privacy of individually identifiable health information. Privacy may be thought of as the right to be free from intrusion, or to be left alone. It also includes the right to select desired care based on personal values and beliefs and to have control over how sensitive information is shared.

Confidentiality deals with not sharing information. People are concerned that exposure to personal health information, especially that related to genetic tests, could result in loss of or denial of health insurance, or could result in embarrassment or discrimination in the work environment. The information technology, for example, faxed materials on which we have come to rely for prompt communications, creates problems in this area even with the best efforts to remain confidential (see Chapter 8).

The American Nurses Association (ANA) has been concerned about this issue for some time. In 1995, the House of Delegates of the organization approved a policy called "Privacy and Confidentiality Related to Access to Electronic Data." In 1998, the Board of Directors endorsed the "Core Principles of Telehealth," intended to regulate telecommunication technologies used to provide long-distance care, education, and patient data. The organization continues to work with other national groups on the issue of privacy and confidentiality. As a student and as a nurse of the future, you will want to remain ever mindful of your responsibility to maintain patient privacy and confidentiality in all matters.

Autonomy

Autonomy involves the right of self-determination, independence, and freedom. It comes from the Latin *auto* meaning "self" and *nomy*, which means "control." Some refer to autonomy as respect for the individual and include the expectations that each individual will be treated as unique and as an equal to every other individual (Davis et al, 1997). Writers may refer to it as the Principle of Individual Freedom (Thiroux, 1998). Other words often associated with autonomy include dignity, inherent worth, self-reliance, and individualism.

When we consider an individual's autonomy, the way we approach a problem may result in the decision-making process becoming more time consuming. It is closely tied to informed consent (see Chapters 8 and 10), which requires that clients be provided clear and sufficient information about their situation to make a rational decision for themselves. Giving consideration to an individual's autonomy also requires that justification be provided for why the patient is not participating in decision-making, if in fact the patient is not. In today's health care delivery system, it is important to respect patients' rights to make decisions about and for themselves, even when we do not agree with those decisions. For example, you may have difficulty supporting the decision of a new mother, who is a Jehovah's Witness and whose life is in danger because of blood loss, to refuse to have a blood transfusion.

As with most other rights, there may be restrictions on the right to choose—autonomy does not mean that individuals can do anything they want. When one person's autonomy interferes with another individual's rights, health, or well-being, limitations may be imposed. Does a patient's right to self-determination allow that individual to choose a certain expensive treatment if that choice would unjustly deny money to another person for another treatment? What if a patient demands a bone marrow transplant that wipes out the health department's entire budget for immunizations? Does the autonomy of a patient with a highly communicable disease take precedence over the right of the community not to be exposed to the disease? If there are to be limitations, what should those limitations be? In what instances should the legal system interfere with personal decision-making?

For some individuals, autonomy may be less important than values related to the family. Is this acceptable? Who decides how much autonomy is "enough"? Once again, we must consider the idea that autonomy is predominantly a Western value. For example, tribal life occurs under more strenuous circumstances than we normally encounter; it requires more cooperation, less variation from the norm. The individual's freedom to do things is far more limited because decisions are directed toward the common good of the community.

Beneficence and Nonmaleficence

Beneficence refers to the obligation to do good, not harm, to other people. It also maintains that we ought to prevent evil or harm (Burkhardt & Nathaniel, 1998). Thus, the concept of beneficence extends from promoting good to **nonmaleficence** (the prohibition of intentional harm). As far back as Hippocrates, physicians were entreated to do no harm. Florence Nightingale stated that the patient should be no worse for having been nursed. The *Code for Nurses with Interpretive Statements* (2001) addresses this issue when it clearly delineates the steps to be taken to remove harm or evil. Some examples include reporting unethical practice of a colleague to appropriate authorities or expressing concern to the individual who is engaged in practices that result in substandard practice.

In health care we recognize that sometimes we unintentionally do harm to individuals. Nosocomial infections, adverse drug reactions, and the side effects of such treatments as irradiation and chemotherapy for cancer are certainly harmful to the individuals who experience them. In some cases, given the alternatives, a patient will opt not to have the treatment (eg, irradiation). The ethical mandate is that we refrain from intentionally inflicting harm. Sometimes it is difficult to accept that a side effect of a particular treatment might result in harm to a patient. Concern for the possible although rare reaction to smallpox vaccination is but one example.

Good is a general term of approval or commendation, and may be defined as that which produces favorable results, is beneficial, effective, honorable, worthy, respectable, proper, valid, desirable, pleasant, or healthy (Neufeldt & Guralnik, Webster's New World College Dictionary, 1996, p. 581). Thus, we tend to think of it as that which promotes life, development, and fulfillment. We view it as "good" when a friend makes a quick recovery from surgery, when a child graduates from high school or college, or when aging parents are able to take that long-awaited trip they have been planning for years.

It is sometimes difficult to decide who will determine what is good for a specific person in a specific situation. In most instances, we expect that people will make their own decisions about what is good for them. But who decides for the infant regarding procedures such as immunizations that inflict some degree of pain, but have long-lasting and positive benefits? Who decides for the individual who is unconscious or is mentally incompetent?

Another problem centers on what is good. Is all life good, or are there situations in which not living is better than life? Is it better to sustain life in the face of disability, or is it better to allow a person to die and have suffering end? If giving good care to one patient means that lesser care will be given to another (a situation encountered more and more frequently in today's health care environment), how can we defend such an action? What if giving good care means violating good nursing economics (cost containment)? There are no simple answers, and the answers are not the same for everyone.

The issue of sanctity of life is of major concern in the health care arena. Some would argue that all life is good. Others would adamantly assert that life is not good when the quality of life is poor; this latter belief has led to serious discussions regarding euthanasia, supported the establishment of such groups as the Hemlock Society, and has resulted in several states initiating legislation supporting assisted suicide. Many people, particularly physicians, believe that the principles of respect for the patient and relief from suffering fail to do justice to the internal values, professional integrity, and norms of medicine (Miller & Brody, 1995). Another example of a situation in which quality-of-life issues also emerge can be seen in an instance in which parents are advised that a fetus has a life-compromising condition such as meningomyelocele. The parents must weigh the quality of the life against the complications inherent in the meningomyelocele if the pregnancy is allowed to go to term. Surrounding all issues dealing with the sanctity of life are religious views and values, particularly those maintaining that all life is sacred. Certainly arguments regarding the "right to life" play a major role in discussions regarding abortion, whether supported by religious beliefs or personal value systems. The "right to life" also affects our personal beliefs about capital punishment.

Thus it can be said that although the topics of medical futility and the sanctity of life are widely discussed, there exists little consensus about them. As a nurse, you will often encounter difficult situations in the care of your patients in which opposing values play against one another. Understanding your own values, which may change over time, is important in these situations.

Critical Thinking Activity

Identify ways in which the concept of beneficence has shaped medical and nursing care provided to patients. Do you believe this is a concept that will have the same impact in years to come? What assumptions are you making? Are your data accurate? What are the implications for the future?

Justice

Justice refers to the obligation to be fair to all people. It looks at the concepts of fairness, just desserts, and entitlements (Edge & Groves, 1999). We must ask, "How is fairness defined?" Does fairness mean that people should be treated the same? In terms of access to health care, is it "just" for one person to receive more resources than another receives? If so, what makes it "just," and how does that relate to the distribution of scarce medical resources? Does age make a difference in what we consider just? Should it? Does justice imply that the government should provide the resources or services individuals are unable to provide for themselves? Can we measure fairness in any objective sense? What should occur when one person's rights interfere with the rights of another? These issues will be discussed in greater detail in Chapter 10.

DISTRIBUTIVE JUSTICE

The concept of **distributive justice** requires the fair distribution of burdens and benefits (Davis et al, 1997). The expectation is that all individuals have an equal opportunity to access scarce resources and requires health care organizations and health plans to provide to individual recipients the care and service each is due. This would include the frail elderly, poor, disabled, and homeless. Providers, managers, and policy-makers struggle with complicated and complex rules that fail to provide guidance in difficult or ambiguous situations (Maddox, 1998).

Armstrong and Whitlock (1998) cite six criteria that define the just distribution of limited resources: need, equity, contribution, ability to pay, effort, and merit. Need involves known medical need, not elective procedures. Equity addresses trying to distribute equally to all in need. Contribution considers what an individual might be expected to give to society at a future date. Ability to pay is self-explanatory, but to deny needed health services because an individual cannot pay contradicts the concepts of charitableness that exist in our society. Patient effort deals with a patient's compliance or noncompliance with medical advice. Merit addresses the potential that exists for benefit from the additional investment of limited health resources. These six criteria have not always provided a strong basis for decision-making, and the ethical issues related to allocation of scarce resources promise to become more complex in the coming years.

ETHICS AND FINANCIAL COMPENSATION

Another issue receiving attention, discussion, and review is the practice of rewarding physicians monetarily or nonmonetarily for limiting care. This process was first seen in the advent of diagnosis-related groups (DRGs) under Medicare that established limits for payment for services (Silva, 1998). Recently, health maintenance organizations (HMOs) have come under fire for rewarding physicians who maintain lower costs of care or for penalizing those who do not. What impact might this have on nurses who are involved in the care of clients who the nurse believes receive less than adequate treatment? How does this affect the nurse's obligation to serve as an advocate for the patient? These and similar issues are yet to be played out in the health care environment, but certainly emphasize the importance of all nurses understanding ethics and ethical principles.

Fidelity

Fidelity refers to the obligation to be faithful to the agreements, commitments, and responsibilities that one has made to oneself and others. Interestingly, it is one of the ethical concepts not addressed specifically in some textbooks of nursing ethics. Fidelity is the foundation of the concept of accountability that we hear about so often in nursing today. What are the responsibilities of health care personnel to individuals, employers, the government, society, and self? When these responsibilities conflict, which should take priority? In reality, which do take priority? Are nurses obligated to provide care to all patients? Under what circumstances, if any, might this be challenged? What are the nurse's promises to society? Would it also cover areas such as competence? Abiding by institutional policies? Operating within the profession's Code of Ethics?

A situation that often challenges us in health care is that of confidentiality. Is maintaining confidentiality one of the promises that nurses make to clients? Is maintaining confidentiality a moral/ethical issue as well as a legal issue? Are there any instances when it is acceptable to violate the principle of confidentiality? If you are working with an impaired colleague, is it appropriate and ethical to violate a confidential situation in the interest of patient well-being? We discuss this issue in detail later in the chapter.

Veracity

Veracity refers to telling the truth or not intentionally deceiving or misleading patients. From childhood, we are all admonished to tell the truth and to avoid lying. When we are children, this seems straightforward. As we become adults, we see more and more instances where the choices are less clear. For example, do you tell the truth (veracity) when you know the truth will cause harm to an individual (maleficence vs. nonmaleficence)? Do you tell a lie when it would make someone less anxious and afraid? You might see this as beneficence (doing good), but then you have abandoned the principle of veracity. Edge and Groves (1999) refer to the lack of truth telling as leading to a slippery slope, because when we conceal the truth to a patient, it teaches all others involved (eg, family members, friends, nursing assistants, housekeeping staff) that health practitioners lie. This deception is later remembered and the concept that one cannot rely on health professionals pervades. In other words, it diminishes one's esteem and reliability.

The Standard of Best Interest

When a decision must be made about a patient's health care and the patient is unable to make an informed decision, it is done in the **standard of best interest**. As the name implies, it is based on what the health care providers or family believe is best for that individual, taking into account tangible factors such as how the patient may be harmed, how the patient may benefit, and physical and fiscal risks. Such decisions are based on the individual's expressed wishes or on documents such as living wills. Health care professionals strive to avoid unilateral decisions made by a health care provider. Unilateral decisions often imply that the decision-maker knows what is best for the patient. When this occurs, it is referred to as **paternalism**, or the deliberate limiting of the patient's autonomy. In instances where parents have denied their children lifesaving care, the courts have, on occasion, overturned the parent's decision on the best-interest standard (Edge & Groves, 1999).

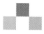

ETHICAL THEORIES

It is not our intent to delve with any depth into the writings of early philosophers. However, because ethical theories are mentioned frequently in the literature that deals with bioethical issues, some background seems appropriate.

An ethical theory is a moral principle or a set of moral principles that can be used to assess what is morally right or morally wrong in a given situation. Over the years, we have called on the theories of philosophers to guide us in our decision-making.

The most widely used theories are presented in Table 9-2. You are encouraged to consider various ethical approaches and discuss with your classmates when each might be used appropriately. For example, an application of **utilitarianism** (or consequentialism) as seen in the health care industry would be the justification of capitation in the managed care organization (MCO). Because the MCO pays a certain amount of money per member per month to a contracted provider, the MCO would argue that it has provided the greatest good for the greatest number of members (Stahl, 1996). An example of **deontology** might be applied to the situation in which all persons involved in a research study have a complete understanding (informed consent) of the study and its purposes. The participant is treated as a moral being with freedom of decision-making and not simply a means to an end. In applying Rawls' (1971) **theory of social justice**, we could not ethically justify using income inequalities or the ability to pay to determine a patient's eligibility for access to health care.

Critical Thinking Activity

Of the ethical theories provided in this chapter, select the one that most appeals to you and describe the aspects of the theory that make it most attractive. Examine factors that bring you to this point of view. What are your biases? What are the consequences of support of this ethical theory on your professional practice?

FACTORS THAT INFLUENCE ETHICAL DECISION-MAKING

Ethical decisions are not made in a vacuum. Many factors influence us as we seek appropriate answers to the dilemmas that we face. As change continues, the realities and new problems confronting us today are challenging the answers that were chosen yesterday.

TABLE 9-2.	MAJOR ETHICAL THEORIES AND THEORISTS	
TITLE OF THEORY (OTHER NAMES)	**THEORIST ASSOCIATED WITH WORK**	**BASIC PRINCIPLES OF THEORY**
Natural Law (Objectivism)	St. Thomas Aquinas (1225–1274)	Actions are morally right when they are in accord with our nature and end and human beings. Good should be promoted, evil avoided, and ethics grounded in our concern for human good.
Deontology (formalistic system, the principal system of ethics, or duty-based ethics)	Immanuel Kant (1724–1804)	Ethical decision-making is based on moral rules and unchanging principles (or motivations that are derived from universal values), considered separately from the consequences. The fundamental principle is called the categorical imperative, unconditional commands that must be applied similarly in all all situations without exception.
Utilitarianism (often referred to as teleology, consequentialism or situation ethics, although there are some differences)	Jeremy Bentham (1748–1832) and John Stuart Mill (1806–1873)	An act is right when it is useful in bringing about a desirable or good end. A second principle allows the end to justify the means. Fits well into Western society's values regarding work ethic and the behavioristic approach to education, philosophy, and life. Applicable to research.
Social Equity and Justice	John Rawls (1921–2002)	Sets forth principles of justice developed in 1971. Allows social and economic positions to be to everyone's advantage and open to all. Introduces a "veil of ignorance" whereby persons making choices would not have any specific information regarding those involved thus choosing the alternative that supported the most disadvantaged person. Supports justice and equal rights for everyone.
Ideal Observer	Raymond W. Firth (1901–2002)	Requires that decisions be made from a dispassionate, disinterested, and consistent viewpoint with full information about the situation and the consequences available.

In determining their own bases for making ethical decisions, some individuals rely on formal philosophic or religious beliefs that define matters in relation to what is believed to be the truth or good or evil. Others make decisions based on personal life experiences or on the experiences of those close to them. Still others rely on professional codes of ethics to give guidance on ethical issues. In reality, ethical decision-making often involves a combination of all of these factors.

In studying ethical issues, it is important for you to understand the many forces that are operating simultaneously in our society. These forces are not independent or mutually exclusive, but act and react with one another in a constantly changing milieu, causing evolutionary changes in all segments of society (Fig. 9-1). The following is a discussion of some of the factors that affect ethical decision-making in the health care environment.

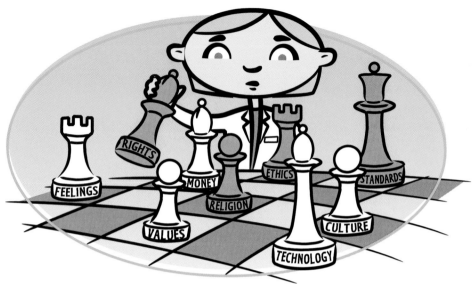

FIGURE 9-1 Decisions made in relation to one aspect of an ethical situation will affect all other aspects of the problem.

Codes for Nurses

Through their professional organizations, nurses have developed some common guidelines to use in making ethical decisions. They are contained in the ANA's Code for Nurses, the International Council of Nurses' Code for Nurses, and the NAPNES Standards of Practice for Licensed Practical/Vocational Nurses. Each attempts to outline the nurse's responsibilities to the patient and to the profession of nursing.

The ANA code is unique among professional codes because it addresses fairly specific issues and does not confine itself to matters of etiquette or broad general statements. Nurses presented tentative codes in the 1920s, the 1930s, and the 1940s. Finally, in 1950, a **code of ethics** was adopted. It has been revised several times since then (Table 9-3). Early versions stated that a nurse had an obligation to carry out a physician's orders; later versions, however, stress the nurse's obligation to the patient. This includes protecting the patient from incompetent, unethical, or illegal practice. The nine primary provisions of the Code for Nurses without explanatory provisions are presented in Display 9-1. You can view the entire Code, including the preface, by accessing it on the ANA Web site, *http://www.nursingworld.org/ethics/chcode.htm* and then clicking on "View the Code Online."

The International Council of Nurses' Code was revised in 1973 and again in 2000. The introductory section of this code addresses the general responsibilities of the nursing profession. Four sections follow, dealing with the more specific concerns of people, practice, the profession, and coworkers. In addition, the International Council of Nurses has written a Pledge for Nurses, which is a statement of affirmation and acceptance of the personal and ethical responsibilities of being a member of the nursing profession. Both of these documents can serve as guidelines for ethical conduct. The International Council of Nurses' Code is presented in Display 9-2.

TABLE 9-3.	CHRONOLOGY OF THE DEVELOPMENT OF CODE FOR NURSES AND DISTINGUISHING CHARACTERISTICS

DATE	CHARACTERISTICS
1896	The Nurses' Association Alumnae of the United States and Canada identify their purposes—the first is to establish and maintain a code of ethics
1921	The National League for Nursing Education appoints an advisory Committee on Ethical Standards. Development of a statement recommended.
1923	Task of developing a Code of Ethics shifted to the American Nurses Association (ANA)
1926	"A Suggested Code" published in August issue of AJN to solicit input. Rhetorical and effusive in style; never formally adopted; discussed moral duties of the nurse and ideal of service.
1940	"A Tentative Code" published, expressing more overt concern for the profession of nursing; input sought from AJN readers.
1950	The Code for Professional Nurses unanimously adopted at ANA House of Delegates. The Code had a preamble and listed 17 provisions; several related to personal ethics of the nurse. Response solicited.
1960	Code revised to reflect social context of increasing assertiveness of nurses and increasing sense of nurses participation in the care of patients (as opposed to subordination).
1968	Code revised. Preamble deleted and provisions reduced to 10. Omits for the first time any reference to the private behavior of the nurse.
1976	Code revised, with greater emphasis on patients participating in their care. Published with Interpretive Statements. Changed the word "patient" to "client."
1985	Code remained basically the same but Interpretive Statements revised to reflect concerns of the day—bioethics, legal language, societal discrimination, effects on the person of technological advances in medicine.
1996	ANA convened a task force to examine the Code. Task force recommended revision of both the Code and the Interpretive Statements.
1998	Revised draft of code presented to the ANA House of Delegates.
2001	Revised code adopted.

Adapted from Fowler, M. (1997).

Since 1941, the National Association for Practical Nurse Education and Service (NAP-NES) has set standards for nursing practice of LP/VNs; they were last revised in 1992. These standards (presented in Display 9-3) also incorporate moral, ethical, and legal components to guide the practice of the practical nurse.

The Patient's Rights

The patient's rights are another consideration in decision-making. Ideally, we have always recognized them in some way. As early as 1959, the National League for Nursing formulated a statement regarding patient's rights. For many years, however, health care professionals assumed that they knew what was best for patients and made many decisions without consulting or considering the rights of the patient. For example, a patient with a specific disease was not offered information about possible treatment alternatives, even when valid alternatives did exist. The patient's physician decided which treatment method was preferable, and that was the only one presented to the patient. This is another example of paternalism, discussed earlier in this chapter.

As the health consumer movement became more active, greater attention was paid to the rights of the patient (see earlier discussion of rights). Today patients may expect to be informed

Display 9-1 PRIMARY PROVISIONS OF THE ANA CODE FOR NURSES

1. The nurse, in all professional relationships, practices with compassion and respect for the inherent dignity, worth, and uniqueness of every individual, unrestricted by considerations of social or economic status, personal attributes, or the nature of health problems.
2. The nurse's primary commitment is to the patient, whether an individual, family, group, or community.
3. The nurse promotes, advocates for, and strives to protect the health, safety, and rights of the patient.
4. The nurse is responsible and accountable for individual nursing practice and determines the appropriate delegation of tasks consistent with the nurse's obligation to provide optimum patient care.
5. The nurse owes the same duties to self as to others, including the responsibility to preserve integrity and safety, to maintain competence, and to continue personal and professional growth.
6. The nurse participates in establishing, maintaining, and improving health care environments, and conditions of employment conducive to the provision of quality health care and consistent with the values of the profession, through individual and collective action.
7. The nurse participates in the advancement of the profession through contributions to practice, education, administration, and knowledge development.
8. The nurse collaborates with other health professionals and the public in promoting community, national, and international efforts to meet health needs.
9. The profession of nursing, as represented by associations and their members, is responsible for articulating nursing values, for maintaining the integrity of the profession and its practice, and for shaping social policy.

Source: Reprinted with permission from American Nurses Association. (2001). *Code of Ethics for Nurses with Interpretive Statements.* American Nurses Publishing, American Nurses Association, Washington, DC.

of all alternatives for treatment and often want to participate in choosing a type of treatment, weighing the possible benefits and risks of the treatment methods presented. The law also has supported the right to informed decision-making. Despite these efforts, a recent study of 1057 audiotaped encounters during routine office visits involving 59 primary care physicians and 65 general and orthopedic surgeons found that informed decision-making was often incomplete (Braddock et al, 1999).

In 1973, the American Hospital Association (AHA) published A Patient's Bill of Rights (AHA, 1992), which outlined the rights of the hospital patient and served as a basis for making decisions about hospitalized patients. Some criticized this document, saying that it is rather innocuous because it simply reminded patients of their rights (such as privacy, confidentiality, and informed consent) but said nothing of hospitals that fail to act in accordance with these rights. The AHA revised this document in 1992 to speak more forcefully to the hospital's responsibility for providing medically indicated care and services and to emphasize the collaborative nature of health maintenance. In April, 2003, the Patient's Bill of Rights was updated with a version titled, "The Patient Care Partnership." This document outlines what patients may expect during a hospital stay and encourages patients to ask questions if they have concerns. The Patient Care Partnership is presented in Display 9-4.

Some groups, nurses' associations among them, also have formulated statements regarding the rights of the health care consumer. In some states, the rights of the health care consumer are being formalized into legal statements.

Display 9-2   **INTERNATIONAL COUNCIL OF NURSES CODE FOR NURSES ETHICAL CONCEPTS APPLIED TO NURSING (2000)**

Nurses have four fundamental responsibilities: to promote health, to prevent illness, to restore health, and alleviate suffering. The need for nursing is universal.

Inherent in nursing is respect for human rights, including the right to life, to dignity and to be treated with respect. Nursing care is unrestricted by considerations of age, colour, creed, culture, disability or illness, gender, nationality, politics, race or social status.

Nurses render health services to the individual, the family and the community and coordinate their services with those of related groups.

Nurses and People

The nurse's primary responsibility is to people requiring nursing care.

In providing care, the nurse promotes an environment in which the human rights, values, customs and spiritual beliefs of the individual, family and community are respected.

The nurse ensures that the individual receives sufficient information on which to base consent for care and related treatment.

The nurse holds in confidence personal information and uses judgment in sharing this information.

The nurse shares with society the responsibility for initiating and supporting action to meet the health and social needs of the public, in particular those of vulnerable populations.

The nurse also shares responsibility to sustain and protect the natural environment from depletion, pollution, degradation and destruction.

Nurses and Practice

The nurse carries personal responsibility and accountability for nursing practice and for maintaining competence by continual learning.

The nurse maintains a standard of personal health such that the ability to provide care is not compromised.

The nurse uses judgment regarding individual competence when accepting and delegating responsibilities.

The nurse at all times maintains standards of personal conduct that reflect well on the profession and enhance public confidence.

The nurse, in providing care, ensures that use of technology and scientific advances are compatible with the safety, dignity and rights of people.

Nurses and the Profession

The nurse assumes the major role in determining and implementing acceptable standards of clinical nursing practice, management, research and education.

The nurse is active in developing a core of research-based professional knowledge.

The nurse, acting through the professional organization, participates in creating and maintaining equitable social and economic working conditions in nursing.

Nurses and Co-workers

The nurse sustains a cooperative relationship with co-workers in nursing and other fields.

The nurse takes appropriate action to safeguard individuals when their care is endangered by a co-worker or any other person.

Display 9-3 **NAPNES STANDARDS OF PRACTICE FOR LICENSED PRACTICAL/ VOCATIONAL NURSES**

The LP/VN Provides Individual and Family-Centered Nursing Care. The LP/VN Shall:

A. Utilize principles of nursing process in meeting specific patient needs of patients of all ages in the areas of:

1. Safety
2. Hygiene
3. Nutrition
4. Medication
5. Elimination
6. Psychosocial and cultural
7. Respiratory needs

B. Utilize appropriate knowledge, skills and abilities in providing safe, competent care.

C. Utilize principles of crisis intervention in maintaining safety and making appropriate referrals when necessary.

D. Utilize effective communication skills.

1. Communicate effectively with patients, family members of the health team, and significant others.
2. Maintain appropriate written documentation.

E. Provide appropriate health teaching to patients and significant others in the areas of:

1. Maintenance of wellness
2. Rehabilitation
3. Utilization of community resources

F. Serve as a patient advocate:

1. Protect patient rights
2. Consult with appropriate others when necessary

The LP/VN Fulfills the Professional Responsibilities of the Practical/Vocational Nurse. The LP/VN Shall:

A. Know and apply the ethical principles underlying the profession.

B. Know and follow the appropriate professional and legal requirements.

C. Follow the policies and procedures of the employing institution.

D. Cooperate and collaborate with all members of the healthcare team to meet the needs of family-centered nursing care.

E. Demonstrate accountability for his/her nursing actions.

F. Maintain currency in terms of knowledge and skills in the area of employment.

The LP/VN Follows the NAPNES Code of Ethics. The LP/VN Shall:

1. Consider as a basic obligation the conservation of life and the prevention of disease.
2. Promote and protect the physical, mental, emotional, and spiritual health of the patient and his family.
3. Fulfill all duties faithfully and efficiently.
4. Function within established legal guidelines.
5. Accept personal responsibility (for his/her acts) and seek to merit the respect and confidence of all members of the health team.
6. Hold in confidence all matters coming to his/her knowledge, in the practice of his profession, and in no way at no time violate this confidence.
7. Give conscientious service and charge just remuneration.
8. Learn and respect the religious and cultural beliefs of his/her patient and of all people.
9. Meet his/her obligation to the patient by keeping abreast of current trends in health care through reading and continuing education.
10. As a citizen of the United States of America, uphold the laws of the land and seek to promote legislation that shall meet the health needs of its people.

Display 9-4 | **THE PATIENT CARE PARTNERSHIP: UNDERSTANDING EXPECTATIONS, RIGHTS, AND RESPONSIBILITIES**

When you need hospital care, your doctor and the nurses and other professionals at our hospital are committed to working with you and your family to meet your health care needs. Our dedicated doctors and staff serve the community in all its ethnic, religious, and economic diversity. Our goal is for you and your family to have the same care and attention we would want for our families and ourselves.

The sections below explain some of the basics about how you can expect to be treated during your hospital stay. They also cover what we will need from you to care for you better. If you have questions at any time, please ask them. Unasked or unanswered questions can add to the stress of being in the hospital. Your comfort and confidence in your care are very important to us.

What to Expect During Your Hospital Stay

- **High quality hospital care.** Our first priority is to provide you the care you need, when you need it, with skill, compassion, and respect. Tell your caregivers if you have concerns about your care or if you have pain. You have the right to know the identity of doctors, nurses, and others involved in your care, as well as when they are students, residents, or other trainees.

- **A clean and safe environment.** Our hospital works hard to keep you safe. We use special policies and procedures to avoid mistakes in your care and keep you free from abuse or neglect. If anything unexpected and significant happens during your hospital stay, you will be told what happened, and any resulting changes in your care will be discussed with you.

- **Involvement in your care.** You and your doctor often make decisions about your care before you go to the hospital. Other times, especially in emergencies, those decisions are made during your hospital stay. When they take place, making decisions should include:

  ➤ *Discussing your medical condition and information about medically appropriate treatment choices.* To make informed decisions with your doctor, you need to understand several things:
  - The benefits and risks of each treatment.
  - Whether it is experimental or part of a research study.
  - What you can reasonably expect from your treatment and any long-term effects it might have on your quality of life.
  - What you and your family will need to do after you leave the hospital.
  - The financial consequences of using uncovered services or out-of-network providers.

  Please tell your caregivers if you need more information about treatment choices.

  ➤ *Discussing your treatment plan.* When you enter the hospital, you sign a general consent to treatment. In some cases, such as surgery or experimental treatment, you may be asked to confirm in writing that you understand what is planned and agree to it. This process protects

(continued)

Display 9-4   **THE PATIENT CARE PARTNERSHIP: UNDERSTANDING EXPECTATIONS, RIGHTS, AND RESPONSIBILITIES (*continued*)**

your right to consent to or refuse a treatment. Your doctor will explain the medical consequences of refusing recommended treatment. It also protects your right to decide if you want to participate in a research study.

➤ *Getting information from you.* Your caregivers need complete and correct information about your health and coverage so that they can make good decisions about your care. That includes:
  – Past illnesses, surgeries, or hospital stays.
  – Past allergic reactions.
  – Any medicines or diet supplements (such as vitamins and herbs) that you are taking.
  – Any network or admission requirements under your health plan.

➤ *Understanding your health care goals and values.* You may have health care goals and values or spiritual beliefs that are important to your well-being. They will be taken into account as much as possible throughout your hospital stay. Make sure your doctor, your family, and your care team know your wishes.

➤ *Understanding who should make decisions when you cannot.* If you have signed a health care power of attorney stating who should speak for you if you become unable to make health care decisions for yourself, or a "living will" or "advance directive" that states your wishes about end-of-life care, give copies to your doctor, your family, and your care team. If you or your family need help making difficult decisions, counselors, chaplains, and others are available to help.

• **Protection of your privacy.** We respect the confidentiality of your relationship with your doctor and other caregivers, and the sensitive information about your health and health care that are part of that relationship. State and federal laws and hospital operating policies protect the privacy of your medical information. You will receive a Notice of Privacy Practices that describes the ways that we use, disclose, and safeguard patient information and that explains how you can obtain a copy of information from our records about your care.

• **Help preparing you and your family for when you leave the hospital.** Your doctor works with hospital staff and professionals in your community. You and your family also play an important role. The success of your treatment often depends on your efforts to follow medication, diet, and therapy plans. Your family may need to help care for you at home.

  You can expect us to help you identify sources of follow-up care and to let you know if our hospital has a financial interest in any referrals. As long as you agree we can share information about your care with them, we will coordinate our activities with your caregivers outside the hospital. You can also expect to receive information and, where possible, training about the self-care you will need when you go home.

Display 9-4   THE PATIENT CARE PARTNERSHIP: UNDERSTANDING EXPECTATIONS, RIGHTS, AND RESPONSIBILITIES (*continued*)

- **Help with your bill and filing insurance claims.** Our staff will file claims for you with health care insurers or other programs such as Medicare and Medicaid. They will also help your doctor with needed documentation. Hospital bills and insurance coverage are often confusing. If you have questions about your bill, contact our business office. If you need help understanding your insurance coverage or health plan, start with your insurance company or health benefits manager. If you do not have health coverage, we will try to help you and your family find financial help or make other arrangements. We need your help with collecting needed information and other requirements to obtain coverage or assistance.

While you are here, you will receive more detailed notices about some of the rights you have as a hospital patient and how to exercise them. We are always interested in improving. If you have questions, comments, or concerns, please contact _____.

Reprinted with permission of the American Hospital Association. Copyright © 2003.

Social and Cultural Attitudes

Changes in the attitudes of society as a whole profoundly influence each of its segments. For example, the changing roles of women, the shifting attitudes toward marriage and the family, and the increasing emphasis on culturally competent care have all required nurses to reexamine their personal feelings and alter their approach to providing nursing care.

Ethical concerns are the by-products of many factors at work in our society today, including the role of the individual and the family. In the health care field, this is most pointedly illustrated by the use of the terminology "health care" as opposed to "medical care." Health care suggests much greater involvement of others and places the patient in the center of the activity, whereas medical care places the physician in the key role. We see similar language being applied to "telehealth" as opposed to "telemedicine." The meaning of "consumer unit" is shifting from an individual to a whole family or even a whole community. The focus of care also has changed from one that was primarily disease oriented to one that focuses on prevention and wellness.

The size of the group being affected by ethical decisions has a bearing on the decision-making process. The smaller the group, organization, or society involved in or affected by the decision-making, the easier the process of arriving at an acceptable alternative. For example, the Oregon Medicaid system limits care for HIV-infected people based on the reasoning that their average life expectancy is short (Hall, 1996). It is unlikely that this decision could have been made if the state had a large population of people who were HIV-infected. The larger the group affected by a decision, the more complex it becomes. Many of our ethical considerations now involve our society as a whole or, in some cases, the world; therefore, solutions are difficult.

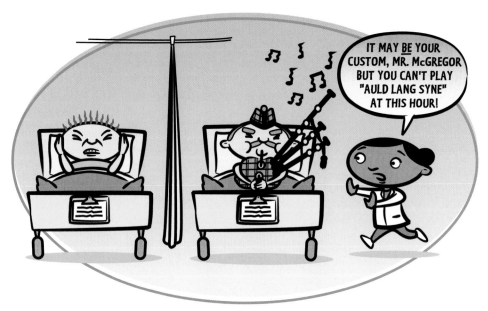

FIGURE 9-2   In providing care, the nurse respects the beliefs, values, and customs of the individual.

The value a society places on the individual or the family directly influences the standard of care (Fig. 9-2). In Western society, we believe in each person's right to exercise choice based on individual beliefs and conscience. We also place high value on preserving individual life; therefore, we often use tremendous resources to try to achieve additional years, months, or even days of life. A society that placed greater emphasis on the community good than on the individual might not choose to use resources in that way. The standard of care might aim for comfort without the use of expensive treatment modalities.

A culture's religious values and belief in an afterlife directly affect ethical issues. The Hindu belief in rebirth after death and the immutability of fate affects decisions about using health care resources. Those who believe that an outcome is predetermined by fate will not choose to commit major resources and efforts toward altering that outcome.

The population, or, more accurately, the overpopulation of a country relative to its resources also may have a direct bearing on the value placed on life. The material resources to provide many health services may not be available. Decisions may be made to eliminate certain costly health care procedures even though they are known to be effective and desired by individuals.

Critical Thinking Activity

Identify two sociocultural factors with which you have had personal experience that could impact ethical decision-making. How is your view of this different than it might have been 5 years ago? In what ways have your views remained the same? Why do you think your views have changed or remained the same? What implications does this have for the way you will view things in the future?

Science and Technology

Scientific advancement and technology have left us wrestling with concerns that would have been considered science fiction 50 years ago. Before the development of kidney dialysis, we accepted the fact that people with nonfunctioning kidneys would soon die. After machines that could filter body wastes became available, a genuine dilemma arose over who would have dialysis and who would not; the number of people needing treatment far exceeded the personnel, time, and equipment available to treat them. As the technology became available, the ethical questions refocused on decisions to end treatment rather than on issues related to initiating treatment.

Other technology has had similar effects. The advent of machines that could artificially breathe for someone challenged the medical and legal professions to examine their definitions of life, and brought into focus problems of whether and when to turn off a ventilator. Heart and lung machines that could adequately perfuse the body while the heart was stopped for surgical procedures enabled operations to be performed that were unheard of 50 years ago. Fetal monitors, which can be attached to women in labor, provide a continuous readout of the status of the fetus. Such monitoring has resulted in a greater number of infants delivered by cesarean section. The transplantation of organs from one individual to another has created untold ethical dilemmas. Stem cell research using embryos challenges us at a national level. Individuals with AIDS have a limited life expectancy even with the best of health care. Should they be encouraged to participate in research that is sometimes risky to advance scientific knowledge and the possibility of future benefit to others? How far should experimentation go? Should it include the transfusion of bone marrow from a baboon? Advances in science and technology continue to offer us some of the greatest challenges.

Legislation

Social change and legislation are constantly interacting. Legislation may follow changes in society's attitudes, converting new ideas into law. For example, a greater acceptance of infants born to single mothers has resulted in legislation that changed the wording of birth certificates and dropped the word "illegitimate." Similarly, attitudes are being challenged regarding parenting by lesbian and gay couples, either through artificial insemination or adoption.

When social change is desired, legislation may be actively sought to require people to behave in new ways. This was true for civil rights legislation. A change in society was desired, and supporters of civil rights sought legislation as one step toward change. Recent legislative action that addresses the needs and opportunities available to the disabled has brought about changes in public policies, procedures, and even architecture.

Judicial Decisions

The judicial system provides a major avenue for debating and trying to solve ethical problems. More issues are being taken to court, and judicial decisions are used more often as the basis for determining appropriate action. As you continue to study this topic, note that we have often cited a landmark decision regarding an ethical issue. The process does not stop there, however. Some people may disagree with a judicial decision and continue to oppose it.

Higher courts may overturn judicial decisions. Meanwhile, the questions regarding the individual's role in carrying out a judicial decision remain. For example, although the law in the past forbade abortions, some physicians believed strongly in the right of the individual to have the procedure done. These physicians were upset by the results of abortions performed by individuals who lacked the necessary education and skill to do it safely, and therefore were willing to perform abortions despite the law prohibiting the procedure. These physicians were, of course, liable to prosecution if it were discovered they were performing illegal abortions, and some were prosecuted. The issues of abortion and government funding of the procedure are still controversial. It is not likely that these issues will be resolved in a way that is satisfactory to everyone.

Funding

The financing of health care represents a major area of conflict that has ethical dimensions. The government has become more involved in providing funds for health care. Some people are asking how much time, money, and energy we should allocate to health care, and how those resources should be divided. How obligated are we as a society to make some form of health care available to all? What is it that health care can and cannot provide? Which is more important, prevention or cure? Health care includes controversial procedures, such as abortion, sterilization, and transplantation. This challenges the basic values of some taxpayers who do not ethically sanction these procedures and do not want their tax dollars used to fund them.

Personal Religious and Philosophic Viewpoints

Your personal viewpoint certainly will be a major factor influencing your ethical decision-making. Achieving self-understanding in values is a lifelong learning task, and undoubtedly your position on various issues will change as you move through life. Values are the product of our life experiences and are influenced by family, friends, religion, culture, environment, education, and many other factors.

RELIGIOUS BELIEFS AND ETHICAL DECISION-MAKING

Religious beliefs form the basis for ethical decision-making for some people; however, a person who is a member of a particular religious group may not ascribe to all of the beliefs of that group. Some individuals make their own decisions regarding each situation, which in some cases may not parallel the doctrines of their religious group. For example, some Muslims maintain that women should be completely separated from men and wear veils when in the presence of men. They would find any health care setting that did not respect this belief to be in conflict with their basic values. Other Muslims do not adhere to this strict interpretation of Islamic law, and women wear modest clothing but need not wear veils. They would be more comfortable in most Western health care settings because they would not feel a conflict with their personal values.

RECOGNIZING THE IMPACT OF PERSONAL VALUES

Nursing offers a variety of job opportunities to the new graduate and you will want to consider your personal values when choosing a position after graduation. You certainly cannot expect to avoid all conflict or problem situations, but you will want to avoid working in an area in which conflict is constant. Before you accept a position, you may want to consider whether it has the potential to conflict with your basic beliefs. For example, if you believe that no individual should be denied life-saving techniques, you might be unhappy working in a research institution where the effects of treatment or no treatment were being studied. In this situation, making your views known and refusing certain assignments after you begin employment might result in termination because the employer may justifiably assert that you agreed to fulfill all the responsibilities of the position when you accepted employment.

Similarly, you might choose to work in an area that supports your personal value system or strong ethical commitment. For example, religious groups who saw value in the life of the dying person began the hospices for the dying in England. Their religious beliefs were and have continued to be part of their approach to care. If you strongly value your own ethnic or cultural approach to health care, you might choose to work in a health care setting where that approach is part of the philosophy.

FACTORS IN THE WORK ENVIRONMENT THAT AFFECT ETHICAL DECISION-MAKING

By virtue of the positions they hold in the health care system, nurses experience special pressures as they try to make decisions. An awareness of these factors may help you as you grapple with personal problems in decision-making.

Status as an Employee

Most nurses are not in independent practice, but are employed by hospitals, nursing homes, community agencies, or outpatient facilities. Pressures divide the nurse's loyalty among patient, employer, and self. You will notice that codes do not speak of responsibilities to the employer, yet, from an ethical standpoint, you have certain loyalties and obligations to the employer who pays your salary and makes decisions regarding your work. It is not unusual for an ethical decision to involve conflict between the best interests of the employer and the patient.

When discussing ethical decisions in the abstract, most people say that, of course, the patient's best interest should be the only priority. In real situations, however, the issues often are not so clearly defined. If a nurse's decision affects the employer adversely, the result may be job loss, poor references, and a severely curtailed economic and career future. For example, one physician was known to routinely require his patients to sign blank surgical permits on admission to the hospital; a staff nurse became upset with this procedure after learning that the patients often did not understand what was being planned. Eventually, she discussed the matter with the physician, pointing out that she did not believe it was ethical to require the patients to sign the blank documents, especially because they were not informed of alternative methods of treatment. The physician became angry and complained to the hospital administration, threatening to take his surgeries elsewhere. This might have created a considerable economic loss for the hospital and, depending on the action of the administrator, the nurse might have been labeled a troublemaker, and even discharged to placate the physician.

Collective Bargaining Contracts

Collective bargaining contracts can protect nurses in making ethical decisions. By formalizing reasons and procedures for termination of employment, and outlining grievance measures to provide a mechanism by which the individual nurse can be protected, a contract may provide greater freedom. Others believe that contracts hamper individual freedom because of the lengthy processes that are required. (See Chapter 12 for more discussion of collective bargaining and grievance measures.)

Collegial Relationships

An excellent climate for ethical decision-making can be provided when nurses who work together support one another, share in decision-making, and present a unified approach to others. All too often such relationships are lacking in health care institutions. Nurses feel alone and are not experienced in seeking and providing support to one another. Greater effort on the part of all nurses in this area might be rewarding and is certainly long overdue.

Authoritarian and Paternalistic Backgrounds

The historically authoritarian and paternalistic attitudes of physicians and hospitals often have relegated nurses, most of whom are women, to dependent and subservient roles. These role differentiations have discouraged nurses from taking independent stands on issues, and they continue to affect relationships in the health care field. In some settings, ethical decisions are made without the participation of nurses, yet nurses are expected to implement the decisions.

More nurses are speaking out against an approach that leaves them out of the decision-making process. Nurses today might expect a physician to discuss the possibly futile treatment of a critically ill patient with the patient, with the family, and with the nursing staff. The patient would be encouraged to express personal needs, the family's views would be included, and the nurses' input would be part of the decision-making process regarding the medical plan of care. The advent of ethics committees, in which nurses have a voice, has created a positive environment for discussions in many institutions.

Ethics Committees in Health Care

Many hospitals for years have traditionally had ethics committees composed of physicians. With a major goal of monitoring physician behavior, they acted when a physician's inappropriate behavior, such as arriving at the hospital intoxicated, was reported to them. Today the scope of ethics committees has enlarged considerably. Membership has grown, and representatives of the hospital administration, the community, and a variety of health care disciplines are being included. An ethicist may serve as a consultant or as a member of the committee. If nurses participate, their membership and attendance allow them to share in decision-making.

With their expertise and experience, the members of ethics committees help individuals who must make ethical decisions to identify whether they have all the relevant information, to determine other options they have not considered, and to compare the situation with basic ethical principles and theories. Often the committee acts in an advisory capacity to medical staff members and families struggling with difficult decisions. Ethics committees also may help institutions establish policies regarding ethical concerns that tend to recur in that setting.

Consumer Involvement in Health Care

With consumer involvement in health care, nurses again may face situations in which they are expected to take action based on the conclusions of others. Many nurses may find this problematic. For example, an elderly diabetic who has gangrene of the foot may refuse amputation, saying, "If I'm going to die, I'm going to die whole." The nurse, recognizing the life-saving benefit of the amputation, may have difficulty maintaining effective communication and rapport with the patient and family, because of his or her own conviction that an amputation is the best treatment. Mental health is another area in health care in which nurses may struggle. Patients may refuse to comply with the recommended treatment and as a result live in a homeless, psychiatrically unhealthy situation. This also is very difficult for family members.

A FRAMEWORK FOR ETHICAL DECISION-MAKING

When faced with ethical decisions, most of us hope to find the "right" answers. Unfortunately, a right answer may not exist for everyone or every situation; such is the nature of dilemmas. However, you can proceed from a basic framework that encourages you to look beyond your first thoughts or feelings to basic issues. A great deal has been written about the decision-making process in the last 2 decades—more in recent years than before. Along with this, several models have been developed to assist us when ethics are involved (Curtin, 1978; Jameton, 1984; Milner, 1993; Thompson & Thompson, 1981). The steps identified below, gleaned from various approaches, offer a process you can use as a guide. In studying it, you will recognize a similarity to the steps of the nursing process with which you are already familiar. When patients and families must make ethical decisions, you may assist them in working through this process within the framework of their own values.

Identify and Clarify the Ethical Problem

To define the ethical concern, you need to review the situation and gain as clear a perception of the problem as possible. Is there something wrong? How deep does the issue go? Are there legal or institutional concerns? What is the decision to be made? You need to clarify information about which you are not certain. Consider what ethical principles might be involved. Are those principles in conflict? Who are the relevant parties to this decision? What are their values? What is your role and relationship to the problem? Is this really someone else's decision, which you should not assume, or is it one in which a collaborative decision must be made? Are there time constraints on making this decision? What other factors influence the decision?

Gather Data

It is important to have as much information about the unique situation as possible. The facts of the situation make a difference in what options are possible. Remember that there is no magic pattern or formula to facts in most situations; they are screened through each person's background and experience. What clearly appears to be a "true fact" to one person may seem to be "opinion" to another. Therefore, seeking other viewpoints may help everyone involved to see the situation more clearly. You need to identify the relevant people in the situation and understand their concerns and perspectives as much as possible. Consider whether legal cases might affect decision-making in this case.

Identify Options

Most ethical problems have more than one possible solution. If only one solution existed, there would be no ethical dilemma, because there would be no choice. In some cases, more than one solution may be satisfactory; in others, none of the options will seem satisfactory. The more options identified, the more likely those involved will find one they can support. What is the range of actions that could be taken? What would be the anticipated outcome of those actions? For each option, consider its impact on each person involved. Also think about the impact on society as a whole if this option were chosen. Consider the ethical theories presented and explore how each option compares with the basic principles of each theory. In this way, you might determine that one option is basically a utilitarian approach (seeking the greatest good for the greatest number), whereas another is clearly supporting a deontologic position of doing one's duty. Which option does the greatest good while at the same time doing the least harm? Which option respects the rights and dignity of all persons involved? Is one approach more appropriate than another in this situation? Is this approach in keeping with your own moral and ethical position? Helping others to explore these questions (without necessarily using the terminology of formal ethical theories) requires personal involvement and interpersonal skill.

Make a Decision

At some point, you have to make a decision. Patients and families, as well as care providers, may find this difficult and, in some instances, painful. However, to not make a decision is, in fact, making a decision. There will never be enough time, enough data, or enough alternatives in some situations. No matter how thorough the analysis or how carefully people weigh all competing claims, there may still be uncomfortable feelings. When dealing with these feelings, you might think ahead to the action you plan to take. If you explained to someone you respect and admire why you chose this option, what would that individual say? This strategy may help patients and families as well.

Act and Assess

Once you have chosen a course of action, you must carry out your decision. This may involve working with others or personally carrying out plans. Patients and families need ongoing support as they carry out their decisions. Assess the outcomes as the processes go forward.

Unforeseen outcomes are common in ethical situations. Share your thoughts and concerns with others as you proceed, and continue to seek new insights into the situation.

As you assess the outcome in any particular situation, consider its relevance for a wider range of situations and concerns. Use this situation as a foundation from which to grow and develop. Ask yourself, "What have I learned from this experience that will be useful in the future?" "What would I do in another situation?" "What would I change?"

SPECIFIC ETHICAL ISSUES RELATED TO THE PROFESSION OF NURSING

Some ethical issues of concern to nurses relate specifically to the nursing profession; others relate to bioethical issues confronting all of society. In this section, we discuss the issues facing nurses through commitment to the patient, commitment to personal excellence, and commitment to the nursing profession as a whole. Bioethical issues that relate to the whole society are discussed in Chapter 10. We present a definite viewpoint regarding ethics in the nursing profession. We feel strongly about the individual nurse's responsibility for nursing practice and place high value on personal integrity in professional relationships.

Commitment to the Patient

Nursing has a strong history of being committed to the well-being of patients who need care. Both the ANA Code for Nurses and the International Code for Nurses, presented earlier in this chapter, clearly point out the nurse's obligation to fulfill this commitment. In the past, this obligation has been used to try to persuade nurses that they must not be concerned for themselves, their working conditions, their salaries, or other aspects of their employment. However, rejection of the handmaiden philosophy and the adoption of more nurse autonomy does not require rejection of a basic philosophy that nursing is focused on providing patients and their families with support for growth toward maximum health and well-being. Patients can never become the objects of nursing care, but must be approached as unique individuals who deserve concern, respect, and culturally competent care.

Commitment to Your Employer

Once you have accepted a position in a health care organization, you have also accepted the responsibilities that the position encompasses. Some of these responsibilities are spelled out in the contract if a formal contract exists between the employer and the employee. Others are more or less taken for granted. It is these latter responsibilities than can present problems.

RESPONSIBLE WORK ETHIC

First of all, it is understood that you will arrive at work on time. When you arrive late you obligate others to remain overtime to assure continuous patient care. If you find yourself in an emergency situation that is going to cause you to be delayed, it is important that you notify your supervisor that you are going to be delayed.

It is also expected that you will not abuse breaks or sick leave. When one extends a break beyond the usual time allowed, it jeopardizes the opportunity for others to have a full break. Likewise, the fact that you have a given number of paid sick days each year does not mean that you are entitled to that many more days off. They are intended for use if you are ill. Often, it is difficult to find replacements when staff members do not report for work. This means that others must pick up additional work assignments and/or that the quality of care provided that day is less than desired.

Many health care facilities operate 24 hours a day, 7 days a week. This means that there are at least two or three different shifts to be covered, as well as weekends and holidays. Be prepared to take your share of weekend and holiday shifts as well as evening and night rotations without grumbling if this is part of the staffing pattern. Most employers have developed some system of rotation, with employees able to make requests for the time that works best for them. Some employees for whom the holiday carries less significance may prefer to work, especially if there is additional pay for those days.

If you are working in an area where you have a fair amount of privacy, it is important to remember that you should not conduct personal business during your work shift. Scheduling appointments, telephoning friends or business associates, writing notes, and similar activities should occur during your break or after you have finished your shift.

When you decide to terminate your employment, it is expected that you will give appropriate notice. Please refer to Chapter 11 for further discussion regarding resignation.

RESPONSIBLE USE OF SUPPLIES

Pilfering includes stealing in small amounts or stealing objects of little value. Many people who are scrupulously honest in other aspects of their lives do not recognize that taking small items from a place of employment is indeed theft. Employees often take home adhesive bandage strips, pens, and other such objects so routinely that they do not even consider whether this is right or wrong. This constant petty theft may total thousands of dollars, the cost of which must be passed on to those who pay the bills—the patients. As a leader in the care setting, the registered nurse (RN) is often in a position to communicate clearly to all employees that pilfering is unacceptable. The nurse can set an example of careful stewardship of the hospital supplies.

Sometimes removing supplies is an oversight rather than a planned action (Fig. 9-3). To make efficient use of time, nurses commonly place many small items such as alcohol wipes, extra needles, and pens in their pockets. One hospital unit found that their yearly supply budget for black pens was almost exhausted in the first 6 months of the year. The simple action of placing a basket in the lounge into which nurses dropped everything from their pockets before leaving cut the pen costs dramatically. Perhaps you can be equally creative in helping to solve such problems in your work setting.

As the costs of health care soar, it is important that everyone associated with health care be mindful of the use of resources. You can help reduce costs by being judicious in your use of resources. For example, supplies that will not be used should not be taken into patient's rooms, only to be discarded later. Using extra linens such as bath towels to clean up spills adds to costs. Determining that a clean glove is acceptable rather than reaching for sterile gloves reduces costs. Assuring that all charges are processed for supplies that are used is also important. Operating equipment in a knowledgeable manner to reduce breakage or repairs is the responsibility of all workers. When all persons do their part, the cumulative effect can be significant.

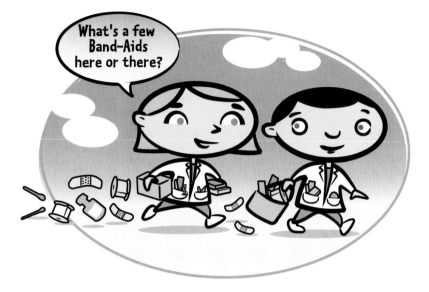

FIGURE 9-3   Many people who are otherwise scrupulously honest do not recognize that taking small items from a place of employment is theft.

Commitment to Your Colleagues

It has been suggested that a strategy to improve the nurse shortage is to improve the quality of the work environment (Bates, 2002). Many factors influence the climate of the work environment. One of the most noteworthy is our relationship with colleagues. As a new graduate, how do you impact this area?

One approach is to model those behaviors that you wish to see in others. Develop a collaborative approach. Maintain a positive attitude, respond to others in a pleasant, courteous manner, be sensitive to others, be a positive ambassador for nursing. Be supportive of others and avoid opportunities to gossip about your colleagues and their activities. Compliment others on things they do well, provide assistance with things they are still learning. This is especially important as you become a more seasoned employee and have responsibility for helping to orient others. Give new employees time to learn skills that are new to them and to become efficient in their execution. Show care and compassion to fellow workers as well as to your clients.

Commitment to Personal Excellence

Each individual nurse must be committed to personal excellence and assume responsibility for maintaining competence. This means that you are willing to engage in genuine self-evaluation in the work setting. You are the one who is best able to identify your weaknesses and practice deficits as well as your strengths. Your careful self-evaluation is the patient's best protection against poor or inadequate care.

When we are truly honest with ourselves in the self-evaluation process, we often uncover areas we wish were not there. These weaknesses, once identified, provide the greatest opportunity for growth and improvement. It is helpful to remember one of the beauties of self-evaluation.

When it is done informally, these weaknesses do not have to be shared with anyone. On the other hand, you should not hesitate to ask for assistance if you think you need it.

Many institutions are now including self-evaluation and the establishment of personal goals in the formal evaluation of employees. In this process, you might be asked to prepare a written self-evaluation that will be shared with your immediate supervisor and may be incorporated into your records.

So how do you proceed? One approach to self-evaluation is the use of the nursing process format. Begin with a thorough personal assessment, objectively gathering data about your own performance. After outlining areas in which you want to gather data, actually keep notes on yourself. For example, if you want to increase your efficiency in carrying out treatments, you may want to time yourself on several occasions to determine how long you are taking and whether you improved with performance.

After data have been collected, you need to give yourself time to analyze it thoroughly. The self-assessment outline includes questions you should ask yourself (Display 9-5); however, the criteria that you use to determine whether your answers reflect the quality of performance you want to attain are not included. Those specific criteria must be individualized to the setting in which you work and the nature of your role in that setting. The breadth of data that represent excellent practice for the nurse in the emergency department differs from what would represent excellence for the nurse working in a rehabilitation setting. The degree to which a patient participates in decisions regarding care differs between the post-anesthesia recovery room and the outpatient clinic. Thus, criteria specific to your work situation are needed.

Your analysis can reveal strengths, weaknesses, and areas for growth or improvement. Congratulate yourself on the strengths identified and then clearly delineate those areas in which you want to change or to improve. As in nursing care planning, clearly identifying and stating the problems or growth needed helps you to plan more effectively.

It is appropriate to establish a plan of action next. The plan is more helpful to you if it contains clearly defined goals. What is a realistic expectation? How long should it take to reach that expectation? Once the goals are set, you are better able to plan appropriate action to meet them. You might consider such things as requesting in-service education, taking continuing education courses, consulting with colleagues, and doing independent reading and study. Some plans need to include specific things related to your daily nursing care. To do this, you may want to request assignments that provide opportunities for practice of the desired skills. Perhaps you are interested in transferring to a specialty area of care. This will involve communication with your immediate supervisor and may involve enrolling in some special classes.

Implementing this plan will require you to remain focused on what you are trying to accomplish. Keeping records on your progress is often helpful. It also provides positive reinforcement when you realize that some of your goals have been met.

Periodic evaluation of your progress is necessary so that you do not become discouraged. Sometimes it is hard to identify gradual change. Any records you have kept are valuable for this purpose. You might even plan rewards for yourself for improvement that occurs. Try not to become discouraged if you do not see the improvement you desire. Remember that just as a reassessment and a new plan are often necessary in patient care planning, a revised plan may be needed in the self-evaluation process. Keep in mind that your overall goal is personal excellence in nursing practice.

Display 9-5   **SELF-EVALUATION PLAN**

Assessment of Patients
- Do I gather enough data about patients and families, including both strengths and deficits?
- Is there sufficient depth and breadth in the data I gather?
- Do I listen closely to the patient and attend to what is being said?
- Do I regularly use all available sources for information about my patients (eg, patient, family, other staff, chart, Kardex)?
- Have I recognized problems quickly so that they did not become worse through inattention?
- Do I recognize physiologic, social, and psychological problems?
- Is my assessment free of personal biases and viewpoints?
- Do I separate relevant from irrelevant data?

Planning for Patient Care
- Do I routinely seek more information on which to base decisions about patient care?
- Are my assumptions correct?
- Do I include the patient in decision making whenever possible?
- Do I consult with others on the health care team when planning?
- Are my written plans clear, concise, and reasonable to carry out?
- Do I take into account the realities of the situation when planning care?
- Are my plans for care sound and appropriate to the individual patient?
- Do I employ principles from the biologic and social sciences in planning?
- Have I considered all alternatives?

Intervention
- Is my work organized and finished on time?
- Do I maintain optimum safe working habits?
- Do I perform technical skills in an efficient and safe manner?
- Do I communicate clearly and effectively with patients, family, and staff?
- Do I use therapeutic communication techniques appropriately and effectively?
- Do I use teaching approaches appropriate to the individual patient and family?
- Do I keep accurate and complete written records?
- Do I understand and perform any administrative tasks that are my responsibility (eg, ordering supplies, planning for laboratory tests)?
- Do I make the effort to learn about new techniques and procedures?
- Do I function as a team player?
- Do I incorporate critical thinking into all of my activities?

Evaluation
- Do I routinely evaluate the effectiveness of the nursing care I give?
- Do I effectively assist in evaluation of the patient's response to medical care and to ordered therapies?
- Do I encourage the patient to participate in evaluating both the process and the outcome of care?
- Have I evaluated all aspects of care fair-mindedly?

(continued)

Display 9-5   **SELF-EVALUATION PLAN** (*continued*)

Personal Growth and Relationships
- Have I established a sound trust and working relationship with coworkers?
- Do I support and assist my coworkers when possible?
- Do I communicate effectively with others on the health care team?
- Do I seek answers to questions for which I have no answer?
- Have I sought opportunities for learning and personal growth?
- Is my attitude helpful and productive?
- Do I have sound working habits (eg, appearing on time, limiting coffee and lunch breaks to the correct time)?
- Is my appearance appropriate to the working environment?
- Do I use appropriate channels of communication within the institution?
- Do I handle criticism constructively?
- Do personal biases interfere with the care that I provide or my relationship with colleagues?
- Am I doing my share in overall professional activities (eg, serving on committees, assisting with development projects)?
- Am I honest with myself, being neither too harsh nor too easy on myself?
- Do I have personal values and beliefs that interfere with providing quality nursing care?

Commitment to the Nursing Profession

Commitment to the nursing profession requires that each individual nurse be concerned not only about personal performance, but also about how nursing is practiced. This involves participation in formal and informal evaluation of nursing care, dealing with poor care, and identifying the impaired nurse. Nurses always have evaluated one another in both formal and informal ways. Some people think that evaluation implies noting error or deficiency. Good evaluation is much broader than this. The main purpose of peer evaluation is to maintain consistent high-quality nursing care. This is an ethical, professional obligation.

FORMAL EVALUATION

Formal evaluation of nursing care is occurring in most settings under the title of quality assurance and quality improvement. Quality assurance is a planned program of evaluation that includes ongoing monitoring of the care given and of outcomes of care. It includes a mechanism for instituting change when problems or opportunities for improvement are identified. Quality assurance programs are required by the Joint Commission on the Accreditation of Healthcare Organizations and by Medicare (see Chapter 2). Special nursing projects such as the work done on nursing outcomes (see Chapter 6) have a focus on the quality of care provided.

All types of evaluation first call for establishing specific criteria to be used in the evaluation. These criteria may refer to process, to outcome, or to both. The creation of the criteria is a professional nursing responsibility.

The process begins by determining if the nursing actions taken are complete and appropriate. Criteria developed to evaluate this aspect are called process criteria. One basis for developing process criteria is the "Standards of Clinical Nursing Practice" developed by the ANA (ANA, 1991). General standards refer to all settings; more specific ones exist for specialty areas of nursing. Some specialty organizations, such as the Intravenous Nurses' Society, also have published standards that refer to their specialty.

Another basis for formal evaluation is the use of outcome criteria for patient care. Outcome criteria are specific, observable patient behaviors or clinical manifestations that are the desired results of care. Typically, nurses working in groups develop the criteria. Nursing literature is consulted so the appropriate criteria are established.

Several methods have been used to evaluate both the process and the outcomes of nursing care. These may include conferences designed to discuss the matter to be evaluated, interviews with either patients or staff, or direct observation of patients. The method that is gaining wider acceptance in nursing is the audit based on review of the patient's record. This chart review involves comparing the patient record with the criteria and is often completed by medical records personnel. The accuracy of the review depends on the adequacy (that is, the completeness) of the charting. If information does not appear in the record (other than situations in which "charting by exception" are employed), then, for the purposes of the audit, the appropriate observations were not made or the actions were not taken.

This is just one of the reasons why you must recognize the importance of your charting and make sure that you maintain a high standard in written records. If audits are being done at your institution, you should become familiar with the criteria being used, which can serve as guidelines in evaluating your own care and record-keeping. The chart review has raised serious concerns, which have resulted in greater attention to documentation and even revision of record systems. Nurses then have taken the initiative to determine the meaning of the data in relationship to enhanced patient well-being. Changes in policies and procedures and in-service education classes often occur. Once remedial action has been taken, re-evaluation is done to determine its effectiveness.

INFORMAL EVALUATION

An important day-to-day evaluation of patient care occurs informally as peers observe the performance of others. Watching other nurses also helps you to grow in your own practice. When you observe coworkers, you need to strive for objectivity. A common mistake is to let personal feelings influence what we see, viewing a close friend in a positive light and seeing only the negative aspects of a nurse with whom we have a poor relationship. We need to remember to examine the results or outcomes of care. Two nurses may use different approaches or techniques in similar situations, but both may achieve positive results. In most instances, you will see good care. Do not hesitate to commend others and share your positive feelings. Everyone benefits from positive reinforcement of skill; it helps nurses to create a good climate for personal growth and sharing.

DEALING WITH SUBSTANDARD CARE

Concern for the welfare of patients requires that nurses acknowledge the existence of substandard care and work toward improving that situation. It is not a matter of whether the nurse should become involved but rather how to most effectively accomplish the goals of better care.

If faced with a situation where patient care is less than desired, you first need to consider whose care you are criticizing. If it is the care of another nurse, or a care provider with less educational preparation than you possess, the situation is more straightforward. If you have questions about medical care delivered or the action of a physician, it becomes more difficult, because medical actions are outside the scope of practice of nursing. You want to be careful about how you proceed, referring to hospital policy manuals, trusted colleagues, your supervisor, or possibly the chief of the medical staff for advice before taking action.

When you observe a colleague practicing what you think is poor patient care, such as poor sterile technique, it is not as difficult. The action you choose to take depends on the seriousness of the situation you have observed.

Suppose you observed a break in sterile technique during a dressing change. Usually the simplest and most effective solution is to go directly to the person involved and to state: "I observed this specific incident, and it seemed to me that it was not in the best interest of the patient because . . . What is your perception of the situation?" With this response, it allows the nurse to give a rationale for the action taken. When you understand the situation more fully, you may have a different point of view. If you disagree with your colleague and the situation is not critical, you might want to state simply that you disagree. If the situation is critical, the two of you will want to seek resources that will outline the best approach. If you observe poor care a second time, and it has been determined that your colleague's care is substandard, you should again approach the person. State what you have seen and note that it is the second time. If the person still disagrees that a problem exists, state that you feel obligated to discuss this with your immediate superior because it is not in the best interest of the patient. You should then follow through on this.

If you have a reputation on the unit for maintaining a focus that enhances the welfare of patients, and you have been quick to praise the good care provided by others, your action in response to poor care will be more readily accepted. Remember that your attitude when approaching another nurse is crucial. Facial expressions and tone of voice, as well as words, need to be considered. If you are perceived as friendly and caring, your comments probably will be accepted in a far different manner than if you are seen as being negative and critical.

However, you cannot always count on this reaction. Many nurses feel threatened by the idea of evaluation, or have had bad experiences in which evaluation only involved pointing out deficiencies. These nurses may be angry and upset with any colleague who considers evaluation part of the colleague role. Therefore, it is wise to have thought out how you will proceed.

A Basic Pattern for Action. The first step in any situation in which you believe substandard care exists is to collect adequate, valid information on behavior that you have personally observed. Do not make decisions based on gossip, hearsay, or a single isolated instance unless the single incident was very serious. If this is the case, be certain of your facts before taking action.

You will also want to be certain you understand both the formal and the informal systems of authority and responsibility within your facility and the laws of the state in which you are practicing. In some states, laws exist requiring that poor practice be reported directly to the relevant licensing board. You need to know which people have the authority to make decisions and changes, what the official prescribed route of change is, and what the hidden priorities of the institution might be. It is most commonly recommended that once you are certain of your data and know how the system works in your organization, you take concerns to your immediate supervisor, who would forward the concern until it reached the individual or body with the authority and duty to act. Many people believe that reporting to a supervisor fulfills your ethical responsibility as well as your legal responsibility.

When you approach a supervisor, you need to give specific information that includes the dates, situations, and the action you took. You should not indulge in generalities or sweeping statements, but should stick to specific observed instances by simply describing what you saw. Let the supervisor know that you have talked with the person under discussion and have informed the person that you would speak with the supervisor. It is important to specify the action you would like to see occur. You might ask the supervisor to discuss the matter with both of you or you might ask the supervisor to discuss the matter with the other nurse or observe the nurse. It is also important to remember that once you have initiated this action, you may also be involved in some follow-up.

If you observe an incident that has the potential to cause a patient danger (eg, an unreported medication error) or one that has legal ramifications (eg, the falsifying of narcotic records), you have a legal as well as an ethical responsibility to go immediately to a supervisor with your information. In a situation that has the potential for legal involvement, it is prudent to keep an exact personal record of your observations and actions. Your record should include times and dates of incidents and of your reporting efforts (see Chapter 8).

Alternative Approaches for Action. At times, the system does not always work as expected. Your concern regarding what you perceive as poor practice may be dropped or ignored at any one of many points. You may never learn what was done, even when positive action was taken, because of the constraints of confidentiality for the affected employee. Occasionally, results emerge only much later, when a change in procedure and policy occurs.

Often there are good reasons for this. Perhaps the persons in authority want to collect more specific data about a situation, with as little general discussion as possible. Sometimes there are aspects of a legal contract or a collective bargaining contract of which you are unaware that must be considered in the actions that are taken. Other times, professional confidentiality may make it seem that nothing is being done, when, in fact, steps have been taken to correct a situation. It is easy as a newcomer to the health care scene to see only part of a picture.

If your initial approach is not effective, a formal route for seeking further change would lead you through the official lines of authority within your facility. After discussing your concern with your immediate supervisor and receiving no satisfactory response, you would tell the supervisor formally that you intend to carry your concern to the next higher authority. Technically you could proceed in this manner until you reached the administrator or even the board of directors, although it is unlikely that this would occur. Informing your supervisor of your plans should help to avoid problems, but you should be prepared to listen to some words of warning from the supervisor or efforts to discourage you from taking action. There are reasons this individual has chosen not to pursue the issue; some of these may be valid.

However, there are times when an alternative approach is more appropriate than formal action. Another route for seeking further change is through designated committees or procedures within your facility. As hospitals move into models of shared governance, this may be your best alternative. Discussing or sharing a problem with a particular committee might require a carefully written and documented report explaining your concern. You then might be called to answer questions that the committee believes are important to ask.

You may volunteer to serve on committees that deal with peer review. If there are no such committees, you may work to have them established, perhaps through a bargaining unit. This route of action will require a considerable investment of your own time and effort, a factor you need to consider.

Another alternative approach is to use the informal system within the facility. You may discuss your concern with a trusted person (or mentor) who has influence within the system. You may learn that you are not alone in your concerns, that efforts toward change are being made, and that your input of data is welcomed. Another approach would be to seek the assistance of another individual with power within the organization. However, we must caution you about using informal systems; informal systems can backfire. Therefore, we suggest that you use these alternative approaches only when the ones suggested earlier have failed to bring about the desired results.

A final alternative to a problem in your work setting is to offer your resignation if a change is not made. Continuing to work in an environment in which poor practice exists may place you in conflict with your ethical standards and values. If you find it necessary to do this, be careful that you do not jeopardize your own future with angry letters or intemperate remarks. Render your resignation in a polite and professional manner even when expressing dissatisfaction with the system.

Reporting directly to a state licensing board or professional organization's disciplinary committee is an avenue of action outside of the employment setting. The licensing board exists to assure the public of safe practice; therefore, these organizations and agencies usually deal with serious problems that represent a breach of the public trust or serious harm. They may not have the capacity or desire to pursue minor (though still important) problems. The same constraints apply when reporting to these organizations. Remember that their investigation and decisions may be done in a judicial or legal manner. This may involve the requirement that you provide legal testimony regarding your complaints.

Personal Risks in Reporting. If you decide to pursue any of these routes, you need to be fully aware of the possible consequences. You may be labeled a troublemaker, or worse. You may lose the opportunity to be promoted because you are seen as being antagonistic to the system. Although officially it should not happen, it is even possible that you could lose your job for raising too many issues. We do not mean to be unduly discouraging, but we want to warn you that the role of change agent is not easy, and you should be aware of and weigh the consequences before you decide to act. And above all, be certain that your perceptions are correct and that your concerns are well grounded.

RECOMMENDING A CARE PROVIDER

Patients and acquaintances may ask you to recommend a physician or other care provider because they believe that, as a nurse, you have special knowledge and insight in such matters. If you have no personal knowledge about the requested information, then you should honestly tell an individual requesting information that you have no personal or professional knowledge regarding a particular care provider. However, if you do have knowledge, you could recommend several competent persons, pointing out characteristics of each that might be factors in personal choice. For example, if you were asked to recommend an obstetrician, you might recommend three. You then could state further that Drs. A, B, and C are all board-certified specialists in obstetrics. You might add some information about their practices: Dr. A is an older physician with a more traditional approach to childbirth; Dr. B is a young and innovative physician who strongly advocates partner participation and the Lamaze natural childbirth method; Dr. C is new in the community but appears to allow patients a great deal of choice in their approach to childbirth. The patient can further research these physicians and make a personal choice.

If you are asked specifically about a physician whose care you believe to be less than satisfactory, you are faced with a different dilemma. Making severely critical statements might leave you open to a legal charge of slander by the physician (see Chapter 8). However, saying nothing is ethically a problem because you are not acting to protect the patient. A safe approach is to state, "I personally would not choose Dr. X as my physician. Instead, I would prefer to see Dr. N or Dr. O." If pressed to give reasons, you are legally more secure if you say that you would prefer not to discuss specifics.

You need to be careful that any recommendations are not based on hearsay or gossip. If you do not have solid information on which to base a referral, do not be drawn into making one. Being a nurse does not obligate you to be an expert on all health care questions.

THE CHEMICALLY IMPAIRED PROFESSIONAL

Chemically impaired professional is a term used to describe that person whose practice has deteriorated because of chemical abuse, specifically, the use of alcohol and drugs. There is a strong possibility that if you remain active in the profession, at some time will find yourself working with a chemically impaired colleague; perhaps you already have.

One would like to believe that nurses, who have studied the physiologic effects of alcohol and drugs on the system, would avoid such abuse. However, this is not the case. In the 1980s, nurses began to be concerned about this problem and data began to be collected (Bissell & Haberman, 1984; Bissell & Skorina, 1987; Sullivan et al, 1988). Sullivan and colleagues conclude that the percentage of chemically dependent nurses is at least as great as the percentage of chemically dependent people in the general population, and it may be that there is a greater percentage in the nursing population, based on accessibility of drugs.

Studies conducted in the 1990s have assessed probable alcoholism among nursing students. Marion and colleagues (1996) reported that the use of alcohol by nursing students paralleled the alcohol consumption of other college students, an age group recognized as demonstrating high usage. Their findings indicate significant drinking problems among the students sampled. Campbell and Polk (1992) also have expressed concern about substance abuse among students, and have encouraged nurse educators to identify students suspected of abuse and to educate students about the problem. Sullivan, Bissell, and Leffler (1990) reported that the addiction process was starting earlier, sometimes even before nursing school, and that younger nurses were more likely to use narcotics, resulting in serious problems in job performance.

Why are nurses affected by this problem? Factors that lead to chemical dependency include the stress of the nursing profession, particularly in intensive care units and emergency departments. Frequent shift changes and staffing shortages add to the situation. Unrealistic personal expectations, frustration, powerlessness, anxiety, and depression contribute to the problem. Once the problem exists, denial is a big part of the disease.

Jefferson and Ensor (1982) provide the following information about addiction:

Addiction is an insidious process that occurs as the result of a) prolonged intake of a chemical, b) processes going on within the individual (including genetic, psychological, and chemical), and c) processes external to the individual (that is, the actions and reactions of family, friends, coworkers, supervisors, and society). . . . Addiction is present any time a chemical interferes with any aspect of a person's life and that person keeps using the chemical.

All areas of the profession are affected by the problem of chemical dependency in nursing. A significant financial impact is realized by institutions that employ nurses with dependency problems in the forms of sickness, absenteeism, tardiness, accidents, errors, decreased productivity, and staff turnover. Early recognition and treatment have been recommended to help offset this problem (LaGodna & Hendrix, 1989). Nurse managers who are confronted with the problem of impaired practitioners may begin to question the efficacy of treatment (Hendrix et al, 1987).

In 1981, the ANA appointed a Nursing Task Force on Addiction and Psychological Disturbance to develop guidelines for state associations in the treatment and assistance of nurses whose practice was impaired by alcoholism, drug abuse, or psychologic dysfunction. These guidelines approached chemical dependency in nursing from a treatment and rehabilitation viewpoint rather than from a punishment viewpoint. In 1990, the ANA developed suggested state legislation to respond to the problems of chemical dependency and drug diversion in nurses that emphasized voluntary treatment and monitoring programs rather than traditional legal proceedings (ANA, 1990).

The concerns about the chemically impaired nurse are twofold. The first is a personal concern for the nurse who is afflicted: the illness may go undetected and untreated for years. The second concern is for the patient, whose care is jeopardized by the nurse whose judgment and skills are weakened.

Because nurses, by virtue of their education, are socialized into caring roles, they have not always dealt with the problem in a straightforward fashion. The impaired nurse was often protected, transferred, ignored, and, in some instances, promoted. None of these actions helped solve the problem. What are some of the behaviors you will notice in a chemically impaired colleague? The following characteristics are commonly seen in alcoholic nurses:

* More irritable with patients and colleagues; withdrawn; mood swings
* Ilogical and sloppy charting
* Excessive errors
* Unkempt appearance
* Social isolation; wants to work nights, lunches alone, avoids informal staff gatherings
* Elaborate excuses for behavior, such as being late for work
* Blackouts: complete memory loss for events, conversations, phone calls to colleagues; euphoric or "glossed over" recall of *unpleasant* events on floor (eg, arguments)
* Frequent use of breath purifiers, drinks high volume of "sodas"
* Flushed face, red or bleary eyes, unsteady gait, slurred speech
* Signs of withdrawal; tremors, restlessness, diaphoresis (Washington State Nurses Association, 1992, p. 10)

Problems related to drug abuse are complicated by the fact that the nurse often is obtaining drugs from the supply available on the hospital unit and is therefore in violation of the Controlled Substances Act. A drug-addicted nurse commonly exhibits the following behaviors:

- Extreme and rapid mood swings, irritable with patients and then calm again (after taking drugs)
- Wears long sleeves all the time
- Suspicious behavior concerning controlled drugs
- Consistently signs out more controlled drugs than anyone else
- Frequently breaks and spills drugs
- Purposely waits until alone to open narcotics cabinet
- Constantly volunteers to be the medications nurse
- Disappears into bathroom directly after being in narcotics cabinet
- Vials/medications appear altered
- Incorrect narcotic count
- Discrepancies between his or her patient reports and others' patient reports on effect of medications
- Patient complains that pain medications dispensed by this individual are ineffective
- Defensive when questioned about medication errors
- Abnormal number of syringes being used or missing
- Frequent use of restroom by the nurse; evidence of broken syringes, bloody pieces of cotton in bathroom (Washington Health Professional Services, 1992)

In addition to personal behavior changes, job performance changes also occur in those with drug and alcohol problems. These job performance changes include:

- Doing the minimum necessary
- Difficulty meeting schedules and deadlines
- Illogical and sloppy charting
- Excessive medication errors
- Excessive incidence of controlled drugs broken or spilled
- Increasing absences without adequate explanation (Washington State Nurses Association, 1992, p. 11)

As an RN, what should you do if you suspect that a colleague has a chemical dependency problem? First of all, you need to know what the law in your state requires of you. In many states, every professional is legally obligated to report a chemically dependent health care professional. This reporting most commonly is done through channels at the place of employment, but also may be done directly to the State Board of Nursing. If you do not know the requirements, you should immediately learn what they are. In some states, failure to report can result in disciplinary action toward you.

When planning to report, you do not have to be sure beyond any doubt that a problem exists. You need to have enough data to represent a reasonable concern. The investigation to clearly establish the problem is the responsibility of the employing agency or the state board.

To establish reasonable concern, collect data and document it, including objective facts, dates, and times that support your concern. For several good reasons, you should not confront the person whom you suspect at this time.

First, the person may become more secretive about the behavior because of the danger of being caught. This will make collection of data more difficult, if not impossible. Personal defenses and denial may become stronger. The suspected person may ask for a transfer to another shift or to a different part of the facility, or, if truly threatened, may seek employment in another facility.

Second, the person may feel attacked and rejected. To ensure that it will not end in a disaster, a confrontation needs the support of an appropriate and knowledgeable health care professional to ensure that the individual is guided to appropriate choices for treatment and rehabilitation. If the person is someone you know well, who confides in you regarding personal problems, you might use those occasions to refer the individual to appropriate resources for personal assistance and counseling.

Another reason you should not confront the suspected person at this time is that you are still collecting data and documenting it. You cannot be sure from a single observation that a problem exists. There are often reasons why things are not what we initially perceived them to be.

Once you feel you have data to support a realistic concern, you should report it to a supervisor to validate your observations. Usually, once you have notified your supervisor, he or she will assume responsibility for the problem, but may ask for your continued assistance with data collection or with confrontation (see earlier discussion on reporting to your supervisor).

Once adequate information has been gathered, agency administrative personnel will notify the State Board of Nursing. In addition, they usually must notify the State Board of Pharmacy if drugs are involved. More investigation will be carried out; records will be examined. If a problem exists, actions appropriate to the situation will be taken. These usually include a carefully planned confrontation by an intervention team, a requirement that treatment be sought, and a presentation of the consequences of not seeking treatment.

The worst thing you can do if you suspect a problem is to ignore it or help a colleague "cover" for inadequacies. The problem will not get better if it is not recognized and treated. The longer the delay, the greater the chance that an innocent patient will be placed in jeopardy.

Fortunately, help and rehabilitation are being made available to those who need it. Many states now have programs to provide treatment of health care professionals with a chemical dependency. These programs usually provide a specific contractual agreement regarding professional practice during the treatment and monitoring period. This is often done without formal disciplinary proceedings. The goal of this process is restoration of the individual to effective functioning.

In some states, the licensing boards may institute formal disciplinary proceedings to suspend a license or issue a license with limitations on practice, and to provide monitoring and supervision while the individual seeks treatment. When treatment is completed, the board may reinstate the license with temporary limitations and continued monitoring and support. The goal is the eventual full rehabilitation of the health care professional to the service of the community. Baldwin and Smith (1994) reported a much higher treatment success rate in nurses than in the general population. These researchers further identified that successful recovery was most likely in those nurses who retained their employment during treatment. Therefore, reporting a chemically dependent colleague may be the most caring action you can take.

If, as a nursing student, you suspect that a fellow classmate (or worse yet, an instructor) has a problem with chemical abuse, you would be wise to discuss your concerns with your instructor (or with the director of the program if you suspect an instructor). Because such problems typically get worse with time, the earlier they are addressed and corrected, the better it is for everyone. Again, it is important that you have accurate information to report, along with times, dates, and examples of the behavior that caused your concern.

Critical Thinking Activity

Assume that you have serious concerns that a colleague is delivering poor patient care because of problems with chemical dependency. Where would you begin? What is your personal responsibility? What is your responsibility to your colleague? What is your responsibility to the patients? What steps should you take? Do you have a personal liability in the situation?

BOUNDARY VIOLATIONS

The term **boundary violations** is used to refer to situations in which nurses move beyond a professional relationship and become personally involved with a patient and the patient's life. It is of particular concern because it represents a violation of the trust relationship that exists between the patient and the nurse. In nurse–patient relationships, the nurse necessarily holds power, creating a vulnerable situation for the patient. The nurse also has access to confidential and privileged information about patients and their families. It is the nurse's responsibility to define the boundaries of the relationships and ensure that they are maintained. The nurse must be warm and empathetic but should not try to be friends with the patient (Fig. 9-4).

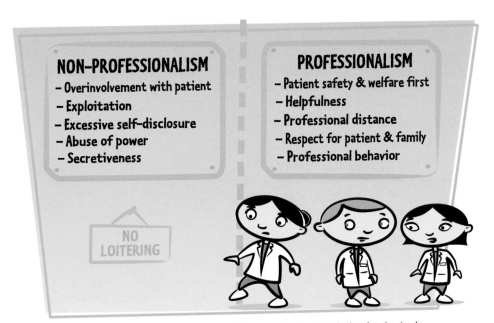

FIGURE 9-4   Everyone benefits when boundaries are clearly established and maintained.

Perhaps the most extreme boundary violation is professional sexual misconduct. Professional sexual misconduct has been defined as "any expression by a nurse or other health care provider of erotic or romantic thoughts, feelings, or gestures that are sexual or may be reasonably construed by the patient as sexual" (Smith et al, 1997). At present, there is no official reporting of the violation of sexual boundaries; however, it is the topic of focus groups and workshops conducted by the National Council of State Boards of Nursing.

Although sexual misconduct is the major focus of this concern, boundary violations expand into other areas of conduct, such as overidentifying with a particular family member or moving into pseudofamily relationships with the patient's family. If this happens, the family may question the nurse's motives, wondering if she is looking for a bequest in a will or other tangible benefit. Such overinvolvement will interfere with the nurse's personal life and even could result in legal actions on the part of the family.

Some early indications that boundaries are beginning to break down include situations in which the nurse spends extended time with a patient beyond assigned duties or visits the patient when not on duty. Showing favoritism or possessiveness of a patient, meeting patients in isolated areas not required in direct patient care, or personal disclosure by the care provider are other indicators that boundaries are being violated (Ellis & Hartley, 2000).

It is important that you are able to recognize situations in which a colleague may cross sexual boundaries. If you believe sexual misconduct is occurring on the unit where you are employed, the steps you would follow are similar to those you learned to use in dealing with chemical abuse. It is extremely important that you document the behavior carefully, noting dates, times, and the names of the individuals involved. Keep your documentation focused on factual information and objective data. You would then share this information with your immediate supervisor.

KEY CONCEPTS

- Ethics is a branch of philosophy referred to as moral philosophy. It seeks to provide answers to some of the questions of human conduct that arise in our life, and attempts to determine what is "right" or "good."
- Inherent in the study of ethics is an appreciation of individual values that are derived from societal norms, religious, and family orientation. We can get in better touch with our own value system through the process of values clarification.
- The basic ethical concepts of beneficence, nonmaleficence, autonomy, justice, fidelity, veracity, and the standard of best interest underlie ethical decision-making and may be in conflict in an individual situation.
- The ethical theories of utilitarianism, deontology, natural law, and social equity and justice may be used to examine the implications of ethical decisions.
- The concept of justice has been expanded to include distributive justice that is applied in situations requiring the allocation of scarce resources. The problems associated with the allocation of scarce resources are expected to increase in the near future.
- Ethical decision-making may be based on personal religious and philosophic viewpoints, but must always be grounded in professional standards seen in the Codes for Nurses and the statements of patient rights.

- A variety of social and cultural factors including attitudes, science and technology, legislation, judicial decisions, and funding all influence ethical decision-making.
- The nurse's status as an employee, collective bargaining contracts, collegial relationships, the authoritarian and paternalistic backgrounds of health care, deliberations of ethics committees, and consumer involvement create pressures regarding ethical decision-making.
- A basic framework for ethical decision-making emphasizes identifying and clarifying the problem, gathering data, identifying options, making a decision, acting, and assessing.
- Nurses have ethical obligations to the patient and to the employer, and must maintain an objective stance regarding other health care providers, and when confronting substandard care. Commitment to personal excellence and to the profession of nursing are also desired characteristics of the professional nurse.
- The chemically impaired nurse is a concern to the profession and a danger to patients. All nurses have an obligation to report those who demonstrate chemical impairment and to assist impaired colleagues in finding treatment and rehabilitation.
- Boundary violations, a situation in which the nurse moves beyond a professional relationship and becomes involved with patients and their families, has become a concern in nursing. Educational programs to increase understanding of this problem and to help avoid its occurrence are being conducted.

RELEVANT WEB SITES

The American Nurses Organization: *www.nursingworld.org/* (Click on Ethics, go to the Center for Ethics and Human Rights)

Boston College, Nursing Ethics Network: *www/bc.edu/nursing/ethics*

John Hopkins University, Bioethics Institute: *www.med.jhu.edu/bioethics_institute*

Midwest Bioethics Center: *www.midbio.org/*

National Catholic Bioethics Center: *www.ncbcenter.org/*

National Reference Center for Bioethics Literature: *http://www.georgetown.edu/research/nrcbl/home.htm*

University of British Columbia, The W. Maurice Young Center for Applied Ethics: *www.ethics.ubc.ca/*

REFERENCES

American Hospital Association. (1992). *A patient's bill of rights.* Chicago: AHA.

American Nurses Association. (1991). *Standards of clinical nursing practice.* Washington, DC: American Nurses Association.

American Nurses Association. (1990). Suggested state legislation: Nursing Practice Act, Nursing Disciplinary Diversion Act, Prescriptive Authority Act (Pub. No. NP-78). Washington, DC: American Nurses Association.

Armstrong, C. R. & Whitlock, R. (1998). The cost of care: Two troublesome cases in health care ethics. *The Physician Executive 24*(6): 32–35.

Baldwin, L. & Smith, V. (1994). Relapse in chemically dependent nurses: Relevance and contributing factors. *Issues 15*(1): 1, 4–5.

Bates, T. J. (2002 [October 14]). Letters of advice. *Mountain West Nurse Week 3*(14): 7.

Bissell, L, & Haberman, P. W. (1984). *Alcoholism in the professions*. New York: Oxford University Press.

Bissell, L. & Skorina, J. (1987). 100 alcoholic women in medicine. *JAMA* 257:2939–944.

Braddock, C. H., Edwards, K. A., Hasenberg, N. M., Laidley, T. L. & Levinson, W. (1999). Informed decision making in outpatient practice: Time to get back to the basics. *JAMA 282*(24):2313–2320.

Buchanan, A. (1996). Judging the past: The care of the human radiation experiments. *Hastings Center Report 2*(13):25–30.

Burkhardt, M. A. & Nathaniel, A. K. (1998). *Ethics & issues in contemporary nursing*. Albany, N.Y: Delmar Publishers.

Campbell, A.R. & Polk, E. (1992). *Legal and ethical issues of alcohol and other substance abuse in nursing education*. Atlanta, GA: Southern Council on Collegiate Education for Nursing.

Curtin, L. (1978). A proposed model for critical ethical analysis. *Nursing Forum 17*(1):12–17. Davis, A. J., Aroskar, M. A., Liaschenko, J. & Drought, T. S. (1997). *Ethical dilemmas & nursing practice* (4th ed.). Stamford, CT: Appleton & Lange.

David, A. J., Arokar, M. A., Liaschenko, J., Drought, T. S. (1997). *Ethical dilemmas in nursing and nursing practice*, (4th ed.). Stamford, CT: Appleton & Lange.

Edge, R. S. & Groves, J. R. (1999). *Ethics of health care: A guide for clinical practice*, (2nd ed.). Albany, NY: Delmar.

Ellis, J. R. & Hartley, C. L. (2000). *Managing and coordinating nursing care*, (3rd ed.). Philadelphia: Lippincott Williams & Wilkins.

Fowler, M. (1997). Nursing ethics. In Davis, A. J., Aroskar, M. A., Liaschenko, J. & Drought, T. S.: *Ethical dilemmas & nursing practice* (4th ed.) (pp. 17–34). Stamford, CT: Appleton & Lange.

Fung, L. (1994). Implementing the Patient Self-Determination Act (PSDA): How to effectively engage Chinese-American persons in the decision of advance directives. *Journal of Gerontological Social Work 22*(1-2): 161–174.

Hall, J. K. (1996). *Nursing ethics and law*. Philadelphia: W.B. Saunders.

Hendrix, M., Sabritt, D., McDaniel, A. & Field, B. (1987). Perceptions and attitudes toward nursing impairment. *Research in Nursing and Health* 10:323–333.

Jameton, A. (1984). *Nursing practice: The ethical issues*. Englewood Cliffs, NJ: Prentice-Hall.

Jefferson, L. V. & Ensor, B. E. (1982). Confronting a chemically impaired colleague. *AJN* 82(4): 574.

LaGodna, G. & Hendrix, M. (1989). Impaired nurses: A cost analysis. *Journal of Nursing Administration 19*(9):13–18.

Lane, S. D. & Rubinstein, R. A. (1996). Judging the other: Responding to traditional female genital surgeries. *Hastings Center Report 26*(3): 31–40.

Maddox, P.J. (1998). Administrative ethics and the allocation of scarce resources. *Online Journal of Issues in Nursing*. [On-line]. Available: *www.nursingworld.org/ojin/topic8/topic8_5.htm*. Accessed December 7, 1999.

Marion, L. N., Fuller, S. G., Johnson, N. P., Michels, P. J. & Diniz, C. (1996). Drinking problems of nursing students. *Journal of Nursing Education 35*(5):196–203.

Miller, F. G. & Brody, H. (1995). Professional integrity and physician-assisted death. *Hastings Center Report 25*(3):8–17.

Milner, S. (1993). An ethical nursing practice model. *Journal of Nursing Administration 23*(3):22–25.

Neufeldt V. & Guralnik, D. N. (1996). *Webster's New World collegiate dictionary*, (3rd ed.). New York: Macmillan.

Rawls, J. A. (1971). *Theory of justice*. Cambridge, MA: Harvard University Press.

Silva, M.C. (1998). Financial compensation and ethical issues in health care. *Online Journal of Issues in Nursing.* [On-line]. Available: at *www.nursingworld.org/ojin/tpc6/tpc6_4.htm.* Accessed October 4, 1999.

Smith, L. L., Taylor, B. B., Keys, A. T., & Gornto, S. B. (1997). Nurse-patient boundaries: Crossing the line. *AJN 97*(12), 26–31.

Stahl, D. A. (1996). Ethics in subacute care—Part I. *Nursing Management 27*(9): 29–30.

Sullivan, E., Bissell, L. & Leffler, D. (1990). Drug use and disciplinary actions among 300 nurses. *International Journal of the Addictions 25*(4):375–391.

Sullivan, E., Bissell, L. & Williams, E. (1988). *Chemical dependency in nursing: The deadly diversion.* Menlo Park, CA: Addison-Wesley.

Thiroux, J. (1998). *Ethics: Theory and practice* (6th ed.). Upper Saddle Drive, N.J.:Prentice Hall.

Thompson, J. & Thompson, H. (1981). *Ethics in nursing.* New York: Macmillan.

Videbeck, S. L. (2001). *Psychiatric mental health nursing.* Philadelphia: Lippincott Williams & Wilkins.

Washington Health Professional Services. (1992). *A guide for assisting colleagues who demonstrate impairment in the workplace.* Olympia, WA: Washington State Department of Health.

Washington State Nurses Association. (1992). *Handbook for working with the chemically dependent nurse.* Seattle: Washington State Nurses Association.

10

Bioethical Issues in Health Care

KEY TERMS

Abortion (spontaneous, therapeutic, elective)	Euthanasia—negative and positive	Patient Self-Determination Act (PSDA)
Advance directives	Family planning	Property rights
Age of consent	Futile treatment	Rationing of health care
Amniocentesis	Gene therapy	
Artificial insemination	Genetic screening	Right-to-die
Assisted death	Genome	Right to refuse treatment
Behavior control	Human Genome Project (HGP)	Sonogram
Bioethics		Stem cell
Chorionic villus sampling (CVS)	Informed consent	Sterilization
	In vitro fertilization	Surrogate mother
Durable power of attorney for health care	Living will	Withdrawing/withholding treatment
	Mature minor	
Emancipated minor	Organ procurement	Wrongful birth
Eugenics	Organ transplantation	Xenotransplantation

 Bioethics is the study of ethical issues that result from technologic and scientific advances, especially as they are used in biology and medicine. This area of study is also called biomedical ethics because of its association with medical practice. It is a sub-discipline within the larger discipline of ethics, which (as discussed in Chapter 9) is the philosophic study of morality, or what is right and what is wrong. Today more than ever, nurses and their patients need to keep pace with the technologic changes occurring in health care. The critical choices that must be made by patients, their families, and members of the health care team are the result of changes that were not a part of our decision-making in earlier times.

This chapter discusses some of the choices with which nurses and their clients must grapple. It should be read, studied, and discussed within the framework of the information concerning ethical decision-making that was provided earlier. The content of the chapter should provide a basis with which you can look at judicial rulings, legal mandates, and social standards, and how they can be used to assist in resolving concerns that face us in health care delivery. You have had some experience in looking at what is right or wrong regarding your personal professional practice. This chapter examines more specifically the issues that apply to the bioethics of patient care.

MAJOR AREAS WHERE BIOETHICS ARE APPLIED

The bioethical issues surrounding the delivery of health care grow in number each year, constantly changing and taking on new scope and proportions. Today, issues related to birth and death, which earlier were the major focus of debates, represent just the "tip of the iceberg." Of equal or greater concern are such matters as universal access to health care and insurance for all, rationing of health care, cost containment and quality of care, where and how federal dollars should be spent with regard to the nation's health, and the obligation of others to assist the homeless. Our media thrive on issues created by recent biomedical research, such as concerns regarding the Human Genome Project, gene therapy, and stem cell research, with one area blurring into another.

Each year the percent of America's gross domestic product (GDP) spent on health care increases. Today it is estimated at 14%, making it a $1.4-trillion industry (Schroeder, 2002). Because of lifestyle changes and medical breakthroughs, more people live today to reach old age, thus placing a greater burden on an already stressed system. Life expectancy has increased a year or 2 in each recent decade. In the United States, the life expectancy for females born today is 79.5 years, and for males it is 74.1, compared with 47 years at the beginning of the 20th century. Diseases such as Alzheimer's and AIDS, for which cures are still being sought, have increased in prevalence. With globalization have come new threats to our well-being, such as that created by the Nile virus. New technologies have led to treatments that were not available 15 years ago. Rather than decreasing health care needs, the new technologies have resulted in increasing needs because these specialized services are available today. Many treatments require use of technologies so expensive that they are priced beyond what an individual or family can afford without help from third-party payers. Finding new and better ways to treat life-threatening conditions challenges medical researchers, and the treatments that become available often invite debate among bioethicists. For example, the use of xenografts (animal-organ transplants) has been suggested to meet the increasing demand for healthy organs to transplant, but many people question this practice and, to date, it is relatively undeveloped.

Some would indicate that the "birth of bioethics" occurred with the publication of a magazine article in *Life* titled "They Decide Who Lives, Who Dies" (November 9, 1962). This article told the story of a group of individuals in Seattle whose duty it was to select patients for the first hemodialysis program to treat chronic renal failure. Many more patients needed treatment than could be accommodated; those not selected would likely die. This event was followed several years later by an article about the ethics of medical research that provided impetus for examining these issues.

Centers for research in bioethics emerged, most notably the Institute of Society, Ethics, and the Life Sciences, located in Hastings-on-Hudson, New York (often called The Hastings Center), and the Kennedy Institute of Ethics, located at Georgetown University in Washington, DC. The Kennedy Institute of Ethics, founded in 1971 by Joseph and Rose Kennedy, is a teaching and research center that provides ethical perspectives on major policy issues. It boasts the largest university-based faculty in the world devoted to research and teaching biomedical ethics. Journals such as the *Hastings Center Report* and the *Journal of Medicine and Philosophy* have come into being, and an encyclopedia, *The Encyclopedia of Bioethics,* has been published. Web sites devoted to the topic of bioethics are so numerous that they cannot be listed in the confines of this textbook. Today, bioethicists are included in many important task forces and special committees.

Entire textbooks have been devoted to bioethical considerations. Initially, most of these were written for medical students, but now just as many are written for nursing students. Some nursing programs include a course in ethics and bioethics in the curriculum. This chapter can only introduce the topic and, we hope, broaden your perspective and deepen your interest. You are encouraged to read about and study these issues further as they affect your nursing practice.

As we mentioned earlier, most of the bioethical issues have evolved as a product of the technologic advances occurring in medical practice and research and were not a concern 15 years ago. Table 10-1 lists some of the significant medical milestones that have occurred

TABLE 10-1.   SOME MEDICAL MILESTONES OF THE 1900S

WHEN	WHO	WHAT
1928	Alexander Fleming	This British bacteriologist noticed that one of his culture plates had grown a fungus and the colonies of staphylococci around the edge of the mold had been destroyed. Because this fungus was a member of the *Penicillium* group, he named it penicillin.
1938	Howard Florey & Ernst Chain	These two pathologists took up the work of Fleming and demonstrated the efficacy of penicillin in treating infection. In 1945, the three were jointly awarded the Nobel Prize for Physiology of Medicine.
1951	Forrest Bird	The first Bird breathing device was developed (Bird Mark 7) and breathing treatment machines were introduced. Inhalation (respiratory) therapy rapidly developed as a health profession (Pilbeam, 1998).
1953	James Watson & Francis Crick	These two geneticists deciphered DNA's double-helix structure. Researchers began to focus on the internal functioning of the cell and molecular biology developed as a specialty.
1954	Physicians in Boston	Transplanted the kidney from one twin to the other, thus moving kidney transplantation from the experimental stage it had occupied since 1902. Kidney transplantations have been the most successful of transplantations (Miller-Keane, 1992).
1955	Jonas Salk	Public health officials began immunizing children against polio with Dr. Salk's vaccine, which contained dead virus.
1957	Albert Sabin	A polio vaccine was developed, which was based on weakened live virus, that could be administered orally.
1967	Christiaan Barnard	This South African surgeon performed the first human-heart transplant.
1972	British engineers	The computed tomography (CT) scanner, which assembles thousands of x-ray images into a highly detailed picture of the brain, was developed in England. It was later expanded to provide scans of the entire body.
1978	English physicians	The process of in vitro fertilization was developed. Louise Brown became the first person to be conceived in a test tube, then implanted into the mother's uterus.
1979	World Health Organization	This group declared that smallpox had been eradicated 2 years after the last known case was identified. This occurred because of world-wide immunization against the disease.
1981	Physicians in San Francisco and New York	Doctors from these two cities reported the first cases of what would later become known as acquired immunodeficiency syndrome (AIDS). To date, no cure exists.
1982	The U.S. Food and Drug Administration	The first drug developed with recombinant-DNA was approved by this group. It was a form of human insulin; its availability saves thousands of lives.
1995	Duke University surgeons	Hearts from genetically altered pigs were transplanted into baboons, proving that cross-species transplantations can be done. Transmission of animal viruses to humans emerges as a serious concern.
1998	James Thomas and Scientists from University of Wisconsin—Madison	Culture embryonic stem cells (cells that are the parent cells of all body tissues) from donated human blastocysts, opening the door to potential repair or replacement of diseased tissues or organs (DHHS, 2001).

* Much of the material for this table was gathered from an article by Sherwin B. Nuland, *Time Special Issue,* Fall 1996.

since 1920, some of which we have come to take for granted (eg, antibiotics and DNA). You readily can see that in 1960 there was no quest for human organs or critical decisions regarding the life status of a possible donor. We were not able to fertilize ova outside the human body and transfer the fertilized eggs in a woman's uterus until 1978. Certain life-saving machines (eg, ventilators) and miracle drugs (eg, some of the chemotherapeutic agents used today) were not available to offer extension of life. Technologies such as magnetic resonance imaging (MRI), which gives us information about the structure of tissues and allows for early diagnosis and treatment, were not available. Positron Emission Tomography (PET) was to follow. As advances occur in medical practice, we must challenge ourselves to think through our own beliefs and feelings about these practices, especially as they relate to quality of life and patients' choices.

BIOETHICAL ISSUES RELATED TO THE BEGINNING OF LIFE

Many bioethical issues with which we wrestle are focused on the process by which conception occurs, the products of conception, and the beginning of life, including whether it should occur. Much of the early debate related to family planning and conception.

Family Planning

Family planning refers to the various methods used to control the size of one's family or to space births. Although we often think of it as synonymous with contraception, in reality it is much broader. For some it could include abortion, for others it might involve adoption. It can employ natural methods, pharmaceutical preparations, or barriers. The religious beliefs and personal values of individuals usually influence the methods and approaches used.

In 1798, in an essay titled, "On Population," Thomas Malthus, a minister in the Church of England, expressed deep concern about a population that was growing faster than were the resources to support it. To offset this problem, he advocated late marriage, no marriage, or sexual abstinence in marriage. No forms of contraception as we know them today were available, although women sometimes developed homemade devices in an effort to prevent pregnancy.

In 1873, the U. S. Congress passed the Comstock Act, prohibiting the sale, mailing, or importing of "obscene literature and articles for immoral acts." All contraceptives and any material teaching about sexuality or birth control were encompassed in this prohibition. Those who continued to import and distribute birth control literature or contraceptives were breaking the law. You may have read about Margaret Sanger (1883–1966), a nurse who championed for contraceptive practices in the early 1900s. Although charged and sentenced for disseminating information on birth control, she went on to establish the National Committee on Federal Legislation for Birth Control, the forerunner of the Planned Parenthood Federation. In 1938, in Sanger's landmark case, a federal judge dismissed this federal law as unconstitutional, thus ending the federal ban on contraceptives. Although some states were more liberal than others, and some changed sooner than others, the state that had prohibitions against contraceptives for the longest time was Connecticut.

It was not until 1965, in the case of Griswold and Buxton vs. the State of Connecticut, that the Supreme Court of the United States overrode the state law forbidding sale or teaching about contraception and established the right of the individual to obtain medical contraceptive advice and counseling. (*http://womenshistory.about.com/library/ency/blwh_comstock.htm*).

Much of the controversy over birth control is related to the theologic teachings of some religious groups, who believe interference with procreative powers is wrong. The Roman Catholic Church has strongly advocated that the natural purpose of sexual activity is to create new life and nothing should try to interfere with that potential.

The members of the Church of Jesus Christ of Latter Day Saints (Mormons), although less adamant in their teachings, also discourage the use of artificial birth control under normal circumstances. Some conservative Protestant Christians and conservative Muslims also advocate allowing God to plan families and do not use birth control methods. Orthodox Judaism has specific rules about when sexual intercourse may or may not occur; these rules have the effect of supporting sexual activity when a woman is fertile. The Orthodox Jewish population is so small in proportion to other groups that the impact is not significant.

The opposite end of the spectrum is found in those who are strong advocates of zero population growth and encourage individuals to limit families to one or two children in all instances. Others are so concerned about population growth and the state of the world that they decide to have no children.

During your career as a nurse, you will care for patients who represent many differing viewpoints. When caring for individuals whose personal beliefs prohibit the use of artificial birth control, you must be knowledgeable about natural methods of family spacing, such as fertility awareness methods, that will meet the patient's needs. If your personal views regarding contraception differ, your values must be set aside as you focus on assisting the patient in selecting a method that is compatible with the patient's personal values and beliefs.

Among the methods of birth control available to those who have no religious sanction against their use, not all methods are acceptable to all people. For example, some find the intrauterine device unacceptable because they believe that interfering with a fertilized egg should be viewed as abortion (researchers are not entirely sure how the intrauterine device works, but some suggest that it prevents the fertilized egg from implanting in the wall of the uterus). Those who find abortion an acceptable method of coping with an unwanted pregnancy represent another set of values.

Central to all discussions of contraception is the issue of freedom of a woman to control her own body. This immediately raises a second question: Who has that right? Is it the woman's right because it is her body? What if the partners disagree about family planning practices? Does one have more say than the other? What if one partner wants to have a family and the other does not?

Abortion

In Pennsylvania in August 2002, a temporary injunction blocked a young single woman from securing an abortion. The injunction was issued in response to a lawsuit filed by her boyfriend (from whom she was estranged), who wanted the pregnancy continued. Appeals were filed. A week later, a judge dismissed the injunction and was critical of the fact that the young woman had experienced emotional distress and possible risk because of the delay. She miscarried (aborted spontaneously) the afternoon of this ruling.

Problems of Consent and Family Planning

The ability to procreate precedes what is generally considered legal age; therefore, we find ourselves grappling with problems related to age of consent, its definition, and the role of the parents and the family. In legal terms, the **age of consent** is the age at which one is capable of giving deliberate and voluntary agreement. This implies physical and mental ability and the freedom to act and make decisions. The age of consent is established state by state and varies from age 14 in Hawaii and Pennsylvania to age 18 in fourteen other states. Most states have established age 16 as the age of consent (*totse.com*, 2002).

Until children reach the age of consent, parents are required to give consent for the care of their children. Implicit in this is the assumption that the parents have the best interests of the child at heart and that they are better qualified than the child to make decisions in the child's best interest. Generally speaking, the parents are responsible for the care (including medical costs) and education of the minor. However, today's trends cloud the issue as we struggle with "rights."

With regard to research, federal guidelines required that children with a mental age of 7 years or older be informed about proposed treatment or research and agree or concur with the decision made by the parent or guardian. This is referred to as *assent.*

Another example is the concept of the **emancipated minor**. As previously discussed, emancipated minors (an individual legally under the age of majority), who are financially independent, married, or in the military, may give consent for medical treatment, including all treatment for sexually transmitted diseases, contraception, and pregnancy-related concerns, regardless of their parent's or legal guardian's knowledge or agreement. Most states recognize some form of emancipation of minors.

Mature minors are "individuals in their mid- to late teens who are considered mature enough to comprehend a physician's recommendations and give **informed consent**" (Judson & Hicks, 1999). Under this definition, most states allow mature minors to seek treatment for sexually transmitted diseases, drug or alcohol abuse, contraception, and pregnancy care without the consent of a parent or guardian. The most liberal legislation applies to the treatment of sexually transmitted disease and is endorsed by most states. Minors of any age can consent to diagnosis and care for sexually transmitted diseases. For more discussion of age of consent and informed consent, see Chapter 8.

In some instances, this autonomy of the mature minor may bring health providers into a conflict between two laws. Although the mature minor may be able to consent to treatment for sexually transmitted disease, if the health provider believes this to have been contracted through sexual abuse of the minor, the provider is required to report that abuse. Most authorities direct that child abuse laws take precedence over privacy laws.

Certainly, there are times when physicians' ethical and moral convictions prevent them from complying with adolescents' requests for care. This occurs most commonly in response to requests for contraceptive pills and abortions. In such cases, physicians often discuss their beliefs with the adolescent, and frequently refer the patient to a medical colleague for assistance.

A major controversy exists around the role of the school in the sex education of high school students and the dispensing of contraceptives through high school health clinics. The advent of emergency contraception in the form of birth control pills taken in high dose for a limited time after intercourse has added another dimension to these ethical issues about birth control and minors. In some states, emergency contraception is available directly from a pharmacy without a physician's prescription. The pharmacist, therefore, is drawn into the decision-making web.

Those who are concerned about the high incidence of teenage pregnancies and sexually transmitted diseases argue that the information must be disseminated, regardless of who does it. Others believe that this promotes erosion of the role of the family, and worry that the indiscriminate dispensing of contraceptives encourages promiscuity among teenagers. Concern about the spread of AIDS has done much to alter thinking, particularly regarding the dispensing of condoms.

Abortion

What has been said about contraception becomes an even greater issue when related to abortion. In medical terms, **abortion** is the termination of pregnancy before the viability of the fetus—that is, any time before the end of the 6th month of gestation. An abortion may occur spontaneously as a result of natural causes (**spontaneous abortion**). A pregnancy may be interrupted deliberately for medical reasons (**therapeutic abortion**), or for personal reasons (**elective abortion**). It is the last two classifications (especially the latter) that induce bioethical debate. Ethically, the entire debate revolves around the definition of human life and when the fetus should be considered a human being. There are two major schools of thought about the nature of the fetus: one supports the belief that new life occurs at the moment of conception; the other contends that human life does not exist until the fetus is sufficiently developed biologically to sustain itself outside the uterus.

The legal aspects of abortion were clarified on January 22, 1973, when the U. S. Supreme Court ruled in the case of Roe vs. Wade that any state laws that prohibited or restricted a woman's right to obtain an abortion during the first 3 months of pregnancy were unconstitutional. In this case, the Supreme Court recognized that, during the first trimester of pregnancy, a privacy right exists that allows an individual woman to make the final decision with regard to what happens to her own body (Roe vs. Wade, 1973). Certain time limitations as to when an abortion can be performed were determined to be necessary, because of the state's interest in protecting potential life. At the period of viability, the state's interest took precedence over the mother's desire for an abortion. Supreme Court Justice Blackmun, in writing an opinion that met with agreement from six other justices in Roe vs. Wade, decided that a woman's decision to terminate a pregnancy was encompassed by the right to privacy, up to a certain point in the development of the fetus (Blackmun, 1981). It was established that this lasted until the end of the first trimester. Thus, the courts ruled that the state could not prevent abortions during the first trimester, but could regulate abortions in the second and third trimesters of pregnancy, at which point the interests of the fetus took precedence over those of the mother. In 1992, the Court reaffirmed the basic principles of the 1973 decision.

Despite these rulings, the issue of abortion continues to surface, with new legislation and rulings being considered each year and the issue being debated each presidential election. In 1977, Congress barred the use of Medicaid funds for abortion, with the exception of those done for therapeutic reasons and in other specific circumstances. However, the legal positions do little to help us deal with bioethical concerns. Many people view termination of life at any point after conception as murder. The Roman Catholic Church firmly upholds its traditional position on abortion. Many conservative Protestant Christian groups also are active in opposing abortion.

Some believe that although abortion is not desirable, under certain circumstances it would be justifiable—for example, in cases of rape or incest, or in instances where amniocentesis indicates that a fetus would be born retarded or genetically defective. Others think that early termination of a pregnancy might be acceptable, but that termination after the 4th month would not be appropriate.

Those who support abortion without restriction usually do so because they believe that women should have control over their own bodies, which is tied to issues of privacy. They further argue that the quality of life of an "unwanted" child, or a child born with a deformity or genetic defect, may be minimal. Interesting and challenging cases have emerged with respect to this concept. These are generally known as **wrongful birth** cases, and are based on the principle that it is wrong to give birth to children (such as those with birth defects or limitations that can be diagnosed or anticipated before birth) who will not have the same quality of life as other children.

As a nurse, these issues present some difficult questions you will need to answer. To what extent do you believe you can personally participate in the abortion procedure? Would the stage of pregnancy and type of procedure make a difference? As a nurse, you have the right to refuse, based on your own ethical beliefs, to be involved in abortion procedures or the care of patients seeking abortion. Employment in certain areas (eg, labor and delivery rooms), however, may rest on the nurse's willingness and ability to assist with abortions and to give conscientious care to the patient who has had an abortion. Some religiously affiliated hospitals have elected to close their labor and delivery services rather than perform abortions.

Although textbooks traditionally have defined the age of viability (the earliest age at which fetuses could survive if they were born at that time) as 20- to 24-weeks' gestation, technology has increased the ability to enable very-low-birth-weight and premature babies to survive. The age of viability is less clear than it once seemed. Attention has been focused on incidents in which an abortion was attempted toward the end of the 5th or 6th month of gestation, and the fetus was born showing signs of life. Is the doctor or nurse obligated to try to keep the infant alive? Is the doctor or nurse guilty of malpractice, or even murder, if he or she does anything to hasten the infant's death? Should this infant be considered a human being? Does the infant have "rights"? Does the mother have legal possession of and responsibility for the child if, in fact, she attempted to abort the fetus? This issue, like so many others, probably will be settled in a court of law while we continue to debate it ethically.

The abortion issue also is complicated by consent problems. Many states have recognized the special problems related to parental consent for teenagers and to health care involving pregnancy and have legislated special exceptions. Nurses practicing in areas that provide abortions to minors must be concerned about parental consent and counseling issues because of the wide variations in state statutes governing abortions (Killion & Dempski, 2000).

In the last few years, the abortion issue has been made more complex by research that would use the fetal tissue resulting from an abortion for stem cell research and therapeutic purposes. We will discuss stem cell research later in this chapter.

As a society, it seems likely that we will continue to debate the issue of abortion. Ultimately, the decision rests with the individual who must make the choice. Certainly the legal entanglements become more complex with each court ruling, and will be limited only by our willingness to challenge other aspects of the question.

Critical Thinking Activity

Select one of the positions taken regarding abortion. Defend your position, providing a strong rationale for your thinking. Examine your thinking for biases. Why did you develop those biases? Discuss the topic of abortion with a classmate who holds a different position, remembering that all persons are entitled to their own viewpoints.

Prenatal Testing

The ability to identify birth defects and genetic disorders of the fetus has created a different dimension in the abortion debates. A major breakthrough in our ability to detect genetic abnormalities in the fetus occurred in the 1970s with the development of techniques to carry out amniocentesis. **Amniocentesis** is performed between 14 and 20 weeks after the woman's last menstrual period. Amniotic fluid is aspirated and analyzed. From these cells, many genetic problems of the fetus can be diagnosed prenatally, including such conditions as Down syndrome (which accounts for about one third of the cases of mental retardation in Western countries), hemophilia, Duchenne's muscular dystrophy, Tay-Sachs disease, and problems related to the brain and spinal column (eg, anencephaly and spina bifida).

The potential for Down syndrome, a condition occurring with higher frequency in mothers in their early 40s and older, is the most common reason for seeking amniocentesis. When amniocentesis reveals a genetic disease, a woman will often choose to have an abortion. Rothstein (1990, p. 39) reports that "termination rates for muscular dystrophy, cystic fibrosis, and alpha and beta thalassemia are nearly 100%; they are 60% for hemophilia; and 50% for sickle cell anemia." Some couples request amniocentesis if they are in an "at-risk" group, but state that they would not abort the fetus under any circumstances; instead, they believe that an additional 5 months will give them time to adjust to the presence of a serious condition before the baby is born. Usually doctors are reluctant to do an amniocentesis under these circumstances, because the risk of performing the procedure, although small, does not seem justified.

Chorionic villus sampling (CVS) involves securing a sample of chorionic villi from the developing placenta. A sample of the placenta is obtained either vaginally or percutaneously and then analyzed genetically. Like amniocentesis, these tests can predict birth defects and certain diseases. CVS can be performed earlier than an amniocentesis, usually in the 10th or 11th week of pregnancy.

Today almost all pregnant women have a **sonogram** (ultrasound). It is most likely used for fetal assessment at least once in a normal pregnancy, more often in those who have a risk factor. The sonogram can detect a number of abnormal conditions in addition to assuring that the pregnancy is progressing normally.

The advent of amniocentesis, CVS, and ultrasound heralded the development of yet another medical specialty: prenatal surgery. Although the specialty is still new, some corrective surgery is being performed on infants while they are in their intrauterine environment.

Some people are concerned about prenatal testing because of where it might lead. Is mass genetic screening a possibility? **Genetic screening** makes it possible to determine if persons are predisposed to certain diseases and whether a couple might have the possibility of giving birth to a genetically impaired child. Ethicists have expressed concern about the possibility of the government making diagnostic amniocentesis and abortion of all defective fetuses mandatory. Others argue against genetic screening, counseling, and amniocentesis because of the stress it places on a marriage, and because of the guilt placed on the partner carrying the defective gene (when that can be determined). They argue that there are some things we are better off not knowing. Genetic screening also may result in at least one of the partners (often the carrier) seeking voluntary sterilization to prevent pregnancies with less than favorable outcomes. Despite concerns, amniocentesis has become a fairly common test offered to mothers who are in an "at-risk" group.

As a nurse, you may care for clients with varying viewpoints regarding prenatal screening and abortion, and you will also have your own values to consider. Will your values conflict with those of your clients? Are you obligated to advocate for a client when the client's request is squarely in opposition to what you believe to be right? Should you try to sway a woman who is indecisive toward either decision?

Sterilization

For years, surgical operations resulting in permanent **sterilization** have been performed for therapeutic purposes, such as the removal of reproductive organs to halt the spread of cancer or other pathologic processes. Although problems may arise for the patient and family as a result of such surgeries, usually they are resolved without serious ethical debate, depending on the family's religious values, the patient's body concept, family plans, and personal values.

With increasing frequency, voluntary sterilization has been requested by individuals to terminate reproductive ability. Although sometimes reversible, patients are counseled that these surgical procedures, whether performed on men or women, should be considered permanent and irreversible. Many people see it as the prerogative of an individual; others find any type of sterilization in conflict with their religious and moral beliefs. Sterilization may pose few problems for those who are satisfied with the number of children they have had or who are adults who have determined that they do not want to have children. People may decide not to have children for a variety of reasons, including personal health status, familial genetic disorders, or simply not wishing to parent. Full and informed consent is required of the person being sterilized; however, health care providers often prefer to obtain assent from the spouse if the person is married to avoid subsequent emotional and family problems. Some people question whether a man or woman should be free to make such a decision without consulting the partner, but doing so is completely legal. A few states still have laws forbidding voluntary sterilization for contraceptive purposes, but these laws may not be enforced. In 1935, Oklahoma passed a law that was not struck down by the U. S. Supreme Court until 1942. It resulted in 13 states' establishing laws specifically permitting sterilization of repeat criminals (Lombardo, 2002).

Chemical sterilization, sometimes referred to as chemical castration, refers to providing drugs that decrease libido, sperm production, and sexual ability. This approach has been used in individuals with a history of repeated rape, who are often incarcerated during the time they are receiving chemical sterilization. In some instances, this has been recommended or even requested by those individuals who were convicted of repeated sexual offenses, particularly those against children. Despite the criminal history, some challenge the ethics of this action.

Because sex crimes are related to power and aggression, and not just to sex drive, this remains a controversial issue.

Eugenics

Eugenics is a term that has had different meanings in different eras but is generally thought of as the study of methods to improve inherited human characteristics. The idea of improving the quality of the human race is at least as old as Plato, who wrote on the topic in his *Republic*. The philosophic beliefs of certain 18th-century thinkers about the notion of human perfectibility were central to the eugenics movement, which is thought to have started in the 19th century. Charles Darwin's cousin, Francis Galton, who created the term eugenics, based his work on Darwin's theory of evolution. When Mendel's law provided a framework for explaining the transmission and distribution of traits from one generation to another, the eugenics movement took hold. Organizations focusing on eugenics were created around the world.

The center of the eugenics movement in the United States was the Eugenics Record Office in Cold Spring Harbor, New York, and its leader was geneticist Charles Davenport. Until the early 1930s, the eugenics movement grew. Eugenicists presented a two-part policy. Positive eugenics encouraged increasing the desirable traits in the population by urging "worthy" parents. "Superior" couples were encouraged to have more children. Negative eugenics advocated the elimination of unwanted characteristics from the nation by discouraging "unworthy" parents.

Negative eugenics included a variety of approaches, such as marriage restriction, sterilization, and permanent custody of "defectives." Many eugenicists were actively involved in other issues of the day, including prohibition, birth control, and legislation that would outlaw miscegenation (ie, marriage between two persons of different races, especially between white and black people in the United States). Indiana enacted the first law permitting sterilization on eugenic grounds in 1907; Connecticut followed soon after. In 1914, Harry Laughlin, who worked at the Eugenics Record Office, published a Model Eugenical Sterilization Law that proposed sterilization of the "socially inadequate," a group that included "feebleminded, insane, criminalistic, epileptic, inebriate, diseased, blind, deaf, deformed and dependent" including "orphans, ne'er-do-wells, tramps, the homeless and paupers." By the time the law was published in 1914, 12 states had enacted sterilization laws; by 1937, 31 of the 48 states had compulsory laws. By 1924, approximately 3,000 people in America had been involuntarily sterilized (Lombardo, 2002). This number increased to more than 60,000. The Immigration Restriction Act of 1924 also was passed at this time, dramatically limiting the immigration of people from southern and eastern Europe on the grounds that they were "biologically inferior." The trend in recent times has been for states to modify, repeal, or ignore sterilization laws.

The eugenics movement also grew in Germany. In 1933, Hitler sanctioned the Hereditary Health Law, or the Eugenic Sterilization Law, thus ensuring that the "less worthy" members of the Third Reich did not pass on their genes. This action resulted in the sterilization of several hundred thousand people and helped lead to the death camps. By the late 1930s, eugenics in the United States began a tremendous decline. Americans became concerned about the concept of a "master race."

When the eugenic movement was rekindled in the 1960s, it had a different focus—one related to genetic counseling and genetic research. Today, a couple giving birth to a child with a congenital anomaly (or who realize that one of them is carrying a genetic trait that could cause a child to have a congenital anomaly) might voluntarily seek genetic counseling, and possibly opt for the sterilization of one of the partners. Again, this approach offends the religious and moral values of some, but generally it is viewed as the couple's prerogative.

Citing a presentation given by Roberts at a bioethics course held in Washington D.C. in June 2000, Burkhardt and Nathaniel (2002) observe that the early birth control movement in the United States became tied to eugenics. This is supported by Randall (2002), who further states that in 1939, the Birth Control Federation of America planned a "Negro Project" to limit reproduction by blacks, who were seen as a portion of the population least fit for parenthood. The first public birth control clinics were established in the South, where poor black women were being coercively sterilized through government welfare programs. This resulted in a lawsuit that prompted federal regulation requiring informed consent and a waiting period before sterilization.

In states that permit sterilization of a person who is not competent to give consent, questions can be raised about who may request sterilization, who may sign the consent, and who must fund the procedure. Some states allow a guardian to make such a decision, but other states specifically prohibit guardians from consenting to sterilization. As the result of a court decision, federal dollars may not be used for sterilization of a person who cannot give personal consent. However, the taxpayer contributes to the cost of institutionalizing people who are not capable of living independently in today's society, and caring for those with severe illnesses and disabilities.

The question must be raised regarding the ability of two individuals who are mentally retarded to care for children they may parent. Therefore, it is not only a personal concern, but also society's concern.

In Vitro Fertilization

In 1978 in England, much attention focused on the birth of the first child who was conceived in a test tube, a process we refer to as **in vitro fertilization** (IVF). Due to a blockage in the mother's fallopian tubes, conception in her tubes was impossible. The ovum was removed from the mother, united with the father's sperm in a laboratory setting, and then implanted in the mother's uterus, where it grew to term and was delivered by cesarean section. Today, IVF and similar procedures (Table 10-2) help many infertile couples.

Many herald this as one of medical science's great advances. For others, it raises many concerns. Several fertilized ova are usually returned to the uterus to assure that at least one will survive. If more than one implant successfully, it is possible for the mother to have multiple births. Multiple births seldom go full term, resulting in financial and emotional costs. When the number of implanted embryos is too great, consideration is given to aborting several of them to improve the chances of full development for the remaining ones; this creates additional ethical dilemmas for the family.

What should be done with fertilized ova that are not returned to the uterus? (There are an estimated 100,000 to 200,000 such embryos in the United States.) Should they be thrown

TABLE 10-2		TYPES OF ASSISTED REPRODUCTIVE TECHNIQUES	
NAME	**INITIALS**	**DESCRIPTION**	**FIRST USED WITH HUMANS**
Artificial Insemination: Homologous	AIH	Husband's semen is collected and then deposited at the cervical os or in the wife's uterus by mechanical means.	United States, 1884
Artificial Insemination: Donor	AID	Donor's semen is collected and deposited at the cervical os or in the woman's uterus by mechanical means.	United States, 1884
In Vitro Fertilization	IVF	After heavily medicating the woman with hormones to trigger ovulation, eggs are harvested and fertilized with father's sperm in a laboratory. Several of the resulting embryos are implanted in the mother's uterus.	England, 1978
Gamete Intrafallopian Transfer	GIFT	Eggs and sperm are inserted directly into the woman's fallopian tubes using a laparoscope. Embryos travel to the uterus for implantation.	United States, 1984
Zygote Intrafallopian Transfer	ZIFT	Eggs and sperm are combined in the laboratory. The resulting zygotes are then inserted into the woman's fallopian tubes and travel to the uterus for implantation.	Belgium, 1989
Preimplantation Genetic Diagnosis	PGD	Egg and sperm are united in the laboratory and the embryo is allowed to develop to 4–8 cells. One or two cells are removed and examined for harmful genes. Defective embryos are discarded; healthy ones are implanted in the woman's uterus.	United States, 1991
Immature Egg Harvest	IEH	Similar to IVF, the eggs are harvested from the ovaries while still immature, are cultured in the laboratory, fertilized, and transferred into the woman's uterus.	South Korea, 1991
Intracytoplasmic Sperm Injection	ICSI	In a laboratory setting, a single sperm cell is injected into an egg and then both are implanted in the woman's uterus.	Belgium, 1992

away? Given to a donor? Used for research? Should tax dollars be used to fund this type of research? If frozen, how long should they remain frozen? What should be done with them at the end of that time? Is discarding the embryos the moral equivalent to having an abortion?

Some couples with embryos to spare have chosen to give the embryos to another infertile couple. The fertilized ovum is implanted into the uterus of the infertile female and often results in a full-term pregnancy. Recently, a $1-million federal program was funded to promote the practice. Although opponents of abortion rights may view this as a better alternative than stem-cell research, in which embryos are destroyed, the moral and legal implications comprise a gray area. Are these embryos people, property, or their own entities worthy of respect? Like other adoptions, should a home study and background check be completed on the family receiving the fertilized ova? Some believe embryo donation is different because most state laws presume that a woman who carries and gives birth to a child has earned the right to be a parent.

Other offshoots of in vitro fertilization allow people who are carrying a severe genetic disease to be assured that their children will not be affected by the condition or carry the defective gene. Fertilized ova are examined for possible disease before being implanted in the uterus; those that are diseased would not be implanted.

EXAMPLE

In Vitro Fertilization

A Louisiana couple decided, after the death of their 3-year-old daughter from Tay-Sachs disease, not to risk having more children. They learned that they both carried one copy of the Tay-Sachs gene, which would result in a 1-in-4 chance of conceiving a child with the disease. Shortly thereafter, the couple were notified that a procedure had been developed through IVF and high-tech genetic testing (known as preimplantation genetic diagnosis [PGD]) whereby technicians can remove one or two embryonic cells from those fertilized in vitro and test for the harmful gene. This allows only healthy embryos to be transferred back to the woman's uterus. This procedure resulted in the birth of a healthy child for this couple, and one who is not a carrier of Tay-Sachs disease.

As wonderful as this may seem, concerns exist regarding what some would call the misuse of IVF. In Italy, a 62-year-old woman became pregnant using donated eggs and IVF before implantation in her uterus. She gave birth by cesarean section in 1994. A 59-year-old woman in England delivered twins by this method. A record was set for what is thought to be the oldest woman to give birth to a healthy infant, when it was announced in April 1997 that a 63-year-old woman had given birth via cesarean section on November 7, 1996. The woman, married and previously childless, is said to have told doctors she was 50 and had medical records attesting to that age. (The medical center where the IVF occurred sets an age limit of 55 on accepting patients.) A donor egg and the husband's sperm were used for the IVF (Roan, 1997).

In some countries, legislation has been passed to prevent such situations. In January 1994, the French Senate opted to prohibit the use of reproductive options in certain cases (Capron, 1994). One can readily identify some of the difficulties in starting the mothering process at age 62 or 63, not the least of which would be living long enough to see the child reach adulthood. Quality-of-life issues also may be involved. If the mother is 62 when the child is born, she will be 67 or 68 when the child starts school and 75 when the child becomes a teenager.

Other concerns focus on the fear that PGD will be used to make "perfect babies" or for sex selection, even when there is not a medical reason (such as hemophilia, Tay-Sachs, or sickle-cell anemia) for such action. A case was reported in Chicago in which a 33-year-old married geneticist used PGD to selectively screen for an embryo that would be free of the gene responsible for early-onset Alzheimer's.

Artificial Insemination

Other discussions revolve around the topic of **artificial insemination**, which is the planting of sperm in the woman's body to facilitate conception. Although we tend to think of this as a fairly new procedure, the first time artificial insemination is said to have been used was in

Philadelphia in 1884. There are two different kinds of artificial insemination: homologous (Artificial Insemination Homologous—AIH), in which the husband's sperm is used, and heterologous (Artificial Insemination Donor—AID), in which a donor's sperm is used. Using the husband's sperm is by far the most common and creates the fewest problems legally, ethically, and morally. In some instances, the sperm from the husband and the sperm from a donor with similar physical characteristics are mixed together. As a result, if conception occurs, the couple could easily believe it was the husband's sperm that was accepted by the ovum.

Although some religious groups may have objections, few concerns arise when the husband's sperm is used. That is not true with donor sperm. If the woman is artificially inseminated with donor sperm without the knowledge and consent of her partner, the problems are multiplied. If conception occurs and the child is not biologically that of the husband, can one say that adultery has occurred? Others suggest that the husband should legally adopt the child. To some extent, this helps to clarify issues of inheritance, child support (if the couple should later divorce), and the legal status of the child.

Single Parents

Another ethical issue has emerged as our society has developed greater acceptance for single-parent families. More single women are trying to adopt children, and some see artificial insemination as a logical solution. In some instances, these women are also lesbians. One of the couple will seek artificial insemination with a donor sperm; the child then is raised as family in the lesbian relationship. Providing a parenting option to lesbians is totally unacceptable to many people. Aside from the emotion that the issue of a lesbian relationship may introduce, there is the argument against the artificial insemination of any unmarried woman on the basis that the traditional two-parent family composed of a man and woman is in the best interests of all children.

Recent years also have witnessed the adoption of children by gay couples. Such instances do not involve artificial insemination but, rather, a formal adoption process through the courts. Again, some of the same arguments are set forth against this process as for lesbian parenthood.

Surrogate Mothers

A **surrogate mother** is one who agrees to bear a child conceived through artificial insemination and to relinquish the baby at birth to others for rearing. This practice has occurred with increasing frequency and in a variety of relationships and presents unique problems. The following represents one such situation.

EXAMPLE

Surrogate Mothering Within a Family

A 47-year-old woman agreed to serve as gestational surrogate for her own daughter, whose uterus had been removed because of disease. The daughter's eggs were inseminated with her husband's sperm and the embryos were then implanted in the mother, who gave birth to triplets when she was 48. Thus, this woman became the gestational mother and the genetic grandmother to triplets.

As you see, these artificial means of reproduction have complicated even the language that we are accustomed to using. The term biologic is no longer adequate for making some critical conceptual distinctions. Macklin (1991, p. 6) states, "The techniques of egg retrieval, in vitro fertilization (IVF), and gamete intrafallopian transfer (GIFT), now make it possible for two different women to make a biological contribution to the creation of a new life." Macklin further believes that the woman who contributes her womb during gestation is also a biologic mother. We find terms such as genetic mother used to refer to the individual contributing the ovum, and gestational mother used to refer to the individual who provides the uterus in which the child develops. In some instances the surrogate mother is both.

Surrogate mothering within a family has caused fewer problems than have been seen when a stranger serves as the surrogate mother. Ethically, carrying a child for a family member out of love and concern and planning to remain in that child's life as part of the family reflect a commitment to a child and respect for the personhood of the child. The majority of serious conflicts have occurred in situations in which a woman has been paid to serve as a surrogate mother. A formal, contractual relationship is usually established. The couple who wish to have the child agree to pay all expenses associated with the pregnancy, and to pay the surrogate mother an agreed sum for her time and involvement. The contract must be carefully drawn up because it is illegal in all states to sell a child.

Many ethicists view parenting for pay as a gray ethical area that may fail to value the personhood of the child. This becomes apparent when things do not go as planned. What happens if the child is born with an anomaly, as occurred with a New York couple in 1982? How are these dilemmas to be solved? What is to happen to the child? Who bears the responsibility?

EXAMPLE

Surrogate Mothering and a Child With an Anomaly

A man paid a woman to be artificially inseminated with his sperm and to carry his child. When the child was born with microcephaly (an unusually small brain), the man rejected the infant, stating that he could not be the father. The surrogate mother and her husband also did not want to accept the responsibility for parenting the child.

Recently, problems associated with surrogate mothering have centered around the surrogate mother's unwillingness to give up the child after birth (Fig. 10-1).

EXAMPLE

Surrogate Mothering and Custody

"Baby M," as the court called her, was born to a surrogate mother after she was impregnated with the sperm of a man for whom she agreed to bear the child. This man's wife, a pediatrician, chose not to bear a child because she had multiple sclerosis. Although signed agreements existed, the surrogate mother broke the contract within days of the baby's birth and asked for custody of the child.

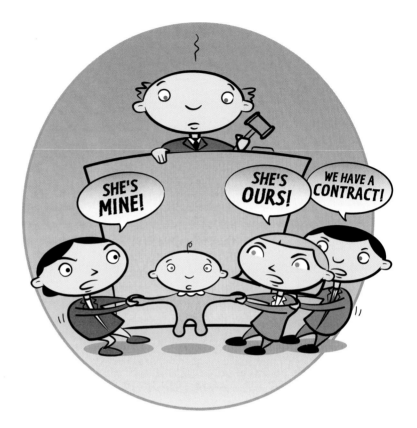

FIGURE 10-1 Complexities arise when surrogate mothers are unwilling to relinquish the infant after birth.

Critical Thinking Activity

What safeguards would you recommend regarding IVF, artificial insemination, and surrogate mothers to ensure respect for the human condition? Be specific about how you believe these safeguards would be effective. Reflect on your proposals. Are there any you would change? Discuss your proposals with a classmate.

Sperm Banks

Another aspect of the artificial insemination issue is that of sperm banks. Sperm banks have been established in different parts of the United States for various reasons. Men who want to have a vasectomy may contribute to a sperm bank "just in case" they change their minds in the future. Men who will be exposed to high levels of radiation in their work, or during treatment of disease, may wish to have sperm stored because radiation may cause mutation of the genes or result in sterility. This allows them to father children at a later date without concern about the effect on the sperm.

In most cases, the medical community establishes sperm banks so that sperm is available for artificial inseminations. In California, a sperm bank was started that contains only sperm of outstanding and brilliant men. The idea was to create children with this sperm who will be genetically endowed with greater intelligence and creativity. Many find this unacceptable because it brings up the issue of creating a super race. Concerns also have been raised regarding the possible number of offspring in a single community who might be genetically related without knowing it.

Are there ethical implications for the man who becomes a sperm donor and is the biologic father of a child, but assumes no ethical responsibility for who receives that sperm or for the resulting child and, in fact, has no knowledge regarding the use of his sperm? Some ask how a man can ethically father offspring and have no responsibility for their well-being.

The Right to Genetic Information

All the issues of artificial insemination using donor sperm, surrogate mothering, single parenting, and sperm banks are further complicated by a recent trend toward providing individuals with information regarding their familial background, makeup, and history. You can readily anticipate the problems that would be created if donor sperm were used for insemination. In some instances, no record has been maintained regarding who donated the sperm.

As society emphasizes the importance of the role of fathers and the rights of children to know their family heritage, will anonymous sperm donation remain an option? How many individuals would be willing to donate sperm if it were to include a detailed background? What might be the ultimate legal involvement? On the other hand, what are the rights of the child to know what genetic factors he or she carries? Whose rights should take precedence? Oregon has passed legislation opening birth records for adults adopted as infants to learn their backgrounds, even though anonymity of the birth mother was guaranteed at the time of the adoption. Will tracking of sperm donors also become a concern in the future?

BIOETHICAL ISSUES CONCERNING DEATH

One of the most important areas of ethical debate revolves around the topic of death and dying. As mentioned earlier, the advent of life-saving procedures and mechanical devices has required redefinition of the term death, caused us to examine the meaning of "quality of life," and created debates about "death with dignity."

Also associated with the issue of death are several companion concerns that did not exist before the technologic advances that occurred in the past 15 years. Some of these concerns relate to euthanasia, the right to refuse treatment, and the right to die. Other concerns relate to organs retrieved from the dying, because of the scarcity of these medical resources. Generally, the demand for donated organs far exceeds the number of organs available to meet the needs. Superimposed on all these issues is that of informed consent.

Death Defined

Until recently, the most widely accepted definition of death was from Black's Law Dictionary, which defines death as the irreversible cessation of the vital functions of respiration, circulation, and pulsation. This traditional view of death served us well until the development of ventilators, pacemakers, and other advances in medical science that made it possible to sustain these functions indefinitely. We also have learned that various parts of the body die at different times. The central nervous system is one of the most vulnerable areas, and brain cells can be irreversibly damaged if deprived of oxygen, while other parts of the body will continue to function.

Newer definitions of death have been built around the concept of human potential—meaning the potential of the human body to interact with the environment and with other people, to respond to stimuli, and to communicate. When these abilities are lacking, there is said to be no potential. Because this potential is directly related to brain function, the method most often used to assess capability is electroencephalography. Brain activity, with few exceptions, is said to be nonexistent when flat electroencephalographic (EEG) tracings are obtained over a given period, often 48 hours. At this point, the person may be considered dead, although machines may be supporting the vital functions of respiration and circulation. Many institutions now accept this definition of cerebral death and use it as a basis for turning off respirators and stopping other treatments. It is also used as a basis for determining death when there is a desire to recover organs from the patient.

Planning for End-of-Life Issues

Increasing emphasis is being placed on prior planning for end-of-life issues. Identifying futile treatments is one aspect of this process. Another important consideration relates to patient self-determination regarding these issues. Many hope that the use of such planning will decrease the ethical dilemmas in end-of-life situations.

FUTILE TREATMENTS

Futile treatments are those that "cannot, within a reasonable possibility, cure, ameliorate, improve or restore a quality of life that would be satisfactory to the patient" (Hudson, 1994b). For example, when an individual is dying of terminal cancer, treatment for a respiratory infection may be deemed futile because it will not alter the fact that the person is dying and will not restore a satisfactory quality of life. Identifying whether further treatment is futile may be extremely difficult. However, Schneiderman and Jecker (1993) suggest that if, in the last 100 cases of the same nature, there was no change in the outcome based on the treatment, it can be considered futile. Others take a position that treatment never can be declared futile. In their thinking, the future cannot be predicted accurately, and if there cannot be absolute certainty about the outcome, then futility cannot be clearly identified.

Other problems may arise when futility is declared. Does a patient have a right to treatment even if it has been identified as futile? What about cost considerations? Should insurance companies be required to pay for treatment that has been classified as futile? What about Medicare or Medicaid? Should there be differences in decisions based on age or quality of life?

Critical Thinking Activity

Do you think that factors such as ability to pay, treatment of children or younger adults versus the elderly, the cost of the treatment, and the percentage of time the treatment is effective should be issues considered when deciding whether treatment is futile? Provide a rationale for each answer. What are your biases?

ETHICAL ISSUES SURROUNDING ADVANCE DIRECTIVES AND LIVING WILLS

When end-of-life concerns arise, the patient is often unconscious or not able to participate in decision-making. This raises the question of obtaining consent. A patient may have left advance directives such as a living will or durable power of attorney for health care, indicating preferences and identifying a substitutionary decision-maker (see Chapter 8). If the patient has not done this, the law in each state specifies who may give consent when an individual is incapacitated. Would the ethical answer to this question be the same as the legal answer? Does everyone involved agree with the decision-maker? Are there others who should be involved? Even the existence of advance directives does not eliminate the ethical concerns surrounding some of these situations.

In an attempt to gain greater control over the area of dying, many people are now completing a variety of documents that have been titled advance directives. An **advance directive** is a legal document that indicates the wishes of an individual in regard to end-of-life issues.

In December 1991, the federal **Patient Self-Determination Act (PSDA)** went into effect. Passed by Congress in 1990, this legislation requires that all Medicare and Medicaid providers inform patients on admission of their right to refuse treatment. The intent of this legislation was to enhance an individual's control over medical treatment decisions by promoting the use of advance directives (see Chapter 8). The entire process has not been without its problems. The time of admission to a health care facility is often filled with anxiety, making it almost impossible to consider such matters. Most patients indicate that they prefer to discuss these matters with a doctor or nurse who is involved in their care, but in some settings, this task is delegated to an admissions clerk (Hudson, 1994a).

In 1995, the American Nurses Association (ANA) revised "A Position Statement on Nursing and the Patient Self-Determination Act," written in 1990. They believe that nurses should play a primary role in implementation of the Act, should facilitate informed decision-making for patients, and should occupy a critical role in education, research, patient care, and advocacy (ANA, 1995b).

A living will is a document that has been widely used as an advance directive (Fig. 10-2). In a **living will**, a person identifies what measures to include in care if he or she becomes terminally ill. The living will is often used to request that no extraordinary measures be implemented, although it can be used to indicate a preference that all possible actions should be taken. Although the living will is not necessarily considered legal consent, it does reveal the desires of the person receiving care. It may help families to make decisions more confidently.

Another approach being used with increasing frequency is the signing of a **durable power of attorney for health care.** In this type of an agreement, an individual (referred to as the "principal") may designate another person to have the power and authority to make health care decisions for the principal should the principal be unable to make those decisions. Durable power of attorney documents may simply name the decision-maker, or may contain detailed preferences of the individual. The durable power of attorney goes into effect after the principal is no longer capable of making decisions, but not until this point is reached. These forms can be purchased in most office supply stores and become valid if signed before a notary public. However, it is best to consult an attorney before entering into such an arrangement (Fig. 10-3).

TO MY FAMILY, MY PHYSICIAN, MY CLERGYMAN, MY LAWYER

If the time comes when I can no longer take part in decisions for my own future, let this statement stand as the testament of my wishes:

If there is no reasonable expectation of my recovery from physical or mental disability, I, _____ request that I be allowed to die and not be kept alive by artificial means or heroic measures. Death is as much a reality as birth, growth, maturity and old age—it is the one certainty. I do not fear death as much as I fear the indignity of deterioration, dependence and hopeless pain. I ask that medication be mercifully administered to me for terminal suffering even if it hastens the moment of death.

This request is made after careful consideration. Although this document is not legally binding, you who care for me will, I hope, feel morally bound to follow its mandate. I recognize that it places a heavy burden of responsibility upon you, and it is with the intention of sharing that responsibility and of mitigating any feelings of guilt that this statement is made.

Signed _____

Date _____

Witnessed by:

_____

_____

FIGURE 10-2 The living will.

Euthanasia

Euthanasia, meaning "good death," may be classified as either negative or positive. The word, as it is generally applied, refers to the act or method of causing death painlessly so as to end suffering.

NEGATIVE EUTHANASIA

Negative, or passive, euthanasia refers to a situation in which no extraordinary or heroic measures are undertaken to sustain life. The concept of negative euthanasia has resulted in what are called "no codes" (also designated as DNR—do not resuscitate) in hospital environments. In these situations, hospital personnel do not attempt to revive or bring back to life persons whose vital processes have ceased to function on their own.

It is difficult to describe what constitutes extraordinary measures, and to determine on whom they should or should not be used. Is it one thing to defibrillate a 39-year-old man who is admitted to an emergency department suffering from an acute heart attack, and quite another to defibrillate a 95-year-old man whose body is riddled with terminal cancer and whose heart has stopped? Often, people who are involved in giving medical and emergency care develop an almost automatic response to life-saving procedures and have difficulty accepting dying as an inevitable part of the life process. It is difficult to know when it is permissible to omit certain life-supporting efforts, or which efforts should be omitted. If the 95-year-old man who is dying of terminal cancer were also to develop pneumonia, should his physician prescribe antibiotics? This brings us to the distinction between stopping a particular life-supporting treatment or machine, and withdrawing treatment or not starting a procedure in the first place—that is, withholding treatment.

[PLEASE NOTE: This is a standardized legal document that may not be appropriate for a person in your particular situation. You should consult your attorney before signing this or any legal document.]

DURABLE POWER OF ATTORNEY FOR HEALTH CARE DECISIONS

I, _____ as principal, domiciled and residing in the State of Washington, hereby enter into a Durable Power of Attorney to provide informed consent for health care decisions pursuant to the laws of the State of Washington.

1. **Designation.** I designate _____ , if living, able and willing to serve, as my attorney-in-fact. If he or she is not living, able and willing to so serve, then I designate _____ , if living, able and willing to serve, as my attorney-in-fact.

2. **Powers.** The attorney-in-fact, as fiduciary, shall have all powers to provide informed consent for health care decisions on principal's behalf.

3. **Effectiveness.** This power of attorney shall become effective upon the disability or incompetence of the principal. Disability shall include the inability to make health care decisions effectively for reasons such as mental illness, mental deficiency, physical illness or disability, advanced age, chronic use of drugs, chronic intoxication, confinement, detention by a foreign power or disappearance. Disability may be evidenced by a written statement of a qualified physician regularly attending me. Incompetence may be established by a finding of a Court having jurisdiction over me.

4. **Duration.** This power of attorney shall remain in effect to the extent permitted by RCW 11.94 notwithstanding any uncertainty as to whether the principal is dead or alive.

5. **Revocation.** This power of attorney may be revoked in writing by notice mailed or delivered to my attorney-in-fact, and by recording the written instrument of revocation in the office of recorder or auditor of the county of my residence.

FIGURE 10-3   Durable power of attroney.

6. Termination.

    a. By Appointment of Guardian. The appointment of a guardian of the person of the principal terminates this power of attorney. The appointment of a guardian of the property only does not terminate this power of attorney.

    b. By Death of Principal. The death of the principal shall be deemed to revoke this power of attorney upon proof of death being received by the attorney-in-fact.

7. Reliance. The designated and acting attorney-in-fact and all persons dealing with the attorney-in-fact shall be entitled to rely upon this power of attorney so long as neither the attorney-in-fact nor person with whom they were dealing at the time of any act taken pursuant to this power of attorney had received actual knowledge or actual notice of the revocation or termination of the power of attorney by death or otherwise, and any action so taken, unless otherwise invalid or unenforceable, shall be binding on the heirs, devisees, legatees, or personal representatives of the principal.

8. Indemnity. The estate of the principal shall hold harmless and indemnify the attorney-in-fact from all liability for acts done in good faith and not in fraud on behalf of the principal.

9. Applicable Law. The laws of the State of Washington shall govern this power of attorney.

10. Execution. This power of attorney is signed on this _____ day of _____, 200 _____ , to become effective as provided in Paragraph 3.

Signature: _____

Print name: _____

STATE OF WASHINGTON)
) ss.
COUNTY OF KING   )

    I certify that I know or have satisfactory evidence that _____ is the person who appeared before me, and said person acknowledged that _____he signed this instrument and acknowledged it to be h_____ free and voluntary act for the uses and purposes mentioned in the instrument.

FIGURE 10-3 *(continued)*

Some ethicists do not differentiate between withholding treatment in the first place and withdrawing treatment once it has been determined to be inappropriate or futile. They would see both as having the same position in terms of right and wrong. Those who support negative euthanasia support both withholding and stopping treatment. The general public often sees these as separate issues and may support withholding treatment, while not supporting the termination of treatment once it has begun. Increasingly, the legal system has supported withdrawing treatment that is determined to be futile. Even the Roman Catholic Church, which has a strong pro-life stance, has supported both the right not to institute heroic treatment and the right to withdraw it once it has begun.

POSITIVE EUTHANASIA

Positive, or active, euthanasia occurs in a situation in which the physician prescribes, supplies, or administers an agent that results in death. In the case (cited later in this chapter) in which parents choose to let a newborn with Down syndrome and an intestinal blockage die, positive euthanasia would have occurred if the doctors had hastened the infant's death with medication. There may well be more instances of positive euthanasia than we know about publicly.

On some occasions, a physician prescribes strong narcotics for a terminally ill patient and requests that the medication be given frequently enough to "keep the patient comfortable." Nurses often are reluctant to administer a medication that they realize has a potentially fatal effect when given in that dosage. In such cases, the ethical intent of the action is often considered. Medications given for the comfort of the dying patient may be ethically justifiable even if they hasten death to some extent. This is based on the ethical concept of double effect, in which the acceptable effect (such as pain relief) is the purpose of the medication and the secondary effect (such as depressing respiration) is not the intended effect. This is not legally considered positive euthanasia. When nursing staff have difficulty with this issue, a patient conference with an oncology specialist or with a nurse skilled in the area of death and dying can help the staff to clarify values and deal with individual feelings.

Right-to-Die Issues

Right-to-die issues are gaining much more attention than in previous years. Kass (1993, p. 37) identifies four reasons for such a right to be asserted:

1. Fear of prolongation of dying due to medical interventions; hence, a right to refuse treatment or hospitalization, even if death occurs as a result
2. Fear of living too long, without fatal illness to carry one off; hence, a right to assisted suicide
3. Fear of the degradations of senility and dependence; hence, a right to death with dignity
4. Fear of loss of control; hence, a right to choose the time and manner of one's death

A great deal of controversy has surrounded the issue of maintaining the lives of persons considered to be in a persistent vegetative state (PVS). Some of the issues that arise are the patient's rights, the family's wishes, and the cost to society. In most cases, the problems emerge when the life of a family member is being maintained through support measures that might be considered extraordinary.

In 1991, St. Francis-St. George Hospital in Cincinnati was sued in one of the first cases of its kind. The suit charged that the nurses should not have resuscitated an 82-year-old man when he suffered a heart attack. In so doing they disregarded the "no code" status of the patient ("Hospital sued . . .," 1991).

WITHHOLDING TREATMENT

Withholding treatment could be considered negative euthanasia. A historic case occurred in 1963.

▼

Withholding Treatment

A couple on the East Coast gave birth to a premature infant who was diagnosed as having Down syndrome, with the added complication of an intestinal blockage. The intestinal blockage could have been corrected by surgery with minimal risk; without surgery, the child could not be fed and would die. The Down syndrome, however, would have resulted in some degree of permanent mental retardation. The severity of the retardation could not be determined at birth, but would range from very low mentality to borderline subnormal intelligence. The parents, who had two normal children at home, believed that it would be unfair to those children to raise a child with Down syndrome and refused permission for the corrective operation on the intestinal blockage. Although it was an option, the hospital staff did not seek a court order to override the decision. The staff believed it was unlikely that a court would sustain an order to operate on the child against the parents' wishes, because the child had a known mental handicap and would be a burden to the parents financially and emotionally, and perhaps a burden to society. The child was put in a side room (an interesting action) and was allowed to die, a process that took 11 days. When confronted with the possibility of giving medication to hasten the infant's death, both doctors and nurses were convinced that it was clearly illegal (Gustafson, 1973).

The situation above stimulates both ethical and legal questions. Would the approach have been the same if the infant had not been mentally retarded? Would the staff have been guilty of murder if the infant had been given medication to hasten death? If a court decision to proceed with the surgery had been requested and granted, who would have been responsible for the costs incurred? What are the rights of the child? Who advocates for those rights if the child is unable to do so?

WITHDRAWING TREATMENT

In some instances, a family has sought to have extraordinary life-support measures discontinued, ie, **withdrawing treatment**. A landmark case is that of Karen Quinlan.

▼

Withdrawing Treatment 1

Karen Quinlan was a young woman left in a vegetative state after suffering severe brain damage from chemical abuse that involved both drugs and alcohol. She was placed on a respirator, and her physicians believed that she would live only a short time if it were to be removed. Her parents requested that the respirator be discontinued, but because she continued to manifest a minor amount of brain activity, their request was refused. After previous petitions to the Supreme Court of New Jersey had been rejected, the courts ruled on March 31, 1976, that her parents could exercise her privacy right on her behalf, and the respirator was discontinued. Much to everyone's surprise, Karen continued to live after the respirator was stopped, although she never emerged from her comatose condition; she died in 1986.

This case represents a situation in which treatment was withdrawn even though the individual was not considered immediately terminal. Such cases represent hard decisions for all involved and evoke legal, moral, and ethical questions in almost all instances. A similar case that attracted much attention was that of Nancy Cruzan.

EXAMPLE

Withdrawing Treatment 2

In March 1988, Joe and Joyce Cruzan requested through the Jasper County, Missouri Probate Court that they be allowed to remove the gastrostomy tube that kept their daughter Nancy alive. Nancy had been in a persistent vegetative state since an automobile accident in 1983. Although the request was granted, Missouri's attorney general appealed the decision, asking for a clear precedent from a higher court. In June 1990, the U. S. Supreme Court effectively denied the request in asking for "clear and convincing" evidence of the patient's view. In reaching this point, a fine line was drawn between initially withholding medical treatment and later withdrawing it. In Missouri, once the family gives initial consent for treatment, they forfeit all power to undo that consent or to stop treatment. No other state has such a law (Colby, 1990). Treatment can be stopped in only two ways: if it can be demonstrated that it causes pain, or if the patient left behind clear and convincing evidence of his or her wishes prior to incompetency. The first was not an option because of Nancy Cruzan's persistent vegetative state. Therefore, her parents presented a state court with testimony from her physician and three friends that Nancy would not have wished to continue existing with irreversible brain damage. The Circuit Court judge ruled that this met the test and Nancy's feeding tube was removed on December 14, 1990. She died on December 26th.

Other cases have reached the headlines as individuals and families have striven to have more voice in determining issues related to the right to die. In all cases, much conflict exists in the arguments put forth by those supporting the right-to-die and right-to-life movements. In 1990, Congress took a major step regarding this issue by passing the PSDA. Increasingly, states have supported the right of appropriate substitutionary decision-makers to both refuse and withdraw medical treatment. Medical treatments include tube feeding, oxygen, medications, and intravenous fluids.

Of particular concern to nurses are their own feelings when a decision is reached to remove life-supporting measures, whether the measures are tube feedings or ventilators. Strong emotional attachments often form between the nurse and patient, even when the patient is in a vegetative state. Nurses who have worked to preserve the patient's dignity have great difficulty "letting go." In some instances, patients are transferred to other facilities to die in an environment where the nurses are not so emotionally involved with the patient.

POSITIONS ON WITHHOLDING AND WITHDRAWING TREATMENT

Several organizations and groups have issued guidelines for their members and others who would find them useful, with regard to the issue of withholding or withdrawing treatment. Key to all of these guidelines is whether the patient is legally competent (able to make decisions for herself or himself), or incompetent (in need of someone else to make those decisions). Table 10-3 outlines the date, organization and major tenets of some of those positions.

TABLE 10-3	POSITIONS ON WITHHOLDING AND WITHDRAWING TREATMENT	
	ORGANIZATION	**POSITION**
1983	President's Commission Report— *Deciding to Forego Life-sustaining treatment*	Focused on the ethical, medical, and legal issues in treatment decisions. Distinguished between withholding (not starting) and withdrawing (stopping after it started) treatment without making a moral distinction between the two. Suggested that withholding may require more justification because the positive effects would not be known.
1986	American Medical Association— *Statement on Withholding or Withdrawing Life-prolonging Medical Treatment*	Stated that life-prolonging medical treatment and artificially or technologically maintained respiration, nutrition, and hydration, could be withheld from a patient in an irreversible coma even if death was not imminent (Fry, 1990).
1986	Office of Technology Assessment of the U.S. Congress—*Life-sustaining Technologies and the Elderly*	Issued the results of its study on the use of life-sustaining technologies on the elderly. Report noted that the most controversial of the technologies was that of nutritional support. Identified that the most troublesome aspect of nutritional support is whether it is intravenous feeding and hydration or a tube feeding (Fry, 1990).
1987	Hasting's Center—*Guidelines on the Termination of Life-sustaining Treatment*	Provided clear definitions of key terms and a general guideline for making decisions regarding treatment. Viewed nutrition and hydration as medical interventions, much as other life-sustaining measures. Placed emphasis on the patient's ability to make decisions and required case-by-case assessment (Fry, 1990).
1988	American Nurses Association— *Guidelines on Withdrawing or Withholding Food and Fluid*	Indicated that there were few instances under which it would be permissible for nurses to withdraw food or fluid from their patients. No distinction was made between withdrawing and withholding (ANA, 1988).
1995	American Nurses Association— *Position Statement on Foregoing Medically Provided Nutrition and Hydration*	Stated that the decision to withhold medically provided nutrition and hydration should be made by the patient or surrogate with the health care team. The nurse continues to provide expert and compassionate care to patients who are no longer receiving medically provided nutrition and hydration. Distinguished between medically provided nutrition and hydration and the provision of food and water (ANA, 1995a).

ASSISTED DEATH

Assisted death involves helping another end his or her life. The activities of a retired Michigan pathologist, Jack Kevorkian, who is alleged to have assisted patients in their suicide, have received much media attention in the past few years. Although eluding criminal charges for a number of years, in March 1999, Dr. Kevorkian was convicted of second-degree murder and the delivery of a controlled substance after CBS televised a video showing him administering lethal drugs. The first case in which he was charged but not convicted involved an Oregon woman with Alzheimer's disease.

In June 1997, the U. S. Supreme Court rendered a decision on physician-assisted suicide. This decision took the position that there was no constitutionally protected right to physician-assisted suicide on behalf of terminally ill patients. In October 1997, the residents of Oregon legalized physician-assisted suicide, despite the Supreme Court decision. Legal debate regarding its continuance has been ongoing.

Statistics compiled by the Oregon Department of Human Services indicated that of the approximately 30,000 Oregonians who died in 2001, 21 used state law to get and take lethal medication. Most of these individuals were suffering from cancer and 76% were hospice patients; all had insurance. As in previous years, they tended to be better educated than average, beyond the traditional retirement age, 62% were female, and 95% were white. In 2001, 44 prescriptions for lethal doses of medication were written, an increase of 5 from 2000. Fourteen died of their underlying illnesses, and 11 were alive at the end of 2001. Some of the 21 who died during 2001 had received the prescription in 2000 ("Oregon suicides steady . . . ," 2002).

In April 2001, The Netherlands became the first nation to fully legalize euthanasia, a process that was 3 years in the making ("Netherlands is first nation . . . ," 2001). A year later in April 2002, Europe's leading human rights court threw out an appeal by a terminally ill and paralyzed British woman who wanted her husband to help end her life. Although suicide is legal in Britain, helping someone else commit suicide is a crime ("European court throws out . . . ," 2002).

The ANA has developed a position statement on assisted suicide in which they state that the nurse should not participate in assisted suicide. Such an act is viewed as a violation of the Code for Nurses (see Chapter 9). It is the position of the ANA that the challenge for nurses should not be in legalizing assisted suicide. Rather, the role of the nurse should be directed toward reversing the despair and pain experienced in the last stages of life, and in fulfilling the obligation to provide competent, comprehensive, and compassionate end-of-life care (ANA, 1994).

THE RIGHT TO REFUSE TREATMENT

The **right to refuse treatment** is an issue closely aligned with the right to die. However, it carries special implications that require separate consideration. Although we discussed some of the parameters of this issue in the previous section on the right to die, other aspects can create even bigger problems for the nurse. The moral, if not legal, precedent for refusing treatment occurred in 1971.

EXAMPLE

Refusing Treatment

Carmen Martinez was dying of hemolytic anemia, a disease that destroys the body's red blood cells. Her life could be maintained by transfusions, but her veins were such that a cut-down (a surgical opening made into the vein) was necessary to accomplish the transfusions. Finally, Martinez pleaded to have the cut-downs stopped and to be "tortured" no more. The physician, fearful of being charged with aiding in her suicide, asked for a court decision. The court ruled that Martinez was not competent to make such a decision and appointed her daughter as her guardian. When the daughter also asked that no more cut-downs be performed, the compassionate judge honored the daughter's request. He decided that although Martinez did not have the right to commit suicide, she did have the "right not to be tortured." She died the next day (Veatch, 1976).

People working in the health care professions often are confronted with such dilemmas. Cases such as one in which a patient refuses to have a leg amputated, even though not having the surgery undoubtedly will result in death, often will make the news. The right to refuse treatment can take on additional implications when the patient, by refusing one type of treatment, is essentially demanding alternative medical management. Our support of the right to refuse treatment is based on a basic belief in and respect for the autonomy of the patient. When the refusal of medical intervention means that the individual is no longer a patient, it is known as a "negative right simpliciter" by bioethicists. In these cases, the patient's physician need only do nothing, as in cases in which the patient discharges himself or herself from the hospital.

When the patient refuses treatment but does not withdraw from the role of being the patient, the matter becomes more complex. An example would be the patient who refuses to have a gangrenous toe surgically removed and demands to have it treated otherwise. These are referred to as positive rights. In the case of a patient with a gangrenous toe, one form of treatment may be more accepted than another, but both may be successful. A case illustrating this right occurred in 1993 in Chicago and attracted national attention.

Refusing a Form of Treatment 1

A Pentecostal Christian mother refused to have a cesarean section when physicians recommended the procedure because her fetus was being deprived of oxygen and would die if delivered vaginally. The courts upheld the patient's right to refuse the surgery. She later gave birth to an apparently healthy boy.

When children are involved, it is even more newsworthy, and again points out that there is as yet no consensus about when minors should be allowed to refuse treatment.

Refusing a Form of Treatment 2

In November 1994, 16-year-old Billy Best made national news when he ran away from home to avoid another 5 months of chemotherapy and radiation. Suffering from Hodgkin's disease, the high school junior was experiencing nausea, aching, and fatigue, as well as hair loss, from the treatment. He stated, ". . . I could not stand going to the hospital every week. I feel like the medicine is killing me instead of helping me." (Dorning, 1994).

Often in such cases, the parents refuse to have the treatment started, many times because of religious beliefs. The courts usually become involved in reaching a decision. A case in Illinois in 1952 is typical.

Refusing a Form of Treatment 3

Eight-day-old Cheryl suffered from erythroblastosis fetalis (Rh incompatibility). Her parents, who were Jehovah's Witnesses, refused to authorize the administration of blood necessary to save her life. The judge in the case ruled that Cheryl was a neglected dependent and overrode the parent's refusal. In such instances, the child is usually made a temporary ward of the court and legal documents are attached to the record authorizing the needed treatment. Such court decisions usually have been based on the premise that the right to freedom of religion does not give parents the right to risk the lives of their children or to make martyrs of them (Veatch, 1976).

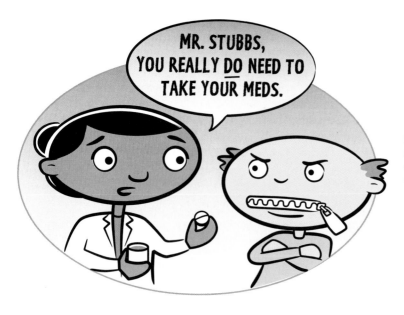

FIGURE 10-4   People working in the health care field are frequently confronted with the dilemma of patients who may wish to refuse treatment.

Sometimes, when time is not a factor, the court will recommend that treatment be delayed until the child is 15 or 16 years old and can make a decision as an older minor. Other judges will rule just the opposite, deciding that it is cruel to place the burden of the decision on this older minor.

Situations like those that have been cited are always difficult for the people involved. Because nurses have the most contact with patients, they must examine their own feelings and attitudes. Nurses must recognize that patients also have the right to attitudes and beliefs. If a nurse decides that his or her feelings are so strong that they might interfere with the ability to give compassionate care, it would be wise to ask to be assigned to other patients (Fig. 10-4).

BIOETHICAL CONCERNS RELATED TO SUSTAINING QUALITY OF LIFE

With the increase in technology, bioethical concerns have expanded significantly to include issues related to maintaining or sustaining the quality of life through such procedures as organ transplantation, xenotransplantation, and stem cell research. We cannot discuss all of these in detail but will provide an overview of the topics.

Organ Transplantation

Developments in the area of organ transplantation have created several issues deserving consideration. **Organ transplantation** is the process by which a tissue or organ is removed and replaced by a corresponding part. Transplants can be done using tissue from one's own body (eg, skin, bone, or cartilage); this is called an autograft. Transplantation using organs from a donor's body is known as homograft or allograft; it might involve organs such as the kidney, liver, pancreas, heart, cornea, or skin of another individual. Some organs (eg, the heart) must be transplanted immediately or they will die. Others, such as the kidney or skin, can be stored for short periods. According to the United Network for Organ Sharing (UNOS), there are more than 80,000 individuals waiting for an organ transplant; 16 Americans die each day while waiting for an organ to become available ("Critical data . . . ," 2002).

Initially, the replacement for a diseased organ was obtained from a donor who had died. More recently, organs have been received from living donors. In 2001, the number of living donors reached an all-time high with 6,485, exceeding the 6,081 donations that were given after death. More than 90% of the donors (5979) gave a kidney, about 500 donated livers, and about three dozen people gave part of a lung ("Most transplanted organs . . . ," 2002).

The supply of organs that can be used for transplantation has not been able to keep up with the demand. This concern resulted in the Secretary of Health and Human Services, Tommy Thompson announcing his "Gift of Life Donation Initiative" in April 2001. This initiative had five major elements to encourage organ donation. Among these was a model donor card, which included provisions for designating whether all organs and tissues may be donated, as well as lines for signatures by two witnesses (Fig. 10-5). This card may be downloaded from the Internet site *www.organdonor.gov/SecInitiative.htm.* Concomitantly, the number of bills in Congress that address the issue of organ transplant continues to grow.

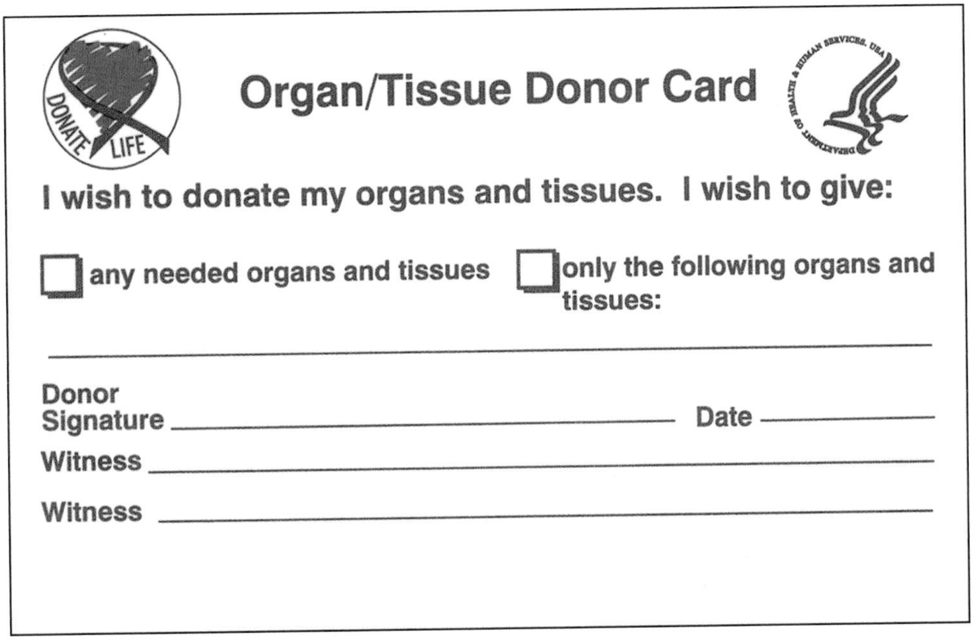

Organ/Tissue Donor Card

I wish to donate my organs and tissues. I wish to give:

☐ any needed organs and tissues   ☐ only the following organs and tissues:

_____

Donor
Signature _____ Date _____

Witness _____

Witness _____

FIGURE 10-5   Organ/tissue donor card.

CONCERNS ABOUT PROCUREMENT

Organ procurement refers to all the activities involved in obtaining donated organs. The idea of consent becomes important when we talk about organ transplantation and procurement. It is preferable to have the consent obtained from the donor. This has been facilitated in many states by the Uniform Anatomical Gift Act, which was drafted by a committee of the National Conference of the Commissions of Uniform State Laws in July 1968, and now by the Model Donor Card. People who are willing to donate parts of their bodies after death may indicate the desire to do so in a will or other written documents, or by carrying a donor's card. Many states also provide a space on the driver's license where individuals can authorize permission for organ donations.

The next-of-kin also must grant permission for the removal of organs after death. However, the time factor is crucial; the deaths are often accidental, and the relatives are often so emotionally distressed that the process of obtaining permission may be uncomfortable. Hospitals that receive Medicare funds are mandated to have required request policies in place. Typically, they have developed a procurement team that has received special preparation related to requesting organ donations. These are persons skilled in recognizing the stress being felt by the family and experienced in providing information that will be important to them. A growing number of hospitals are designating a nurse as transplantation coordinator to facilitate this process.

An interesting and controversial case related to obtaining necessary material for transplantation occurred in California in 1990.

EXAMPLE

Transplantation

An 18-year-old woman, an only child, was diagnosed as having chronic myelogenous leukemia. Although this form of leukemia responds favorably to bone marrow transplants, no compatible donor could be found after testing the girl's family and contacting the National Marrow Donor Program. In desperation, the parents decided to have another child with the hope that the new baby would have genetically matching tissue type. This required that the father have a vasectomy reversed and that the mother, age 43, go through another pregnancy, which terminated in a cesarean section. The baby proved a good match and was able to provide donor tissue for her sister.

The case drew considerable attention as medical ethicists voiced concern about creating one child to save another. Citing Immanuel Kant, they argued that the baby was conceived, not as an end in itself, but for utilitarian purposes. Some medical ethicists argued in favor of the rights of the individuals involved, saying that it is not the concern of biomedical ethicists to intrude into matters affecting private citizens, especially when that intrusion approaches "intruding into a couple's bedroom." Still others say that striking cases must be brought before the public because an obligation to inform society exists.

Children and young people experience the most critical need for human organs. This has caused us to challenge previous decisions. A good example is that raised when considering organs removed from an anencephalic infant. An anencephalic infant is one born with only enough brain to support such vital functions as heartbeat and respiration. It has been estimated that about 60% of these infants are stillborn, and of those born alive, only about 5% will live more than 3 days. Because anencephaly affects only the brain, other organs can be used for transplantation if the infant is kept alive on a respirator until an organ recipient is located. This challenges our definitions of death. How can current definitions of "brain" death be applied to a condition in which there is no brain as we normally recognize it?

ARTIFICIAL ORGANS

Other problems also arise regarding organ transplantations, especially because more people need organs than there are organs available. The skill of modern technology has resulted in the development and implantation of artificial organs such as the heart. Such technologic advances once were viewed as science fiction. As a result, historic cases such as the implantation of an artificial heart in Barney Clark in 1982 received a great deal of publicity. Over the years, the use of artificial organs has not proven effective for long-term use, but artificial organs have made it possible for individuals to live with the hope that a transplantable organ will become available. Work and research to develop better organs continues and recipients are living longer, although the promise is far less than that with donated organs. The use of artificial joints, heart valves, and other prostheses continues to grow and to be successful.

MINORITY GROUPS AND ORGAN DONATION

Another issue that has emerged is that of minority differences regarding organ donation. Of the persons awaiting an organ for transplantation, approximately 42% represent minorities (National MOTTEP, 2002). The risk of end-stage renal disease for African Americans and Native Americans is three to four times higher than for the white population (Kasiske et al, 1991). Although minority groups donate in proportion to their population distribution, minority organ donations lag behind those from the white population, with more than 74% of cadaver donations coming from whites, 12.4% from African Americans, 10% from Hispanics, and 1% from Asians (National MOTTEP, 2002). One of the reasons this presents a concern is that minorities form more than half of the kidney transplant waiting list. More minority donors are needed to increase the chances that a well-matched organ will be available to minorities awaiting transplants.

Several factors may impact reticence of minorities to donate organs. Some groups have identified religious beliefs and cultural customs as forbidding organ donation, although no major Western religion prohibits organ donation. Religious objection often stems from the high value attached to keeping the body intact ("Body and soul," 2002). African Americans listed distrust of the medical community, fear of premature death, and racism as major barriers. Hispanics experienced language barriers and identified the importance of having the entire extended family involved in all decision-making regarding donations. Puerto Ricans verbalized denial of death and fear of mutilation of the body as critical factors. Barriers to organ donation in Asian American cultures included the belief that the body should remain intact to the grave and lack of respect during the handling of the body after death. Although Native Americans are theoretically supportive of organ donations, their rate of donation is low, probably due to lack of knowledge (Wheeler & Cheung, 1996). Although no single approach to organ donation fits all groups, efforts to decrease barriers to donation are being instituted.

The first national program specifically designed to empower minority communities to become involved in education activities to increase the number of minority donors and transplant recipients has been started. The National Minority Organ/Tissue Transplant Education Program (MOTTEP) now has 15 sites across the country and represents African American, Hispanic/Latino, Native American, Asian, Pacific Island, and Alaskan Native populations. MOTTEP includes a health promotion and disease prevention component designed to reduce the incidence of conditions that can lead to organ failure. It can be reached at the Web site *http://www.nationalmottep.org*

Critical Thinking Activity

Have you signed an organ donation card? If not, discuss the reasons why you have chosen not to do so. If you have, discuss the reasons why you have. Is there a possibility you will change your mind? Why or why not? What solutions can you suggest to help the nation deal with the shortage of organs needed for transplantation?

CONCERNS ABOUT ALLOCATION

How will we determine who receives donated organs? Does "elitism" exist in their distribution—that is, does a white-collar worker have a better chance to receive an organ than a blue-collar worker? Medicaid and most insurance policies refuse to pay for the cost of many organ transplants, although Medicare usually covers the costs of corneal transplants and kidney transplants. Transplants are expensive procedures, often running into several hundreds of thousands of dollars. If money is required "up front," as it sometimes is, where can the needy person procure such funds? Other questions involve both donor and recipient. Should the donor or the donor's family have the right to say who will receive the organ? How can one "get in line" for an organ, and how can that need be made known? What about selling a healthy organ, such as a kidney?

Much has been written about the problem of selecting recipients for organ transplantation when the number of applicants exceeds the number of available organs. Many criteria have been suggested, and as one might anticipate, these criteria have arguments both pro and con; the criterion requiring medical acceptability is probably the only exception. Many transplants require that compatibility exist in the tissue and blood type of donor and recipient. It would not be logical to give a much-needed organ to a person whose body would automatically reject it.

The criterion of the recipient's social worth is probably one of the hardest to defend, although it was used in the Pacific Northwest in the early 1960s to decide who should be allowed to live by kidney dialysis. Social worth, including past and future potential, was considered, and even such factors as church membership and participation in community endeavors were considered.

Some suggest a form of random selection, once the criterion of medical acceptability has been met. This could be either a natural random selection of the first-come, first-served variety, or an artificial selection process such as a lottery. A criticism of this method is that it removes rational decision-making from the process.

We offer no suggestions to solve this problem but merely demonstrate the difficulty it presents. Even the issue of who should serve on the decision-making committee can be touchy. The problem of personal biases is a big concern.

In an effort to gather donations and disseminate information about individuals who need various organs, an Organ Procurement Program was started in Pittsburgh, Pennsylvania. This program was established to facilitate the matching of donor with recipient and to provide a central listing agency for those in need of transplants. Today, organ procurement agencies are located in all regions of the country. These groups carry out many activities related to organ procurement, including establishing groups for individuals who have received donated organs and their families, publishing newsletters, developing educational materials, increasing public awareness of the need for organs, and serving as a clearinghouse for organ procurement and matching. They are connected through the federally funded United Network for Organ Sharing.

CONCERNS ABOUT INDIVIDUAL PROPERTY RIGHTS

Concern for an individual's **property rights** regarding human tissues also has attracted attention. Developments in biotechnology allow profit-oriented companies to use human tissue to generate lucrative products, such as drugs, diagnostic tests, and other medically related materials. The modern legal system has consistently held that no property rights are attached to the human body (Swain & Marusyk, 1990).

EXAMPLE

Human Body Property Rights

In 1990, a Seattle man sued the University of California, two researchers, and two biotechnology and drug companies, because in 1976, he had sought treatment for hairy cell leukemia and subsequently had his spleen removed (which is the standard treatment). It was later discovered that the removed spleen contained unique blood cells that produced a rare blood protein, which then was used experimentally in the treatment of certain cancers and possibly AIDS. The patient was never told that his cells had great potential value, although he was brought from Seattle to Los Angeles frequently for blood and other tests. His cells were then developed into a self-perpetuating cell line to mass-produce the rare blood protein. The patient's suit claimed that the defendants wrongfully converted to their own use his personal property (ie, the blood cells) and that this was done without his consent.

Xenotransplantation

Xenotransplantation refers to the practice of using animal organs, cells, and tissues for transplantation into human beings. Some scientists believe that having a reliable supply of organs from pigs or other animals could solve the great shortage from human donors. It is in the stage of experimentation around the world.

Xenotransplantation usually involves organs or tissues from pigs and nonhuman primates. One case receiving national publicity was that of an AIDS patient in San Francisco who received the transplant of baboon bone marrow to bolster his weakening immune system. Since 1906, some 55 animal-to-human whole organ transplants have been attempted; none was successful (Fano et al, 1999). Cases that received particular attention were the 1984 transplant of a baboon heart into Baby Fae (who died 20 days later) and the 1992 transplant of a baboon liver into a 35-year-old man (who also died).

In addition to the obvious problems associated with immune system rejection, of particular concern to some is the possibility of transmitting serious animal viruses and other microbes, so-called zoonotic diseases, to people. Fano and associates (1999) report more than 20 known, potentially lethal viruses that can be transmitted from nonhuman primates to humans. This has prompted the use of pigs as the "donor" of choice, and has led to attempts to alter pigs genetically so that tissues would be more adaptable to transplantation. In August 2002, a British biotechnology company announced the creation of the first so-called "double knock-out" pigs, genetically engineered to lack both copies of a gene that causes rejection ("Cloned pigs . . . ," 2002).

Concerns in England over the communicability of bovine spongiform encephalopathy through the ingestion of meat from ill animals has prompted the discussion of the potential for all animal organs to transmit diseases that would appear only years later. Even raising animals in a sterile environment has its limitations because it is now being discovered that some diseases are transmitted from mother to fetus in utero. Some groups in England are urging the xenotransplantation project be abandoned and that research into xenotransplantation be stopped because of the social cost and because of on-going suffering of animals inherent in such an approach.

In September 1996, the federal government proposed strict safeguards to provide protection. Representatives from the Food and Drug Administration (FDA), the Centers for Disease Control and Prevention (CDC), and the National Institutes of Health (NIH) developed the guidelines. The guidelines urged that patients and their families be fully informed of potential risks, and further required that any planned procedure be thoroughly screened and approved by a series of local institutional review boards, and by the FDA. The recommendations also require that transplants take place at a clinical center associated with an accredited biology and microbiology laboratory.

The Human Genome Project

A **genome** may be defined as all the DNA in an organism, including the genes that carry information for making the proteins required by all organisms. These proteins determine such things as how the organism looks, how well its body metabolizes food and fights infection, and sometimes even how it behaves. Genomes have been studied for many reasons, including disease prevention, determination of the effects of radiation and chemicals on living species, and more recently, genetic therapy. DNA is made up of four similar chemicals called bases and abbreviated A, T, C, and G, and are repeated millions or billions of times throughout a genome. The order of As, Ts, Cs, and Gs is important because the order underlies all of life's diversity, including whether an organism is human or of another species.

The **Human Genome Project** (HGP) was first proposed by Nobel prize-winning virologist Renato Dulbecco in 1986. Coordinated by the Department of Energy (DOE) and the NIH, the project started in October 1990 and involved at least 18 countries in the international effort. The project was planned to last for 15 years; effective resource and technologic advances have accelerated the expected completion date to 2003. Several types of genome maps have already been completed, and a working draft of the entire human genome sequence was announced in June 2000. The analysis was published in February 2001.

The goals of the project are to:

- Identify all the approximate 30,000 genes in human DNA
- Determine the sequences of the 3 billion chemical base pairs that make up human DNA
- Store this information in data bases
- Improve tools for data analysis
- Transfer related technologies to the private sector
- Address the ethical, legal, and social issues (ELSI) that may arise from the project (Human Genome Project Information, 2002).

An additional part of the HGP includes parallel studies being carried out on several non-human organisms, including the *Escherichia coli* bacterium, the fruit fly, and the laboratory mouse. Studying nonhuman organisms' sequences can lead to an understanding of their natural capabilities, which can be applied toward solving challenges in health care, energy sources, agriculture, and environmental cleanup.

It is anticipated that knowledge about the effects of DNA variations among individuals can lead to new ways to diagnose, treat, and someday prevent the thousands of disorders that affect us. This could unlock a plethora of bioethical concerns. Once this technology has been developed, where does it end? How is the information handled regarding issues of privacy and confidentiality? What is the impact if third-party payers gain access to the information? What might be the advantages and disadvantages of knowing the diseases to which you are susceptible? With whom should that information be shared? What would be the effects of manipulating stature, intelligence, or sex? Does this project represent eugenics revisited? Who among health care providers will provide access to patients? Will the responsibility fall to the family practitioner, who will most likely be the first contact for those with a genetic disorder? How prepared are family practitioners for this type of care delivery?

In a study of family physicians' perspectives on genetics and the HGP conducted in the midwestern United States, many family physicians indicated that they felt educational opportunities to learn about genetics had been inadequate, and some indicated reluctance to gain the additional education that would be required. Will we see the advent of a new medical specialty in structural genomics? Will molecular medicine teams be developed in our society? Will new and expensive technology result, such as a program of high-throughput X-ray crystallography aimed at developing a comprehensive mechanistic understanding of normal and abnormal human and microbial physiology (Burley et al, 1999). The DOE and the NIH have devoted 3% to 5% of their annual HGP budgets toward studying these concerns. A few that have been identified include:

- Fairness in the use of genetic information by insurers, employers courts, schools and others
- Privacy and confidentiality of genetic information
- Psychological impact and stigmatization due to an individual's genetic differences
- Reproductive issues, including adequate informed consent for controversial procedures, reproductive rights, and use of genetic information in reproductive decision-making

- Clinical issues, including the education of doctors and other health service providers, patients, and the general public
- Uncertainties associated with gene tests for susceptibilities and complex conditions
- Conceptual and philosophic implications regarding human responsibility, free will versus genetic determinism, and concepts of health and disease
- Health and environmental issues concerning genetically modified foods and microbes
- Commercialization of products, including property rights and accessibility of data and materials (Human Genome Project Information, 2002b).

More information regarding these issues can be obtained from the Web site: *http://www.ornl.gov/hgmis.*

Gene Therapy

An estimated 4,000 disease genes have been identified that reside with the genome. Identification and isolation of defective genes, and their replacement with functional genes (gene therapy), could result in the elimination of diseases that have plagued society for generations. Several significant conditions currently under study are cystic fibrosis, Huntington's disease, myotonic dystrophy, gout, and adult polycystic kidney disease.

In the genetic lexicon, the gene is a length of DNA that codes for a particular protein. The average human gene is a little more than 1,000 nucleotides long and, in many inherited disorders, only one or a few of these nucleotides is incorrect. For example, in sickle cell anemia, a single nucleotide causes the structural deformity that results in the characteristically distorted shape of the sickled red blood cell that prohibits the cell from adequately carrying oxygen to the body's organs and tissues. Seventy percent of the cases of cystic fibrosis may be due to the deletion of three nucleotides (Kmiec, 1999).

Theoretically, **gene therapy** can take the form of somatic (body) or germ (egg and sperm) cells. Somatic gene therapy results in the recipient's genome being changed but the change is not passed down to the next generation. With germline gene therapy, not being actively investigated at the present time, the goal is to pass the change on to offspring. The genetic testing of eggs and the sex selection of embryos mentioned earlier in this chapter are a matter of selection; no cells are altered or changed.

Decisions on clinical applications of gene-therapy approaches are under the oversight of the federal government. The Office of Recombinant DNA Activities Advisory Committee (OAC) evaluates protocols and makes suggestions for approval to the director of the NIH. Gene therapy policy conferences and gene therapy conferences designed to provide public information regarding research progress have been instituted.

To date, gene therapy is primarily experimental and has experienced far more failures than successes. Positive results in mice do not necessarily promise positive outcomes for humans. Many of the basic problems with gene therapies have not been worked out. Finding a mechanism to insert the new gene into the body needs to be found. Scientists need a better understanding of how genes function. The problems associated with multigene disorders must be solved. Questions regarding the repair of genes versus the replacement of genes are yet to be answered. The high costs associated with this new technology present another concern.

However, gene therapy offers a wide array of possibilities and undoubtedly will gain momentum in the near future.

Stem Cell Research

A **stem cell** is a special kind of cell that is able to renew itself and give rise to specialized cell types. These cells, unlike most other cells in the body, such as those of the heart or skin, are not committed to conduct a specific function. The cell remains uncommitted until it receives a signal to develop into a specialized cell. Scientists are now looking at a type of stem cell that is called *pluripotent* because the cells have the potential to develop almost all of the more than 200 different known cell types. These cells, which originate from early human embryos, may have the potential to generate replacement cells for a wide array of tissues and organs, including the heart, the pancreas, and the nervous system (DHHS, 2001). Thus, they offer hope for patients with diseases such as Parkinson's disease, diabetes, chronic heart disease, end-stage kidney disease, liver failure, cancer, multiple sclerosis, Alzheimer's disease and those with spinal cord injuries. Many of these conditions shorten lives and no effective treatments have been found. In heart disease, for example, numerous heart cells are destroyed and the body cannot replace them. Doctors hope to inject patients with stem cells and then signal them to grow into new heart tissue ("The stem cell debate . . . ," 2001).

As progress was being made with tissue from early embryos, research was being conducted on adult stem cells. An adult stem cell is an undifferentiated cell that occurs in a differentiated tissue, renews itself, and becomes specialized. These adult stem cells are capable of making identical copies of themselves for the lifetime of the organisms. Sources of these cells include bone marrow, blood, the cornea and retina of the eye, brain, skeletal muscle, dental pulp, liver, skin, the lining of the gastrointestinal tract, and pancreas. They are rare and often difficult to identify (DHHS, 2001). Because of this, the stem cells of human embryos are considered by some to be more desirable.

However, to retrieve the needed cells, the embryo is destroyed because the needed cells lie in the center of the blastocyst, a cluster of about 150 cells has developed about 1 week after the ova is fertilized by a sperm. Thus we find ourselves with the same ethical question raised earlier in this chapter: Do blastocysts equal human life? Many people, including antiabortionists, believe the answer is yes. Others find the benefits to be so great they tend to view the blastocysts as potentially human but not quite there yet.

Because research of this nature needs federal funding and approval to move forward, stem cell debate is a national issue. In August 2001, President Bush approved federal funding of some human embryo-related research, but not for studies that allow any more embryos to be destroyed, stating that the government would pay only for experiments using stem cells that already had been drawn from embryos or that used adult stem cells. Although this pleased the National Right to Life Committee, it greatly disappointed prominent scientists who see stem cell research as the single most promising avenue of medical research ("Stem cell stalemate . . . ," 2001). The concern is that the existing lines of embryonic stem cells are too limited to achieve the desired research objectives and that adult stem cells do not have the same potential. Those who want to see this research pushed forward want to use some of the thousands of leftover frozen embryos in storage at fertility clinics. The frozen embryos were created by couples who intended to use them for in-vitro fertilizations. The embryos can be left frozen for potential later use, donated to someone else who wants to have a child, or thrown out. Some privately funded research and research in other countries may continue with embryonic stem cells.

This is another issue to which there are no easy answers. However, as powerful and well-known individuals such as Nancy Reagan, Michael J. Fox, Mary Tyler Moore, and Christopher Reeve push for legislation to support research, we can be assured of hearing more about the retrieval of embryonic stem cells for research.

Critical Thinking Activity

Given the arguments for and against stem cell research, what position would you take? Why do you hold this position? What are your biases? Discuss your position with someone who holds the opposite point of view. What are that person's strongest arguments?

OTHER BIOETHICAL ISSUES

Although our discussion cannot be exhaustive of the topic, certain events occur frequently enough in the health care delivery system that we would be remiss in not mentioning them.

Truth-Telling and Health Care Providers

The issue of "to tell" or "not to tell" may not carry the emotional and bioethical impact that one experiences with concerns such as euthanasia, but it is often encountered in the health care environment. Although informed consent has forced a more straightforward approach between physician and client, the problem of having the patient fully understand the outcome of care still exists (see Chapter 9). Sometimes the question about telling the client the expected outcome of care results from a request made by a close relative, but most of the time it results from the persistence of past medical practices.

In such instances, the physician operates in a paternalistic role in relation to the client. Under this model of care, the locus of decision-making is moved away from the client and resides with the physician. "Benefit and do no harm to the patient" is the dictum often cited as the ethical basis for this approach. It rationalizes that complete knowledge of his or her condition would place greater stress on the client. More recent discussions of medical ethics explore the rights of clients, particularly their right to make their own medical decisions. These discussions emphasize that in our pluralistic society, which also has fostered medical specialization to keep up with advances in knowledge and technology, physicians may be unable to perceive the "best interests" of their clients and to act accordingly.

Physicians do not agree on how much information should be provided to patients regarding their conditions. We usually experience a major controversy relating to this issue when a client has a terminal diagnosis such as cancer. Physicians may be concerned that sharing bad news will result in unhappiness, anxiety, depression, and fear, and that the client suffering from a terminal illness will "give up." In some cultures, such as Japan, this approach is widely considered appropriate and both physicians and families strongly believe that those who are ill should be protected from bad news.

Physicians who argue the other side of the issue state that there exists a common moral obligation to tell the truth. They believe that the anxiety of not knowing the accurate diagnosis is at least as great as knowing the truth, especially if the truth is shared in a humane manner. These physicians also argue that one needs to have control over one's life and, if the news is bad, to have time to get personal affairs in order.

Regulations regarding informed consent and more aggressive treatment for all life-threatening conditions have minimized situations in which patients are not provided full knowledge of their condition. However, these situations still arise. Sometimes care providers are challenged as to the best ethical and legal approach when a family is from a different cultural background and strongly disagrees with giving full information to a patient.

Thus far, we have discussed situations in which information regarding a terminal illness may be shared with the client and family. At least one other circumstance that involves telling the truth is worth mentioning, although many examples could be included. One that we often see in the obstetric area of the hospital deals with sharing information with the parents of a newborn who is critically ill or who has a malformation. Sometimes physicians may want to spare the mother unpleasant news until she is stronger. This occurs frequently enough for obstetric nurses to have labeled it *spare-the-mother syndrome*. In some instances, the physician may want to delay giving information until suspicions can be validated. If the doctor is waiting for the return of laboratory tests to confirm suspicions of genetic abnormalities, several days may be required. If good communication exists between nurse and physician, so that the nurse is well informed, the nurse can provide emotional support and meet the client's need for information.

Although to tell or not to tell (or to delay telling) is a problem that exists between client and physician, nurses often become involved. Because the nurse is in contact with the client for a more extended time, he or she may be put on the spot by the client's questions. The nurse may feel that hedging on a response compromises the ethics of nursing practice. In such instances, a conference, whether formal or impromptu, that would involve the physician, nurses, and other appropriate members of the health team, may help everyone deal with the situation. The nurse who is a novice in the health care system should realize that anyone may initiate a client care conference, although appropriate channels of communication should be followed in organizing it.

The question of whether "to tell" or "not to tell" has been applied to another issue in the health care delivery system in recent years. That controversy pits the rights to privacy of the individual who is HIV positive against society's right to be protected. Dr. Cary Savitch, who has treated AIDS patients since 1981, advocates universal testing. Dr. Savitch (1996, p. 140) states, "Controlling the epidemic is the only means to limit needless suffering and death. Controlling the epidemic will not come at the hands of a vaccine or miracle drug. Controlling the epidemic requires prevention. Prevention requires knowing who is communicable. Knowing who is communicable requires universal testing."

Many express concerns about privacy and confidentiality. If universal testing for AIDS is mandated, what would be next? Others argue that if health care providers exercise proper precautions, little danger exists. Still others would find the cost of universal testing too great to make it realistic. There is no agreement among health care providers, activists, civil libertarians, and all concerned citizens regarding this issue, and the controversy is certain to continue.

Ethical Concerns and Behavior Control

Many people experience extreme discomfort when contemplating research into human behavior and **behavior control**. Although it may be one thing to work with atoms, molecules, and genes, it seems quite another to look at the science of human behavior.

Some of the problem seems to center around the fact that people define "acceptable behavior" in different and sometimes conflicting ways. When is behavior deviant? When is the client mentally ill? An excellent example is that of homosexuality, which the American Psychiatric Association at one time listed as a mental illness. Although many people may not approve of homosexuality, they would not classify all homosexuals as being mentally ill. Increasingly, society looks on sexual orientation as a personal matter.

The world has benefited from the work of many people whose behavior might not be looked upon as normal. Van Gogh cut off his ear; Tchaikovsky had terrible periods of depression; Beethoven was known for his uncontrollable rages. Some have suggested that Florence Nightingale's flights into fantasy could better be described as neurosis. Should this behavior have been changed? If so, by what methods?

We now can change behavior by several methods. Certainly one of the most common methods in which nurses will be involved is the administration of pharmacologic agents. Psychotropics are now one of the largest classifications of drugs in the United States. Many of these such as antianxiety agents and antidepressants are prescribed for people who wish to modify their feelings and behaviors. Other chemicals, such as alcohol, marijuana, cocaine, and lysergic acid diethylamide (LSD), also change mood and/or behavior. Some of these are considered socially acceptable, whereas others are not. Some are socially acceptable to some people or to some cultures yet unacceptable to others.

Electroconvulsive therapy (ECT), known earlier as electric shock therapy (EST), has been used for years to treat severe depression. Although antidepressant drugs are more commonly used today, ECT is still used in many areas of the country for depression that does not respond to drugs. Opponents of this form of therapy, who see it as inhumane, are becoming an organized political force. Proponents point out that with the current safeguards, it can be an effective therapy.

Psychosurgery—for example, frontal lobotomy (portrayed in *One Flew Over the Cuckoo's Nest*)—was used in the 1930s. This is undoubtedly one of the most criticized treatment modalities because of its effect on the person. It is rarely used today, although another type of brain surgery is now being suggested for obsessive–compulsive disorder.

Psychotherapy can change other behaviors. Techniques include verbal and nonverbal communication between the client and the therapist. Although psychotherapy requires considerable time, it is widely used.

When are any of these methods justified? Who makes the decision? What behavior is beyond the realm of acceptability? Who determines this? How does behavior control mesh with our beliefs about the autonomy of the individual or with concepts of self-respect and dignity? The issues of power and coercion pose a concern at this point. Problems related to involuntary commitment have moved this from the arena of ethics to that of legal determinants.

Halleck (1981, p. 268) has defined behavior control as treatment "imposed on or offered to the patient that, to a large extent, is designed to satisfy the wishes of others. Such treatment may lead to the patient's behaving in a manner which satisfies his community or his society."

Halleck goes on to point out that the question of behavior control has become more critical because newer drugs and new behavior therapy (such as aversive therapy and desensitization) make it possible to change specific behavior more rapidly and effectively. Traditional psychotherapy, which works slowly, offers the patient time in which to contemplate the change and reject it if it is unacceptable.

Dworkin (1981, p. 278) has proposed a set of guidelines that preserve autonomy in behavior control, as briefly stated here. Although these guidelines are almost 20 years old, they continue to be recognized for the direction they provide.

- We should favor those methods of influencing behavior that support the self-respect and dignity of those who are being influenced.
- Methods of influence that destroy or decrease a person's ability to think rationally and in his or her own interest should not be used.
- Methods of influence that fundamentally affect the personal identity of the person should not be used.
- Methods of influence that deceive or keep relevant facts from the person should not be used.
- Modes of influence that are not physically intrusive are preferable to those that are (eg, drugs, psychosurgery, and electricity).
- A person should be able to resist the method of influence if he or she so desires, and changes of behavior that are reversible are preferable to those that are not.
- Methods that work through the cognitive and affective structure of a person are preferable to those that "short-circuit" his beliefs and desires and cause him to be passively receptive to the will of others.

Critical Thinking Activity

Review the guidelines for ethical treatment of psychiatric conditions. Which do you believe are the strongest, and why? Are there any that you question; if so, why? Are there any that you think should be added?

Rationing of Health Care

Perhaps no issue in health care will receive more attention in the next few decades than the **rationing of health care**. Technology has allowed people to live longer. New treatment modalities have become more expensive. Dollars do not exist within our current social system to make all forms of health care available to all who wish to receive it. What should be treated and what should not? Who should receive the treatment and who should not? Should age be a factor? Mental status? Ability to contribute to society?

Rationing is restricting the availability of some desired commodity to limited allotments. Most consider rationing to be a planned, thoughtful approach to a limited supply. Some would argue that we currently ration health care by restricting its availability to those with the financial means to pay, although none would argue that this is a carefully planned approach.

Some states have begun to address these issues. In 1989, the Oregon legislature passed several statutes that, among other things, created a process to establish health care priorities so that Medicaid and state-encouraged private coverage could provide the most cost-effective and beneficial forms of care for the largest number of persons. Explicit in this legislation was the involvement of the public in the process of building consensus on the values to be used to guide health resource allocation decisions. Oregon has continued to lead the nation in health care reform, especially at the consumer involvement level.

In Vermont, a statewide public education and discussion project was initiated to explore public attitudes and values that underlie health care and the public's priorities in the allocation of health resources. The project focused on the need for individuals to make known their preferences with regard to personal treatment.

In New Jersey, a Citizens' Committee on Biomedical Ethics has taken the position that citizens have the right and responsibility to insist that their preferences and values influence the development of health care policies and the allocation of medical resources. They have launched a community health program to clarify the ethical and social issues surrounding the provision of health care in that state.

Other states are following these examples. Citizens are being asked to make informed decisions regarding health care. As a nurse, you have a vital role to play in the sharing of information regarding the delivery of health services. It is critical for you to anticipate some of the questions you may be asked and to analyze your own values (Fig. 10-6).

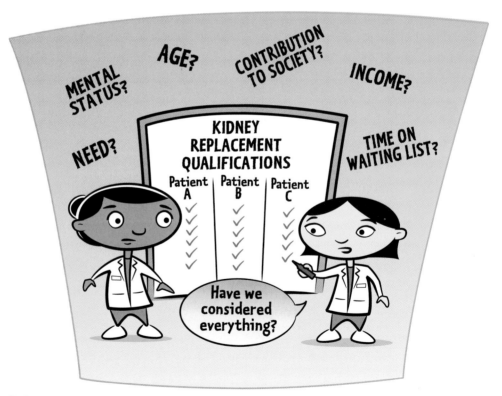

FIGURE 10-6   It is critical that you analyze your own values.

Critical Thinking Activity

What do you see as the major issues regarding the rationing of health care? Develop a list of the major health conditions for which you believe care should be funded. Identify those that should receive partial funding. List those that you believe should not be funded. Give a rationale for placing the various conditions on one of the three lists.

KEY CONCEPTS

- Bioethics is the study of ethical issues that result from technologic and scientific advances, especially in biology and medicine. The number of bioethical issues surrounding the delivery of health care is growing.
- Many bioethical issues can be divided into two major categories: those related to the beginning of life and those related to the end of life.
- Family planning (and the associated concern regarding age of consent) is one issue related to the beginning of life. Personal preferences and religious beliefs are critical determinants, and nurses should be prepared to meet the needs of all clients without imposing their personal values on clients.
- Abortion, amniocentesis, chorionic villus sampling, prenatal diagnosis, genetic screening, sterilization, the concept of eugenics, in vitro fertilization, artificial insemination, surrogate mothers, single parents, sperm banks, and the right to genetic information are additional topics presenting concerns.
- Fundamental bioethical issues concerning death are the changing definition of death and the decision about when it occurs.
- End-of-life issues include identifying futile treatment and establishing patient self-determination.
- Although many courts, based on individual circumstances, have accepted negative euthanasia, positive euthanasia remains very controversial.
- Surrounding the discussion of right-to-die are many issues, including those related to withholding treatment, withdrawing treatment, assisted death, and the right to refuse treatment.
- Bioethical concerns associated with the process of organ transplantation include procurement of organs, availability of organs for minorities, allocation of organs, individual property rights, and the appropriateness of xenotransplantations.
- The area of human genetic research has raised many ethical questions, including how this knowledge should be used, rights to privacy, and who in the health care delivery system carries the responsibility for making testing, diagnosis, and cost-effective care available to patients.
- Stem cell research, which holds great promise for diseases and conditions for which there is no cure, is also laden with bioethical concerns, particularly those related to whether a blastocyst should be considered a human life.
- Debate and controversy have long surrounded determining what degree of information should be shared with clients and their families.

- The area of behavior control is subject to bioethical review, and guidelines have been established to preserve autonomy in behavior control.
- Rationing of health care commands major attention now. Many states have begun to establish citizen committees to respond to this concern.

RELEVANT WEB SITES

American Journal of Bioethics, Bioethics Network: *www.bioethics.net*
Boston College, Nursing Ethics Network: *www.bc.edu/nursing/ethics*
Georgetown University, The Kennedy Institute of Ethics, National Reference Center for Bioethics Literature: *www.georgetown.edu/research/nrcbl/*
International Society of Nurses in Genetics: *http://nursing.creighton.edu.isong.*
John Hopkins University, Bioethics Institute: *www.med.jhu.edu/bioethics_institute*
Medical College of Wisconsin, Center for the Study of Bioethics, Bioethics Online Service: *www.mcw.edu/bioethics/*
Midwest Bioethics Center: *www.midbio.org/*
National Catholic Bioethics Center: *www.ncbcenter.org/*
National Coalition for Health Profession Education in Genetics: *www.nchpeg.org.*
President's Council on Bioethics: *www.bioethics.gov/*
Understanding Gene Testing: *www.accessexcellence.org/AE/AEPC/NIH*
United Network for Organ Sharing Transplantation Information Site: *www.unos.org/*
University of British Columbia, W. Maurice Young Centre for Applied Ethics: *www.ethics.ubc.ca/*
University of Southern California, Pacific Center for Health Policy and Ethics: *lawweb.usc.edu/Pacific_Center/*

REFERENCES

American Nurses Association. (1995a). *Position statement on foregoing medically provided nutrition and hydration.* Washington, DC: American Nurses Association.

American Nurses Association. (1995b). *Position statement on nursing and the Patient Self-Determination Act.* Washington, DC: American Nurses Association.

American Nurses Association. (1994). *Position statement on assisted suicide.* Washington, DC: American Nurses Association.

American Nurses Association. (1988). *Guidelines on withdrawing or withholding food and fluid.* Washington, DC: American Nurses Association.

Blackmun, H. (1981). Majority opinion in Roe vs Wade. In T. A. Mappes & J. S. Zembaty, *Biomedical ethics* (2nd ed.) (pp. 478–482). New York: McGraw-Hill.

"Body and soul." (2002 [October 27]). *Seattle Times,* p. A3.

Burkhardt, M. A. & Nathaniel, A. K. (2002). *Ethics & issues in contemporary nursing* (2nd ed.). Albany, NY: Delmar.

Burley, S. K., Almo, S. C., Bonanno J. B., Capel, M., Chance, M. R., Gaasterland, T., Lin, D., Sali, A., Studier, F. W. & Swaminathan, S. (1999). Structural genomics: Beyond the human genome project. *Nature Genetics 23*(2):151–157.

Capron, A. M. (1994). Grandma? No, I'm the mother! *Hastings Center Report 24*(2):24–25.

"Cloned pigs raise transplant hopes." (2002 [August 22]). [On-line]. Available: *http://news.bbc.co.uk/2/hi/ science/nature/2210306.stm.*

Colby, W. H. (1990). Missouri stands alone. *Hastings Center Report 20*(5): 5–6.

Critical Data: U. S. Facts About Transplantation. (2002). UNOS Critical Data Main Page. [On-line]. Available: *http://www.unos.org/Newsroom/critdata_main.htm.* Accessed September 26, 2002.

Department of Health & Human Services. (2001 [June]) "Stem cells: Scientific progress and future research directions, executive summary". [On-line]. *http://www.nih.gov/new/stemcell/ scireport.htm.* Accessed October *12*, 2002.

Dorning, M. (1994 [November 13]). Teen-agers refusal of treatment stirs debate. *San Diego Union Tribune* A-8.

Dworkin, G. (1981). Autonomy and behavior control. In T. A. Mappes & J. S. Zembaty. *Biomedical Ethics* (2nd ed.) (pp 273–280), New York: McGraw-Hill.

"European court throws out appeal for assisted suicide." (2002 [April 30]). *The Seattle Times*, p. A-12.

Fano, A., Cohen, M. J., Cramer, M., Greek, R. & Kaufman, S. R. (1999). Of pigs, primates, and plagues: A layperson's guide to the problems with animal-to-human organ transplants. [On-line]. Available at *www.mrmcmed.org/pigs.html.* Accessed December 22, 1999.

Fry, S. T. (1990). New ANA guidelines on withdrawing or withholding food and fluid from patients. In C. A. Lindeman & M. McAthie: *Readings: Nursing trends and issues.* (pp. 499–507). Springhouse, PA: Springhouse.

Gustafson, J. J. (1973 [Summer]). Mongolism, parental desires, and the right to life. *Perspectives in Biology and Medicine*, p. 529.

Halleck, S. L. (1981). Legal and ethical aspects of behavior control. In T. A. Mappes & Zembaty J. S.: *Biomedical ethics* (2nd ed.) (pp. 267–273). New York: McGraw-Hill.

"Hospital sued for 'wrongful life'." (1991). *American Journal of Nursing, 91*(5):111.

Hudson, T. (1994a). Advance directives: Still problematic for providers. *Hospitals and Health Networks 68(*6): 46, 48, 50.

Hudson, T. (1994b). Are futile-care policies the answer? *Hospitals and Health Networks 68*(4):26–32.

Human Genome Project Information. About the Human Genome Project (2002a). [On-line]. Available: *www.ornl.gov/ hgmis/project/about/html.*

Human Genome Project Information. Ethical, legal, and social issues (ELSI) of the Human Genome Project. (2002b) [On-line]. Available at *www.ornl.gov/hgmis/elsi/elsi.html.*

Judson, K. & Hicks, S. (1999). *Law & ethics for medical careers* (2nd ed.). New York: Glencoe/ McGraw-Hill.

Kasiske, B. L, Neylan, J. F., Riggio, R. R. et al. (1991). The effect of race on access and outcome in transplantation. *New England Journal of Medicine* 324:302–307.

Kass, L. R. (1993). Is there a right to die? *Hastings Center Report 23*(1):34–43.

Killion, S. W. & Dempski, K. M. (2000). *Legal and ethical issues.* Thorofare, New Jersey: Slack, Inc.

Kmiec, E. G. (1999 [May-June)]. Targeted gene repair. *American Scientist,* [On-line]. Available at *www.amsci.org/amsci/articles/99articles/Kmiecrepair.html.* Accessed September 19, 2002.

Lombardo, P. (2002). Eugenics sterilization laws. [On-line]. Available at *http://www.eugenicsarchive.org/html/eugenics/essay_8.html.*

Macklin, R. (1991). Artificial means of reproduction and our understanding of the family. *Hastings Center Report 21*(1): 5–11.

"Most transplanted organs from live donors, U.S. says." (2002 [April 23]). *The Seattle Times*, p. A2.

National Minority Organ Tissue Transplant Educational Program. Statistics: MOTTEP Facts and Figures. (2002). [On-line]. Available at *http://www.nationalmottep.org.ststs.html.*

"Netherlands is first nation to fully legalize euthanasia." (2001 [April 11]). *The Herald*, p. 3A.

Nuland, S. B.(1996). An epidemic of discovery. *Time Special Issue*, Fall: 8–13.

"Oregon suicides steady, still sharply divisive." (2002 [February 10]). *The Seattle Times*, p. B1, 4.

O'Toole, M. (Ed.). (1992). *Miller-Keane encyclopedia and dictionary of medicine, nursing, and allied health* (5th ed.). Philadelphia: W.B. Saunders.

Pilbeam, S. P. (1998). *Mechanical ventilation: Physiological and clinical applications* (3rd ed.). St. Louis: Mosby.

Randall, V. R. (2002). Basis of distrust. [On-line]. Available at *http://academic.udayton.edu/health/05bioethics/slavery02.htm.*

Roan, S. (1997 [April 24]). Woman gives birth at 63: Ethical questions raised. *Los Angeles Times*, A1, A31.

Roe v. Wade, 410 U.S. 113 (1973).

Rothstein, M. A. (1990). The challenge of the new genetics. *National Forum 69*(4): 39–40.

Savitch, C. (1996). *The nutcracker is already dancing: The HIVs and the HIV-nots.* Ventura, CA: Teague House Press.

Schneiderman, L. F. & Jecker, N. (1993). Futility in practice. *Archives of Internal Medicine 153*:437–440.

Schroeder, S. (2002). Steven Schroeder reflects on the uninsured. Roberts Woods Johnson Foundation. [On-line]. Available at *http://www.rwjf.org/newsEvents/healthPolicy2.jhtml.*

Stem cell stalement. (2001 [August 10]). *The Herald*, p. A1.

Swain, M. S. & Marusyk, R. W. (1990). An alternative to property rights in human tissue. *Hastings Center Report 20*(5):12–15.

"The stem cell debate hinges on when human life begins." (2001 [August 10]). *The Herald*, p. A11.

totse.com. Age of consent in every state. [On-line]. Available at *http://www.totse.com/en/law/justice_for_all/aoc.html.* Accessed 10/16/02.

Veatch, R. M. (1976). *Death, dying and the biological revolution.* New Haven, CT: Yale University Press.

Wheeler, M. S. & Cheung, A. (1996). Minority attitudes toward organ donation. *Critical Care Nurse 16*(1):30–34. *http://womenshistory.about.com/library/ency/blwh_comstock.htm.* Accessed 10/16/02.

Career Opportunities and Professional Growth

The final unit in this textbook is devoted to topics that will assist you to move into the world of employment as a registered nurse (RN). Information is provided about the competencies needed for the wide variety of opportunities available to nurses today. Chapter 11 describes how to set short- and long-term goals, write resumés, and compose letters of application and letters following up on interviews.

Strategies you can use to prevent reality shock and cope with the realities of the work world (including workplace violence) are included. As you move toward employment in one of the health care environments, it is important to understand organizational structure, including the purpose of missions, organizational charts, chains of command, and approaches to governance. You will find this information in Chapter 12.

This chapter also discusses the forms of nursing care delivery, collective bargaining in nursing, and the purpose of and what to expect in a contract. The pros and cons of having a professional nursing association serve as the bargaining agent for nurses concludes the unit.

All RNs have responsibilities in regard to leading and managing others. Understanding the leadership and management role of the nurse is the focus of Chapter 13. You will find helpful information about how power is distributed and used in the health care system. The chapter concludes with a discussion of time-management issues.

As a leader in the health care system, nurses have specific responsibilities regarding delegation within the nursing team, and interacting with the transdisciplinary team. Nurses also have responsibilities regarding the implementation of the medical plan of care, which necessitates the exploration of physician–nurse relationships, including both positive aspects and problem areas. Helping you to navigate these aspects of the system is the focus of Chapter 14.

11

Beginning Your Career as a Nurse

After completing this chapter, you should be able to:

1. Describe a variety of employment opportunities available to nurses today and the educational requirements of each.

2. Explain the competencies needed by the new graduate as outlined by the job analysis study that is the basis for the NCLEX-RN examination.

3. Analyze the eight common expectations employers have of new graduates and relate them to your own background and education.

4. Develop a list of your personal short- and long-term career goals.

5. Design strategies to maintain your competence in nursing.

6. Formulate a plan for beginning your career, including developing a personal resumé; sample letters of application, follow-up, and resignation; and your possible responses in an employment interview.

7. Construct strategies to prevent or alleviate reality shock.

8. Analyze your own values and life situation in relationship to your personal potential for burnout, and adapt personal stress management techniques to control your work stress.

9. Discuss ways racial, ethnic, and sex discrimination have affected nursing.

10. Discuss the various hazards to the health of employees in the health care workplace and ways that you can act to protect yourself and others.

K E Y   T E R M S

Burnout	Long-term goals	Resumé
Competency	Novice to expert	Sexual harassment
Cover letter	Occupational hazard	Short-term goals
Criticality	Proficiency	Stereotype
Discrimination	Quality assurance report	
Incident report	Reality shock	

When you graduate, one of your first objectives will be obtaining employment as a registered nurse (RN). You probably look forward to practicing in the nursing role you have spent so long attaining. You may even envision the "perfect" nursing position and have thought no further ahead than this first job. For other new graduates, the desire for a job is initially general, rather than specific, in view of student loans to be repaid and the desire to move into a lifestyle different from the student one.

Unlike graduates of the hospital programs of the past, you will have spent fewer hours working in the patient care setting. Although some new graduates have worked as unlicensed assistive staff or practical nurses during their education, others' contact with health care settings may have been as students rather than as employees. You may not have experienced all of the many settings in which RNs are employed. You may have questions regarding employer expectations and your own role as an RN employee.

In the past, the expectations of most new graduates were simple, but a nursing career is now much more complex. In this chapter, we try to assist you as you survey the RN job market and plan for a successful approach to obtaining that important first position. We also try to provide suggestions to help you find satisfaction and growth after your initial employment.

EMPLOYMENT OPPORTUNITIES TODAY

In the 1990s, the pressures of a changing health care system and cost containment created many changes for nursing. Hospital stays shortened so dramatically that hospital censuses decreased across the country. The nursing shortage appeared to end abruptly as hospitals began reassessing their needs. Some hospitals closed; many downsized. In addition, many hospitals restructured to employ more unlicensed assistive personnel. These factors contributed to layoffs of nurses from hospitals. Long-term care and home care increased, although funding of home care remained a problem.

Now as we enter a new century, a nursing shortage is again present. The client of the downsized hospital is more acutely ill and older than before. To maintain short stays and early discharge, patient teaching and planning for discharge have assumed more importance than before. Hospitals that downsized too abruptly found that they needed to replace RNs. As the population ages, with an expected increase of 54% in those 65 and older, the demand for RNs is expected to increase in all settings with an overall increase in demand of 40% between 2000 and 2020 (Projected Supply, 2002).

Concerns that the nursing shortage will continue and even grow more acute are based on the convergence of several factors. The RN workforce is aging, with a majority of nurses over 45 years of age. This trend is expected to continue until 2020 (Projected Supply, 2002). The workload is high and the pace is demanding. As a consequence, older RNs often choose to work less than full time or retire early, further depleting the supply. Positions for those with baccalaureate and higher degrees and for those with specialty training, such as intensive care or operating room nursing, are growing faster than the job market in general. There are also regional differences in the nursing supply (Spratley et al, 2000).

Meanwhile, the number of new graduates entering the employment market decreased during the second half of the 1990s. Some programs failed to meet targets for admissions and, subsequently, graduations from nursing schools declined. Although this trend is now reversing, the supply of new RNs is expected to increase by only 6% by 2020 if no actions are taken to increase the number of spaces in nursing schools (Projected Supply, 2002). Thus, as a new graduate, you will find yourself in high demand as an employee.

Most new graduates choose to begin their careers in structured health care settings that offer support for the novice in making the adjustment to the RN role. In its trend study, the National Council of State Boards of Nursing (NCSBN) identified changes over time in the work environments, employment characteristics, and job activities of newly licensed nurses through surveys conducted every 3 months, beginning in January 1998. The survey indicated that in July 1999, 82% of the new graduate RNs were working in acute care environments, 10% were in subacute or long-term care, and 8% were in community-based care (NCSBN, 1999). Acute care hospitals employ approximately 62% of RNs (Projected Supply, 2002).

The growth of autonomy for the RN has been even more marked outside the hospital setting than in it. Community health nurses have always operated much more independently than hospital nurses. Many positions in the community require a baccalaureate degree or specialized educational programs. Although these settings once required that new graduates have experience in a structured setting before beginning practice in such an independent setting, the shortage has caused some employers to begin recruiting new graduates. The new graduate in these settings needs to be assertive in obtaining the necessary support to make the transition into the role.

The number of positions for RNs in many settings other than those providing client care also has grown. Health care-oriented businesses, such as insurance companies and medical equipment supply companies, have found that it is easier to teach nurses about business than to teach business people about health care. As a result, nurses are being employed in what some individuals see as non-nursing positions. Others argue that these, too, should be considered nursing positions, because the expertise that makes the individual successful is nursing expertise. Although experienced nurses usually hold these positions, moving into these positions may be a part of a career plan of the new graduate.

The number of men in nursing, which remained relatively small for many years, is beginning to grow as society reassesses its attitude toward labeling jobs as women's or men's work. Only 5.4% of practicing nurses are men, but the percentage of men in nursing has been increasing steadily (Spratley et al, 2000). Men have been attracted by the career opportunities and improving economic picture of nursing.

The economic position of the nurse has improved for several reasons. One reason is the extension of laws governing fair labor practic   o nonprofit institutions and the advent of collective bargaining. Another major factor affecting the economic position of nurses was the nursing shortage of the 1980s. The demand for nurses rose faster than the supply, and employers began increasing salaries and benefits to attract nurses. This trend was especially notable in urban communities.

Although wages have increased substantially since the 1980s, the study regarding supply and demand concluded that inflation accounts for most of the increase. Real wages in terms of purchasing power have risen only slightly (Spratley et al, 2000). Nurses have expressed concern that high wages quoted in some settings often reflect large amounts of overtime pay that increase the stress of the job.

All of these factors bring you, as a new graduate, into a world of uncertainty, but one also filled with opportunity and promise. As we enter a new century, the nursing shortage is acute. Now you must determine your place in this world.

COMPETENCIES OF THE NEW GRADUATE

Recently you may have heard the term **competency** used a great deal, especially as it applied to you as a student. Competency, as used here, refers to the ability of the person to effectively and safely perform specified nursing skills, including the application of critical thinking skills. Some have differentiated "competency," which is an entry-level expectation, and "**proficiency**," which is expected of the experienced nurse (Fig. 11-1).

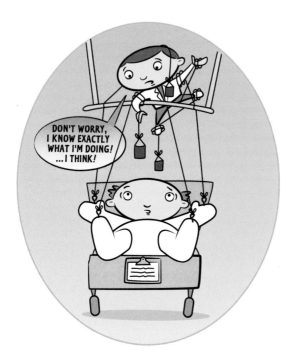

FIGURE 11-1 New graduates are expected to know both their own abilities and when to seek appropriate help.

Competencies Identified by Nursing Organizations

The most definitive statements on the competencies needed by the newly licensed practical nurse (PN) and the RN have been developed by the NCSBN, based on its job analysis studies, which serve as the basis for the NCLEX-RN and NCLEX-PN licensing examinations.

In these studies, activities reported by a stratified random sample of newly licensed, entry-level nurses were examined. Both the frequency of the nursing activities and their criticality were studied. **Criticality** refers to activities that cannot be delayed or omitted without a "substantial risk of unnecessary complications, impairment of function, or serious distress to clients" (NCSBN, 2002). The most recent RN study was completed in 1999; the results of that study supported the continuation of the current test plan and passing score (NCSBN, 2002). The most recent PN study was completed in 2001 (NCSBN, 2001).

Activities expected of newly licensed RNs that led the list for criticality were:

- Use appropriate infection-control measures
- Report significant changes in the client's condition
- Perform cardiopulmonary resuscitation
- Perform Heimlich maneuver/abdominal thrust
- Provide emergency care for a wound disruption
- Recognize the occurrence of hemorrhage
- Manage a medical emergency until a physician arrives
- Implement measures to prevent circulatory complications (eg, embolus, shock, hemorrhage)
- Respond to symptoms of fetal distress

Activities were studied further in terms of the frequency with which they were expected of newly licensed RNs. In all settings, nurses were expected to:

- Coordinate care through working with others on the health care team and supervising delivery of care by assistive personnel
- Preserve the quality of care through such activities as advocating for needed changes in care, documenting errors or problems, and intervening in situations involving unsafe or inadequate care
- Maintain the safety of the client as exemplified by verifying, identifying, and reporting unsafe equipment, and following infection-control guidelines
- Prepare clients and families for care that is to be done, including procedures and treatments, and help them to understand expected outcomes
- Carry out procedures in a safe, effective manner

Physiologic and psychosocial integrity were supported by many individual nursing actions. Some, such as assessing vital signs, seemed almost universal. Others, such as monitoring for side effects of radiation therapy, were needed in a small minority of settings. Allowing clients to talk about their concerns and assisting them to communicate effectively were almost universal activities.

Nursing process continues to be a strong expectation for RNs. In the 1999 study, newly licensed RNs indicated that they spent 30% of their time on assessments, 12% on analysis, 14% on planning, 30% implementing client care, and 14% on evaluation. Seventy-eight percent stated that they were required to know nursing diagnosis, and 70% used it in their current position (NCSBN, 1999).

In addition to the National Council, other organizations have explored the issue of competencies of new nursing graduates. The various educational councils of the National League for Nursing have developed statements regarding competencies of new graduates. The NLN Council of Associate Degree Programs approved a new set of competencies of the associate degree graduate in 1999 (NLN, 1999). The American Association of Colleges of Nursing developed a document titled "Essentials of Baccalaureate Education for Nursing," which includes expected competencies. Additionally, some states have developed statements of competencies for graduates of the nursing programs in those states. This often has been part of a process to improve articulation between programs at different levels.

Similarities and patterns have emerged from all of these statements. The outline of theoretic knowledge and functioning regarding the nursing process seems to be the most consistent. The most divergent opinions seem to be in the area of specific skill or task competency.

Employers' Expectations Regarding Competencies

Employers often ask for further clarification of competence. Have these graduates only the necessary theoretic knowledge of the skill? Have they actually performed the skill? If so, was it in a practice laboratory only, or was it in a client care situation? Does competence mean that the new graduate can function independently, or will some supervision still be needed?

Further complicating the picture is the confusion surrounding competencies of the graduates of the three types of nursing education programs that prepare individuals for RN licensure: the hospital-based diploma program, the associate degree program, and the baccalaureate degree program. Although statements by several organizations have distinguished among levels of functioning, many employers do not differentiate expectations. Some employers state that new graduates from different types of programs have not clearly demonstrated differences in competencies. This has created confusion in the minds of nurses, employers, and the public over the role of the RN prepared in each type of educational program.

What is expected of the new graduate varies in different health care agencies and in different geographic areas. Expectations are affected by factors in the community, such as whether there are nursing programs in that community and whether new graduates come from one or from many different schools. The acuity of the client care load and the types of services offered by an agency also may affect expectations. The Joint Commission on the Accreditation of Healthcare Organizations (JCAHO) has a criterion requiring that accredited institutions monitor and assure the competence of their staff. This requires that an institution identify expected competencies for staff and then design an assessment method. As institutions move to comply with this standard, most are directing their initial efforts toward technical skills because these are more easily identified and assessed. Other competencies will be more difficult to assess.

Based on the NCSBN job analysis studies, some general patterns of employer expectations can be seen.

1. **Possess the necessary theoretic background for safe client care and for decision-making.** For instance, the new graduate should understand the signs and symptoms of an insulin reaction, recognize the reaction when it occurs, and know what nursing

actions should be taken. The new graduate must know when an emergency or complication is occurring and secure medical help for the client when that is needed. Many employers believe that new graduates today are very competent in their theoretic foundations for practice.

2. **Use the nursing process in a systematic way.** This includes assessment, analysis, planning, intervention, and evaluation. New graduates should be able to develop plans of care and follow plans, such as care pathways, that have been developed by the agency.

3. **Recognize own abilities and limitations.** To provide safe care, the nurse must identify when a situation requires greater expertise or knowledge and when assistance is needed. Employers may be able to assist if nurses ask for help and direction, but cannot accept the risk to clients created by nurses who do not know or accept their own limitations.

4. **Use communication skills effectively with clients and coworkers.** In every setting, there are clients and families who are anxious, depressed, suffering loss, or experiencing other emotional distress. The nurse is expected to respond appropriately to these individuals and to facilitate their coping and adaptation. Effective communication skills are essential to the functioning of the entire health care team. Often, the nurse is expected to help coordinate the work of others, and this cannot be done without effective communication skills.

5. **Work effectively with assistive personnel, delegating and supervising nursing care tasks in an appropriate manner.** In most settings, assistive personnel are a part of the nursing team. The RN nurse, and, in some instances, the PN, is expected to identify what can be delegated and do so in a way that contributes to appropriate patient care outcomes.

6. **Understand the importance of accurate and complete documentation.** Employers generally recognize that the new graduate must be given time to learn the documentation system used in the facility. However, the new graduate is expected to recognize the need for recording data. It is anticipated that the nurse will keep accurate, grammatically correct, and legible records that provide the necessary legal documentation of care.

7. **Possess proficiency in the basic technical nursing skills.** This is an area in which a wide variety of expectations may be present. In most settings, proficiency in the basic skills required to support activities of daily living is expected. These skills include transferring, giving baths, and performing general hygienic measures. In some settings, nurses will be carrying out these tasks, whereas in others they will be directing or teaching others who do them, such as nursing assistants or family members. In either case, proficiency is essential to evaluating the care provided. The technical skills or tasks that are reserved for the RN represent the area of widest diversity in the identification of essential skills. The settings in which nurses practice are wide-ranging, and therefore technical skills may be needed in one setting but not in another. Some facilities provide extensive orientation programs in which every skill is checked before the new graduate is allowed to proceed independently. Other employers expect the new graduate to perform the skill if able, and be checked off as required, or to ask for help if unable to be independent. Often

employers are flexible in their expectations, so that it may be acceptable if an individual seems to have competency in a reasonable percentage of the skills required by that agency; further development of skill competency will be supported by the institution. Other employers have a list of skills in which competency is mandatory at the time of hire, although speed may not be expected. Also, there may be a difference between what the employer would wish and what the employer will accept.

In addition to these professional responsibilities as a nurse, employers also speak of their concern for worker-related competencies they want to see in all health care workers. These include:

8. **Understand and have a commitment to a work ethic.** This means that the employee will take the responsibility of the job seriously and will be on time, take only the allowed coffee and lunch breaks, and will not take "sick days" unless truly ill. It also means that the new graduate recognizes that nurses may be needed 24 hours a day, 365 days a year, and that this may require sacrifices of personal convenience, such as working evening shifts or on holidays.

9. **Function with acceptable speed.** This is another area in which expectations differ greatly. Most employers state that they expect the new graduate will be slower; however, they may vary in how much slowness is acceptable and how soon they feel that nursing actions should become more time efficient. Generally, an orientation period is planned—although, with the pressures on health care agencies, this often has been shortened considerably. An acceptable speed of function is reflected by the ability to carry out a usual RN assignment within a shift. Thus, if the usual client assignment for an RN is the care of four to six moderately ill clients, the new graduate is expected to accomplish this by the end of the orientation period.

PERSONAL CAREER GOALS

In caring for clients, you are involved in the process of goal setting. Many nurses recognize the value of this in client care but never transfer the concept to their personal lives. Nursing as a profession offers many career options. Without carefully setting goals, you might drift for years.

Focusing Your Goals

You may want to focus on a broad area of clinical competency, such as pediatric nursing, or on a more restricted area, such as neonatal care. Clinical areas available for concentrated effort become more varied as health care becomes more complex. Emergency care, coronary care, neurologic and neurosurgical nursing, and specialties in the care of persons with ear, nose, and throat disorders are just a few of the clinical possibilities. Nurses specialize in aerospace nursing, enterostomal therapy, and respiratory care, as well as operating room nursing and postanesthesia care. Opportunities for additional education and for practice in most clinical specialties are now available for any experienced RN, regardless of the person's initial educational background.

Some specialty positions are in the primary care field, such as the woman's health care specialist, the family nurse practitioner, and the pediatric nurse practitioner. Increasing numbers of these specialties require a master's degree for certification. Although some educational programs preparing primary care nurses require the BSN for entry, many will accept an individual with an ADN and a bachelor's degree in another field.

Another approach may be to focus your goals on the setting in which care is delivered, such as acute care, long-term care, or community care. As health care needs expand, these separate realms of care delivery are all demanding more specialized knowledge. Even within the individual area of focus, differences are present. For example, within the community are ambulatory care settings, public health nursing agencies, occupational health nursing departments, and day care facilities.

Yet another way of focusing your goals is according to functional categories. Although nurses are initially thought of as direct care providers, they are needed in many other positions. For example, there is need for those who would move into supervisory and administrative capacities, those who teach, and those who conduct nursing research. Nursing also lends itself to writing, to community service, and even to political involvement.

You may decide to set your goals in relation to all three foci. That is, you might identify a clinical area, a care setting, and a functional category.

Setting Your Goals

The first step in setting personal career goals is a thorough self-assessment. Determine how your abilities and competencies correspond to your own expectations and to those of employers. Other factors to explore are your likes and dislikes and the situations or types of work you particularly enjoyed as a student. Also, it is important to recognize the area in which you were most comfortable. Were there areas in which you or your instructor felt that you were an above-average student? Consider your health and personal characteristics in relation to types of work. Do you have physical restrictions? Do you prefer working independently or with others? How do you respond to close supervision or to relative freedom in the job setting? Do you prefer a work environment that is relatively predictable, or do you thrive in a situation that changes frequently? Do you work well with **long-term goals** and a few immediate reinforcements, or do you need to see results quickly? Another factor to consider is your own geographic mobility: would you be willing to move or travel as part of a job? Both your personal responsibilities and preferences operate in this arena.

As you plan ahead, you need to examine many of the options offered by nursing. What types of jobs and opportunities are open to you? What education and personal abilities are needed in these areas? Are you interested? Does the education you have meet the educational requirements? Are avenues for additional education available to you? All of these considerations are important as you plan for the future. Career goals need to be both short- and long-term. They will help you to plan your future constructively. This does not mean that goals are static. Just as client goals must be realistic, personal, and flexible, so must your own goals.

Short-term goals encompass what you want to accomplish this month and this year. What do you want to do and what do you want to be in the immediate future? For example, one recent graduate stated that her short-term goal was to have 2 years of solid experience in a busy metropolitan hospital.

Long-term goals represent where you want to be in your profession 5 to 10 years or even farther into the future from now. The long-term goal of the graduate referred to above was to work in a small, remote community in which she would have the opportunity to function autonomously.

Although both long- and short-term goals will be revised as your life evolves, they guide you in making day-to-day decisions more effectively. In today's world of rapid health care change, you may need to keep your goals somewhat broad and flexible. Be ready to consider alternative goals and a variety of pathways to one goal. These approaches will be of value as you enter a system in transition.

Critical Thinking Activity

Write out your short- and long-term professional goals, with a brief plan on how you can achieve these goals. Think critically about the obstacles you will need to overcome to reach these goals. How will you deal with the obstacles?

Maintaining and Enhancing Your Competence

Every nurse has an obligation to society to maintain competence and continue practicing high-quality, safe care. Continuing education may occur through learning on the job, reading professional publications, or online or in-person classes. There are television courses, programmed instruction programs, and examinations related to journal articles. Any of these avenues may be appropriate, depending on the circumstances. Some nurses may want to advance through specialty or higher education. Included in your goal setting should be an approach to maintaining and enhancing your competence.

MAKING GOALS REALITY

Philosophic questions regarding goals must be resolved by practical approaches. As a new graduate, your first goal simply may be to get a job in nursing. Some new graduates, who recognize that there is a severe nursing shortage, assume that there is no need to make an effort to make a positive impression on employers. After all, the employer will be glad to have any RN. Although this is true, you should keep in mind that you are not only applying for any entry-level job. If you have identified a specific clinical area in which you wish to work, a specific employer you prefer, or a long-term goal that requires moving from one position to another, then you need to do those things that will obtain your preferred position, not just any position. Additionally, when applying for your first job you may also be making an impression that will affect later promotions or requests for educational opportunities. Those who interview you for an entry-level position, may be making decisions about future job assignments. The impression you make initially will carry over into other situations.

Whatever the situation, you are more likely to realize your goals if you are prepared to present yourself in the best possible way to a prospective employer. Many of you have held different jobs in the community as students and as adults. You may be familiar with and competent in the job search process. Others have never applied for the kind of job that truly could be considered the beginning of a career. Employers and prospective employees may hold different expectations in such a situation.

Identifying Potential Employers

To begin your job search effectively, you need to identify potential employers. You might begin your review with those more familiar to you and gradually move outward in an ever-widening circle to identify others.

The clinical sites where you had experiences as a student or where you worked when a student are good places to begin. You may know these agencies, be familiar with the type of care provided, and already be oriented to many of their policies and procedures. Your prior association with these agencies may provide you with ready access to their hiring procedures. If you worked as an employee in a health care setting before graduation, you may be given preference in hiring. This is one reason for seeking health care employment during your nursing education process.

Another source of potential jobs is the classified section of the local newspaper. There you are more likely to find single jobs in small facilities, as well as general recruitment announcements from larger facilities. However, just because an agency does not advertise does not mean they will not be hiring any employees. Advertising is expensive and may not result in the desired outcome. Therefore, some health care agencies do not advertise and rely on those who independently seek them out as potential employers.

Job fairs for health care employers are becoming more common. Each employer participating provides a booth or table to provide information on job openings in their agencies. An individual looking for employment may explore a variety of employers, learning about job openings, benefits, and opportunities in a brief time without the difficulty of searching out each employer. The employer may see many potential employees in a focused period. Thus, job fairs benefit both employers and potential employees. Job fairs may be held in the community, attracting experienced health care workers as well as students and new graduates. Some colleges arrange job fairs on campus. Nursing programs or nursing student clubs also may arrange job fairs.

The "Yellow Pages" of the telephone directory may help you to locate smaller employers in your community. You could look under "Nursing Homes," "Home Care," "Nursing Care," and other such headings. This may help you to identify health care providers you were not aware of. Do not hesitate to call or even personally visit these settings to obtain information for a job application.

If you have the flexibility to move from your local area, you may expand your search for possible positions. The major nursing journals have sections in the back pages devoted to advertisements. Some of these advertise nursing positions. If you have a specific area in mind, you might visit your local library and consult the newspaper and the telephone directory for that area. Your nursing program may receive advertising magazines that are designed to present job opportunities for new graduates. These magazines provide a few articles about relevant job search topics, such as interviewing, as well as advertisements from health care agencies. These advertisements present information on the agency itself and how to contact them for an application.

Additional sources of potential jobs are available via the Internet. Many governmental job openings also are posted on-line. Using your search engine, look for "employment opportunities," "jobs," or "careers" combined with the term "nursing." Some on-line service providers have additional support services for a job search that might include career guidance (for a fee), or sample documents such as resumés and **cover letters**.

Letter of Inquiry or Application

Writing a letter of inquiry is an excellent way to approach many prospective employers (Display 11-1). This letter is often termed a "cover letter" because it is sent with your resumé (see next page). You can present yourself positively through a well-written letter. In addition, a letter may be dealt with at the recipient's convenience, whereas a telephone call may interrupt a busy schedule. There are fewer chances for misunderstanding if your request is in writing and if you receive a written reply.

Before you write your letter, you should make sure you have information about the prospective employer. What kind of facility is this? What types of clients do they serve, and what special services do they offer? It makes a poor impression to write to a prospective employer stating that your goal is to work in pediatrics when that facility does not provide any pediatric services. Some agencies maintain a Web site with information regarding their mission, goals, and services. You might obtain this information by calling the human resources department of the facility or by contacting a public information office. In a small agency, you may simply speak with a receptionist or secretary. Be honest and straightforward in explaining that you are considering applying for employment and would like information about the agency before making that decision. The cover letter is sent to the nurse recruiter (if the agency has one) or to the human resources department. If you are not sure to whom to address your letter, ask when you call to inquire about the agency itself.

Another part of your advance planning is identifying how you will focus your letter on your special qualifications and what you want to highlight. You will want to focus on the skills or accomplishments related to the position you want. Your letter should be no more than one page in length but should be planned to present all essential information. Introduce yourself and your purpose for writing in the first paragraph so that the reader immediately understands why you are writing. You may want briefly to state your reasons for applying for a position with this particular employer. The more specific the reasons, the better the impression you are likely to make.

Briefly highlight your qualifications for the position. This should not be a simple recitation of what is in your resumé, but should either present the information in a slightly different light or add pertinent detail that is not in the resumé. If you are responding to an advertisement, you should respond to each of the qualifications listed in the advertisement. You might include personal qualities that would make you an effective employee in the position. You should relate your skills and abilities to the needs of this particular agency. If your health care experience is limited, you should point out skills you have gained from other jobs that would be useful in nursing. These might be interpersonal skills, management skills, or adaptability.

In the final paragraph, make a summary statement indicating why you want to work for this employer and ask for an appointment for an interview. Be sure to indicate the times you can be available and how and where you can be contacted if the employer so wishes. It is also

Display 11-1 **LETTER OF APPLICATION**

Maribeth Wilson
3428 1st Ave. N.
Seattle, WA 98103
(206) 274-5978
e-mail: maribethw@email.com

January 30, 2004

Joyce Montgall, R.N.
Nurse Recruiter
Seattle General Medical Center
321 Heath Blvd.
Seattle, WA 98101

Dear Ms. Montgall:

Enclosed please find a copy of my resumé, along with my application to Seattle General Medical Center's New Graduate Residency Program. I will graduate from Shoreline Community College's associate degree nursing program on May 28. I expect to acquire my registered nurse license by the end of June. I am extremely interested in a medical-surgical nursing position within your upcoming residency program.

I believe that I would bring many strengths to a new graduate position. I have worked here at Seattle General as a nursing assistant for the past year, and my experience has given me an excellent foundation in understanding the philosophy and mission of the Medical Center. During this time I have been assigned to several different units, including 4 West and 4 Center, where new graduate positions are available. The nurses at Seattle General have been generous in their mentoring and have helped me to increase my understanding of the patients' conditions. They have been supportive as I developed increased problem-solving and decision-making skills.

Within my nursing student educational experience, I have had the privilege of working in a wide variety of health care institutions throughout the city. From these experiences I would bring an understanding of the community standards of care as well as a unique appreciation of the position of Seattle General in the health care community.

I hope that I will be selected for an interview and look forward to hearing from you. My phone number, email address, and home address are at the top of this letter. If I do not hear from you within the next two weeks, I will contact your office to ascertain the status of my application.

Sincerely,

Maribeth Wilson

Maribeth Wilson

wise to indicate that you will contact the person to whom the letter is addressed to request an appointment. This allows you to maintain some initiative in the process. Thank the person for considering your application, and close.

Another point to remember is that the letter's appearance and its content both represent you. You will be judged on spelling, grammar, clarity, and neatness, in addition to content. Be cautious about relying on the spell-checking function on your computer. An incorrect word may pass the spell check but be clearly seen as an error by the careful reader. Your letter of application should be written in standard business format on plain white or off-white business paper. Make it brief and clear. Ask a friend or family member to check your first draft if you have any questions about its correctness.

Preparing an Effective Resumé

A **resumé** is a brief overview of your qualifications for a position. (Display 11-2). Its purpose is to provide the employer with a way to identify quickly whether you have the basic qualifications for a position, and to present you in the most positive light to be considered for the position in which you are interested. Resumés are used primarily to screen applicants for interviewing; therefore, you will want to make an impression that is good enough to result in an interview. In most instances, you will want to include your resumé with your initial letter. In some situations, you may want to leave an additional copy of your resumé with a unit manager at the end of your interview because your original resumé is retained in the human resources office.

APPEARANCE

The appearance of your resumé is important because it initially presents your image to the prospective employer. You want its appearance to reflect a competent, professional image. It is not necessary to have a professionally produced resumé. Nursing employers, when asked, have indicated that it neither adds to nor detracts from their impression to read a resumé that has been produced by some professional printing method. The important point is that it be a somewhat formal, standard, informative document that is neat and without errors. In today's business world, a computer-produced resumé is standard.

Display 11-2 **QUESTIONS TO HELP YOU PLAN A RESUMÉ**

1. What educational institutions have you attended? Dates? Degrees or certificates?
2. What credentials do you have that might be useful in a nursing employment setting?
3. What jobs have you held that you want to highlight? Were any of them health care related?
4. What specific skills did you apply in your workplace that would be transferable to nursing?
5. What skills, abilities, or personal characteristics do you want to draw the employer's attention to?
6. Have you had volunteer or community experiences that demonstrate positive personal attributes?
7. Have you had any awards or recognition that identify your positive abilities or attributes?

Your resumé should be on standard-sized (8.5" × 11"), white or off-white, good-quality paper so that it is easy to handle, file, and read. A resumé that is individually printed (or reproduced well enough so that it appears to be) usually will be received more positively than a poor-quality photocopy. If you have access to a computer and word processing, you will find it valuable to create a resumé and save it to a disk. In this way, you will be able to revise it easily, and you may even be able to tailor it to an individual job situation. In addition to the capabilities of standard word processing software, there are inexpensive software programs especially designed to facilitate the production of a well-organized and formatted resumé.

To achieve legibility, use wide margins, spacing, indentation, bullets, and numbering to separate different sections and topics. You might want to underline or bold print important items or highlight them with an asterisk or bullet to draw swift attention. When an employer is reviewing many such documents, anything that facilitates review and makes you stand out is an advantage. Ask someone to review the appearance of your resumé and identify those areas that first caught their attention. This helps you to evaluate its appearance.

CONTENT

The content of your resumé is critical. It always begins with your name, address, and telephone number (including area code). If you will be moving, indicate the date the move will be effective and provide an alternate method of contacting you after that date. A permanently settled relative or friend who would be willing to forward your mail would be appropriate. Employers are not permitted to ask about age, marital status, and dependents, and you do not need to include this information. An e-mail address is very helpful to employers. If your e-mail address is an informal phrase such as "lovedub" or "prettygirl," plan to set up an e-mail address for business use. This can be done for no cost through one of several Internet mail providers such as Yahoo®, Juno®, or Hotmail®. Use a simple derivation from your name that gives you a more professional appearance.

Objective. You should include a personal goal or objective. This may include both a short-term goal such as "employment as a registered nurse on a general medical unit" and a longer-term goal such as "with eventual move to employment in coronary care." Be sure that your goal is realistic and does not imply that you are not really interested in a beginning-level position. If you state that your goal is to work in an emergency room and you do not have the experience for this kind of position, your application usually will be discarded. If you state that you want to work in maternity nursing and the only position available is in medical-surgical nursing, you may not be considered for the medical-surgical position that you would have accepted although it was not your first choice. You may wish to write an objective that is tailored to a specific employer.

Credentials. You will want to include information regarding your licensure and other credentials. Indicate the date your license will be effective and whether you have a temporary permit to work as a nurse. Your nursing license or permit number should be listed after you have it. If you do not have a license at the time you are preparing your resumé, you may choose to put information about when you expect to have your license in your letter of application.

Employment History. Work experience is of critical importance, and you should provide a meaningful employment history. If using a traditional format, for each job you held include address, dates employed, position, and duties. The prospective employer would be especially interested in a previous nursing assistant position or any other position that demonstrates your knowledge of or experience in some area of health care or the assumption of responsibility. Other positions also may be important if you are clearly able to identify skills used in those settings that are transferable to nursing.

If you have had only one or two part-time jobs during your educational program, it would be appropriate to include them in detail. However, if during your educational program you held 15 part-time jobs, it is appropriate to list significant ones that offered valuable experience. In one line, write "Various part-time jobs to finance schooling: clerk and waitress. Individual names provided on request." Include the overall dates for this period.

You may choose a more skill-focused resumé and not include details of all your previous positions. For individuals who are older and have an extensive employment history, a resumé focused on skills and types of positions rather than a chronologic list of employers is often the most effective. To keep your resumé on one page, you should consider how you might most effectively present employment history. In a skill-focused resumé, you can emphasize the responsibilities you had within positions rather than each specific position. Be sure to include language proficiency if you are fluent in more than English. Computer literacy is also a valuable skill.

Regardless of the organizational format of your resumé, we suggest that you focus on accomplishments and use active verbs to describe skills. Words such as supervised, designed, managed, developed, analyzed, coordinated, documented, planned, delegated, created, completed, and operated give life to your resumé and create interest in the reader. If you were part of a team that accomplished a significant project or task, you might indicate that. However, be careful not to take personal credit for team accomplishments. See the accompanying display for a list of active verbs you might use (Display 11-3).

Education. Educational background should form another section and cover your nursing education and any specialized courses or postgraduate work you have done. It is appropriate to note any college-level work. Do not include high school information unless you entered your nursing program directly from high school. Then you might indicate your high school and graduation date on one line of your educational information. In each group of information, list the most recent items first. The most common approach is to group information in the categories just mentioned. See Display 11-4 for an example of this type of resumé.

Another approach is to identify specific skills that you possess. These might come from other jobs or life experience (Display 11-5). You might also highlight specific experiences in an area that especially relates to the position for which you are applying. For example, you might have had a senior leadership practicum on an orthopedic unit—this would be particularly relevant to an application for a nursing position in orthopedics. If you had a practicum in the facility or agency to which you are applying, indicate this in some way. Your familiarity with their policies and procedures would be a valuable asset. If you attended any special workshops, include those in a separate section. Information included in this part of the resumé can be used to demonstrate your ability to meet deadlines, produce good work, and relate to people in ambiguous situations.

Additional Experience. Volunteer or community work and awards and honors form two sections when you have these experiences. You also might want to add a section for special

Display 11-3   POWER VERBS FOR RESUMÉS

- Use of verbs without subjects will be more concise and space conserving.
- Use of active, not passive, voice, such as "advanced to" rather than "was promoted to," "earned" rather than "was given," indicates a person who does things rather than receives them.
- Use of "-ed" or "-ing" as verb endings can both be effective.

accompanied	demonstrated	generated	mastered	proposed
achieved	designed	governed	mediated	proved
acquired	detailed	graduated	motivated	provided
activated	determined			
administered	developed	headed	negotiated	reconciled
advanced to	devised		nominated	reduced
advised	diagnosed	identified		regulated
analyzed	directed	implemented	obtained	related
arranged	discovered	improved	officiated	reorganized
assembled	displayed	improvised	operated	reported
assessed	doubled	increased	ordered	represented
assisted		induced	organized	researched
	earned	influenced	originated	
balanced	educated	informed	overcame	satisfied
budgeted	employed	initiated		secured
	enacted	innovated	participated	served
clarified	encouraged	inspired	perceived	simplified
composed	engineered	installed	perfected	solved
conceived	established	instructed	performed	structured
concluded	evaluated	insured	piloted	succeeded
conducted	executed	integrated	pioneered	supervised
constructed	exhibited	intensified	placed	
consulted	expanded	interviewed	planned	trained
controlled		invented	prepared	transferred
converted	facilitated		presided	transformed
coordinated	financed	led	processed	
counseled	formalized	located	procured	unified
created	formed		produced	
	formulated	maintained	progressed	verified
decided	founded	managed	promoted	won
delegated		marketed	prompted	wrote

skills such as computer familiarity or experience with special types of equipment. Choose the items you list under volunteer and community work carefully. If you are older, the fact that you were student body president in high school would probably be considered irrelevant. However, if you went from high school directly into a nursing program, this information could be important in demonstrating your leadership ability. If you are an older student, your participation in any community organizations, such as the Parent–Teacher Association, and service in any leadership roles might be significant to an employer.

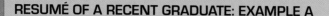

Display 11-4 **RESUMÉ OF A RECENT GRADUATE: EXAMPLE A**

Sarah Mitchell

5714 31st Ave. N., Seattle, WA 98117 • (206) 733-8934 • e-mail: *sarahmit@email.com*

Objective

An entry-level registered nurse position in an acute care hospital.

Experience

2000-present   Seattle General Medical Center   Seattle, WA
Patient Care Technician, Medical-Surgical Units
- Provide basic care and ADLs with attention to psychosocial needs for acutely ill medical-surgical patients. Assist R.N. with procedures and carry out delegated duties.
- Work collaboratively with nursing team, assuring prompt response to patient needs.
- Effectively manage time to support seven patients on evening shift.
- Document care on computerized system, maintaining accuracy and confidentiality.

1999–2000   Health Choice Urgent Care Center   Seattle, WA
Nursing Technician, Urgent Care Clinic
- Interviewed clients, took vital signs, initiated documentation, and prioritized care for urgently ill and injured adults and children.
- Under RN supervision, performed assessments, dressing changes, ECGs, nebulizer treatments, and hospital admission processes.
- Attended to psychosocial needs of family and others accompanying a sick or injured individual.

1997–1998   First United Bank   Lynnwood, WA
Bank Teller
- Maintained excellent customer service by following detailed bank policies and procedures.
- Utilized a variety of computerized systems to assure accurate and detailed documentation of all activities.
- Incorporated information from employee training classes into job skills to assure up-to-date function.

Education

1999–2001   Shoreline Community College   Seattle, WA
AAAS Nursing, to be awarded June, 2001

Display 11-5 RESUMÉ OF A RECENT GRADUATE: EXAMPLE B

Joseph M. Sanchez

1298 Avenida Diaz
La Quinta, CA 92252
(619) 524-4321

OBJECTIVE: A beginning Registered Nurse position that will provide the opportunity for professional development and advancement toward critical care nursing.

SKILLS:

- Work effectively in a multicultural environment
- Communicate in a positive, supportive way with co-workers, clients, and families
- Bilingual Spanish/English
- Strong work ethic and experience in working multiple shifts/floating positions
- Excellent critical thinking and problem-solving developed in a wide variety of occupations as well as in the nursing context

EDUCATION:

College of the Desert, Palm Desert, CA
Associate in Science in Nursing, June 2001

EXPERIENCE:

Manor Care Center, Palm Desert, CA
Nursing Assistant, Certified: 1998–Present

- Maintained function and dignity of dependent elderly adults by providing direct care, strong interpersonal relationships, and effective collaboration with nursing and allied health.
- Earned promotion to position of mentor for new hires and team leader for a group of nursing assistants. Facilitated team performance to accomplish assigned responsibilities.

Northrup Corporation, Los Angeles, CA
Machinist: 1988–1997

- Performed precision skills with accuracy and attention to detail.
- Followed precise written protocols and procedures to assure quality.
- Led a team in a program of total quality management within our department.

AWARDS:

- College of the Desert Merit Scholar 2000
- Golden Acorn Award for Leadership of Parent Involvement
  Cactus Valley Elementary School PTA, LaQuinta, CA

In some instances, you may want to list briefly the skills or abilities gained from a particular volunteer activity. For example, if you worked as a volunteer for a Planned Parenthood clinic, you might specify that your duties included individual client counseling in relation to family planning methods. Simply stating that you were a volunteer would not communicate the level of responsibility you assumed. This is an area that you might want to individualize to target the particular skills you think are important to the position for which you are applying. For example, you might use your volunteer experience to demonstrate past success in the skill of organizing, managing or coordinating people and events, and in effectively delegating responsibilities. It also might be used to highlight public relations skills or ability to work within or control a budget. If you have served as the coach of a Little League baseball team or a soccer team, or as a Girl or Boy Scout leader, it would be an opportunity to focus on your ability to direct, coach, and teach others.

List awards, honors, and professional associations (such as NSNA) that would demonstrate your competence or leadership ability. This provides an opportunity to show responsibility in directing the activities of others, public speaking, and, perhaps, for motivating people. You may omit this section if you feel that you have nothing pertinent to enter.

Personal References. References are typed on a separate page and given to the prospective employer if they are requested, or copied onto an application form. Be selective in choosing the people you list as references. Consider the people who know you and would be able to speak positively of you to a future employer, and who would have credibility with the employer.

A primary reference should be an instructor from your basic educational program. This person would be able to affirm your ability in the nursing field. Some agencies request two instructor references, so be prepared for that. Another reference should be someone who has employed you and who can describe your work habits and effectiveness as an employee. If you have had any health care work experience, this would be the best work reference. Also look at the position in which you assumed the most responsibility. This should be reasonably recent (within the last 10 years). Again, some employers ask for two work references. You should have available, as one reference, someone who has known you personally for a relatively long time and who could attest to your ability to relate with others and to such attributes as personal integrity. Not all employers are interested in personal references. Some agencies indicate the type of references they want. If this is the case, supply the names of references that comply with the agency's request. Include full names with titles (if any), addresses, and telephone numbers, so that the employer will be able to contact the references easily.

Seek the person's permission before giving an individual's name as a reference. When seeking permission to use someone as a work reference, you might outline what you would like the person to emphasize if contacted—for example: "If you are contacted, I would particularly like you to provide information about my work habits and effectiveness as an employee."

Employers express differences of opinion about the value of a standardized letter of reference addressed "To Whom It May Concern." Some employers may consider this a useful initial presentation of your qualifications. Other employers want the reference to address the specific position needs or the qualifications outlined on a reference form. One advantage of the general letter is that you might be able to obtain this reference from a part-time faculty member or supervisor who may no longer be employed by the institution. If you do obtain this type of letter, be sure to preserve the original carefully (perhaps in a clear, plastic sleeve) to show to a potential employer; you then would provide a good-quality photocopy for the employer to place in your file. Even when an employer accepts this as an initial reference, your references probably will be personally contacted as well.

Critical Thinking Activity

Create an effective resumé and samples of letters to employers that present you as a positive addition to their staff.

Successful Interviewing

The interview should be a two-way conversation in which you will gain as well as give information. Typically, the employer has three major concerns for which they seek answers in the interview: they want to know if you have the required knowledge and skills to do the job; if you possess an attitude toward the job and the organization that is compatible with what they are seeking; and if your personality and style will fit with the image the organization wishes to put forth. They are going to be interested in what you can do for them and, at this point, are more interested in what you can do than in what you think.

Think through the situation before going to the interview, and outline information that you want to obtain and questions that you want answered. It is helpful to write out your questions so that they are clearly stated, and so that you do not forget items in the tense atmosphere that often exists in an interview situation.

Time spent reflecting on your personal views in advance will be valuable for the interview. Remember that an interview is a chance to sell yourself to an employer, a chance to present yourself as a valuable addition to their nursing staff, and an opportunity to determine how you will fit into that work setting.

When planning for an employment interview, consider your appearance, your attitude and approach, and what the content of the interview will be. Your personal appearance is likely to evoke some response from the interviewer. Consider what you would like that response to be and dress appropriately. This means that what you wear when applying for one type of job might be inappropriate when applying for another type of job. For example, if you were applying for a position at a hospital, you would wear businesslike clothing, such as dress pants and shirt, or a suit or dress. Being neat and well groomed contributes to a businesslike atmosphere. If you were applying for a position in a walk-in health care clinic that offered services to persons who are uncomfortable in a traditional environment, it might be appropriate to wear the casual clothing worn by the workers at the clinic. Casual clothing does not include attire with a bare midriff, shorts, or pants with holes in the legs. In all instances, your hair should be clean and neatly styled. Although wild colors and styles that include spiking may be the style in some circles, they are out of place in a professional interview. You need to make a conscious decision about the impression you want to create. Although some may wish that appearances had no effect on the opinions of others, remember that, in reality, appearance often does make a significant difference.

Take a copy of your resumé with you to the interview. In addition, be prepared with the names, addresses, and telephone numbers of all references, and your Social Security number. If you have already received your nursing license, take that with you. Take along a black pen to fill out any forms, and a note pad with your questions listed and a place to make personal notes of important information obtained during the interview. This can increase your self-confidence if you have forms to fill out or if questions about statements on your resumé arise during the interview.

Plan to arrive at an interview early. This gives you time to check your appearance and focus your thoughts. When you arrive at an interview, be sensitive to the problems and concerns of the interviewer. If it is apparent that unplanned events are demanding the interviewer's attention, state that you are aware of the difficulty and ask whether it would be more convenient if you made another appointment. Your sensitivity to the interviewer's cues is evidence of your sensitivity to clients' cues.

Your manner in the interview is also important. Although the employer expects an applicant to be nervous, he or she will be interested in whether your nervousness makes you unable to respond appropriately. Follow common rules of courtesy. Wait to be asked to sit down before you take a chair. Avoid any distracting mannerisms, such as chewing gum or fussing with your hair, face, or clothes. If you carry a cell phone, turn it off during the interview. Be serious when appropriate, but do not forget to smile and be pleasant. The interviewer is also thinking of your impact on clients, visitors, and other staff members.

When you prepare your responses, try to anticipate possible questions from the interviewer. To do this, you must know the role of the person interviewing. In large agencies, your first interview might be with a human resources department employee, not a nursing employee. If you are successful at this stage, you might be recommended for an interview in the nursing department.

Role-playing an interview situation with a friend or relative may help you to feel more confident in your responses. Another technique is to visualize the interview situation in your mind and mentally rehearse responses to questions. Some interviewers focus on asking questions about your past experiences and your future plans. Others focus their questions on specific accomplishments and problems encountered in your past nursing experiences. Presenting hypothetical problems for you to consider and asking you to provide appropriate nursing responses is common. See Display 11-6 for a list of questions you might reflect on as you prepare.

In most instances, be sure to answer questions that are asked rather than skirting them. However, if the interviewer asks a question that is illegal, such as a question regarding age or marital status, you might want to redirect the question to address what appears to be the concern of the interviewer. For example, in response to a question about your age you might say, "Perhaps you believe that I appear to be young and inexperienced. I want to assure you that I have demonstrated my maturity and responsibility both in my nursing education and in my position with (name of employer)." In response to a question about marital status or children, you could reply, "Perhaps you are concerned about how long I plan to stay in my first position? I want to assure you that whatever my personal situation, professionally, I am looking for a position in an organization where I can be a long-term employee and plan for advancement within the organization." Avoid simple yes or no answers, but try to describe or explain to give a more complete picture of yourself.

Display 11-6   QUESTIONS TO HELP YOU PREPARE FOR A JOB INTERVIEW

Nursing Philosophy and Beliefs
- What is your philosophy of nursing?
- Is there a nursing theorist that you use as a basis for your nursing practice?
- What do you believe is the most central concept to support excellence in nursing?

Personal Goals and Planning
- Where do you see yourself in 1 year? 5 years? 10 years?
- Have you developed any professional goals? If so, would you share those with me?
- Why do you want to work here?
- What plans do you have for continuing education in nursing?
- What do you see as your weakest area in nursing?
- What do you see as your strengths in nursing?

Your Experiences
- What experience in your nursing education did you find the most rewarding? Why?
- What experience in your nursing education did you like the least? Why?
- In what kind of settings did you have an opportunity to work as a nursing student?
- What other job experiences have you had? What skill did you develop there that will be useful in nursing?

Problem Solving
- Identify a problem in patient care that you encountered as a student and explain how you solved that problem.
- Describe a difficult patient with whom you worked. Include why you found that patient difficult and how you managed the situation.
- Identify a situation in which you were involved in a conflict and describe how you handled that situation. If you had it to do over again, what would you do differently?
- Explain how you would use the nursing process in patient care.
- A problem may be presented to you for your solution. Plan ahead to approach it in a systematic manner.

Technical Skills
- What technical nursing skills do you feel comfortable peforming?
- What skills will you require assistance with?
- What do you do when you encounter a technical skill you have not performed before?

The Employment Setting
- In what type of unit do you wish to work?
- Why do you want to work here?
- Why do you think we should hire you for this position?

An interview usually covers a wide variety of subjects. The interviewer may direct the flow of topics or may encourage you to bring up the ones that concern you. Applicants who focus initial attention on the issues of wages and benefits may be viewed as more concerned about themselves than about nursing. Therefore, if you are asked to present questions, ask professional questions first. Make sure your questions are appropriate for the interviewer. In the human resources department, you might ask about the overall mission and philosophy of the organization, its organizational structure, and how authority and accountability are determined. With a nursing interviewer, demonstrate that you are concerned about how nursing care is given and by whom, where responsibility and authority for nursing care decisions lie, the philosophy underlying care, the availability of continuing education, and where you would be expected to fit into their overall picture. However, before you leave, be sure to cover such topics as hours, schedules, pay scales, and benefits.

Some interviews are conducted by a group of interviewers. This might include a person from nursing administration, a unit manager, and a staff development nurse. For an applicant to sit across the table from three to five individuals can be unnerving. You will need to look around the group, being sure to make eye contact with each individual. Make sure that you understand the role of each person present. You might actually write down individual names and roles on your notepad. This would allow you to direct a question to a specific individual or to use an individual's name when replying to a question. While replying to the person who asks the question, you might also glance at others as you make your point. Be sure that you do not ignore any individual, even if one of the interviewers does not seem to ask questions or to be as active in the process as the others. Interviews of this type are often longer than interviews with one person.

Some interviewers are less skilled than others; in these situations the questions may seem less focused and more vague. You may sometimes feel at a loss as to exactly what is being asked. Before proceeding you should seek clarification, but be careful that your manner of asking for clarification does not offend the interviewer. You might ask, "Would you give me an example of the type of situation you were thinking about?" Another clarifying approach is for you to state clearly what you perceive to be the central question before continuing, "Let me clarify. You would like me to identify a situation in which I believe I responded effectively to a problem. Is that correct?" In this situation, you may have to take the initiative to be sure that you have an opportunity to present your strengths and skills.

If you are unfamiliar with the interview process, you might benefit from reading books on the topic. Reading several different books will give you a variety of viewpoints and might provide you with strategies that are comfortable for you.

Follow-up Strategies

You should always follow up after your initial inquiry. If you were granted an interview, you would follow up with a letter, as described below. If you did not obtain an interview, you should continue to contact the potential employer at intervals to learn of other job opportunities and to indicate that you are still seeking a position. When a new position opens, employers do not necessarily go back through previous employment files. They are more likely to interview a person who appears to be currently searching for a position than one who was searching several months previously.

After your interview, you should write a brief thank-you letter to the person who interviewed you. If a group interviewed you, direct the letter to the person who seemed to be in charge. In that letter, thank the individual for the time and attention to your questions and concerns. Restate any agreement you feel was reached. For example, "I understand that I am to call your office next week to learn whether I have been scheduled for an interview with the maternity unit manager." Close your letter with a positive comment about the organization. Even if you are not offered a job or do not choose to work at that facility, you are leaving a positive impression. You can never tell when that will be important to you in the future (Display 11-7).

Display 11-7 **INTERVIEW FOLLOW-UP LETTER**

Maribeth Wilson
3428 1ˢᵗ Ave. N.
Seattle, WA 98103
(206) 274-5978
e-mail: maribethw@email.com

February 9, 2004

Joyce Montgall, R.N.
Nurse Recruiter
Seattle General Medical Center
321 Heath Blvd.
Seattle, WA 98101

Dear Ms. Montgall:

I want to thank you for meeting with me today to discuss your new nursing graduate residency program at Seattle General. I am particularly interested in the medical-surgical positions available on 4 West and 4 Center, although I am certainly willing to consider another unit.

My educational background, clinical experience, and commitment to excellent patient care appear to make me an ideal match with Seattle General. In addition, I feel very "at home" in the Seattle General environment, having worked there as a nursing assistant for the last year.

Again, I hope that you will consider me for one of the medical-surgical positions in the June graduate program. I am available to meet with any of the unit managers, which I understand is the next step in your hiring process. I can be contacted at the above telephone number or by e-mail. I do have an answering machine and would promptly return your call if I were not there to receive it. If I have not heard from you within two weeks, I will check with your office regarding the status of my application.

Thank you again for your time and consideration.

Sincerely,

Maribeth Wilson

Maribeth Wilson

Do not let this letter be your last contact with that potential employer. Call back as agreed. One of the main reasons for not getting a position is the failure to ask for it. Even if you do not get a position at this time, you might ask that your application be kept on file because you are still interested in employment with that particular agency. Then continue to call back every 2 or 3 weeks to find out if any other positions are available.

Setting up your own record-keeping system often enhances managing a job search. You should have a record of when you contacted an agency, in what manner (letter or telephone call), interviews—including the interviewer's name and the content of the interview—and dates and times of any follow-up letters or calls. Have a place to record your own notes or impressions. This will enable you to keep track of details when you manage an extensive job search. By keeping this type of record, you will not forget to call an agency to recheck on job availability, or mistakenly send an inquiry letter and resumé twice to the same agency.

Resignation

When you decide to leave a nursing position, it is important that you provide the employer with an appropriate amount of time to seek a replacement. The more responsible your position, the more time the employer will need. For a staff nursing position, you should strive to provide a month's notice, unless an urgent matter requires that less notice be given. Notice of resignation should be in a letter that is directed to the head of your department, often to the Director of Nursing. Copies should be sent to other supervisory people, such as the unit manager and the supervisor.

The letter of resignation is important in concluding your relationship with the employer on a cordial and positive basis. The feelings left behind when you resign will influence letters of recommendation and future opportunities for employment with that agency. Give a reason for your resignation and the exact date when it will be effective. If you have accrued vacation or holiday time and want to take the time off or be paid for it, clearly state that. Comment about positive factors in the employment setting and acknowledge those who have provided special support or assistance in your growth.

If you are resigning because of problems in the work setting, you may find it wiser to address those in person, separately from your letter of resignation, to not affect future recommendations. However you address problems, do so in a clear, factual, unemotional way. Avoid attacking anyone personally and do not make broad, sweeping negative comments. Try to make any written statement a clear and reasonable presentation of your position as a professional (Display 11-8).

PROBLEMS EXPERIENCED BY NURSES IN THE WORKPLACE

For many of you, graduating from a nursing program and becoming an RN is the realization of a long-cherished goal. You have spent years preparing for this status and now it is here! What you have viewed as an ideal state, freed from financial pressures that you felt as a student, liberated from the tyranny of the examination, may prove to be quite different from what you had expected. Let us consider some of the problems that may occur as you make this transition from student to professional.

Display 11-8   LETTER OF RESIGNATION

1546 Avenida Escuela
Palm Desert, CA 76321
February 14, 2004

Marvin Short, R.N., Unit Manager
Transitional Care Unit
Desert Hospital
509 Desert Highway
Palm Desert, CA 76320

Dear Marvin:

It is with mixed feelings that I am submitting my resignation to be effective March 23. I will be moving to Oregon and returning to school full time beginning spring quarter.

My two years here at Desert Hospital have been an excellent foundation for my future career. The nurses were supportive of me as a new graduate and have always encouraged me to think of my career as a lifetime opportunity for growth.

The last day I plan to work will be at the end of this pay period. My understanding is that my unused vacation and holiday pay will be included in my final paycheck.

Thank you again for all of your help.

Sincerely,

John Webster

John Webster, R.N.

cc: Maria Gonzales, Vice President for Patient Care Services

Moving From "Novice to Expert"

The path from **novice to expert** is a challenging one. Benner's (1984) work in this area has provided a basis for understanding and research into this process. She related this path to the Dreyfus Model of Skill Acquisition (1980) in which the individual moves from novice, to advanced beginner, to competent, to proficient, to expert. Throughout this progression she identified exemplars of nurses performing in six different roles:

1. The helping role
2. The teaching–coaching function
3. The diagnostic and monitoring function
4. Effective management of rapidly changing situations

5. Administering and monitoring therapeutic interventions and regimens
6. Monitoring and ensuring the quality of health care practices and organizational and work-role competencies.

Through interviews with nurses, she described the depth of nursing skills and abilities found in the expert nurse. This expertise is forged over time and results from personal experience and personal knowing. One of the challenges for beginning nurses is pressure to function as an expert without this background of growth.

As you look for a first nursing position, learn about the mechanisms the employer has in place to facilitate your transition to the RN role. Is there an orientation program specially designed for new graduates? Will you have an individually assigned preceptor or mentor for support? How long will you be given support before being expected to function independently? If you feel you need more time to be independent, will the employer accommodate this need? As a new graduate, will you be expected to float to different units, or will you be helped to become competent in one area before asked to go to another? Is there assistance with and support for continuing education for nurses? As you answer these questions, you will begin to develop a broader picture of the employer and be able to evaluate whether this job is a fit for your personal journey from novice to expert.

Reality Shock

One problem confronted by the new graduate is the seeming impossibility of delivering quality care within the constraints of the system as it exists. You may feel powerless to effect any changes and may be depressed over your lack of effectiveness in the situation. Marlene Kramer was the first to call the feelings that result from such a situation **reality shock** (Kramer, 1979). She noted that the new graduate often experiences considerable psychological stress and that this may exacerbate the problem. The person undergoing such stress is less able to perceive the entire situation and to solve problems effectively (Fig. 11-2).

CAUSES OF REALITY SHOCK

With all of the uncertain expectations and demands, the new graduate often feels caught in the middle. As a student, you may think that you are expected to learn a tremendous amount in an alarmingly short time. The expectations may seem high and in some ways unrealistic. Then, as a new graduate suddenly thrust into the real world, you may feel unsure of yourself without the security of the instructor's availability. You may think that your educational program did not adequately prepare you for what is expected of you. On one hand, you are expected to function like a nurse who has had 10 years of experience, but, on the other hand, your new ideas may not be considered because you have so little experience. You may become frustrated because you do not have time to provide the same type of care you gave as a student. For example, you may not have adequate time to deal with a client's psychosocial problems or teaching needs.

As a student, you are taught that the "good nurse" never gives a medication without understanding its actions and side effects, and that evaluating the effectiveness of the drug is essential. As a staff nurse, you may find that the priority is getting the medications passed correctly and on time and that there is little or no time to look up 15 new drugs. As for evaluation, that

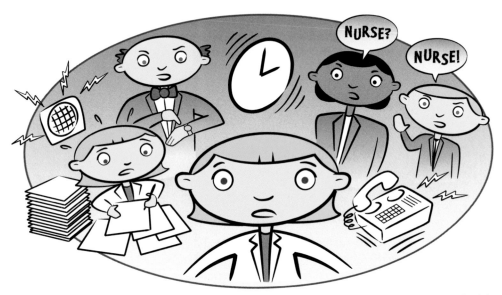

FIGURE 11-2   Some new graduates are disillusioned by the working conditions that they find on their first job.

becomes a dream. How can you evaluate the subtle effects of a medication in the 2 minutes spent passing the medication to a client you do not know? The individually and meticulously planned care that was so important to you as a student may become a luxury when you are a graduate. Often the focus is on accomplishing the required tasks in the time allotted, and it is efficiency in tasks that may earn praise from a supervisor.

Bradby (1990) suggests that reality shock is part of the passage from novice to experienced nurse. She suggests that it be treated as a normal transitional process, with a focus on the growth that can occur. This can best occur if you understand what is happening and are prepared to address the problem.

EFFECTS OF REALITY SHOCK

When reality shock occurs, some nurses become disillusioned and leave nursing altogether. Others begin to "job hop" or return to school, searching for the perfect place to practice perfect nursing as it was learned. Some push themselves to the limit, trying to provide ideal care and criticizing the system. This may result in their being labeled nonconformists and troublemakers. Still others give up their values and standards for care and reject ideals as impossibly unrealistic expectations that cannot be fulfilled in the real world. These persons simply mesh with the current framework and become part of the system.

FINDING SOLUTIONS FOR REALITY SHOCK

There is an alternative to these nonproductive coping methods. It is possible to create a role for yourself that blends the ideal with the possible—one in which you do not give up ideals but see them as goals toward which you will move, however slowly. To do this, you need to be realistically prepared for the demands of the real world.

One way of meeting the challenge is to assess yourself as you approach the end of your educational program. Consider what your competencies are. Think about the areas of expectation that were discussed earlier in the chapter:

1. Theoretic knowledge for safe practice
2. Use of the nursing process
3. Self-awareness
4. Communication skill
5. Delegation
6. Documentation
7. Skill proficiency
8. Work ethic
9. Speed of functioning
10. Interpersonal skills and cultural sensitivity

Second, gain information about what the employers in your community expect from new graduates. You can do this by talking with experienced nurses, meeting with faculty, and contacting recent graduates who are currently employed. Try to get specific information. If you have a nursing student organization, setting up a forum for speakers from various agencies might be one avenue to gaining this insight. Once you are applying for a position, you could explore this issue in an employment interview.

After you have gathered this information, try to correlate it with a realistic appraisal of your own ability to function in accordance with an employer's expectations. If you identify any shortcomings, the time to try to remedy them is before graduation. If you identify a lack in certain technical skills, you might register for extra time in the nursing practice laboratory to increase your proficiency. You could even time yourself and work to increase speed as well as skill. You might consult with your clinical instructor to arrange for experiences that would help you gain increased competence, especially in procedures with which you have had little experience. Having met an objective is far different from skillfully and efficiently carrying out a procedure. If you recognize that you consistently have difficulty functioning within a time frame, you might obtain employment in a hospital or other health care facility while still in school; this will give you more experience in organizing work within the time limits that the employer sees as reasonable.

As you plan for your first job, you can examine the psychological challenges to be met. Understanding that you are not alone in your feelings of frustration is often helpful. It may be useful to form a support group of other new graduates, who meet regularly to discuss problems and concerns and seek solutions jointly. You also can gain valuable reinforcement from other nurses in your work setting. Many have dealt successfully with the problems you face and are able to provide support and help. This "mentor" relationship is an important one and needs to be cultivated.

When confronted with areas of practice that you would like to see changed, weigh the importance of an issue. Use your energies wisely. The "politics of the possible" is important to you. Learn how the system in which you are employed functions and how to use that system for effective change. You, as a person, are important to nursing, so it is important that you neither burn yourself out nor abandon the quest for higher-quality nursing care; you should be able to continue to work toward improving nursing and bringing it closer to its ideals (see Chapter 14 for more information on change).

Some hospitals attempt to help new graduates deal with reality shock by making orientation programs more comprehensive and by providing an experienced nurse to work as a preceptor to the new graduate. Nurse internships or residencies in some settings have been created to provide a planned and organized transition time during which the new graduate participates in a formal program, including classes, seminars, and rotations to various units of the hospital. In some settings, the new graduate is required to be more self-directed in identifying needs and the ways that those might be met within the constraints of the system.

Some hospitals provide an opportunity for nursing students to work during the summer before the last year of their basic program to become familiar with the hospital and the nursing role. In this type of program, the nursing student may be employed as a nursing assistant but participate in a planned program that introduces the role of the RN. In other instances, nursing students work as nursing assistants, and the orientation to the nursing role in the agency depends upon the initiative the individual takes. You may wish to inquire whether hospitals in your area have developed any of these or other programs to assist you when you are a new graduate.

Critical Thinking Activity

With a group of nursing students, develop personal strategies for managing reality shock. Discuss your rationale for any strategy you propose.

Burnout

Burnout is a form of chronic stress related to one's job. This problem arises after you have been in practice for a period of time. It can be identified by feelings of hopelessness and powerlessness, and accompanied by a decreased ability to function both on the job and in personal life. Burnout is more frequent in nurses who work in particularly stressful areas of nursing, such as critical care, oncology, or burn units. It also occurs in other areas when staffing is inadequate or interpersonal relationships are strained. The downsizing of nursing staff and the rapid changes in the health care environment have contributed to burnout in some settings.

SYMPTOMS OF BURNOUT

Symptoms of burnout include both physical changes and psychological distress. Exhaustion and fatigue, frequent colds, headaches, backaches, and insomnia all may occur. There may be changes in disposition, such as being quick to anger or exhibiting all feelings excessively. Individuals experience a decreased ability to solve problems and make decisions as burnout progresses. This frequently results in an unwillingness to face change and a tendency to block new ideas. There may be feelings of guilt, anger, and depression because one cannot meet the expectations for doing a "perfect job."

In response to these feelings, some nurses quit their jobs and move on to other settings that may not even be in nursing. Others remain in their jobs but develop a personal shell that tends to separate them from real contact with clients and coworkers; they may become cynical about the possibility of anyone doing a good job and may function at a minimal level. A few become more and more unable to function and find themselves in jeopardy of losing their positions.

CAUSES OF BURNOUT

Many causes of burnout have been discussed in the literature. Prominent among them is the conflict between ideals and reality. Just as this is a problem for the new graduate, it is also a problem for the experienced nurse. In trying to achieve the ideal, the nurse drives harder and harder and becomes critical of the environment and of himself or herself. Nurses see themselves as being responsible for all things to all people and often take on more and more responsibility, thus increasing their own stress level.

Another cause of burnout is the high level of stress that results from practicing nursing in areas that have high mortality rates. Continually investing oneself in clients who die can take a tremendous toll on personal resources. In addition, the demand is constant for optimal functioning.

Inadequately staffed institutions may also place great stress on nurses. The clients are in need of care, the nurse has the skills to provide the care, and yet the clients do not receive good care. The nurse typically tries to accomplish more, staying overtime, skipping breaks and lunch, and running throughout the shift. Despite this effort, there is little job satisfaction because the things that are left undone or that are not done well seem to be more apparent than all the good that is accomplished.

PREVENTING BURNOUT

As an individual nurse, you can take actions to prevent burnout. These are the same general actions that are designed to control stress in any aspect of life. Paying attention to your own physical health is an important preventive measure; this includes maintaining a balanced program of rest, nutrition, and exercise. Another important point is not to subject yourself to excessive changes over short periods of time, because changes increase stress. You may decide, for example, not to move at the same time you change to a different shift. A period of "wind-down" or "decompression" after work helps you to avoid carrying the stress of the workplace into your private life; this period may involve physical exercise, reading, meditation, or any different activity. The activity you choose should not create more demands and increase stress. An important resource is someone who is willing to listen while you ventilate your feelings and talk about your problems. Sometimes this is a family member or personal friend, but it may be more appropriate for this to be a coworker or counselor.

Rotating out of a high-stress area, such as a burn unit or pediatric oncology, before you become "burned out" may allow you to rebuild resources and return to the job with enthusiasm. This can be done only if there is no stigma or blame attached to the need to rotate and if other nurses are available for replacement. In client care areas that are known to be stressful, it is helpful to have a counselor available for nurses. Consulting with this counselor should be viewed by the staff as a positive step and not as an admission of some lack or fault. The counselor needs to be someone who understands the setting and who has the skills to assist people in coping with stress.

Another strategy is to focus on those positive aspects of nursing that drew you to it initially. Much is being written about cognitively reframing situations and settings to focus on those parts that are positive and affirming. The art of nursing reflects that positive view of nursing. Lindeman (1999) suggests that the art of nursing is composed of three central aspects. The first, informed caring, refers to behaviors that make a difference for patients;

attending to what patients say, analyzing and synthesizing information; and acting as an advocate for patient and family. The second aspect is thoughtful doing. She characterizes nursing practice as a "continuous, interactive, unbroken spectrum of thought and action" (p. 3). The third aspect is lifelong learning. Lifelong learning is an essential foundation for the informed caring and thoughtful doing that are the first two components. Looking at the art of nursing and focusing your energy and attention on this may help you surmount the everyday pressures you encounter.

The most effective prevention of burnout is an institution-wide stress-reduction effort to prevent burnout involving the nursing staff, supervisory personnel, the hospital administration, and other health care workers. The most important objective seems to be bringing burnout into the open and acknowledging the existence of the problems. This alone helps the individual nurse move away from the feelings of separation and alienation that often accompany burnout. Whatever the problems, they seem less frightening if they are defined as "normal" and if the individual nurse does not see himself or herself as the only person not performing as the "perfect nurse." You might investigate the resources that a prospective employer has to assist nurses in preventing burnout.

Another approach may be initiated by individual nurses but requires the cooperation of the institution; this includes establishing group discussions during which nurses can share feelings and specific concerns in an accepting atmosphere. This sharing may lead to concrete plans to reduce the stress created by the setting. For example, if one source of stress is conflicting orders between two sets of physicians involved in care, a plan might be developed whereby the nurses no longer take responsibility for the conflict but refer the problem to some authority within the medical hierarchy. This type of resolution is possible only when the whole health care team is addressing the problem of burnout. However, it also requires that nurses give up trying to control "everything."

Giving nurses more control over their own practice often decreases stress. Assuming more control is limited by the constraints of the setting, but it may involve flexible scheduling, volunteering for specific assignments, and participating in committees that determine policies and procedures.

Critical Thinking Activity

Compare burnout with the stress response you have studied in relation to client care. Compare the strategies that you have taught clients with those suggested for preventing burnout.

DISCRIMINATION IN NURSING

Discrimination relates to treating others differently based on **stereotypes** about groups of people. Discrimination may occur regarding racial or ethnic background, gender or sex, sexual orientation, and/or age.

Racial/Ethnic Discrimination

Racial and ethnic discrimination remain problems in society as a whole and, unfortunately, health care systems are not immune to these problems. Although there are indications that nurses have moved into greater acceptance of all individuals in advance of some other portions of society, concerns about discrimination remain. Historically, the American Association of Colored Graduate nurses united with the American Nurses Association (ANA) in 1952, before the general civil rights movement in the United States. There have always been prominent nurses of color, such as the past president of the ANA, Beverly Malone, and past president of the National League for Nursing, Rhetaugh Dumas, and the current president of Sigma Theta Tau, May Wykle, who are all African-American women who have been leaders for all of nursing throughout their long and distinguished careers. They are just three of the many ethnic/racial minority nurses who have made significant contributions to nursing.

However, the number of minorities in nursing does not reflect the number of minorities in the general population. Spratley et al (2000) reported that 12.3% of nurses represent minority groups. This contrasts with a general population that has 17% racial/ethnic minorities (U.S. Census Bureau, 1999). This difference may stem from many causes, but is of concern because a workforce that reflects the population is more likely to meet the health care needs of that population in a culturally sensitive manner. Some of the root causes of the lower participation of minorities in nursing have to do with access to education, support for high career goals, economic status, the image of nursing, institutionalized racism, and other general societal problems.

A survey of minority nurses published by the ANA indicated that many believe that they have been adversely affected by discrimination in the nursing profession. Some concerns cited were the perception that others questioned their capabilities and that they were passed over for promotions. To combat these issues, several organizations for ethnic nurses have joined together to create the National Coalition of Ethnic Minority Nurses Associations (Bessent, 2002).

Nurses are challenged to examine this situation and be a part of the solution. All of us need to recognize and welcome diversity in the nursing profession. We need to acknowledge that a diversity of views and life experiences will enrich nursing as a profession and support excellence in patient care. When we see discrimination occurring, whether in education or in the workplace, we each need to speak up as agents for change. The National Student Nurses' Association (NSNA) has supported a program called Breakthrough to Nursing, in which nursing students mentor minority individuals in nursing education. These and similar efforts help nursing to move forward as a profession that welcomes and provides opportunities for all.

Discrimination Against Men

Men in nursing also have expressed concern about sex discrimination. Their concern is not monetary, but is related to being allowed to practice in all areas of nursing and being accepted within the profession.

Anti-male sexism of nurses in the United States was brought to the forefront by the research of Kus (1985), who pointed out that society stereotypes men just as feminists have criticized that it stereotypes women. He made a strong case for the importance of nurses examining the stereotypes they hold about men. Stereotypes narrow our thinking and interfere with people being able to develop to their fullest potential. It is important for women in nursing to examine their own behavior and identify whether they have been guilty of perpetuating outmoded stereotypes of the nurse and supporting a type of discrimination toward men that they would fight to eliminate for women.

In some facilities or areas, men are not allowed to care for women clients, or if they are allowed to care for women, restrictions are placed on them in terms of obtaining consent for care from each client. Those who support the limitations on the practice of men in nursing state that it is a matter of providing for the modesty and privacy of female clients. This position was upheld by a court decision in favor of a hospital that refused to assign a man to a nursing position in labor and delivery ("Arkansas judge . . . ," 1981). The argument was made that the client did not have free choice of a nurse but, rather, was assigned a nurse for care, and therefore the restrictions were appropriate.

In an article in *The American Nurse*, Ketter (1994) presented the situations of men who have felt discrimination in the workplace based on their gender. One of these men has filed three complaints with Equal Employment Opportunities Commission (EEOC) regarding discrimination in employment in obstetric/gynecologic settings in the 3 years he has been in nursing. His case is expected to end up in federal court.

In an interview, Luther Christman, PhD, RN, discussed the discrimination that he encountered throughout a long and prestigious career in nursing. His career began with his graduation from a diploma program in 1939 and extended through doctoral studies and a joint position as dean of Rush University and vice-president of nursing for Rush-Presbyterian-St. Luke's Medical Center in Chicago. He identified overt acts that excluded him from positions and covert acts that tried to undermine his influence. He identified this as being in issue of power and control just as is sex discrimination against women (Sullivan, 2002).

Those who oppose limitations on the practice of men in nursing state that, as a professional, a nurse (whether a man or woman) should always consider the privacy and modesty of a client of either gender. This can be done without excluding anyone from providing care in any area. By careful assessment, the nurse can determine the true needs of the client and plan for appropriate avenues to deliver that care. Furthermore, the point has been made that men physicians have not been excluded from any branch of medicine and this has not created problems. The client does not always choose physicians, either. House staff are assigned, referrals are made to specialty physicians, and many group plans designate a physician to provide care. Female nurses care for male clients in all situations. This has been accepted because women are seen in a nurturing, mothering role that the public associates with nursing.

The American Assembly for Men in Nursing provides a forum for the concerns of men in nursing and those who are concerned about the problems of sex discrimination. This organization seeks to educate people and opposes any limitations on opportunities available to men.

Critical Thinking Activity

Review the advertisements for nursing positions in three current journals and analyze them for gender bias.

Harassment and Violence

Harassment and violence are often discussed together because they are both rooted in the same issues of the abuse of power. "Violence isn't limited to the kinds of incidents that make headlines. It includes a range of behavior from verbal abuse, threats, and unwanted sexual advances to physical assault and at the extreme, homicide." (ANA, 1994).

Sexual harassment has been identified as behavior of a sexual nature that creates a work environment that is perceived as hostile and unduly stressful. Sexual harassment may take the form of comments about an individual's body, persistent unwanted attempts to initiate a personal relationship, the ongoing use of suggestive or obscene language, unwanted touching, or direct sexual advances. Both men and women may be the objects of sexual harassment. Issues of sexual harassment have been in the news in many ways in the last few years. Sexual harassment is a concern in nursing. Because nurses are involved with personal care of individuals of the opposite sex, there is sometimes the unspoken assumption that they will not be offended by sexual comments, jokes, or innuendo.

Harassers in the health care workplace may be clients, coworkers, or physicians. According to Kaye (1996) and Williams (1995), most harassers in the health care workplace are physicians; this follows the general data showing that sexual harassment is a demonstration of personal power over others. Traditionally, physicians have had the most power in health care environments. While recognizing the problem, it is important not to stereotype physicians, because the majority of physicians are professional and appropriate in their relationships.

Individuals should take steps to stop sexual harassment by giving clear, direct verbal messages indicating that the behavior in question is unwanted, unpleasant, and must stop. Sometimes this action alone stops inappropriate behavior. If clear, direct messages are not successful, the individual then should report the matter in writing to an immediate supervisor. Any individual who believes that he or she has been the victim of sexual harassment would be wise to keep personal records of the behavior and of all attempts to stop the behavior in question. Most organizations and agencies have an individual designated to deal with issues related to sexual harassment. If you encounter problem behavior, you should discuss your concerns with this person. If you belong to a collective bargaining group, that group can serve as a resource to assist you. In some instances, it may be necessary to seek independent legal counsel to force resolution of the problem.

Employers are legally and ethically responsible for having clear policies that prohibit sexual harassment, and for providing an appropriate work environment. If an employer fails to respond appropriately, the employer may be legally liable. These policies should be publicized so that everyone is aware of them. The courts support the responsibility of the employer to maintain a work environment free of sexual harassment (Neuhs, 1994; Wolfe, 1996).

Verbal abuse also occurs in health care settings. In efforts to increase retention of nurses, hospitals have begun asking why nurses leave specific hospitals and nursing altogether. An important factor is the extent to which nurses see themselves as disrespected and verbally abused in the workplace. In a study conducted by Rosenstein and reported in the *American Journal of Nursing* (2002), nurses were asked to categorize the types of disruptive behavior they either witnessed or experienced. Most frequently cited were yelling or raising the voice, disrespect, condescension, berating colleagues, berating patients, and use of abusive language. In the past, these often were tolerated from physicians because other health professionals knew that they did not have the power to change these behaviors. Bruder (2001) speaks of this as the "elephant in the dining room" of health care. Everyone knows it occurs but no one addresses it directly.

Not all verbal abuse is vertical, moving from more powerful to less powerful. Some verbal abuse is horizontal—nurses verbally abusing one another, saying things to one another that would be clearly inappropriate if said to a patient. Verbal abuse may also come from patients who become demanding.

Why does verbal abuse continue? There are many theories regarding the exercise of power, oppressed group behavior, and others. The bottom line must be that regardless of "why" it happens, verbal abuse must be stopped. How can that occur? Bruder (2001) suggests the following strategies. Nurses must assess themselves and identify their own feelings about self worth. Nurses must recognize their own potential for verbal abuse toward others and deal ethically with one another. He further suggests that nurses start with expecting respect in the use of names. If physicians are calling nurses by their first names, then nurses should call physicians by their first names. If physicians insist on being called "Dr. X," then nurses should be addressed as "Nurse X" or "Ms. X." This helps to diminish the power differential.

Nurses must work together to not succumb to intimidation. Some hospitals have initiated a "code white," in which others come to be observers when an individual begins a temper tantrum or tirade. These people are witnesses and provide emotional support to the recipient of abuse. Administrators and other physicians must also learn not to turn their backs to abuse occurring in the environment. They have both ethical and legal (in the case of administrators) responsibilities for the workplace.

Most nursing students think of hospitals as places where victims of violence are helped. Rarely do they think of themselves as potential victims of violence in their own workplace. According to Occupational Safety and Health Administration (OSHA), two thirds of nonfatal workplace assaults happen in health and social services facilities. The majority of these are assaults by clients on nursing staff, and more occur in psychiatric mental health settings than in other settings. Assaults on staff by visitors and outsiders also occur; most of these take place in emergency rooms. Health care workplace violence is not confined to industrialized societies. The World Health Organization has identified violence as a worldwide problem, which threatens the effective delivery of health care (WHO, 2002). In the United States, violence is also very costly. While the average cost for an injury in terms of lost time and medical treatment was $5,719, costs can go higher than $100,000 for those with permanent injuries. In addition to monetary costs, there are cost in terms of psychological damage and loss of individuals to the profession of nursing (Worthington, 2002). Not included in these estimates were less severe injuries, injuries to patients or property, and the long-term physical and psychological costs of trauma.

OSHA has issued guidelines for use by facilities trying to establish a safer workplace. These are not enforceable rules but may represent what is termed the "General Duty" clause in the OSHA Act. The guidelines call for clear programs designed to protect workers. These programs would include an assessment and analysis of the workplace for hazards and a plan for prevention of problems. One form of prevention is to train employees in the management of hostile and violent behavior. Ways of identifying hostile and assaultive clients should be developed so that staff can be warned to take extra personal safety precautions. Other important environmental safeguards include the use of such devices as metal detectors, panic buttons, and bulletproof glass, where appropriate. Adequate staff to manage potentially violent behavior is of particular concern in psychiatric/mental health settings. The addition of security personnel is important in some environments. There should be an attitude throughout the institution of zero tolerance for abusive or assaultive behavior.

In addition to preventing and managing problem situations, there should be clear guidelines for reporting both verbal and physical abuse and following through on all complaints. Health care institutions should work with law enforcement professionals when abusive or assaultive behavior occurs to assure that legal procedures are carried out correctly.

Those who report incidents should receive support and assistance and be assured that there will be no reprisals or blaming. Some nurses have been reluctant to report verbal and physical abuse or assault because of personal and institutional beliefs that health care staff should be able to handle these behaviors independently. Another common belief in health care environments is that all behavior has meaning for the individual and that staff should accept inappropriate behaviors on the part of clients. Social constraints and adverse consequences related to inappropriate behavior are a valuable ally in redirecting the behaviors of those who are cognitively impaired, mentally ill, or developmentally delayed. Nurses need support from their work environments in accessing these avenues to protect themselves.

Critical Thinking Activity

Formulate an appropriate response to experiencing sexual harassment in the workplace. Include specific statements you would use and each step you would take if the harassment continued.

WORKPLACE SAFETY AND HEALTH FOR NURSES

Nurses have expressed concern regarding safety in the working environment for many years. Employees have a right to expect their employers to provide the safest working environment possible. Some hospitals employ an occupational health nurse to examine the working environment, and use employment practices to promote health and safety on the job. Nurses themselves, however, often have been lax in recognizing on-the-job hazards and acting for self-protection; this can be likened to the response of those who continue to smoke despite their knowledge of the health hazards of smoking, or those who fail to wear seatbelts even though statistics show fewer fatalities in automobile accidents when seatbelts are worn. Some people continue to do those things that they know are detrimental to their health and well-being. Unfortunately, nurses are no exception.

The Bureau of Labor Statistics tracks and reports data related to **occupational hazards**. Reports have identified that hospitals have an incidence of work-related illness or injury of 11.8 per 100 full-time workers. Nursing homes are even more hazardous, with an incidence of 17.3 per 100 workers. Nurse aides were even more at risk than registered nurses ("RNs facing . . . ," 1995). Personal awareness is the first step in attempting to control this growing problem.

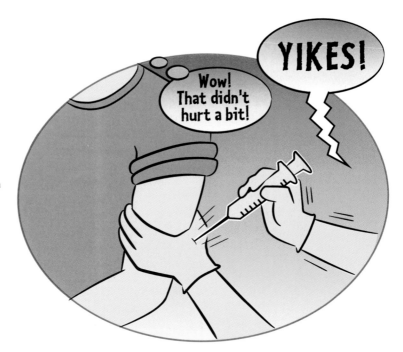

FIGURE 11-3 Needlestick injuries are a major concern in all health care environments.

Infection as an Occupational Hazard

Transmission of infection is a major concern when caring for infected clients. The presence of resistant organisms causes extra concern and makes treatment difficult. All hospitals have an infection-control officer, usually an RN, who has the expertise to guide the staff in planning appropriate infection-control procedures. Staff in other settings may not have access to such an expert.

The hidden danger for nurses lies in those clients who have not been diagnosed as having an infection and for whom specific infection-control measures have therefore not been prescribed. Universal precautions have been mandated by OSHA for use with all clients in all settings (that is, universally) to protect staff from blood-borne pathogens. These precautions prevent the spread of HIV, hepatitis B, and other such blood-borne pathogens. Nurses who have frequent contact with blood and blood products, and those engaged in intravenous therapy, have a special risk for exposure to hepatitis B. OSHA has developed standards that require employers to pay for hepatitis B immunization for those employees with significant exposure to blood and body fluids that can transmit blood-borne organisms.

AIDS has created a reevaluation of all approaches to infection control and of health care workers' obligations to provide care for those with communicable diseases. AIDS remains a serious concern for all health care workers. One of the first employer actions toward preventing AIDS and other blood-borne diseases was the provision of "sharps" containers wherever needles were used. Another important employer responsibility is the provision of a supply of gloves and protective eyewear for employee use. OSHA mandates these measures as part of universal precautions. However, not all cases of transmission of blood-borne pathogens can be prevented by universal precautions. Needlestick injuries—especially those with large-bore needles (eg, bone-marrow aspiration needles)—continue to be the most frequent transmission source. Wearing gloves does not prevent these injuries (Fig. 11-3).

More attention is now being given to designing needles and other sharp devices in new ways that prevent needlestick injuries. For example, a needle with a protective plastic housing is available for injections. These needles are unlikely to injure an individual even if they are not handled properly. Needleless intravenous connections are also available. Syringes are available that have a protective cover into which the needle retracts immediately after use. To participate knowledgeably in decisions regarding needle systems and devices, nurses need to seek information about what devices are available. OSHA does mandate that health care facilities have in place a plan to reduce the risk of needlestick injuries through using safe devices. ANA has been active in workplace advocacy related to needlestick injuries and supports a Web site devoted to this topic, *http://needlestick.org.*

Blood-borne pathogens are not the only pathogens of concern in the health care environment. The Standard Precautions recommended by the Centers for Disease Control and Prevention (Garner, 1996), often referred to as Body Substance Precautions, are used in many places, but they are not required by OSHA. These precautions protect clients and staff from infections that might be transmitted by any body substance. When these Standard Precautions were being formulated, OSHA indicated that regulations would likely be changed from the current requirement for Universal Precautions to a requirement for the more extensive Standard Precautions. Because of the antiregulatory stance of Congress through 2002, OSHA did not proceed with formulating new requirements for employers. This may occur in the future.

The incidence of tuberculosis is again on the rise, with drug-resistant strains of the organism appearing. Although rooms with special ventilation and special masks that are impervious to the tuberculosis organism are available, individuals with the disease may be in contact with health care providers long before they are clearly diagnosed. Should nurses in high-risk areas, such as the emergency room, wear special masks during all client contact, or is this unrealistic? These are important questions to consider.

Although the details of infection control are beyond the scope of this text, we remind you that you hold the key to protecting yourself in many ways. Health care workers often become lax in their attention to the use of gloves or eye protection because these measures are inconvenient. It is your responsibility to use the very best techniques for self-protection. Nurses must assume responsibility for their own protection by conscientiously carrying out appropriate measures at all times. Employers must be held accountable for providing the supplies and environment to make this possible.

Hazardous Chemical Agents

Anesthetic gases can increase the risk of fetal malformation and spontaneous abortion in pregnant women who are exposed to them on a regular basis. Standards exist for waste-gas retrieval systems and the allowable level of these gases in the air. Nurses working in operating rooms should seek information on the subject and expect hospitals to provide a safe work environment.

Chemotherapeutic agents used in the treatment of cancer are extremely toxic, and nurses who work in settings where such agents are prepared and administered should seek additional education regarding their administration, not only in relation to the client's safety but also in relation to personal safety. The employer is responsible for providing the equipment needed to maintain safety when handling these agents. In many settings, protocols now require the routine use of personal protective equipment when handling chemotherapeutic agents.

Contact with many medications, especially antibiotics, during preparation and administration may cause the nurse to develop sensitivity. This can create transitory problems (eg, a hand rash), and may be a threat if treatment for a serious infection is compromised later. Other medications are absorbed through the skin and may produce an undesirable effect. Nurses must take personal responsibility for their own safety regarding these agents. Nurses who understand these hazards handle all drugs with discretion and are careful not to expose themselves to these agents.

Cleaning agents and disinfectants used in the hospital also may be hazardous if used improperly. Employers are now required by OSHA to maintain a list of all chemicals used in the work environment, along with information on their possible effects, and the appropriate treatment if individuals are accidentally exposed to them. If you work with these agents, you should seek out this information, found in the Material Safety Data Sheets (MSDS), and be sure that you handle chemicals correctly.

Back Injuries

Because nursing includes providing direct care to incapacitated individuals, back injuries are a common occupational hazard. Back injuries in general are a serious concern because they interfere with the working life of people in their most productive years. Nursing assistants in long-term care facilities have the highest incidence of back injuries. As staff numbers are reduced, remaining staff often feel pressure to move and lift people and equipment without essential assistance. Back injuries then increase ("RNs facing . . . ," 1995).

In November of 2000, OSHA established ergonomic standards that addressed back injuries in the health care workplace. These were to take effect in January, 2001. Although these standards had been in preparation for 10 years, the Congress disapproved the standards in March, 2001 and included language that assured that OSHA could not address the ergonomics issue through new regulation for at least 6 years.

Voluntary efforts by employers have been developed in some settings. Some institutions provide instruction in lifting, transfer, posture, body mechanics, and other back-saving strategies to help prevent injury. Mechanical lifting devices provide a means of moving clients without danger to staff. More types of lifting devices are now available, and more employers are open to purchasing equipment to prevent these costly injuries. You need to be aware of the potential for back injury and examine your own work habits. Some nurses feel that they must accomplish certain tasks even if the necessary assistance is not available, and therefore carry out actions of danger to themselves. Nurses need to continue to work toward safer workplaces for all health care providers. Nurses must learn to be assertive regarding their own safety.

Critical Thinking Activity

Research the occupational health program offered by a local employer of nurses. Evaluate that program in relation to health hazards in the workplace of which you are aware.

Workers' Compensation

If you believe that you have a work-related injury or illness, you must follow the policies and procedures prescribed by your facility or by state regulation. This includes reporting the injury as soon as possible after it happens. In most institutions, this is done on an **incident report** or **quality assurance report**. A common error is to delay reporting in the belief that you should report something only if you know it will be serious or require medical care. By the time you know this, it may be much more difficult to prove that the problem was work related.

Employers may seek to have workers' compensation claims disallowed to limit their financial liability. Because back injuries are the most common work-related injuries, and often have no clear objective evidence of damage even when pain is present, stigma frequently is attached to those who have back injuries. HIV and hepatitis B are transmitted through needlestick injuries, but they are also transmitted through other unsafe behaviors. These factors may underlie attempts by an employer to disallow claims for care and time lost from work due to these work-related illnesses or injuries. Prompt, thorough reporting is essential to future claims.

You also should have any injury assessed by an appropriate health care provider. If your agency has an occupational health nurse, you may be required to be seen by him or her for initial screening. One concern is whether you may receive care from the provider of your choice or whether you must receive care from a designated provider. This varies based on the regulations governing work-related injury and illness in your state. You should ask this question of your employer and then research it through your state workers' compensation office. If the laws allow the employer or a state agency to designate the provider and you go to another of your choice, you may not be reimbursed for expenses incurred.

Compensation for time off work is another concern when a work-related problem occurs; you usually are required to use your sick leave, but additional time may be available through the workers' compensation program. In general, these programs do not match your working salary, so your income will be lessened. This is one reason why many individuals choose to have private disability insurance that provides replacement income when they cannot work because of illness or disability.

The Americans With Disabilities Act requires that employers seek ways to provide reasonable accommodation for individuals with disability so that they can continue to work. This might include transferring an individual to a different position or modifying the work environment to provide a setting in which the individual can function. Employers have been known to refuse to make accommodations and to try to terminate an individual who has an ongoing disability. Those with work-related illness and disability do have legal rights within the system. Sometimes it requires considerable effort to sustain those rights.

KEY CONCEPTS

* Throughout the history of nursing, employment patterns have changed, moving from a focus on the home and the community in the first part of this century to a focus on acute care institutions.

- In today's health care world, the percentage of nurses employed in hospital inpatient settings is diminishing as more outpatient, home care, long-term care, and community settings are established for the delivery of care.
- Competencies needed by the newly licensed registered nurse can be categorized by criticality and by frequency.
- Employers have expectations in eight basic areas: theoretic knowledge for safe practice and decision-making; ability to use the nursing process; self-awareness; communication skills; understanding the importance of documentation; commitment to a work ethic; proficiency in specified technical skills; and speed of functioning.
- Developing a successful career pathway involves setting personal short- and long-term goals and developing a plan for maintaining and enhancing your own competence.
- To obtain a nursing position, you will need to identify potential employers, develop a professional resumé, write appropriate letters to employers, and interview effectively.
- Reality shock occurs when an idealistic new graduate enters the real world of practice and has difficulty with the expectations and demands found there. You can prepare for this transition by attending to your own expectations and developing personal strategies for coping.
- Burnout is a stress response experienced by nurses and others who work in occupations that make many emotional demands. Burnout may be alleviated by planned actions, but it may be necessary to change job settings when stress accumulates.
- Nurses may see discrimination in the workplace manifested as racial/ethnic discrimination, wage discrimination against women, job opportunity discrimination against men.
- Violence and harassment in the workplace are found in health care settings as well as the rest of society. Nurses working individually and collectively can develop strategies to combat these serious concerns.
- Occupational safety and health are special concerns for nurses because of the infectious nature of the illnesses with which they come in contact, the toxicity of some chemicals in the nursing environment, and the potential for back injury and violence.
- Nurses who experience a work-related injury must carefully follow all relevant rules and regulations for reporting the injury, completing appropriate forms, and seeking care to assure that they receive assistance for any medical care and lost wages.

RELEVANT   WEB   SITES

American Nurses Association, Occupational Health and Safety Issues:
www.nursingworld.org/dlwa/osh/index.htm

American Nurses Association, RN No Harm/Pollution Prevention:
www.nursingworld.org/rnnoharm/

American Nurses Association and Nursing World Online Health and Safety Survey (2001):
http://www.nursingworld.org/surveys/hssurvey.htm

Bureau of Labor Statistics, U.S. Dept of Labor, Occupational Outlook Handbook:
http://www.bls.gov/oco/ocos083.htm

Nurse Advocate: Nurses and Workplace Violence: *www.nurseadvocate.org*

Occupational Safety and Health Administration: *www.osha.gov*
Safety and Health in Nursing Homes: *www.osha.gov/SLTC/nursinghome/*

Employment Agencies and Classified Advertisements

Absolutely Health Care Web Site: *www.healthjobsusa.com/index.html*
Advanced Resource Solutions, Inc.: *www.arsjobs.com/*
American Nurses Association Online Classified: *www.nursingworld.org/market/classifi*
4 Nursing Jobs: *www.4nursingjobs.com/*
Lippincott Williams & Wilkins Career Center Online: *www.nursingcenter.com/careercenter*
Med Hunters: *www.medhunters.com/*
Nurse JobZ: *www.nursejobz.com/*
Nurse Options USA: *www.nursingjobs.org*
RN magazine, Career Search: *www.rnweb.com*
RN Wanted.com: *www.rnwanted.com*

REFERENCES

American Nurses Association. (1994). Workplace violence: Can you close the door on it? [Brochure]. [On-line]. Available at *http://www.nursingworld.org/dlwa/osh/wp5.htm*. Accessed October 12, 2002.

"Arkansas judge rules male nurse out of labor/delivery." (1981). *AJN 81*(7):1253.

Benner, P. (1984). *From novice to expert*. Menlo Park, CA: Addison-Wesley.

Bessent, H. (2002). *Minority nurses in the new century*. Washington, D.C.: ANA Publishing.

Bradby, M. (1990). Status passage into nursing: Another view of the process of socialization into nursing. *Journal of Advanced Nursing 15*(10):1220–1225.

Bruder, P. (2001, Fall). Verbal abuse of female nurses: An American medical form of gender apartheid? *Hospital Topics*. 4(79):30–34.

Dreyfus, S. E., & Dreyfus, H. L. (1980). A five-stage model of the mental activities involved in directed skill acquisition. Unpublished report supported by the Air Force Office of Scientific Research (AFSC), USAF (Contract F49620-79-C-0063), University of California at Berkeley, 1980 (as reported in Benner P, *From Novice to Expert*, Menlo Park, CA: 1984)

Garner, J., HICPAC. (1996). Guidelines for isolation precautions in hospitals. *Infection Control and Hospital Epidemiology*. 17:53–80.

Kaye. J. (1996). Sexual harassment and hostile environments in the perioperative area. *AORN J 63*(2):443–446, 448–449.

Ketter, J. (1994). Sex discrimination targets men in some hospitals. *American Nurse 26*(4):3, 24.

Kramer, M. (1979). *Reality shock*. St. Louis: CV Mosby.

Kus, R. J. (1985). Stages of coming out: An ethnographic approach. *Western Journal of Nursing Research 7*(2):177–194.

Lindeman, C. (1999). The art of nursing. *Creative Nursing 5*(3):3–4.

National Council of State Boards of Nursing. (2000). Linking the NCLEX-PN National Licensure Examination to Practice. Chicago: NCSBN.

National Council of State Boards of Nursing. (2001). Test plan for the NCLEX examination for registered nurses (2001). Chicago: NCSBN.

National Council of State Boards of Nursing. (2002a). Test plan for the NCLEX examination for practical nurses (2002). Chicago: NCSBN.

National Council of State Boards of Nursing. (2002b) Report of findings from the 2001 RN Practice Analysis Update. Chicago: NCSBN.

National Council of State Boards of Nursing. Employment and work environment trends in newly licensed nurses: Findings from the January 1998 Survey. [On-line]. Available: *www.ncsbn.org/research/studies/qja9801.asp*. Accessed January 21, 2000.

National Council of State Boards of Nursing. Employment and work environment trends in newly licensed nurses: Findings from the July 1999 Survey. [On-line]. Available: *www.ncsbn.org/research/studies/employment9907.asp*. Accessed January 21, 2000.

National League for Nursing. (1999). Educational outcomes of associate degree nursing programs: Roles and competencies. Publication No. 23-2348. New York: National League for Nursing.

Neuhs, H. P. (1994). Sexual harassment: A concern for nursing administrators. *Journal of Nursing Administration 24*(5):47–52.

Projected Supply, Demand, and Shortages of Registered Nurses: 2000–2020. (2002). U.S. Department of Health and Human Services, Health Resources and Services Administration, Bureau of Health Professions, National Center for Health Workforce Analysis. [On-line]. *http://bhpr.hrsa.gov/healthworkforce/rnproject/report.htm*. Accessed October 18, 2002.

"RNs facing new danger at work." (1995). *AJN 95*(10):78, 81.

Rosenstein, A. H. (2002). Nurse–physician relationships: Impact on nurse satisfaction and retention, *AJN 102* (6): 26–34.

Spratley, E., Johnson, A., Sochalski, J., Fritz, M., & Spencer, W. (2000). Findings from the national sample survey of registered nurses. DHHS, Bureau of Health Professions. [On-line]. *http://bhpr.hrsa.gov/healthworkforce/rnsurvey/rnss1.htm#T1*, Accessed October 17, 2002.

Sullivan, E. (2002). In a women's world. *Reflections on Nursing Leadership 28*(3), 10–17.

U.S. Census Bureau. (1999). Statistical Abstract of the United States, National Data Book 1999. [On-line]. Available: *http//www.census.gov/prod/www/statistical-abstract-us.html.*

Williams, M. (1995). The prevalence and impact of violence and sexual harassment of registered nurses in the workplace. *Chart 92*(4):5–6.

Wolfe, S. (1996). Legally speaking: If you're sexually harassed. *RN 59*(2):61–64.

World Health Organization. (2002). New research shows workplace violence threatens health services. [On-line]. Available: *http://www.who.int/inf/en/pr-2002-37.html.*

Worthington, K. (2002). Violence in the health care workplace. *AJN 100*(11), [On-line]. Available: *http://www.nursingworld.org/AJN/2000/nov/Issues.htm*, Accessed 10/12/02.

12

Preparing for Workplace Participation

LEARNING OUTCOMES

After completing this chapter, you should be able to:

1. Discuss the purpose of mission statements.
2. Analyze the relationships among organizational charts, chains of command, and channels of communication within the structure of organizations.
3. Delineate the characteristics of shared governance, analyzing the advantages of a shared governance approach.
4. Describe various patterns of nursing care delivery, identifying the major characteristics of each.
5. Discuss the history of collective bargaining as it applies to nursing.
6. Analyze the processes through which resolution is achieved in collective bargaining issues.
7. Identify at least four professional concerns that should be addressed in a contract for nurses.
8. Compare and contrast the characteristics of a grievance with those of a complaint.
9. Discuss the concerns nurses have regarding membership in a collective bargaining group and the reasons for each of these concerns.
10. Outline the advantages and disadvantages of having the state nurses' association serve as a bargaining agent for nurses.

KEY TERMS

Agency shop

Arbitration/arbitrator

Authoritative mandate

Bargain in good faith

Binding arbitration

Bureaucratic

Case management

Case method

Centralized/
Decentralized/Matrix

Chain of command

Channels of
communication

Clinical ladder

Collective action division

Collective bargaining

Common interest bargain-
ing

Concession bargaining

Constructive adversarialism

Contract

Cross-training

Deadlock

Division of labor

Final offer

Functional method

Government seizure

Grievance/Grievance
process

Impasse

Informational picketing

Injunction

Job description

Lockout

Mediation/mediator

Mission statement

Modular care

National Labor Relations
Act

National Labor Relations
Board

Negotiate/Negotiation

Organization

Organizational chart

Organizational hierarchy

Path of authority and
accountability

Pathways—Care, Critical,
Clinical

Policy

Primary care

Procedure manual

Professional collectivism

Protocol

Ratify

Reinstatement privilege

Role transition

Shared governance

Span of control—broad,
narrow

Standards of care

Statements of philosophy

Strike/Strike-breaking

Structure of an organiza-
tion

Team nursing

Total patient care

Unfair labor practice

Union busting

Unions

Organizations surround us. Wherever you look you will find organizations. And, like most other new nursing graduates, when you complete your studies, you probably will seek employment in an organization—a health care organization. This may be in an acute care hospital, a long-term care facility, an intermediate care facility, a clinic, an outpatient unit, or a variety of other organizations that offer challenging opportunities. Accepting employment in a health care organization requires that you are knowledgeable about and become accustomed to the policies and procedures established by that organization. You will go through what we refer to as **role transition**, the process of assuming and developing a new role. This process occurs most comfortably when you have a basic understanding of the organization, how it operates and functions, and how you can participate effectively in the activities of that workplace. It is also helpful to be able to anticipate some of the frustrations you may encounter. When you can anticipate things that may occur, they can be handled with greater ease and with greater adeptness.

This chapter presents content that we believe can assist you in your transition from student to employee. We begin with a brief discussion of the structure of organizations and some of the most common conditions of employment, and then present the most common avenues through which employees participate in workplace decisions. Because we can only touch on these topics, students are encouraged to gain greater depth in this area by reading books devoted to this topic.

UNDERSTANDING ORGANIZATIONS

An **organization** may be defined as a formally constituted group of people, with identified tasks, who work together to achieve a specific purpose defined by the organization. All organizations have structure and purpose. Large organizations that have the delivery of health care as their primary objective, such as hospitals and medical centers, usually are considered **bureaucratic** organizations, which means that they operate and are administered through a number of departments and subdivisions, with designated individuals responsible for carrying out various functions.

The Mission Statement and the Philosophy

All organizations have a purpose, or a reason for existing. This purpose typically is expressed in the form of a **mission statement,** which outlines what the organization plans to accomplish. Sometimes mission statements incorporate **statements of philosophy** (beliefs), purpose, and goals or objectives into a single statement; other times the philosophy, purposes, and goals are addressed in addition to the mission statement. These statements serve as a benchmark against which an organization's performance can be evaluated. A large research hospital might incorporate into its mission statement obligations for research, teaching, and the care of clients with complex problems. A smaller community hospital may reflect a goal of meeting the health care needs of citizens of the community in its mission statement. The hospital's ability to meet these goals would be reviewed as part of the overall evaluation of the organization.

Critical Thinking Activity

Based on your perception of the needs of the community in which you live, write a mission statement for a hospital that would serve the needs of the area. How did you arrive at the decision to offer the services you outlined? What facts support this decision? What services did you not include? Examine your response for personal biases.

Organizational Structure

To continue operation, any organization must make enough money to meet expenses and to improve and develop; some also seek to provide a profit return to investors. This is as true in health care as it is in Wall Street businesses. A central goal of most organizations is to seek an organizational structure that is efficient while providing maximum cost effectiveness. As the values and priorities of our society change and as new technology becomes available, health care organizations also must make adaptations. Thus, today we encounter a health care system experiencing tremendous transformation (see Chapters 1 and 2).

In organizational theory, the concept of management is associated with structure. The **structure of an organization** may be defined as "the sum total of the ways its labor is divided into distinct tasks and then coordination is achieved among these tasks" (Huber, 1996, p. 226). In other words, the structure of an organization refers to the way it is "put together" to accomplish its goals. Breaking work into pieces or tasks, which are assigned to various individuals or groups, is known as **division of labor**. Size, age, services, technical components, and environment influence the structure of an organization.

Types of Structure

The power to make decisions is a key factor in the structure and function of any organization. With regard to the decision-making process, organizations may be described as having a centralized (or tall) or a decentralized (or flat) structure. An organization is depicted as **centralized** when the authority to make decisions is vested in a few individuals (Fig. 12-1).

Conversely, when the decision-making involves a number of individuals and filters down to the individual employee, the organization is said to operate in a **decentralized** fashion. Currently, many organizations are going through a process of restructuring to embrace a transformational approach to decision-making that places the responsibility for finding solutions to problems at the site where the activity is occurring. Later in this chapter we discuss the concept of shared governance, which embraces a decentralized structure and function (Fig. 12-2).

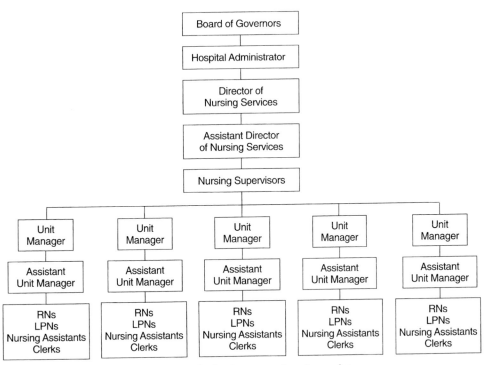

FIGURE 12-1 Centralized (tall) organizational structure of nursing service.

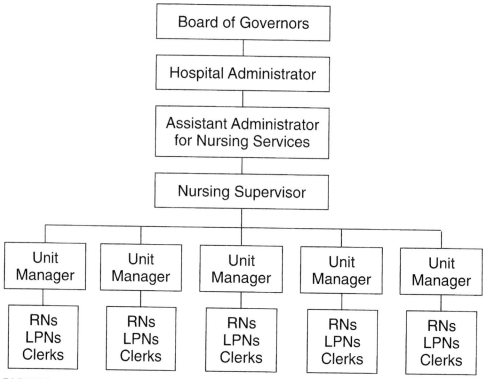

FIGURE 12-2   Decentralized (flat) organizational structure of nursing service.

Another type of organizational structure, the matrix structure, may be either flat or tall. The unique characteristic of the **matrix** structure is that a second structure overlies the first, creating two directions for lines of authority, accountability, and communication. The relationship that exists among individuals is outside the regular **chain of command**. We typically see the matrix structure in very large, multifaceted organizations. Individuals with special expertise or authority in an area serve as resource persons for several departments, all of which can benefit from the knowledge. For example, in Figure 12-3, three different types of expertise (financial services, planning and marketing, and quality assurance) are demonstrated to cross all aspects of this large hospital corporation, which includes acute care, long-term care, and home care. Another example of a matrix-type relationship could be illustrated when a nurse with expertise in gerontologic nursing provides assistance, advice, and information to employees in each branch of this hospital organization.

ORGANIZATIONAL RELATIONSHIPS

When examining organizational function, it is important that you identify relationships among people and departments and realize where the authority is placed within that

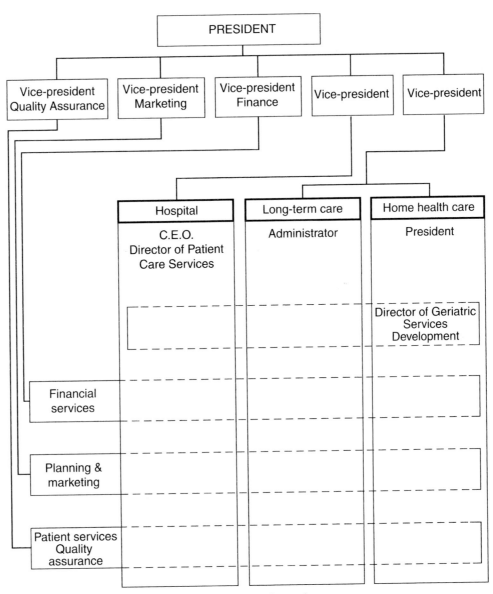

FIGURE 12-3   Matrix organizational structure of nursing service.

organization. Most organizations have several ways of expressing and defining the relationship of one worker to another. Organizational charts, chains of command, channels of communication, job descriptions, and policies and procedures provide different views of organizational relationships.

Organizational Chart

The structure of any large group comprises both a formal and an informal organization. The formal organization can be seen on an organizational chart. The **organizational chart** is a graphic, pictorial means of portraying roles and patterns of interaction among parts of a system. It identifies formal chains of command, communication channels, and the authority for decision-making. In most groups, we also find an informal organization, sometimes called the "grapevine," that represents informal or social relationships. The informal organization is not depicted on an organizational chart or formally acknowledged in any specific manner, but it can often have a profound effect on how an organization functions.

The organizational chart typically is represented by boxes stacked in a pyramid-shaped chart. The greatest authority exists at the top of the chart (often a single box), and authority declines as you move toward the base (many boxes). Persons occupying jobs at the top of the organizational chart are considered administrators, executives, or "the management," and individuals with jobs closer to the base are considered employees or staff. Located between these two levels is an area known as "middle management," comprising those who coordinate and control activities of specified groups of workers.

The organizational chart may take one of several forms, reflecting the type of administration operating within that organization. One term used to describe these forms is **span of control**, which refers to the number of employees supervised by a manager. A **narrow** span of control exists when a manager has responsibility for only three to five subordinates. If, however, the organization operates with a **broad** span of control, it places authority and responsibility for decision-making in the hands of fewer individuals, with each manager supervising a large number of employees. The larger the number of individuals to be supervised, the more difficult it is to control each worker through direct observation. If two organizations of equal size were to exist—one with a narrow span of control and the other with a broad span of control—the organization choosing to implement a narrow span of control would have more managers.

Chain of Command

All organizations have a chain of command. The chain of command represents the **path of authority and accountability** from individuals at the top of the organization to those at the base of the organization. It is often referred to as the **organizational hierarchy**. Thus, in hospitals we typically find that the nursing administrator gives directions to and evaluates the performance of the assistant administrator, who, in turn, gives directions to and evaluates the performance of the nursing unit manager, and so forth. When we look at this process from the base of the organization to the top, we often use the language "reports to"— indicating that the unit manager is accountable to the assistant administrator, and the assistant administrator is accountable to the nursing administrator. Similarly, we find the registered nurse (RN) giving direction to and overseeing the activities of the practical (vocational) nurse and the nursing assistant. The length of the chain of command varies depending on the size of the organization.

Almost without exception, the salaries commanded by persons at the top of the organizational hierarchy are greater than those of persons close to the base. Accordingly, the experience, educational requirements, hours worked, and responsibilities are greater for persons with positions near the top of the organizational chart.

Channels of Communication

Channels of communication are, as the name implies, the patterns through which messages are delivered within an organization. The channels of communication usually reflect the chain of command; they run up and down the organizational chart, moving from one level of responsibility and authority to the next. Thus, the nurse manager communicates concerns and information to the assistant administrator, who may have the authority and responsibility to deal with the problem, or who relays the concern to the nursing administrator. The nursing assistant reports her concerns to the staff nurse, who may have the authority to deal with the issue, or who reports it to the head nurse or clinical manager. For a nurse manager to report a concern directly to the administrator is referred to as "looping" the system; it is generally considered improper and inappropriate to skip or bypass any level in the communication system. For example, if a staff nurse disagrees with a pharmacy technician who delivers medications to the unit, and takes this problem directly to the supervisor without first discussing it with the unit manager, this is considered "looping" the system. You readily can see how this would put the unit manager at a distinct disadvantage, should the supervisor ask about the incident.

Job Descriptions

Job descriptions form another important aspect of any organization. **Job descriptions** are written statements, usually found in policy manuals, that stipulate the duties and functions of the various jobs within the organization, and the scope of authority, responsibility, and accountability involved in each position. Job descriptions should explain the role of each individual working for the company or organization, from the chief executive officer to the janitor.

Sometimes job descriptions are very specific; other times they are more broadly stated. If broadly stated, policy and procedure manuals may help to specify a task or responsibility. Job descriptions provide the foundation for performance standards for each position and should provide the basis for evaluation. Job descriptions also may include competencies expected of employees and can provide the basis for Competency-Based Orientation (CBO). As the RN delegates more and more care to those with lesser educational preparation, it is critical that job descriptions provide sufficient description of the competencies of various workers, so that the document can be used to guide delegation activities (see Chapter 14 for more information on delegation).

Job descriptions also are important when cross-training is used in the organization. **Cross-training** involves teaching one member of the health care team to perform functions usually associated with another position. For example, a respiratory therapist might learn to perform basic patient care skills and, when not needed for respiratory therapy treatments, be available to answer lights and respond to patient needs. Cross-training is viewed by some administrators as a method by which costs can be reduced through the efficiency of having an individual able to do more than one set of tasks within the organization. The effectiveness of cross-training between different disciplines has not been well documented. However, cross-training of nurses between differing specialties has become common, and many nurses welcome the employment flexibility this provides.

Job descriptions also may describe clinical ladders. A **clinical ladder** differentiates and defines the skills and performance expected of nurses in terms of advancing levels. Typically, three or four levels of performance are defined, with each higher level having greater responsibility and authority than the previous one. A new graduate usually enters the system as a Clinical Nurse One (or similar title), moves to Clinical Nurse Two, and then to Clinical Nurse Three as that individual becomes more proficient. Salary increases typically accompany movement from one level to another, as does the responsibility the individual is expected to assume.

Sometimes additional formal education or continuing education is required for advancement. Through this process, the nurse is supported and encouraged to develop greater clinical expertise. The clinical ladder also serves as a mechanism for recognizing and rewarding nurses who wish to remain in direct care positions rather than seek administrative positions.

Policies, Protocols, Procedures, and Standards of Care

A **policy** may be defined as a designated plan or course of action to be taken in a specific situation. In organizations, the governing board holds the responsibility and authority for assuring that appropriate policies are adopted. The governing board usually delegates the development of policies to the chief administrative officer. The administrator usually delegates the responsibility for development of policies for a specific department to individuals or groups in the department that will be most affected by the policy. Once their work is completed, the policy is returned to the governing board for review, possible revision, and adoption. The management within the organization is responsible for assuring that the policies are followed and that more specific policies are developed if necessary.

Written copies of all policies usually are placed in a policy manual that is available in each department, or a current copy may be available on-line in the institution's computer network. On-line policy manuals assure that all departments are referring to the most current policy and that the information is always available. Depending on the area in which you are employed, you will find varying needs for referring to the policy manual in your role as a new employee. As you might anticipate, the need for special policies related to occurrences in an emergency department, delivery room, or a critical care unit is greater than in a general medical or surgical unit in a hospital. When you are confronted with a new nonclinical problem to solve and you are unsure of what action to take, always check your policy manual to see if it offers guidance.

Special unit policies are sometimes termed **protocols**. For example, the protocol for dealing with a patient seen in the emergency department suffering from a dog bite determines which local authorities should be notified, who is responsible for seeing that they are notified, and perhaps general management of the wound.

Procedure manuals contain the written instructions describing the accepted method for satisfactorily performing a particular nursing activity (procedure), often describing it in a number of steps. Procedure manuals should be found in each unit or department. For example, in the manual, you could find a procedure for changing the dressing on a central intravenous line, for administering chemotherapy agents, and for doing many other procedures, such as catheterizations.

Institutions are giving nurses more responsibility for developing institutional policies and procedures, and serving as representatives to various committees that monitor, review, and update policies and procedures. As hospitals move to broader spans of control and to greater involvement of all employees in decision-making, grassroots participation in policy formation is becoming more common. The nature of a policy and the breadth of its scope will determine whether it needs further review within the organization.

Standards of care are authoritative statements that describe a common or acceptable level of client care or performance that have some similarity to policies and procedures. Thus, standards of care define professional practice. In 1991, the American Nurses Association (ANA) formulated general standards and guidelines for nursing practice. They apply across the nation and are broad and general in nature. They are now in their second edition and represent more than 20 areas of specialty practice. (The standards can be purchased from ANA as a package or for single specialty areas.) Similarly, state practice acts contain language describing the standard of practice that applies to all nurses licensed in that state.

Each agency also may develop standards of care for patients with selected health care problems. These more detailed and specific standards may take the form of standard nursing care plans. Some standards are being incorporated into documents termed **care pathways, critical pathways or clinical pathways**. These are intended to serve as guides to direct the health care team in the daily care. It organizes and sequences the care and describes the care required for a patient at specific times in the treatment. It involves a multidisciplinary approach and identifies both the care activities and the outcomes for each 24-hour period of hospitalization. These specific standards of care become the basis for evaluation of care, quality improvement within the organization, and cost analysis.

SHARED GOVERNANCE

Few industries have felt the impact of technology as much as health care. Ranging from new systems of information and communication to different administrative structures, to changing approaches to systems of evaluation, to highly technical equipment, the health care delivery system has seen a radical acceleration in all forms of technology. In the realm of administrative structure, one of the more important changes has been the recent move to a pattern of shared governance within health care agencies.

Shared governance is a professional practice model in which the nursing staff and the nursing management are both involved in decision-making, as opposed to the administrative decision area being controlled by management. It originated during the mid-1980s and gained status and recognition as an alternative to bureaucratic management during the 1990s. This structure allows nursing staff to make major decisions within the organization and attempts to get the decision-making process as close to where the action is occurring as possible, typically through the development of internal councils. Often, this pattern of organization is paired with the concept of total quality improvement (TQI), which has as its hallmark emphasis on the customer. Alexander et al. (1994, p. 283) states "TQI and shared governance (1) empower all employees, (2) encourage decision making at the appropriate level within the organization, (3) promote teamwork with consensus and shared responsibility, (4) encourage and recognize employee contributions, and (5) provide opportunities for personal growth."

There is no single model for shared governance. The shared governance format may take several approaches, including a councilar model in which committees and councils have defined authority and functions, a congressional model that involves an elected representative system, or an administrative model consisting of committees or forums in which people communicate and share ideas (Porter-O'Grady, 1987). The committees or councils result in staff actively participating in management, and, as a consequence, gaining autonomy, control over the work environment, and greater job satisfaction. Often, councils report to a nursing executive board that serves as a coordinating and approval body. Within this framework, the nurse is held to greater accountability within the context of peer-defined and peer-operated parameters (Porter-O'Grady, 1990). The traditional role of the supervisor as one who hires, evaluates, promotes, and fires becomes a thing of the past. The inability to make this change has been a major impediment to the success of shared governance. Many managers find their new and changing role difficult to accept.

The shared governance model has become widespread in hospitals. Its implementation requires that staff nurses participate in professional development sessions that increase nurses' understanding of the decision-making process, team building, group dynamics, leadership, and budgeting.

Many have questioned the continuance of shared governance models in today's health care system. The re-engineering and restructuring of the health care delivery system, which has resulted in multihospital systems, consolidations, mergers, and the use of nurses as primary care providers and case managers, also may result in the demise of shared governance, or in its assuming a different format. The time involved in shared governance is costly to an organization, and the cost-effectiveness of shared governance in terms of patient outcomes is being questioned.

Critical Thinking Activity

Interview some nurses who are working in a shared governance environment. Identify what they find satisfying about shared governance. How would they like to see it changed? If shared governance is not used in your area, interview nurses about the concept of shared governance and how they believe it would improve patient care.

PATTERNS OF NURSING CARE DELIVERY

The nursing department of any health care institution carries major responsibility for the quality of nursing care delivered. Throughout the years, the structure of the delivery of care has taken many different formats. Perhaps you will note that the particular pattern of care that is in vogue has changed about every 20 years. Among the factors influencing the delivery pattern selected in each era were the types of patients served, the type of care provided, the cost of the care, the structure of the hospital, and the number and education level of potential employees. Perhaps a wider variety of patterns of care is being used today than at any other time in nursing's history. In the following section we describe the typical implementation of several patterns of care delivery. However, it is important to remember that you might find a particular pattern of care practiced a little differently in different settings.

Case Method

The **case method** was the first system used for the delivery of nursing care in the United States (around the beginning of the 20th century) and should not be confused with the term "case management" practiced today (see Chapter 2 and discussion later in this chapter). With the case method, the nurse worked with one patient (or case) only and was expected to meet all of that patient's needs. The nurse often lived in the patient's home and was expected to assume other household duties, such as cooking for the patient and family and light house-keeping, when not busy with the patient. Nurses worked long hours and were poorly paid. Advancing technology and increasing costs made this type of care delivery impractical, but vestiges of its structure can be seen in today's home health nursing. However, the role of the RN in home health care is typically one of assessment, planning, skilled intervention, super-vision of care provided by a home health aide, and evaluation of the client's progress.

Functional Method

The **functional method** of care delivery emerged during the Great Depression of the 1930s. This method allowed for the care of greater numbers of patients in hospitals and for use of advancing technology. At this time, the industrial model of narrowly defined and frequently repeated tasks was revolutionizing manufacturing. The idea that this would transfer into all types of work environments was widely accepted.

Typically, the head nurse assigned nursing tasks to the various persons employed on the unit, according to the level of skills required for performance. One nurse might take all tem-peratures, another would do all dressings, while yet another administered all medications, charted them, and provided a list of replacement needs to the head nurse. Assignments varied depending on the size of the unit, the number of personnel available, and the skill level of the personnel. The head nurse gave a report to the next shift.

Although economical and efficient, this system of care delivery had the disadvantage of fragmenting care—no single individual was responsible for the planning of the care. Patients were confused about who was caring for them, and communication among caregivers was lacking. Individual nurse–patient relationships were limited. Nursing care came to be viewed as a list of procedures and tasks. This pattern of care still may be used in long-term care facil-ities or subacute units, largely because of the educational preparation of the care providers. Some nurses are concerned that the economic push in today's health care institutions may see many hospitals returning to functional approaches to care.

Team Nursing

The concept of **team nursing** was introduced in the early 1950s, with the promise that it would result in more patient-centered care. It was also responsive to the nursing shortage that fol-lowed World War II (see Chapter 4) and the involvement of nurse aides and licensed practical (vocational) nurses in patient care. This approach to care was based on the premise that each unit would have two or more teams composed of variously educated care providers. For exam-ple, a team might be composed of two nurse aides, an orderly, a licensed practical (vocational) nurse, and an RN. A more experienced RN would be the "team leader." Team members worked

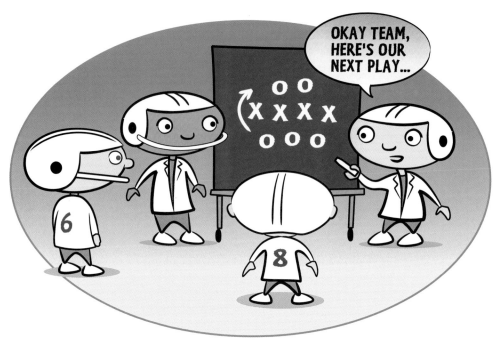

FIGURE 12-4 Team conference, planning, and communication are critical elements of team nursing.

together, each performing those tasks for which they were best prepared. The team leader made assignments, had overall responsibility for the care of patients on the unit, might give all medications, and gave a report to the team that followed on the next shift. An important part of this form of nursing was the "team conference," at which members of the team met to communicate about the needs of their patients and to plan for care. Without the conference and the communication, team nursing might be little different from functional nursing. Today, as we see more health care facilities decreasing the number of RNs and adding more unlicensed assistive personnel, team nursing may again become a prevalent method of care delivery (Fig. 12-4).

Total Patient Care

During the late 1970s and early 1980s, many hospitals returned to a **total patient care** type of assignment, in which an RN or licensed practical (vocational) nurse is assigned for all care needs. A nurse is assigned to the care of a group of four to six patients, depending on how acutely ill each patient is, and depending on patient needs. This returns a greater sense of control to nurses, gives them a greater sense of autonomy, and fosters a greater sense of involvement in the whole spectrum of care and patient outcomes. This type of care focuses on the total person (from which its name is derived) rather than on a collection of tasks or procedures.

This approach to care has the disadvantage of being costly. An individual with less training could satisfactorily complete many of the tasks performed by the RN and at a lesser cost.

Additionally, the continuity of care may be at risk as nurses, who have the right to change care plans, replace one another on shifts and alter the original plan of care.

Primary Care Nursing

In a pattern of **primary care**, which came into popular application in the 1980s, one nurse is assigned the responsibility for the care of each patient from the time the patient is admitted to the hospital until that patient's discharge. The primary nurse is responsible for initiating and updating the nursing care plan, patient teaching, and discharge planning. An associate nurse works with this same patient on other shifts and on the primary nurse's day off, carrying out the plan of care developed by the primary nurse.

Obvious benefits of this method include the continuity of care for the patient and job satisfaction for the nurses because they have more autonomy and control. Whether this method is more expensive has been the subject of debate. Health care administrators argue that the salary costs for RNs make this a more costly approach to care. However, recent studies demonstrating the relationship between nurse–staffing levels and quality of care in hospitals would question this conclusion. Needleman et al. (2002), in examining the outcomes of more than 6 million medical surgical patients in 799 hospitals in 11 states across the country, determined that hospitals with the higher proportion of care delivered by RNs and the greater number of hours of care per day by RNs resulted in better care for hospitalized patients. When the proportion of care given by RNs was greater, complications such as pneumonia, bleeding, blood clots, urinary tract infections and cardiac arrest were fewer. This data would indicate that decreased complication rates, shorter length of stays, and decreased readmission rates for patients, plus the employment of fewer assistive personnel who have greater turnover rates, offset the additional direct care costs. This is consistent with other studies that have resulted in similar findings (Brown, 2001; Domrose, 2002).

Under this system, every nurse is a primary nurse for a few patients and an associate nurse for others. Sometimes the nurse functioning in an associate role has difficulty following the plan of the primary nurse or may disagree with the established plan of care. The patient's condition also may change rapidly, requiring the plan to be changed without consulting the primary nurse. Another concern is the level of expertise and commitment required of all nurses, and the fact that nurses who work autonomously with patients soon forget how to delegate responsibilities.

Modular Care

Modular care gained popularity in the mid-1980s. Patient care units were divided into modules and the same team of care providers consistently was assigned to a particular module. An RN served as team leader of each module, with licensed practical nurses (LPNs) and nursing assistants making up the team. In this sense, modular nursing looked a lot like team nursing. Each module was stocked with its own linens, medications, and supplies.

This form of care delivery has the advantage of offering continuity of care because the same team cares for the same group of patients each day; of involving the RN in planning and coordinating care; and of more efficient communication because of the geographic closeness of the unit. The disadvantages center on the increased costs of stocking each unit, and the fact that many hospitals, with long corridors and halls, do not lend themselves architecturally to a modular design (Komplin, 1995).

Case Management

Case management, although not a system of care delivery in the sense that we have mentioned earlier, involves nurses in the role of managing patient care and bears mention here. Case management refers to a system in which the health care services are controlled and monitored carefully to ensure that policies are followed, that neither too much nor too little care is provided, and that costs are minimized. A key to case management is the identification of a critical pathway for care and treatment that includes specific timelines and protocols. The case manager typically follows the patient from the diagnostic phase through hospitalization, rehabilitation, and back to home care, ensuring that plans are made in advance and that the patient receives care that will achieve the most positive outcomes. The case manager may not provide direct care but is responsible for managing the patient's interaction with the entire health care system. For a more detailed discussion of case management, please refer to Chapter 2.

Registered nurses are the health care professionals who most often act as case managers. In some settings, social workers also act as case managers. Case managers may be employed by third-party payers (such as insurance companies) or by health care agencies (such as hospitals or long-term care facilities). Case managers employed by a particular institution also might be involved in wellness programs (such as blood pressure management, stress management, smoking cessation programs, and exercise classes).

Some objections to this form of care delivery come from physicians, who see the role of the case manager as an infringement on their historic rights of autonomy in decision-making. Providers may also believe that the case manager is more concerned with cost factors than with what is best for the individual, arguing that quality is sacrificed to cost containment.

Critical Thinking Activity

Compare the various patterns of nursing care delivery with the pattern being used in a facility where you currently receive clinical experience. Analyze the pattern in current use and evaluate whether another pattern of care delivery would be more or less effective. Provide a rationale for your answer.

COLLECTIVE BARGAINING

Collective bargaining consists of a set of procedures by which employee representatives and employer representatives negotiate to obtain a signed agreement (contract) that spells out wages, hours, and conditions of employment that are acceptable to both. A key word in this definition is *negotiate*. The goal of the negotiations is to obtain a signed agreement, which is a legal contract that spells out in writing the decisions that are reached. Colosi and Berkeley (1994, p. 3) define **negotiation** as "a process which affords the disputants an opportunity to exchange promises and make binding commitments in an effort to resolve their differences."

These authors divide collective bargaining into two phases: promise-making (contract negotiations) and promise-checking (contract administration).

Because of nursing's long history as a profession of dedication, altruism, and service, initially, collective bargaining was a controversial issue within nursing. Some saw this process as detracting from the professional role of the nurse and ethically improper.

Today, however, nurses are vitally concerned about contracts, services, third-party payers, comparable worth, patients' rights, shared governance, staffing ratios, and a host of issues that can be discussed at the bargaining table. Nurses believe that people who choose nursing as a career should have the opportunity to have some voice in patient care assignments, length of the work day and week, fringe benefits, and wages, without losing face with the public at large, members of the medical profession, or other colleagues.

History of Collective Bargaining

As early as the 1850s, Horace Greeley, a reformer, publisher, and politician, was generating interest in and giving impetus to collective bargaining issues in his editorial columns in the *New York Tribune.* During the early part of the 20th century, efforts by workers to organize were met with opposition from employers, government officials, and some members of the public. After the Great Depression, which immobilized the United States in the late 1920s and early 1930s, several laws were enacted to help improve workers' conditions. Franklin D. Roosevelt was elected president in 1932, and his New Deal administration saw the passage of the National Industrial Recovery Act. One result of this act was the creation of the National Recovery Administration, whose purpose was to administer codes of fair practice within given industries. The nation was called on to accept an interim blanket code that established a 35- to 40-hour workweek for workers, minimum pay of 30 to 40 cents an hour, and prohibition of child labor—all issues that had long been advocated by nurses.

PASSAGE OF THE NATIONAL LABOR RELATIONS ACT

On July 5, 1935, the **National Labor Relations Act** (NLRA) became the national labor policy of the United States. Also known as the Wagner Act, for Senator Robert F. Wagner (who introduced the legislation), the NLRA gave workers federal protection in their efforts to form unions and organize for better working conditions. It listed as unfair practice any actions on the part of employers that would interfere with this process. Senator Wagner wanted management and labor to resolve their mutual problems through a system of self-government. This act also created the **National Labor Relations Board** (NLRB), a quasi-judicial body that was to ensure proper enforcement of the conditions of the legislation.

The NLRB has the responsibility for administering the NLRA. In addition, it has two primary functions: to conduct secret-ballot elections that will determine that the majority of employees of a unit desire the representation of a given union in collective bargaining procedures, and to prevent and rectify unfair labor practices committed by employers or unions. It also has the responsibility for determining to which of the eight bargaining units established for health care workers various employees will be assigned. This is important to nurses because it enables them to have a separate unit and, therefore, to deal with issues important to their role in health care delivery.

The original NLRA used the term labor organization, which was defined in language that could be interpreted to exclude nursing and several other professions, such as teaching and medicine, that were organized through professional organizations. These early labor unions often were viewed negatively by the public—an image that was reinforced in movies, in newspapers, and on radio. Often portrayed as rowdy, aggressive, and hostile, unions did not seem to fit well in nursing.

In 1947, the original NLRA was amended through the Taft-Hartley Act (also known as the Labor Management Relations Act). Because of heavy lobbying by hospital management, the act was written in such a way as to specifically exclude nonprofit hospitals from the legal obligation of bargaining with their employees. Although the administrations of some hospitals chose to negotiate salaries and working conditions with their employees, many did not, and no legal action could be taken to force the process.

ACTIVITY OF THE AMERICAN NURSES ASSOCIATION

By 1931, the American Nurses Association (ANA) was publicly recognizing its obligation regarding the general welfare of its members, and developed within its organization a legislative policy addressing this concern. Some suggest that this effort was spurred by the fact that other groups, particularly the Service Employees International Union (SEIU), an affiliate of the American Federation of Labor/Congress of Industrial Organizations (AFL/CIO), were actively working to organize health care workers. Other factors also were important. Before 1930, most nurses were employed in public health, visiting nurse, or private duty positions. Students, aides, and orderlies, under the direction of a head nurse, delivered much of the care in hospitals. As more care was delivered in the hospital setting, the number of nurses employed by these facilities grew. The existing working conditions affected more people.

The ANA has worked constantly since those early years to provide leadership and support to nurses as they negotiate salaries, working conditions, benefits, and governance opportunity. Table 12-1 summarizes those activities that eventually led to the establishment in 1999 of a separate arm of ANA, with the sole mission of collective bargaining.

TABLE 12-1.	HIGHLIGHTS OF ANA ACTIVITIES RELATED TO COLLECTIVE BARGAINING
YEAR	**ACTIVITY**
1931	Developed within its organization a legislative policy addressing general welfare concerns of its members
1945	Appointed a committee to study employment conditions
1946	Established the ANA Economic Security Program as an outcome of the 1945 study. State nurses' associations encouraged to act as exclusive bargaining agents for their memberships.
1947	Collective bargaining between nurses and hospital administrations implemented in several states with negotiated contracts in effect
1950	No-strike policy adopted officially by ANA due to concern for the image of nursing
1967	ANA identified as the bargaining agent for nurses in Veterans Administration hospitals
1968	No-strike policy rescinded
1991	ANA embarked on a Workplace Advocacy Initiative to improve the work environment of nurses
1999	United American Nurses established as an autonomous arm of ANA to bargain for nurses

Federal legislation passed in 1962 enabled employees of federal health care institutions to participate in collective bargaining. In 1967, investor-owned hospitals and nursing homes also were included, and the ANA was identified as the bargaining agent for the nurses of the Veterans Administration hospitals. Legislation passed in 1970 included nonprofit nursing homes in the collective bargaining process. Concurrently, SEIU and other labor-related organizations were also bargaining for nurses.

THE TAFT-HARTLEY LAW AMENDED

Finally, on August 25, 1974, Public Law 93-360 was put into effect. It amended the Taft-Hartley Act to provide economic security programs for those employed in nonprofit hospitals, and brought health care facilities and their employees under the jurisdiction of the NLRB. Nonprofit hospitals were legally required to bargain with nurses for better wages, hours, staffing conditions, patient–nurse ratios, and a voice in hospital governance. To ensure that the public would be protected from strikes or work stoppage, several amendments were attached to the NLRA passed in 1974, including the requirement of longer notification periods and provisions mandating participation in mediation.

Understanding the Basic Concepts

Intelligent and effective bargaining begins with an awareness of the process itself. The information that follows is designed to provide a better understanding of the terms and processes involved in bargaining collectively to achieve an agreed-upon contract.

BARGAINING AND NEGOTIATING

To **negotiate** means to bargain or confer with another party or parties to reach an agreement. To bargain implies that there will be discussion of the terms of the agreement and suggests that there will be give and take—that neither party will obtain all items asked for in the contract. Ideally, negotiations would proceed in a somewhat philosophic vein, moving toward reasonable compromises that would allow each side to achieve many of the conditions it requested, but this does not always occur.

Common interest bargaining refers to a process in which the employer and employee representatives begin by identifying those areas in which they agree and those goals or values held by both parties. Based on shared values and goals, the two parties then begin to work out their differences regarding specific policies and conditions. Although relatively new as an approach to collective bargaining, common interest bargaining is gaining attention as a less adversarial process, which may preserve effective working relationships and lessen feelings of alienation between supervisory personnel and employees involved in the union.

UNIONS AND COLLECTIVE ACTION

Collective bargaining allows employees working together as a union to negotiate; employees must choose a union that will represent them. Thus, a **union** is a legally authorized, organized group of employees that negotiates and enforces labor agreements. This usually is done through an election. The major concern of the union is improvement in the wages, hours, and working conditions of its members. Three conditions must exist for unions to become organized: (1) a group of employees in an institution must sense a difference between employees and managers regarding policies, practices, or personalities; (2) the group must have unsatisfied concerns but retain a sense of commitment to the job and to the employer; and (3) a supportive legal environment for unionization must exist in the organization (Colosi & Berkeley, 1994, p. 11).

When a branch or part of a professional association assumes the role and responsibility of a union, as often occurs in nursing, the negotiating group may be known as a **collective action division**. The activity of the group may be referred to as **professional collectivism**, which supports the premise that the quality of patient care is directly tied to working conditions and that collective action is a professional responsibility. Nursing collective bargaining units point out that while shared governance provides input from nurses, especially regarding issues related to patient care, that position can be unilaterally changed by administration. A contract can provide a legal commitment to including the voice of nursing in decisions.

A professional organization must work under the same legal constraints as a union. It provides legal counsel and representatives to assist with negotiations, may lobby on behalf of issues, or may participate in other activities that would further the economic welfare of nurses. It oversees the development of the contract.

CONTRACTS

The conclusion of the bargaining process should result in a signed contract that converts to writing the agreements that have been reached. A **contract** is "an agreement between two or more people to do something, especially one formally set forth in writing and enforceable by law" (Neufeldt, 1996 [Webster's], p. 302). This signed contract is enforceable under law and cannot be changed by either party acting unilaterally.

Some would suggest that the contract is the most important product of the collective bargaining process because it converts to an agreement on all issues that have been discussed. It provides the foundation for further activities. In most instances, a contract need not be in writing, but it is much easier to implement when written and signed by all involved. The contract remains in effect until breached or terminated. Most negotiated contracts define the period of time—usually 2 or 3 years—during which the established conditions are effective.

Before being put into effect, a contract must be **ratified**. This means that the members of the bargaining group must accept the terms of the contract. This is usually done by a vote of the membership. Factors to be considered in a contract will be discussed later in this chapter.

RULES GOVERNING LABOR RELATIONS

When two parties agree to begin the negotiation process, it is understood that both will **bargain in good faith**. Bargaining in good faith is a poorly understood concept, but generally it means that the parties will meet at regular times to discuss (with the intent to resolve) any differences over wages, hours, and other employment conditions. Failure to carry out these activities could lead to an unfair labor practice.

An **unfair labor practice** is any action that interferes with the rights of employees or employers as described in the amended NLRA. It is not possible to discuss all of these in detail; however, some examples follow. An employer must not interfere with the employee's right to form a union or other organized bargaining group, join the group, or participate in the group's activities. The employer may not attempt to control a group, once organized, or to discriminate against its members regarding hiring or tenure. Most important, the employer must bargain collectively and in good faith with representatives of the employees.

Likewise, labor organizations have constraints placed on their activities. They, too, must bargain in good faith. They must not restrain or coerce employees in selecting a bargaining group to bargain collectively. They may not pressure an employer to discriminate against employees who do not belong to the labor organization.

One of the issues frequently brought up in negotiations that usually results in a dispute is that of agency shop. When an **agency shop** clause is in effect, all employees are required to pay dues for membership. The obvious advantage of this requirement, from the workers' point of view, is encouraging membership in the union. The union is required to represent all employees, both members and nonmembers. Negotiating a contract, monitoring compliance with its provisions, and facilitating the grievance process may be costly. The union, therefore, desires to have a greater percentage of paying members to support these activities. There are several variations in provisions related to agency shop. If, because of religious or philosophic beliefs, employees are unwilling to pay dues to the bargaining group, provisions may be made to pay the same sum to a nonprofit group, such as a church or foundation. In some instances, those who are already members of the union are required to remain members for the life of the contract, although no one is required to become a member. In some states, laws referred to as "right to work laws" forbid the establishment of an agency shop.

Settling Labor Disputes

When labor disputes arise, several actions can be taken to help resolve the differences. Initially, of course, the parties continue to negotiate, and may agree to extend the negotiation period if progress in settling differences is being made. When the two parties doing the negotiating cannot come to agreement on an issue, they are considered to be **at impasse**, or are **deadlocked** on the issue.

MEDIATION AND ARBITRATION

Perhaps the most commonly used method of seeking agreement between parties when negotiating has not been successful is through **mediation** and **arbitration**. A **mediator** is a third person who may join the bargainers to assist the parties in reconciling differences and arriving at a peaceful agreement. Although the mediator may join the parties at any point in the negotiations, due to the cost of mediation, most negotiation proceeds until things are at an impasse. Mediation involves finding compromises, and the mediator assists with this. He or she must gain the respect of both parties and must remain neutral to the issues presented.

An **arbitrator** is technically defined as a person chosen by agreement of both parties to decide a dispute between them. The primary difference between a mediator and an arbitrator is that the mediator assists the parties in reaching their own decision, whereas the arbitrator has the authority to actually make the decision for the parties if necessary. However, the terms mediator and arbitrator and mediation and arbitration often are used interchangeably; in fact, a mediator may also serve as an arbitrator (Fig. 12-5).

Arbitration may take several forms. It may be mediation-arbitration, in which a third person joins the parties in the negotiation process before any serious disputes arise. This person's

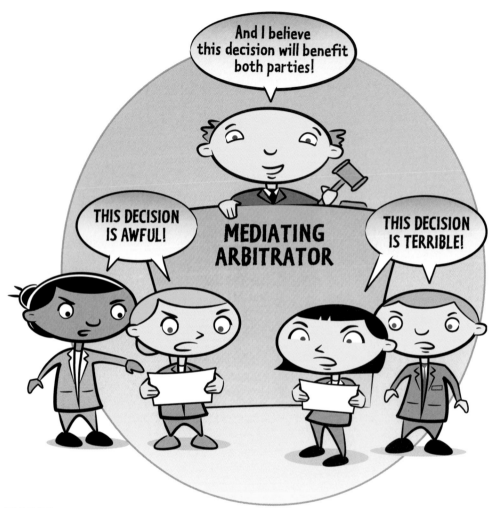

FIGURE 12-5   The arbitrator's decision may not really please either side.

role is to act as a mediator, who attempts to keep the parties talking, suggests compromises, and helps establish priorities. If an agreement is not reached by a specified date, or if it appears that the issue is deadlocked, with neither party willing to compromise, the mediator then assumes the role of an arbitrator and makes a decision based on the information gained in the role of mediator.

Another form of arbitration is called **binding arbitration**. This means that both parties are obligated to abide by the decision of the arbitrator. Some people see this as the least desirable alternative in settling disputes because it may result in a decision that is not satisfactory to either side, but one by which both must abide. It has been suggested, in instances in which binding arbitration is used, that the parties spell out exactly which of the issues are to be decided by the arbitrator. Binding arbitration has the advantage of resolving deadlocked issues without a strike. It also encourages both parties, knowing that the arbitrator's decision may not please either side, to reach a compromise on their own.

One type of binding arbitration uses a **final offer** approach. Employer and employee bargaining representatives reach agreement on as many issues as possible. The deadlocked issues and a final position (final offer) from each side are then presented to the arbitrator, who is obligated to select only the most reasonable package. The arbitrator may not develop a third alternative, which would "split the difference." The final offer approach encourages both sides to come up with a fairly realistic package and serves to close the gap on issues, as each side seeks to maintain some control over the outcome of the deliberations.

One criticism of any type of arbitration is the expense involved. Arbitrators must be paid for their services. Arbitration is also criticized because it undermines voluntary collective bargaining and allows parties to avoid unpleasant confrontation with their own difficulties by shifting that responsibility to a public authority. However, it is useful in preventing the disruption of services.

Arbitration may be requested from the American Arbitration Association or from available state, public, and private mediation and conciliation services. The American Arbitration Association is a nonprofit, nonpartisan organization that, for a nominal fee, can provide a list of qualified arbitrators. Most states have available groups, such as the Public Employees Relations Commission, that also can provide a list of mediators and arbitrators.

STRIKES AND LOCKOUTS

When the negotiation process breaks down, lockouts and strikes are likely to occur. A **lockout** occurs when an employer refuses to allow the employees to work. This is done to force employees to agree to the terms offered by the employer. The employer may close a place of business, or the employer may choose to remain open, discharge the workers, and use replacement workers. One readily can see how undesirable this would be in the health care system, but it has occurred in rare instances.

A **strike** occurs when workers refuse to continue to work until certain demands are met, thus imposing economic hardship and pressure on the employer. When the negotiation process breaks down, employees may use the strike to emphasize the need to improve their own working conditions, salaries, and benefits. The most recent strikes by nurses, however, have been over issues related to patient care rather than those related to the economic status of the nurses.

Striking places a serious economic hardship on employees and therefore is not undertaken lightly. Sometimes a strike is used to gain public attention to the labor dispute and to create public pressure for a settlement. This is only successful if the public agrees with the position of the striking workers.

At one time, nurse's strikes were viewed by some as unprofessional and detrimental to the health of the community and, as indicated in Table 12-1 at one time were *forbidden* by ANA policy. When strikes occurred, they drew major media attention and it was feared that they would damage the image of nurses and nursing. Today that thinking has largely changed, strikes have become more common, and less attention is drawn to the strikes other than in nursing publications.

Strikes in nursing are undertaken only with advance notice, to enable patients to be transferred to another facility and to make other plans for care of individuals in the community.

Typically, arrangements are made with another hospital to admit patients during the strike, and all elective procedures are canceled. The striking nurses may also agree to provide staffing to critical care, labor and delivery, and emergency departments of the facility in which the strike is occurring. Often the notification that nurses intend to strike on a certain date is sufficient incentive to move negotiations to the point of settlement, as occurred in Hawaii at the end of 1999.

REINSTATEMENT PRIVILEGE

A **reinstatement privilege** is a guarantee offered to striking employees that they will be rehired after the strike as positions become available, provided that they have not engaged in any unfair labor practices during the strike, and provided that the strike itself is lawful. The hospital may replace a striking nurse during the strike. If strikers agree unconditionally to return to work, the employer is not required to rehire a striking nurse at that time. However, recall lists are developed, and if the nurse cannot find regular and equivalent employment, he or she is privileged to recall and preference on jobs before new employees may be given employment.

Nurses may lose their reinstatement privileges because of misconduct during a lawful strike. For example, strikers may not physically block other nurses and personnel from entering or leaving a struck hospital. Strikers may not threaten nonstriking employees and may not attack management representatives. These types of activities usually do not occur in strikes conducted by nurses, but are not outside the realm of possibility.

OTHER METHODS OF INFLUENCING SETTLEMENT

There are a wide variety of methods by which solutions can be reached in the negotiating process. The following discussion briefly addresses the more formal and far-reaching of these activities.

One method of reaching solution is to employ an **authoritative mandate**, in which a president, secretary of labor, or other high-ranking or influential person encourages a peaceful settlement. This is usually employed when the situation becomes critical and when continuance of a strike would cause problems for a great number of people.

Another technique is **informational picketing**, which involves employees carrying informational signs outside of the institution. Informational picketing is not designed to stop work, but rather to inform the public of the concerns under dispute and to create public pressure on behalf of the union and the employees; it is seen frequently. Other methods of obtaining community support also may be employed. These include newspaper editorials, letters to the editor, and even paid advertisements. Rallies and marches may be used to draw public attention to the issues.

In some instances, an **injunction** may be requested. This results in a court order that requires the party or parties involved to take a specific action or, more commonly, to refrain from taking a specific action. Employers may use this measure to forestall or end a strike. Unions may use this measure to stop a lockout.

In still other instances, an institution or company may be subjected to **government seizure** and operation. Government employees are then used to run the plant, firm, or industry in question. This is seldom seen in the health care industry, for obvious reasons. However, this option was used in Montana in 1991, when state employees decided to strike. The National Guard was called in to replace striking state patrolmen.

What to Look for in a Contract

The negotiation process should ultimately conclude in the development of a written contract that is signed by both union and management representatives. The contract establishes guidelines for working conditions such as overtime, floating, work schedules, job security, and retention and recruitment of staff (Boisvert, 1991). It usually spells out certain other privileges to be provided to employees, such as in-service education, leaves, health and safety provisions, committee participation, and tuition reimbursement (Flanagan, 1992). The contract also may provide guidelines for the grievance process. (The grievance process will be discussed later in this chapter.)

A contract must meet certain specified criteria to be legally binding. It must result from mutually agreed-upon items arrived at through a "meeting of minds." Something of value must be given for a reciprocal promise, that is, professional duties for an agreed-upon sum. Contracts can be enforceable whether written or oral, but it is easier to work with those that are written. Written contracts are also considered "formal" contracts (Killion & Dempski, 2000).

Although each agreement will differ, most contracts have a fairly general format that includes:

- A preamble stating the objectives of each party
- A statement recognizing the official bargaining groups
- A section dealing with financial remuneration, including wages and salaries, overtime rates, holiday pay, and shift differentials
- A section dealing with nonfinancial rewards, that is, fringe benefits such as retirement programs, types of insurance available, free parking, and other services provided by the employer
- A section dealing with seniority in respect to promotions, transfers, work schedules, and layoffs
- A section establishing guidelines for disciplinary problems
- A section describing grievance procedures
- A section that may explicitly state codes of conduct or professional standards

Several other areas that are negotiable are important and should be incorporated into a contract for nurses. These may be included in the section dealing with professional standards or nursing care. The following are generally accepted as items that should be considered in a contract involving professional nurses.

First, the contract should provide for shared governance—that is, professional staff and administration who work jointly on the policy should develop professional policy decisions. This often takes the form of a nursing practice council or a professional performance committee. The committees should be identified, duties described, and benefits and rights clarified.

Second, the contract should provide for individual professional accountability. It establishes the guidelines for such issues as floating, overtime, and scheduling. It should include areas related to evaluation, such as peer evaluation of a practitioner's competence. It also should assure job security, stipulate retention and recruitment efforts, and deal with issues of promotion or dismissal.

Third, the contract should define the collective professional role. This spells out the responsibility of RNs as professional practitioners and describes their part in the planning of patient care. The purpose of this is to strengthen nurses' influence on the quality of care. It should discourage the encroachment of non-nursing staff into nursing practice and might include guidelines for staffing ratios.

Other items that should be included in contracts relate to health and safety provisions, in-service education or continuing education, tuition reimbursement, and leaves of absence. All of these affect the quality of the work experience.

It is important that, as a new graduate, you know whether there is a contract in effect in the institution in which you seek employment or in the community in which you plan to work. You should also be knowledgeable about the terms of the existing contract so that you might best fulfill your obligations, and recognize and benefit from the provisions to which you are entitled. The organization to which you are applying for employment can provide you with a copy of the current contract. The state nurses' associations can be contacted for information regarding the organization that represents nurses in a particular hospital or facility. They can also provide a copy of any contracts that have been negotiated for which they represented the nurses.

Critical Thinking Activity

As a new employee in a hospital, how will you explore the matter of learning whether there is a contract? Whom will you ask? How will you obtain a copy of the contract? What will you do if the contract includes language that you do not understand? What would you do if you were in total disagreement with some of the stipulations of the contract?

The Grievance Process

Effective contracts include, in addition to wages, hours, working conditions, and other items, a section that spells out the grievance procedure. A **grievance** is a circumstance or action believed to be in violation of a contract (or of policies if a contract is not in place). The **grievance process** represents an established and orderly method to be used in the adjustment of grievances between parties. In this sense, it represents a problem-solving mechanism.

The steps to be used in mediating grievances are usually included in the collective bargaining contract. Some organizations that lack formal collective bargaining agreements have developed internal policies that outline grievance procedures. Perhaps you are aware of grievance processes from your student handbook, where the processes in place in an educational program are shared with students.

Grievances usually are related to interpretations of a contract. They may occur as a result of a misunderstanding or difference of opinion about the contract or its language, or as a result of direct violations of the contract. Although either the management or an employee can file grievances, in most instances, it is an employee who initiates the case.

The grievance process spells out in writing a series of steps to be taken to resolve the area of dissension and a timeline for accomplishing those steps. Initially, the employee and the immediate supervisor attempt to resolve the disagreement through an informal talk. If no resolution occurs, the discussion moves to the steps of the grievance process, involving others within the organization. The steps include providing notifications and responses in writing,

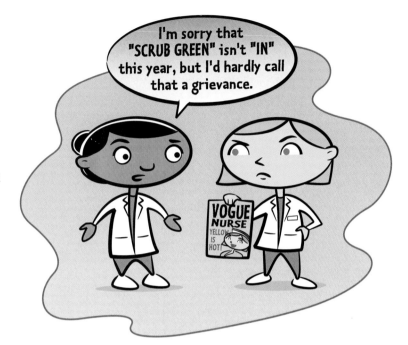

FIGURE 12-6   It is important to discriminate between complaints and grievances.

adhering to strict time lines for action, and eventually involving people at higher levels within the organization (eg, representatives from the bargaining unit, a grievance chairman, the personnel director, and administrative representatives). Perhaps the services of an arbitrator will be needed toward the end of the dispute. Failure of either side to comply with the time lines that are in effect regarding their own actions or responses ends the process. If an arbitrator is involved, that person's decision is usually binding.

It is important to differentiate between complaints and grievances (Fig. 12-6). Employees may have complaints that are not violations of the contract. For example, Nurse No. 1 may object that she was required to float from the postpartum unit to the nursery; she had been oriented to the nursery but preferred to work in the postpartum unit. Nurse No. 2 was required to float from a medical unit to a surgical unit to which she had not been oriented. If the contract in this hospital stipulates that no one would be floated to a unit to which he or she had not been oriented, Nurse No. 1 had a complaint, whereas Nurse No. 2 had a grievance.

At one time, the absence of grievances was thought to be an indication of an effective, well-managed organization; however, that may not be the best indicator of the organization's health. It is entirely possible that problems are not being addressed. On the other hand, a high number of grievances may indicate problems within the organization. These problems also may relate to the language of the contract or the education of the employee regarding the conditions of the contract. Another barometer of the health of an organization is the level at which the grievances are resolved. It is most desirable to settle most grievances at the informal level, without the involvement of an arbitrator.

The grievance procedure may sound like many steps that take a great deal of time, and indeed this is true. Although most grievances are settled short of arbitration, they are still time and energy consuming. Grievances can best be avoided if everyone has a good understanding of the terms of the contract and if sound personnel policies are developed and applied consistently and equitably. A part of the orientation of new employees to an organization should be spent reviewing and explaining the contract. Open discussions between the employees and management to review mutual concerns and share information help reduce the number of grievances. Mutual respect is a critical element in any organization.

Critical Thinking Activity

What are the reasons that grievance processes need to be spelled out in a contract? How would you determine whether an issue is a grievance or a complaint?

Issues Related to Collective Bargaining and Nursing

Four major issues of collective bargaining affect the nursing profession. The first of these relates to the fact that some nurses see collective bargaining as unprofessional. The second is the issue of which bargaining group will represent nursing when nurses participate in collective bargaining. The third issue is an individual one and relates to the question of whether to join a union when one exists; and the fourth deals with the role of the supervisor.

These issues may take on greater or lesser importance depending on the area of the country involved, the length of time the nurses in that area have been participating in collective bargaining, and the group chosen to represent the nurses at the bargaining table. As a staff nurse, you may, at some time, have to make a decision regarding whether to strike. In making this decision, you want to be well grounded in the issues at hand, and knowledgeable about the arrangements that have been made for continuance of services in emergency situations and in special hospital areas, such as labor and delivery.

COLLECTIVE ACTION AND PROFESSIONALISM

The strain that exists between professionalism and collective action has probably received more space in recent nursing literature than any other issue related to collective bargaining. The argument against unionism has its roots in the history of nursing itself. Nursing was perceived by many, including nurses, as a selfless, all-serving, altruistic calling. The act of caring for others, even if that meant subordinating the individual to the goals of that care, was to be compensation enough for the services rendered. The strong religious influences that pervaded the early development of nursing added to this concept of the profession. Early leaders in nursing espoused this dedication to its arts.

Another factor that has hampered the strong development of unionization in nursing is the fact that nursing is primarily a woman's profession. Although more men now enter nursing, currently less than 8% of the RNs in the United States are male.

Early social beliefs that a woman's role should be submissive, supportive, and obedient were extremely compatible with the expectations that our society placed on nurses. The paternalism that has existed in the health care delivery system has also made the process of collective bargaining for nurses a slow one (see Chapters 4 and 5). The combination of the role of women and the role of the nurse under earlier paternalistic practices had the nurse caring for the "hospital family," looking out for the needs of all (from patient to physician) and being responsible for keeping everyone happy (Ashley, 1976). The tendency to see the physician as the father figure in the health care system, the nurse as the corresponding mother figure, and the patients as the children has done little to promote the autonomy of nursing as a profession. A quote by Campbell (1980, p. 1286) illustrates this historical use of the family concept in health care: "If we are to keep unions out of the profession we, as nurses, must make every effort to build loyalty and a family feeling among our fellow nurses."

Despite nursing's history of ambivalence toward union negotiations, today we see nurses involved in collective bargaining in greater numbers than ever before. Several factors are responsible for this change. Wilson and colleagues (1990) have identified these as: the focus on the continued high cost of health care and the need to examine this rise; the scrutiny that has been placed on employee's salaries as part of this process; the fact that nurses constitute the largest number of employees in hospitals (nearly half); and changes in the NLRA allowing nurses to bargain collectively. Various sources differ with regard to whether unionization of hospital employees results in higher hospital costs.

In the early years of collective bargaining by nurses, there was some reticence to use the term union or unionism. Much of the nursing literature surrounding the issue used appropriate and less emotionally charged synonyms. Today the term union is used openly. When entering the Web site for the United American Nurses (UAN), AFL-CIO at *www.nursingworld.org*, one is greeted with a welcome and the words "the union for nurses by nurses." This certainly reflects a change in sentiment, supporting the belief that nurses should be involved in collective bargaining and also reflecting the general acceptance of the process by the public at large.

Many have come to believe that the collective action of nurses provides one of the best avenues for achieving professional goals and exercising control over nursing practice. As nurses are called on to assume greater responsibility for complicated decisions, collective bargaining through a professional organization may provide the means to implement the concept of collective professional responsibility.

The manner in which the bargaining is conducted greatly influences how it will be perceived. Nurses as a group need to develop the skills necessary to communicate to the public the importance of their role in health care delivery. They must be able to handle conflicts and work toward resolution while maintaining integrity and dignity. Nurses need to become enlightened and informed, and they need more than a superficial understanding of the process of collective bargaining.

Of greater concern to some nurses is the issue of whether nurses should participate in strikes activities if negotiations break down. Many nurses believe that the withholding of services from patients is unprofessional, and therefore, personally unacceptable. Others view the strike as a final method for bringing attention to the needs of the nurse as a citizen. Fortunately, as bargaining groups representing nurses become more knowledgeable and skilled in the process, strikes occur less frequently. Disagreements at the bargaining table are more commonly resolved through mediation and arbitration, much to the relief of many professionals.

Critical Thinking Activity

Do you support the concept of nurses becoming members of a union? If so, should all employees of an organization be required to pay membership fees? Analyze your response to this question and provide the rationale to support your views.

REPRESENTATION FOR NURSES

Significant controversy currently exists regarding which organization should represent nurses at the bargaining table. This is determined by elections that are supervised by the NLRB. To become the certified collective bargaining representative of a group of employees, the organization in question must receive 50% of the votes cast, plus one.

When nurses first began to organize, the ANA, through the state nurses' associations, was the bargaining representative. This group still represents more nurses than all other organizations combined. In 1991, across the country, state associations represented more than 139,000 RNs through more than 840 bargain units (Fuller-Jonap, 1994). However, there has been a strong movement on the part of other organizations to vie for the representative position. It has been estimated that more than 30 labor organizations represent health care workers (Miller, 1980). The ANA has been representing nurses since 1946. The National Union of Hospital and Health Care Employees (representing nurses since 1977) and the SEIU have voted to unite, creating something of a "super union" for health care workers. The Federation of Nurses and Health Professionals began organizing nurses in 1978. Other groups representing nurses in various parts of the country include the United Food and Commercial Workers, the Teamsters Union, and the American Federation of Teachers.

Nurses face a difficult decision when trying to decide which group can represent them best. In recent years, this decision has occupied perhaps more time and effort on the part of nurses than has the actual bargaining. Those who have strong allegiance to the ANA contend that only RNs should bargain for RNs. One of the reasons given for this position is that in collective bargaining, nurses face different issues than other workers. In addition to concerns about salary, benefits, working conditions, and the like, nurses also want to negotiate questions pertaining to staffing, patient care concerns, and participation in joint hospital committees. Many believe that only nurses can effectively negotiate such items. These people contend that hospital administrations, fearing the power of labor unions, will bargain more constructively and positively with nurses themselves. They also believe that the ANA will be a stronger, more united organization if it serves as both the professional association and the bargaining agent.

Others believe that nurses compromise their collective bargaining powers when the recognized union is a group other than the state nurses' association. They think that when nurses do not bargain for themselves, the "organization shrivels and their influence on health care weakens" (Mallison, 1985, p. 943).

Some parts of the country are experiencing a trend toward having an organization other than the professional nurses' association represent nurses. Chief among the arguments for bargaining conducted by another group is the issue of supervisor membership in the professional association (discussed later in this chapter). Proponents of this position also would contend that it is not realistic for one group to work with the professionalism aspect of nursing as well as with the issues of wages, benefits, and working conditions.

In most states, the state nurses' association serves as a collective bargaining agent. To do this, they must organize in such as way that the collective bargaining is separated in terms of finances and control from the other activities of the organization. Those who are members but not part of a collective bargaining unit pay lesser dues than those who are part of a collective bargaining unit. Only those who are part of bargaining units have a vote regarding collective bargaining issues. At the national level, the UAN is formed by the state association collective bargaining units and has been made completely separate from the other activities of the ANA. In addition to helping the state organizations work together, the UAN can also act as a collective bargaining agent for multistate healthcare organizations and for states that do not have a collective bargaining arm. Thus, the ANA and its constituent state organizations have tried to address the concerns of those who believe one organization cannot fulfill both roles.

Some nurses prefer two organizations—one to represent issues related to professionalism and another to negotiate salaries. This results in cost factors, because both organizations would collect dues. Many consider the cost of belonging to the ANA and to the state association to be very high, with dues of approximately $350.00 per year. Additional, equally expensive membership dues in another organization might be prohibitive. Second, many believe that the union would become the dominant force between the two groups, because money and working environment issues both speak strongly.

There are no easy answers to this question, and it will certainly be one of the biggest issues facing nurses in the future.

Critical Thinking Activity

If the collective bargaining agent in the hospital in which you worked was other than the state nurses' association, would you belong to both organizations? What factors would you use to support your decision? Why are these factors important to you?

TO JOIN OR NOT TO JOIN

Once an individual nurse has gained an understanding of collective bargaining and has developed a personal philosophy about the professional role of the nurse, he or she is ready to make a decision regarding membership in the bargaining unit.

In working with students who are soon to embark on professional careers, we find that it is easier for them to decide whether to bargain collectively than it is to decide to part with the money that is required for membership. Many nurses want better working conditions and higher salaries, but are all too willing to let someone else fund these endeavors and work to achieve them.

It is in response to these concerns that many "agency shop" clauses have been added to contracts. Those who are members and are active in the negotiation process believe it is inappropriate for some to benefit from the labors of the bargaining process without having contributed, at least financially, to the effort. The presence of agency shop clauses may serve as either an asset or a deterrent to recruitment, depending on the applicant's viewpoint.

THE SUPERVISOR AND COLLECTIVE BARGAINING

In 1994, a nursing home argued before the Supreme Court that the LPNs in its employ were supervisors (because of their role in directing nursing assistants in patient care) and, therefore, were not protected by the National Labor Relations Act. The Supreme Court, in a 5 to 4 decision, ruled in favor of the nursing home. Nursing organizations engaged in collective bargaining have expressed serious concern about the implications of this ruling for all nurses. Labor groups expect to lobby for legislation that would alter this interpretation of the NLRB ("Striking at bargaining . . . ," 1994).

This issue was again addressed in February 1996, when the NLRB ended nearly 2 years of deliberation by ruling that charge nurses at Alaska's Providence Medical Center could not be called "supervisors" simply because the role requires some direction of other workers. The Board stated that the essence of the nurse's role was "judgment," and went on to explain that authority that arises from professional knowledge is distinct from the authority of a front-line manager ("NLRB to the Supreme Court," 1996). The issue continues to occur with surprising frequency.

Changing Trends With Regard to Collective Bargaining

At one time, economic concerns and working conditions may have been the principal motivators for collective action. However, by the mid-1980s, subtle, and at times not so subtle, changes were occurring throughout the United States regarding collective bargaining, unionism, and labor-management relations.

Some working in the area of contract management have reported a shift from the adversarial relationship that historically had existed between the employee and the employer (which focused on salaries, work hours, and the like) to one that placed greater emphasis on the quality of work life.

THE CONCEPT OF UNIONISM

As we move into the 21st century, the perilous state of our economy and the enormously competitive global environment would warn us that it is a time for increased cooperation between unions and employers (Colosi & Berkeley, 1992). The country is not in a good position to deal with the reduced efficiency and productivity in the workplace. Perhaps this contributes to the drop in the percentage of employed workers with union affiliation between 1994 and 2000 ("Union decline," 2001).

An approach to labor-management issues referred to as **constructive adversarialism** is encouraged, which supports mutual cooperation without undermining the legitimate roles and rights of both the management and the union. The union encourages wholehearted employee participation by its members while exercising flexibility on issues. With this approach, the union should have input into the managerial decision-making process through representation on committees at every level of the organization. Unions should be expected to be cooperative with management but not be co-opted. The union exists to represent, protect, and advance the interests of the employees. Management must be fair with the union, neither seeking to destroy the union nor meekly acquiescing to every union demand (Colosi & Berkeley, 1994).

THE THRUST OF COLLECTIVE BARGAINING IN NURSING

The focus of collective bargaining issues changed during the 1990s. Originally focusing on wages and benefits, today the major concern of nurses is often staffing patterns, involvement in decisions affecting patient care, cross-training, the use of unlicensed assistive personnel, and workplace safety. This shift in emphasis reflects the general acceptance of the process of collective bargaining by nurses and the fact that significant headway has been made through this process regarding basic issues. This change of thinking is borne out by a vote of the House of Delegates of the American Medical Association to develop an affiliated national labor organization, under the NLRA, which would support the development and operation of local negotiating units to represent employed physicians. Self-employed physicians were barred from joining collective bargaining units by antitrust laws ("Docs vote . . . ," 1999).

CONCESSION BARGAINING

Concession bargaining is a process in which there is an explicit exchange of reduced labor costs for improvements in job security. This has been occurring with increasing frequency. An example would be a shift in emphasis from one that asks for increases in salary to one that focuses on eliminating the practice of calling nurses and telling them not to report for work because the census has dropped (on such days, the nurses do not receive salary). These are issues that seriously concern nurses today.

"UNION BUSTING" AND STRIKE BREAKING

A trend seen in health care institutions during the 1980s, and persisting in some areas today, is an effort toward "union busting." Although technically illegal when referring to methods used to eliminate an existing union, the term **union busting** has been expanded to include a wide range of legal activities that slow down collective bargaining. Pressured by rapidly esca-lating health care costs, and influenced by the changing attitudes toward work, hospital administrators have hired consultants and law firms to assist and advise in discouraging and impeding organizational activities. This is also a counteraction to the courting by unions of the expanding groups of previously unorganized professionals, such as physicians and nurs-es. Antiunion organizing campaigns usually are aimed at strategies that will delay and thus drag down the momentum of organizing efforts. This could include challenging union mem-bership, attempting to decertify elections, and failing to bargain in good faith—thus drawing out the negotiating process (Ballman, 1985).

Strike breaking refers to efforts directed at causing employees on strike to cease the strike without having reached an agreement. In an effort to break a strike, employers hire tem-porary nurses at very high wages plus living stipends to entice them to come to work. One temporary agency specializes in providing nurses as strike breakers. In Portland, Oregon, the temporary nurses were housed in a hotel and transported to and from the hospital in a bus with blacked-out windows. Their salaries (without the cost of transportation and stipends) were significantly higher than the maximum requested by the striking nurses. That strike was final-ly settled by the intervention of the governor of the state as a mediator, and a contract agree-ment was finally reached.

Additional Issues Addressed in Collective Bargaining

As nurses have become more comfortable and knowledgeable about the bargaining process, their energies have been directed toward many issues. These include such concerns as pay equi-ty, discrimination against female employees, comparable worth, and the rights of employees to know the hazards within a work environment (see Chapter 11). In some instances, discriminatory practices against male nurses also have been an issue.

CHANGES IN THE NUMBER OF BARGAINING UNITS

Within hospitals are many different positions and job titles, ranging from professional staff through office staff to those responsible for hospital maintenance. In nursing alone, there are groups of RNs, LPNs, and nursing assistants. As these groups have been granted authority to organize into bargaining units, concern has been expressed about the number of unions with which any hospital administration must bargain at any given time. Some fairly elaborate estimates have been made regarding the amount of time demanded by the collective bargaining process.

When the NLRA was first passed in 1974, the NLRB specified that seven employee bargaining units would exist within the health care industry (Wilson et al, 1990, p. 37). The seven groups were RNs, physicians, other professional employees, technical employees, business office or clerical employees, and skilled maintenance employees.

In 1984, the NLRB determined that bargaining units would be decided on a case-by-case basis. This resulted in reducing the number of bargaining units to three: all professionals, all nonprofessionals, and guards.

In 1989, the NLRB proposed a new rule that resulted in the establishment of eight collective bargaining units. At this time, it was also determined that the rule would apply to hospitals of all sizes. In response, the American Hospital Association (AHA) sought and obtained a permanent injunction against the rule. Subsequently, "all-RN" units were legally approved. The latest activity regarding this issue occurred in April 1991. The U. S. Supreme Court upheld the NLRB in its authority to define bargaining units for health care workers in acute care hospitals, and allowed for all-RN bargaining units ("Supreme Court okays . . . ," 1991). As might be expected, the AHA and the ANA occupied opposite points of view regarding this issue.

THE IMPACT OF SHARED GOVERNANCE ON COLLECTIVE BARGAINING

Although the greater involvement of staff nurses in health care agency decision-making may have a significant impact on the collective bargaining process, the number of nurses represented by collective bargaining is increasing. When both collective bargaining and shared governance are present, there is a separation of those issues that are the purview of the union and those issues that can be decided within the shared governance structure. If there is a union, it has the responsibility and authority to negotiate those things that fall under wages, benefits, and working conditions, such as the use of agency nurses, work load, and policies regarding floating from one unit to another. The shared governance committees work with clinical standards. Each nurse has greater accountability for participation in decision-making outside of the bargaining process and for implementing decisions that have been made.

THE NUMBER OF GROUPS THAT REPRESENT NURSES

As collective bargaining has become accepted for those in the nursing profession, the number of groups that seek to represent nurses at the bargaining table has constantly increased. As mentioned earlier in this chapter, more than 30 groups now bargain for nurses. Although the

UAN represents more nurses than does any other group, a large number of nurses are also represented by the American Federation of Teachers, the SEIU, or Teamsters. In some instances, as with the SEIU, this organization represents other workers employed in the organization. This may be favored by hospital administration, which often expresses frustration with the number of groups with whom they must carry out negotiations. However, when the SEIU is bargaining for all employees, it has the distinct disadvantage of diluting the ability of nurses to include professional issues in the negotiation process.

KEY CONCEPTS

- One of the critical elements of any organization is its mission statements. Mission statements explicitly outline the purpose of the organization and may also contain the philosophy and goals of the group. These statements serve as a benchmark against which an organization's performance can be evaluated.
- Organizations may be structured a number of different ways. Some are tall and centralized, where the authority to make decisions is vested in a few individuals. Others are flat and decentralized, with a number of individuals involved in decision-making.
- All organizations have chains of command, channels of communication, and spans of control that describe lines of authority and accountability. These can be depicted in organizational charts, which represent the formal organization and are a pictorial means of portraying roles and patterns of interaction among parts of a system.
- Organizations have developed written job descriptions that outline the responsibilities of all employees, and policies and protocols to guide the activities of the employees. Job descriptions are a necessary and vital part of any organization.
- Many hospitals are now using a shared governance process, a form of practice model that involves shared decision-making by nursing staff and management. It results in a decentralized organization and often results in greater job satisfaction for nurses.
- Many patterns of nursing care delivery have existed over the years. These include the case method, the functional method, team nursing, total patient care, modular care, and primary nursing. Nurses are also involved in case management.
- Since 1974, it has been possible for nurses to bargain collectively for salaries, working conditions, and fringe benefits. This process also allows for their participation in committees focused on improving patient care and patient care standards.
- The collective bargaining process culminates in a contract that places in writing the decisions reached at the bargaining table. As a new graduate, you should know whether the health care agency at which you are seeking employment has a contract in effect.
- A contract usually includes a section that spells out the process to be used in a grievance. Should a grievance arise, it is essential that all steps be followed as outlined in the contract. Nurses need to be able to distinguish between issues that are grievances and those that are simply complaints.
- One of the issues surrounding nurses and collective bargaining is related to which group should do the bargaining for nurses. Many believe this process is best conducted by a professional nursing organization; others believe they are served best by an organization that has collective bargaining as its major focus.

- Trends regarding the collective bargaining process include constructive adversarialism, concession bargaining, "union busting," strike breaking, issues of discrimination, and changes in the number of bargaining units.

RELEVANT WEB SITES

Unions:
AFL-CIO: *http://www.nursefriendly.com/unions*
American Nurses' Association: *www.nursingworld.org.* Click on United American Nurses
Support:
http://www.Nursinghands.com

REFERENCES

Alexander, M. K., Bourgeois, A. & Goodman, L. R. (1994). Total quality improvement: Bridging the gap between education and service. In O. L. Strickland & D. J. Fishman: *Nursing issues in the 1990s* (pp. 280–289). Albany, NY: Delmar Publishers.

Ashley, J. A. (1976). *Hospitals, paternalism and the role of the nurse.* New York: Teachers' College Press.

Ballman, C. S. (1985). Union busters. *AJN 85*(9): 963–966.

Boisvert, S. C. (1991). Collective bargaining: Another view. *Maine Nurse 78*(4):5.

Brown, S. J. (2001). Research evidence linking staffing and patient outcomes. *Orthopedic Nursing 20*(1): 67–68.

Campbell, G. J. (1980). In Opinions: Is bargaining unprofessional for nurses? *AORN Journal 31*(6):1289.

Colosi, T. R. & Berkeley, A. E. (1994). *Collective bargaining: How it works and why.* New York: American Arbitration Association.

"Docs vote for unionization." (2000). [On-line]. Available: *www.nursingworld.org/tan/julaug99/inbrief.htm.*

Domrose, C. (2002 [August 12]). Changing tides. *Nurse Week, Mountain West Ed. 3*(11):17–19.

Flanagan, L. (1992). How collective bargaining benefits nurses. *Directions: American Nurse Supplement.* October: 8–9, 22.

Fuller-Jonap, F. (1994). Collective bargaining in nursing: Benefits, issues, and problems. In O. L. Strickland & D. J. Fishman, *Nursing issues in the 1990s* (pp. 33–45). Albany, NY: Delmar Publishers.

Huber, D. (1996). *Leadership and nursing management.* Philadelphia: WB Saunders.

Killion, S. W. & Dempski, K. M. (2000). *Legal and ethical issues.* Thorofare, NJ: Slack, Inc.

Komplin, J. (1995). Care delivery systems. In P. S. Yoder Wise. *Leading and managing in nursing,* (pp. 411–435) St. Louis: Mosby.

Mallison, M. B. (1985). Weathering the economic climate. *AJN 85*(9):943.

Miller, R. U. (1980). Collective bargaining: A nursing dilemma. *AORN Journal 31*(6):1197. Needleman, J., Buerhaus, P. Mattke, S., Stewart, M. & Zelevinsky, K. (2002 [May 30]). Nurse-staffing levels and the quality of care in hospitals. *New England Journal of Medicine, 346*(22):1757–66.

Needleman, J., Buerhaus, P. Mattke, S., Stewart, M. & Zelevinsky, K. (2002, May 30). Nurse-staffing levels and the quality of care in hospitals. *New England Journal of Medicine, 346*(22):1757–66.

Neufeldt, V. (Ed.). (1996). *Webster's new world dictionary* (3rd ed.). New York: Macmillan.

"NLRB to the Supreme Court: Labor law protects nurses." (1996). *AJN 96*(4):67, 72.

Porter-O'Grady, T. (1990). Nursing governance in a transitional era. In N. L. Chaska, *The nursing profession: Turning points (*pp. 432–439). St. Louis: CV Mosby.

Porter-O'Grady, T. (1987). Shared governance and new organizational models. *Nursing Economics* 5(6):281–286.

"Striking at bargaining rights, court says RNs are supervisors." (1994). *AJN* 94(7):67, 70–71.

"Supreme Court okays all-RN unit." (1991). *American Nurse* (June):1.

"Union decline." (2001 [March 26]). *The Herald*, pp. C1, C2.

Wilson, C. N., Hamilton, C. L. & Murphy, E. (1990). Union dynamics in nursing. *Journal of Nursing Administration* 20(2):35–39.

13

Initiating the Leadership/ Management Role

LEARNING OUTCOMES

After completing this chapter, you should be able to:

1. Compare and contrast the skills involved in leadership and management.
2. Differentiate between the terms authority and accountability.
3. Discuss the major theories regarding leadership.
4. Compare and contrast the three prevailing leadership styles.
5. Analyze the factors that have resulted in the development of transformational leadership.
6. Describe how power and empowerment relate to leadership.
7. Identify ways an individual can empower another.
8. Analyze methods by which the development of leadership style can be enhanced.
9. Describe the basic characteristics of effective communication.
10. Analyze the communication strategies that are essential for effective leadership, identifying the critical role of each.
11. Describe the elements of an effective performance-appraisal system, including the conduct of the interview.
12. Analyze the importance of time management and evaluate methods that will help overcome major time wasters and procrastination.

KEY TERMS

Accountability

Authority

Autocratic/authoritarian
leadership style

Charisma

Coercive power

Communication

Connection power

Democratic/participative
leadership style

Empowerment

Expert power

Informational power

Job description

Laissez-faire/permissive
leadership style

Leadership

Leadership/management
style

Legitimate power

Management

Mentor

Motivational power

Multicratic leadership
style

Performance appraisal

Procrastination

Referent power

Responsibility

Reward power

Standards

Theories of leadership

Time management

The novice in the area of health care administration can easily be dazzled by the many terms devoted to the topics of leadership and management that populate the literature. Words such as authority, responsibility, accountability, team building, empowerment, coaching, mentoring, motivating, and collective power are but a few of those incorporated into articles, monographs, and books addressing the topic of successful leadership and management. What do these terms mean to you as you begin reading this chapter? What will they mean to you when you finish this course? In what ways will the meanings gain greater significance as you begin your career as a staff nurse? What will they mean as you begin to assume a leadership role in patient care?

UNDERSTANDING LEADERSHIP AND MANAGEMENT

Although the terms leadership and management are often used interchangeably, differences exist in how each is practiced in the work situation. Gaining an understanding of each will help you be effective in either role. Let's explore the differentiations and how they are applied in the work situation.

How Leadership and Management Differ

Management refers to activities such as planning, organizing, directing, and controlling, with the purpose of accomplishing specific goals and objectives within an organization. Essentially, it involves organizing and directing a group of people to accomplish specific tasks. Management positions often are ones to which one is appointed or are ones to which one is hired after a competitive job application and interview. From this appointment, the manager is granted the power to direct others and is responsible for assuring that certain tasks within the organization are completed effectively and efficiently. In other words, the authority to act is gained by virtue of the position one holds within the organization.

Leadership, on the other hand, refers to the ability to persuade others to follow your direction, to motivate, to inspire, and to instill vision and purpose. To provide leadership, one must be able to influence the beliefs, opinions, or behaviors of others. This can be accomplished in a number of different ways, referred to as leadership styles, that we will discuss later.

Although managers may not always be leaders, the very best managers also are leaders. Conversely, not all leaders are officially managers in the sense we have defined it. Individuals may become leaders because of the way in which they inspire others to follow them. Can you think of a situation in which an individual was a leader but did not have the role of manager? Similarly, can you think of any situations in which the manager lacked the ability to lead a group of people? Can you recall situations in which the manager also was a leader?

UNDERSTANDING ACCOUNTABILITY AND AUTHORITY

We frequently hear three terms associated with leadership and management roles: accountability, responsibility, and authority. Are you clear about the definitions of each of these terms?

Accountability and **responsibility** are terms with similar meanings. They refer to the obligation to answer for one's actions and to accomplish what you have agreed to do. For example, the team leader assigns you the care of four patients and you agree to that assignment; therefore, the patients' care is your responsibility. You have an obligation to provide timely care to that group of patients to achieve the desired outcome regarding that care.

By virtue of the state nurse practice acts, nurses are held responsible or accountable for their actions. This means they must provide the necessary care competently and in compliance with accepted standards, using sound judgment, thinking critically, and delegating wisely. Failure to perform in a responsible manner could result in legal action being taken against the nurse if harm occurs to the patient.

Nurses have always been accountable for the care they give from both a personal and a professional standpoint. However, as we have witnessed the rapid technologic, fiscal, and operational changes that have occurred within the health care system, the term now carries stronger legal implications. Patient involvement in health care decision-making, consumer rights, and public availability of records has created more legal vulnerability for the nurse. Nurses must be aware of the legal aspects of nursing and of the laws that protect the client. Legal aspects of care are discussed in greater detail in Chapter 8.

Accountability flows upward in the organizational hierarchy. Individuals are accountable for their own actions and also for some of the actions of those they supervise. Thus, we see that tasks can be delegated but accountability cannot be. Nurses who delegate tasks to assistive personnel continue to be accountable for that care (see Chapters 7 and 14). For example, if you ask the nursing assistant to check the vital signs of four of your patients, you are asking the assistant to act in your place. You are still accountable for that activity; that the vital signs are accurately measured, reported, and documented. This accountability has become a sensitive issue for nurses as, in an effort to contain costs, more unlicensed assistive personnel are hired to replace licensed staff.

The word **authority** can be defined as the power or right to give directions, to take action, to make decisions (Neufeldt, 1996). Traditionally, we have considered it the manager's job to command or make decisions. In this sense, the manager "authored" all critical decisions. As you read further, you will note that in today's work environment, authority is more often being shared. And along with this shared authority and decision-making is a mutual responsibility for outcomes. We will discuss this concept in greater detail after we have talked about leadership.

In the ideal work situation, workers are given the amount of authority needed to carry out the responsibilities expected of them. However, many nurses experience frustration because they must be accountable for activities yet have no authority to impact the situation or create change. For example, an evening charge nurse has the responsibility of assuring that all patients receive competent care, but the nurse may have no input into the performance appraisal of nursing assistants working on that shift. Therefore, the nursing assistants may not be as responsive to the charge nurse's instructions as they should be. Or perhaps a nurse has the responsibility for seeing that there are adequate supplies on a unit but has no opportunity to affect the unit's budget.

Critical Thinking Activity

Think for a moment of behaviors you noted in your clinical experiences this past week. What behavior did you observe that was a clear demonstration of authority? What were the characteristics that made it so? Can you recall a situation in which a registered nurse (RN) accepted responsibility for an action that had been taken? How was this done?

Theories of Leadership

Let's talk briefly about the various **theories of leadership** (Table 13-1). Just as theories of nursing help us to understand nursing (see Chapter 5), leadership theories help us to describe and understand the processes of leadership. As a society, we have studied leadership theory since about the mid-20th century, and a number of theories have been set forth, far too many to discuss in detail in this text. The theories of leadership listed in Table 13-1 are those most frequently cited as helpful in understanding specific situations.

Current emphasis in most management literature is placed on transformational leadership. Today's work environment relies on teamwork and shared decision-making. In this environment, the goals of the organization are most likely to be met if transformational leadership is employed.

As a student preparing for graduation from your nursing program, you may wonder how all the information on leadership theories relates to you. Health care represents one of the largest, if not the largest business in the United States. Historically, the administrative structure in hospitals has been a predominately bureaucratic one, with few decision-makers and many followers. That situation is changing as more and more hospitals adopt a pattern of transformational leadership. But that will not be true in all organizations nor will it reflect the attitudes of some of the individuals with whom you will work. Having basic knowledge of the various approaches to leadership will help you understand the environments in which you work and will help you determine the leadership approach you wish to develop.

TABLE 13-1.	MAJOR THEORIES OF LEADERSHIP
GENERAL CLASSIFICATION, THEORY AND THEORIST	**ESSENTIAL CHARACTERISTICS AND COMMENTS**
Trait:	Focuses on certain characteristics of the leader.
Great Man theory	Promotes the concept that certain people were born to be leaders because they inherited a set of special characteristics qualifying them for such responsibilities. Because leaders are "born," this theory suggests that leadership cannot be developed.
Attribution theory	Suggests that leadership relates to personal attributes people tend to characterize leaders as having, such as height, social background, creativity, assertiveness, initiative, integrity, ability, intelligence, etc.
Charismatic theory	Often listed as a quality of other theories, this theory relates to a special charm or allure possessed by the leader that inspires others to follow and give allegiance.
Attitudinal:	Based on attitudes of the leader that result in the leader's behavior
Ohio State Leadership Studies	Describes leadership behavior as related to initiating structure and consideration of employees
Michigan Leadership Studies	Describes leader behavior as employee oriented or production oriented
Managerial Grid (Blake and Mouton [1964])	Identifies 5 management styles best described on a grid, in which each style combines elements of concern for production and concern for people
Situational:	Leadership is based on the situation or environment and on behaviors of leaders that occur in response to the situation.
Contingency theory (Fred Fiedler [1967])	Examines factors in the situation, particularly the skills of the leader and that individual's position of power in the organization, as determinants of leader effectiveness
Path–Goal theory (Robert J. House [1971])	Relates effective leadership to leader's ability to minimize obstructions to goals, identify outcomes workers want to achieve, and reward the followers for high performance and achievement, thereby increasing worker satisfaction and productivity
Transactional leadership (J. M. Burns [1978])	Examines leadership in terms of striking a bargain in which there is a mutual exchange between leaders and followers of benefits for work. Leader is a caretaker and focuses on day-to-day operations.
Contemporary Theories:	Theories most commonly in use at the present time
Transformational leadership (Heinrich von Pierer [1994])	Places emphasis on the collective purpose and mutual growth of both the leader and the follower and de-emphasizes differences in the roles of the leader and followers. Leader activities include creating a vision, building relationships, developing trust, and building self-esteem. Leader makes subordinates aware of how important their jobs are, helps them build skills, and motivates them to work for the good of the organization.

Leadership/Management Styles

Lewin (1951) described three prevailing types of behavior observed in leaders/managers that we refer to as **leadership** or **management styles** (Display 13-1). Sometimes these also are listed among the behavioral theories of leadership. The focus of these three styles is the amount of control the manager assumes over the actions of the workers and the beliefs of the leader/manager about the nature of workers. (That is why they may be referred to as behavioral theories.) You will note that the extremes extend from situations in which the manager makes all the decisions to situations in which virtually no direction is given to workers. In addition to

Display 13-1   LEADERSHIP/MANAGEMENT STYLES

Autocratic/Authoritative
Majority of decisions determined by the manager
Dictates work to be done and who will do it
Provides little opportunity for input or suggestions from followers
Gives little feedback or recognition for accomplishments
Communication flows downward, with emphasis on completing the task
Works well in emergency situations where time is of the essence
May be preferred style when working with unskilled or uneducated employees

Democratic/Participative
Input to decision-making encouraged among workers
Leaders see themselves as coworkers
Communication, consensus, and teamwork stressed
Leader leads by providing information, suggesting direction, supporting coworkers
Communication flows both up and down
Human relationships important
Considered the preferred style in the majority of work situations

Laissez-faire/Permissive
Little or no direction or guidance provided
Coworkers develop their own goals, make their own decisions, and take responsibility
Decision-making dispersed throughout the group
Provides maximum freedom for individuals and motivates workers to perform at high levels
If used inappropriately, a leadership vacuum may occur, in which an informal leader may arise

Multicratic
Combines the positive features of authoritative, participative leadership styles
Leader provides a maximum of structure when the situation requires it
Leader provides maximum group participation when needed
Support and encouragement provided to subordinates at all times

the individual characteristics of the leader, several other variables will determine the type of manager a nurse might be. The type of organizational structure will influence the leadership styles. How authority is centralized or dispersed throughout the organization also affects leadership styles. The communication patterns, which are directly tied to organizational structure, also will influence leadership styles. Equally important is the situation at hand.

Autocratic or **authoritarian leadership** may be essential in emergency situations that call for immediate action. When faced with life-threatening conditions, as we see frequently in emergency departments, the leader may be in the best position to make judgments and decisions. Little time exists to contemplate and build consensus regarding the best approach or to allow discussion for alternative actions.

Laissez-faire or **permissive leadership** is at the other extreme and provides the least structure and control. It is highly effective in situations in which coworkers can develop their own goals, and make their own decisions and take responsibility for their own actions. An example might be seen in an inpatient psychiatric unit in which a certain amount of autonomy and self-direction are an important part of the unit's operation.

Democratic or **participative leadership** represents the middle ground. The democratic leader focuses on involving subordinates in decision-making. There are a variety of different methods to accomplish this, such as asking for input, developing a consensus, voting, or delegating decisions to others. It is most effective when the decision or task at hand does not require urgent action and when subordinates have the ability to make meaningful contributions.

A fourth leadership style not identified by Lewin is probably the one that is most frequently used in health care. **Multicratic leadership** combines the most favorable aspects of all styles as mediated by the circumstances at hand. A multicratic leader is able to provide maximum structure and direction when the situation calls for it and provides for maximum group input into decision-making when conditions are conducive to such an approach. Support, encouragement, and recognition of subordinates and their contributions are always present. Learning when to use each of the various approaches is something that a new graduate will need to study and to practice, just as with other nursing skills.

Critical Thinking Activity

In addition to the examples provided in the text, identify a health care-related situation in which each of the styles of leadership would be appropriately employed. Provide the rationale for choosing that particular leadership style in the situation. What are the advantages of that style of leadership? What are its limitations?

Transformation of Leadership

Nothing operates in isolation or in a vacuum; approaches to leadership are no exception. As you may surmise from the information in Table 13-1 and Display 13-1, the leadership systems have changed as societal values and norms changed.

As a society, we have experienced tremendous growth in information systems and technology, which has resulted in individuals at all levels within an organization having access to data. Access to information is no longer reserved for a few selected individuals at the top of an organizational chart but is now available to many. Employees at all levels within an organization are knowledgeable about goals, operations, rewards, and critical areas. The information explosion also has brought a more intelligent and informed customer to the health care arena.

Today, more informed workers are developing into self-directed teams. This has resulted in managers spending time developing the abilities of others rather than directing them. Approaches to leadership have moved away from authoritarian styles to a more collaborative leadership style, with the individuals closest to the problem helping to find solutions to it. This concept is demonstrated in a statement attributed to Colin Powell, "The people in the field are closest to the problem. Therefore, that is where the real wisdom is." (Harari, 2002).

The strategies used for developing human resources have shown significant changes (Avolio, 1997). Many organizations, health care facilities included, are encouraging employees to be involved in decision-making. The leadership required for this type of organization must be much different from that seen in the 1950s, when the manager instructed and directed and the worker acted and followed. Avolio (1997, p. 3) describes leadership today as being "visionary, developmental and service-oriented, ethical, stimulating, facilitative, and clear in establishing expectations." He also suggests that leadership is more widely distributed in organizations today as more people demand a role in making decisions and solving problems.

THE CONCEPT OF POWER

Power, as we refer to it in a leadership sense, is "the ability to do, act or produce; the ability to control others" (Neufeldt, 1996, p. 1098). In other words, power refers to the ability an individual has to get things done. The concept of power forms a basis for action in transformational leadership.

Types of Power

French and Raven (1959) identified five types of power based on the source of that power (Display 13-2). You can find all of these types of power at work in nursing. The most obvious of these forms can be seen in such positions as Clinical Director of Nursing or Director of

---

Display 13-2   **TYPES OF POWER**

Legitimate power:	Power based on an official position within the organization. Often referred to as authority, in which manager has the right to direct others and workers are obligated to respond. Activities typically include making decisions on behalf of the organization and acquiring or controlling human and material resources.
Referent power:	Power an individual has because others identify with the leader or what that leader symbolizes or represents. It also exists because others see the leader as powerful, as in the case of political figures.
Reward power:	Power achieved by having the ability to grant favors or give rewards to others. Rewards might be in the form of praise, commendation, respect, or support.
Coercive power:	Power that occurs because of the ability to place sanctions on another individual in the form of verbal threats, withholding pay increases, undesired assignment, or warnings. The opposite of reward power, it is based on the fear of punishment.
Expert power:	Power gained through the possession of special knowledge, skills, or abilities that are respected by others.
Informational power:	Power that is gained by having information or data that is important to others.
Connection power:	Power that represents the cumulative effect of more than one person working toward a goal; for example, people working together to bring about a change or influence legislation.
Motivational power:	The ability of the leader to stimulate the interest, enthusiasm, or participation of others with regard to a common goal.

Coordinated Care Management. Individuals carrying out these responsibilities enjoy **legitimate power**—that which occurs by virtue of the position held in the institution.

Referent power can be observed when one selects a mentor or an individual after whom he or she wants to model behavior. Mentoring has gained much popularity in the past few years, and new graduates are encouraged to find a mentor when they begin their careers. We will discuss mentors in more detail later in this chapter. A term frequently associated with referent power is charisma. **Charisma** is the power that draws one person to another and includes such behaviors as the way the leader acts, talks, walks, and relates to others. It is sometimes listed separately as a theory of leadership and also is included often in the list of traits in the Trait theory.

Reward power can be seen anytime one individual rewards another with positive statements, compliments, or other ego-boosting comments. It is also seen in promotions, salary increases, and awards. Even beginning nurses will find reward power available to them if they focus on giving recognition to others' strengths and accomplishments.

Coercive power involves using threats of punishment to enforce desired behaviors. Coercive power also has its place in nursing. If you fail to practice safe, competent nursing after you are licensed, the Board of Nursing has the power to compel you to change behavior by the threat to revoke your license to practice (see Chapter 7). For example, if unsafe practice is the result of chemical abuse, an employer can force an individual to enter treatment for chemical dependency, with the threat of job loss for failure to do so.

Expert power involves having specialized skills and abilities that serve to accomplish desired goals or influence others to follow one's leadership. Expert power is observed every day on hospital units. As nursing becomes more and more specialized, the individual with particular skills, knowledge, and ability will have power in the area where these skills are important.

Two other forms of power have been added to those originally identified by French and Raven. **Informational power** (Heineken & McCloskey, 1985) exists when an individual possesses information that others need or want to accomplish a goal. An example would be an individual who has access to information about the unit's budget or one who is more informed about policies that guide behavior of others.

Connection power is the cumulative effect of more than one individual working toward a goal. Connection power is responsible for the effectiveness seen in networking. Nurses who work collaboratively are developing connection power. Connection power also can occur by working with persons who command power, respect, or access to desired positions or places. You will observe nurses using connection power as they work with other professionals in the health care system. You will also see nurses who are politically involved exercising connection power.

Motivational power is a fairly new term. It refers to one's ability to arouse in others an excitement and enthusiasm for what they are doing. Because of its inherent or internal nature, motivation must be generated by the individual as opposed to being provided from outside. Motivational power, therefore, refers to the ability of the leader to stimulate the interest, enthusiasm, or participation of others with regard to a common goal. It involves recognizing the elements that drive individuals or creates satisfaction for them. McGregor's (1966) Theory X and Y, Ouchi's (1981) Theory Z, Herzberg's (1959, 1966) Satisfiers and Dissatisfiers, and Maslow's (1954) Hierarchy of Needs are all examples of approaches to motivation (see Chapter 14). In transformational leadership, motivational power is seen when the leader shares information, involves others in decision-making, recognizes accomplishments, and rewards behavior (Fig. 13-1).

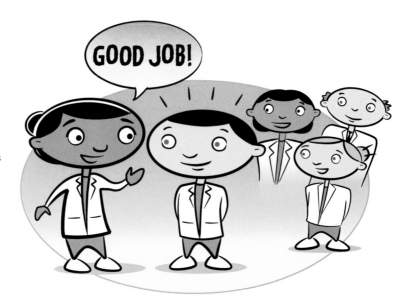

FIGURE 13-1 Motivational power is seen when the leader recognizes the accomplishments of others.

Thus, we see that power is derived from a variety of sources and is used in a number of different situations. It is important for all nurses to realize that they have a power base and to seek positive ways to use it to bring about improvements in the health care system that will benefit patients and society as a whole.

Empowerment

The concept of empowerment has received a great deal of discussion in the last decade. **Empowerment** refers to the process by which one individual who has power is able to share it with another. It involves making others partners in the decision-making process by providing them the necessary knowledge and reinforcement. Perhaps you have already learned about empowering your patients. Transformational leaders seek to empower their followers and thus transform the work environment. Blanchard, Carlos, and Randolph (1999) state, "The real essence of empowerment comes from releasing the knowledge, experience, and motivational power that is already in people but is being severely underutilized."

Transformational leaders openly share information with workers so that everyone is aware of problems and the need for action. The leader provides a vision of what is to be accomplished and helps workers to understand that they are an integral part of the group. Workers are delegated authority for decision-making and for helping to find solutions to problems. Transformational leaders work at developing the skills of workers, who then develop a strong sense of self and are motivated toward achievement. Empowered workers have a greater sense of satisfaction derived from goal achievement. None of this could occur if initially workers were not empowered.

Empowerment is not easily achieved. Some organizations do not support empowerment of employees. Supervisors themselves may not be empowered within the organization. Some supervisors lack the self-confidence necessary to empower others and fear loss of control if workers assume greater responsibility in decision-making. In other instances, the supervisors may have moved into their roles while working in hierarchical organizations and may find it difficult to shift their approach to management in a new setting. Some employees do not want the accountability and responsibility that are required of the empowered individual.

ORGANIZATIONAL CHARACTERISTICS

Senge (1994, p. 51) refers to organizations that support empowerment as "learning organizations" and identifies a number of characteristics of the learning organization. He includes the following among these characteristics:

* People feel they are doing something that matters and that all individuals are growing and enhancing their capacity to create. Values and visions are shared.
* The belief exists that people are more intelligent together than they are apart and that visions of the organization emerge from all levels.
* The knowledge in the hearts and minds of employees is one of the organization's greatest resources.
* Employees are encouraged to learn what is going on at every level within the organization.
* People feel free to inquire about another's values and assumptions and mutual respect and trust exist among individuals, thus freeing people to take risks and openly assess results.

Empowering Others

As we indicated earlier, if the organization does not support the empowerment of people, it is much more difficult to accomplish. If you want to work in an organization that empowers its employees, you will want to set this as one of your goals when seeking employment following graduation (see Chapter 11). An organization that is involved in transformational leadership styles will also support (and require) the empowerment of employees. The two are intricately interwoven.

As you move into positions of responsibility, what are the behaviors and characteristics that you must possess to empower others? How can you motivate others to assume more responsibility and accountability for their actions? Display 13-3 provides a list of personal characteristics that are critical to being able to empower others and identifies some behaviors that help to create those characteristics. How many of those characteristics do you currently possess? Which ones will you need to develop?

Empowering others can be accomplished through a variety of strategies. These are appropriate for any situation where the goal is to give others power and control over a situation.

For a person to gain more control over a situation, that individual must be knowledgeable. So a first step in empowering is often the open sharing of information. Everyone must be aware of the underlying situation, the nature of the problems, and why change is needed. Sharing information with others also is an important aspect of gaining the trust of your followers. Without information, others cannot act responsibly. They need to know how the organization works and the factors that impinge upon a situation.

Display 13-3 **PERSONAL ATTRIBUTES THAT SUPPORT EMPOWERING OTHERS**

Is trustworthy
- Honest in relationships with others
- Honors commitments, follows through on promises
- Can be relied upon
- Is predictable with regard to responses to others

Possesses integrity
- Accepts responsibility for own actions
- Gives credit to others for things done well
- Is fair and just in relationships with others
- Is sincere
- Possesses sound moral values

Demonstrates self-confidence
- Knows one's abilities and limitations
- Models the values and behaviors desired of others
- Maintains a confident body language
- Is able to control one's own feelings and behavior
- Is not arrogant, conceited, or boastful

Is sensitive to others
- Is kind and thoughtful in interactions with others
- Actively listens to others
- Recognizes things that are important to others
- Is free of cultural and racial biases

Displays intelligence
- Is reasonable in decision-making
- Learns from experience
- Able to respond quickly and successfully to new situations
- Maintains keen approach to problem solving
- Seeks new information regularly

Exhibits good communication skills
- Communicates clearly and concisely
- Listens to others
- Knows when not to talk
- Maintains positive body language
- Is sensitive to nonverbal cues
- Does not interrupt others when they are speaking

Once individuals are aware of the problems and situations being faced, they can be involved in setting the goal or developing a vision of what is to be accomplished. Through this process, the employee becomes more vested in achieving the desired outcome and "buys in" to the excellence expected and the productivity needed to accomplish it. Along with this, team members need to know the ranges or boundaries within which they can act (Blanchard, Carlos, & Randolph, 1999).

Another characteristic of empowering others is involving them in finding solutions to the problems once they are aware of the problems being encountered. This is where the collective intelligence of the group is useful. Rather than support the belief that only the leader can propose workable solutions, empowered employees are respected for their contributions and for their first-hand knowledge of a situation. Ideally, employees will become involved in the development of strategies to accomplish the goal or vision.

Reaching this point in any organization requires that the leader has been able to help workers develop their skills. It involves teaching, team building, and coaching abilities on the part of the leader (see Chapter 14). Workers must gain confidence in their ability to make correct decisions and take appropriate action. Employees need to be able to see themselves as members of influential teams, with the ability to discover new resources. Recognizing the accomplishments of others, sharing credit, valuing honesty and openness, and rewarding behavior are important aspects of this development. As a result of feeling empowered, employees understand the valuable contribution they make.

Like many other endeavors, empowering others has no straight line to success; some days are good, others not so good. Do not expect too much success too early. Being successful requires that you maintain an optimistic attitude, persevere in your goals and activities, and remain steadfast in your commitment to them. Continual assessment of yourself and the situation is essential. Be honest with yourself, and at the same time avoid being overly critical of your own human behavior. Remember that the art of empowering others, like other skills you have mastered, can be learned.

Critical Thinking Activity

Think of a situation you have experienced or observed in which an individual was empowered. What were the factors that resulted in the individual being empowered? How did that individual respond? What additional actions might have made the empowerment even greater? Which of the behaviors that helped empower the person would you want to use? Which ones would you not use? Why did you choose these behaviors?

DEVELOPING YOUR LEADERSHIP STYLE

In today's health care environment, all professional nurses will find themselves involved in working conditions that require some leadership skills. Both acute and long-term care facilities are using assistive personnel who have less educational preparation and who require direction from RNs. This trend will increase as the shortage of RNs becomes more keenly felt. As you move into the world of employment, you will want to think about your own leadership style. What approach will you use when directing others? How will you develop those skills? The following suggestions may help to enhance this process:

- *Continue to learn and to grow.* You will be expected to demonstrate competence and knowledge. These can be developed and maintained only when you continue to seek and find answers to problems you encounter, many of which you may not have studied in your nursing program. Subscribe to a nursing journal that focuses on content related to your area of practice so that your clinical knowledge continues to grow. Attend meetings and participate in committees so that you learn more about the organization in which you work.
- *Seek out a role model or a mentor.* A **mentor** is a more experienced individual who is willing to support and guide an individual who is new to a work environment and who systematically develops a subordinate's abilities through tutoring, coaching, and guidance. In selecting a mentor, you should look for someone whose abilities and career accomplishments you admire and who is willing to make the extra effort required to assist in your growth. The mentor will help you navigate through the system until you are capable of doing so on your own. The mentor can provide counsel and guidance regarding issues that concern you. This person can also suggest committees or groups in the workplace that create opportunities for you to learn and excel. The mentor can coach you to perfect your performance and can provide a sounding board when one is needed. This person can protect you by helping to deal with negative feedback and teaching you about rules that are not written in any policy manual. The mentor helps you seek solutions, provides inspirational motivation, and individualized consideration. It is a fortunate novice who has a good mentor.
- *Maintain your personal physical resources.* One of the significant criticisms levied at today's health care environment by those who are employed in it is the high level of stress encountered on a day-to-day basis. This stress can best be managed when a person is physically and mentally fit. Everyone needs a time to unwind, to relax and rest, and to find the time and energy to reflect on work activities. It is important to maintain outside interests and relationships that help to round out life and provide diversion from the stresses of work. As you move into the world of employment, be certain that your life style includes a healthy diet, exercise, rest, and relaxation.
- *Retain an open mind and develop flexibility.* Individuals who are open to new ideas and who can cope with unpredictable circumstances have an advantage in the workplace. Remember that there is often more than one way to approach a problem. Locking into only one way of viewing things or one method of dealing with a situation limits one's growth, can create tension in the workplace, and may result in using the wrong approach to solve a problem. Learn as much about the organization in which you are employed as you can. Developing a broad view of how the organization functions will help you to see where you and your unit fit in. Be willing to compromise and to negotiate; these skills are critical to any good team player. Ask questions when you are not sure.

- *Demonstrate respect and consideration for others.* All individuals bring unique perspectives and contributions to the workplace that should be valued. Sometimes encouraging others to do their best requires patience and understanding. Help others to grow just as you want others to assist you. Observe the basic behaviors considered to be "good manners." Practice common courtesies and etiquette. Address people by the name by which they wish to be addressed. Be polite and considerate to others and generally you will find they will return this behavior. Be sensitive to things that may be distressful to those with whom you work. Trust people and exercise faith. Share information—it helps others to know you believe in them.
- *Believe in yourself.* Develop your own self-confidence. Give yourself credit for the things you know you do well. Identify the things that you need to learn more about and do so. Develop a body language that inspires confidence in others; walk tall. Maintain good grooming and dress. Become articulate in your communication patterns and remember the importance of being a good listener. Review the language you use in reference to yourself. Don't discount your own skills and abilities or minimize your accomplishments. In others words, develop a professional demeanor.

COMMUNICATING EFFECTIVELY

After reading the above material, you have an appreciation for how important effective communication is to your ability to provide leadership. The concept of **communication** is not new to you. In previous studies, you learned that communication involves the sending and receiving of a message from one person to another. Let's list some of the other things that you know about the communication process.

- Communication occurs in four different settings: intrapersonal, interpersonal, group, and societal. Intrapersonal occurs when you "talk to yourself." Interpersonal occurs between two or more individuals. Group communication takes place when a number of persons are involved. Societal communication relates to an entire society or culture.
- Communication takes several forms, notably verbal, nonverbal, and written. Verbal communication occurs in the use of words. Nonverbal involves one's body language and dress and includes facial expressions, body positions, eye contact, boundaries, and body movements. Written communication is that which is recorded, as in charts, memos, letters, and the like.
- Verbal and nonverbal communication systems interrelate, and either may complement one another or contradict one another. For example, if you say, "It doesn't matter to me" and at the same time shrug your shoulders, the messages complement one another. However, if you say, "Please tell me more" but look away, you have given two different messages. Looking away can suggest you don't really care.
- Certain skills can facilitate the communication process and result in therapeutic communication or communications that are goal-directed. Therapeutic communication has a purpose and direction and employs processes to achieve established

objectives. It focuses on the needs of the other person and involves active listening and observation.

- The words we use when communicating can mean different things to different individuals. Chief concerns include the use of figures of speech, jargon, slang, and idioms with which not everyone is familiar, such as "She heard it straight from the horse's mouth" (meaning from a reliable source) or "Up a creek without a paddle" (meaning in a difficult situation without a means of exiting the situation). Another example is abstract messages that use vague terms, such as asking a patient in an urgent care center, "What brings you here?" when inquiring about symptoms and receiving the reply, "A car."
- Communication involves feedback that allows us to know which messages were received and understood as intended and which messages need correction. Feedback performs a regulatory function and helps us to evaluate the communication process.
- Communication is influenced by a variety of factors, including a person's perceptions and values. Words represent generalized symbols that may vary from individual to individual. Your perceptions can be altered by crises and anxiety-producing situations.
- Blocks to communication occur when responses are made that are not helpful, such as generalizing, labeling feelings, making judgmental statements, or changing the subject. Blocks to communication can involve such things as telling the individual how to do something he has already learned. Belittling others' feelings, disagreeing, disapproving, refusing to admit that a problem exists, or being defensive are other examples of blocking communication.
- Communication is culturally sensitive and culture-bound as a result of impressions we learned at an early age about how the world is structured. This applies to both verbal and nonverbal behavior. For example, not all cultures maintain eye contact during communication in the manner we do in Western culture. In other cultures, such as Native American, some Hispanic, African American, Appalachians, Indochinese and Asian Americans, it is not acceptable to make eye contact when talking because it is a sign of disrespect (Videbeck, 2001). Touch, which is a nonverbal form of communication, may be viewed differently by different cultures. Although it may be comforting to some, others may see it as an invasion of personal space.

In the past few decades, electronic devices have significantly affected our communication systems. The computer, e-mail, faxes, the Internet, cell phones and personal digital assistants (such as the Palm Pilot®) have greatly increased the ease and speed with which we can communicate with one another. At the same time, it has resulted in ethical concerns about the sharing of information, how it is stored, and who has access to it. Increasingly, the care provided to clients is recorded electronically.

USING COMMUNICATION SKILLS IN THE LEADERSHIP ROLE

The importance of being able to use communication skills effective in a leadership role cannot be overemphasized. Swansburg and Swansburg (2002) state that 80% of a higher-level manager's time is spent on communication, with 9% of the time spent writing, 16% of the time spent reading, 30% speaking, and 45% listening. To be an effective leader, one must possess an adequate understanding and application of communication techniques. The following are some basic guidelines for skillful communications:

- *Communications should be clear.* A message being given to others should be free of ambiguities, and the person receiving the message should have no difficulty interpreting what is meant. If messages are not understood, the individual being addressed should ask for clarification. However, in the health care environment, we often work with nursing assistants who come from other cultures. They may have difficulty questioning a superior, partially because they may not want to offend someone in a position of authority. Sometimes they do not want to acknowledge that they do not understand because they fear it will cost them their job. Instead, they may nod, smile, or give other nonverbal cues that suggest understanding. In such situations, it is important that you ask to have instructions repeated back to you, or ask such clarifying questions as, "Can you tell me how you are going to do that?" Or, "Now tell me in your own words, how you will know if it is okay to get Mr. Jones up?"

- *Communications should be concise.* This applies to both verbal and written messages. We should work at stating the necessary information as briefly as possible while still providing enough data to be clear. The longer messages become, the more extraneous information is included, and the longer it takes for someone to receive the communication. Learning to communicate in a concise and clear manner is another learned skill that will improve as we try to become more proficient.

- *Communications should maintain a positive approach or perspective.* When problems arise, individuals respond better to communications that give positive direction, are not faultfinding or accusatory, and that focus on finding a solution rather than on the problem itself. When people become defensive, their energy is diverted to self-protection rather than to problem resolution, and they become stressed. This detracts from accomplishing the goals.

- *Communication should recognize and accommodate diversity.* Any work environment presents a variety of personalities, cultures, educational experience and capabilities, and gender differences. Maintaining an open mind and being willing to listen to others will help in difficult situations. While being sensitive to cultural values, it is equally important not to stereotype; for example, assuming that all Hispanic Americans demonstrate emotion more easily. Recognizing and acknowledging that differences often occur in the communication patterns of men and women is also important. For example, men tend to communicate with a purpose to achieve a particular goal and as a tool to deliver information. Women, on the other hand, more often value the role communication plays in relationships (Cherry & Jacob, 1999).

- *Communicating effectively involves active listening.* Active listening tells others that you value both what they have to say and their membership in the team. Active listening involves hearing the facts in the verbal message but also listening for feelings, values, and opinions and observing the nonverbal cues. A busy work situation may not lend itself to this type of communicating. You may need to assess the situation as to its urgency. If it is not urgent, you can arrange to meet later to discuss the concern. When time is available, remember to use the communication skills you have learned earlier: accepting, focusing, reflecting, clarifying, questioning, paraphrasing or restating, and summarizing. Listen for vocal cues such as pressured speech or slow, hesitant responses. This will assist you to understand the context of the situation. A major deterrent to active listening is the fact that we often begin to formulate a response to the individual with whom we are communicating before that person has finished talking. This prevents us from listening to all the cues in an individual's message to us.

It is difficult to think of any time in nursing when one would not use communication skills, but certainly some of the situations calling for the effective use of communication skills include conflict management, negotiations, delegation, assessment, discharge teaching, documentation, and any situation involving interviews. In addition to the interview that is part of data collection from clients and the interviews commonly used in employment activities (see Chapter 11), the interview plays a significant role in performance appraisals.

PERFORMANCE APPRAISAL

Performance appraisal represents a formal process by which an individual's performance is reviewed and evaluated against established standards, most commonly a job description. It might also be appropriately referred to as performance evaluation, performance review, or performance assessment. At all times, the focus should be on the performance and not on personality characteristics of the individual being evaluated. Accreditation standards established by various private, federal and state agencies that review health care organizations require regular performance appraisal as part of the approval process.

The primary objectives of performance appraisal are to maintain or improve employee performance and to enhance the development of employees. As a result of the performance appraisal, the employee should know how he or she has been performing and what he or she can expect in the coming months (McConnell, 1993). The standards used to evaluate the performance must be clear, objective, and known in advance by the employees being evaluated. The process should be consistently applied and the rewards and disciplinary actions understood by all involved (Display 13-4).

Display 13-4	**CHARACTERISTICS OF AN EFFECTIVE PERFORMANCE APPRAISAL SYSTEM**

- The appraisal system has administrative support
- Evaluation is based on job description or other well-defined criteria
- Clear criteria exist for the evaluation used
- Employees know who will be evaluating them
- Evaluation procedures are consistently applied
- Evaluations are conducted in a timely fashion
- Evaluators are well trained in the use of the appraisal system
- The appraisal interview is a two-way communication
- All individuals know the related rewards or disciplinary action
- The final disposition of the evaluation is known to the employee

Often those responsible for conducting the performance appraisal as well as those being evaluated have an aversion to the process. Some of the reasons managers dislike the process relate to the amount of time it consumes, the fact that unpleasant messages may have to be transmitted (many persons are hesitant to criticize others), and fear of legal repercussions. Persons being evaluated may dislike the process because it feels much like receiving a report card or because the process is intimidating. As a new graduate, you should find the process very similar to the end-of-the-term clinical evaluation conference you experienced with your clinical instructors. Hopefully, they helped you to grow and to improve your performance, just as performance appraisals in the work situation should help you grow professionally.

Criteria for Evaluation

All performance evaluations, whether formal or informal, should be based on appropriate standards of performance. This could include the **job description** as mentioned earlier, or policies and procedures. Job descriptions contain statements that describe the duties for which the employee is responsible and should be up-to-date and clearly written to avoid ambiguous interpretation. Policies and procedures should be taught as part of the employee orientation processes and relate to patient care activities, as well as to timeliness, absenteeism and participation in agency committees.

Standards are "authoritative statements that describe a level of care or performance common to the profession of nursing by which the quality of nursing practice can be judged" and that reflect the values of the profession. (Dochterman & Grace, 2001, p. 235). Standards of practice reflect expectations for the behaviors of professionals in relationship to specific areas of practice and may be developed by professional organizations such as the American Nurses Association. Standards of care, which reflect expected processes and outcomes that should occur for individual patients, may be developed by health care agencies or by regulatory groups.

Instruments Used in Performance Appraisal

Instruments used for performance appraisal should include aspects of standards of care or standards of practice and relate to the job description for the position the individual fills in the organization. A number of different instruments can be used for the performance appraisal. Table 13-2 identifies some of the more commonly used approaches. In nursing, a rating scale is frequently employed. It has the advantage of being fairly easy to use and does not require a great deal of time to complete. The most critical aspect is that the assessment methods and the instruments used should focus on what the person actually does as opposed to personal characteristics of the individual.

In addition to knowing the basis of the performance appraisal, the person being evaluated should know who is going to be doing that assessment and when it will occur. In some organizations, the appraisal process may also include a self-evaluation. In such instances, the employee and the manager would use the same instrument to guide the evaluative process and would compare ratings during the appraisal interview.

TABLE 13-2. COMMONLY USED PERFORMANCE-APPRAISAL SYSTEMS	
SYSTEM	**DESCRIPTION**
Rating scales	Composed of a list of behaviors or characteristics to be evaluated and a rating scale to indicate the degree to which the criterion is met. Rating scales may be numeric (1–5), lettered (A–E), graphic (always, frequently, seldom, never), or descriptive. Rating scales are a widely used type of evaluation instrument in nursing.
Checklist	Describes the standard of performance; the evaluator puts a check-mark in a column (usually yes or no) as to whether the employee demonstrates the behavior. Behaviors can be weighted based on importance.
Essay or narrative	Evaluator writes several paragraphs outlining the employee's strengths, weaknesses, and potential. The evaluator may be provided with a guide for development of the narrative.
Critical incident	Requires that the evaluator observe, collect, and record specific instances of the employee carrying out responsibilities critical to the job. Incidents must be recorded regularly.
Group appraisal methods	May take one of two forms. The first involves using multiple judges. Several people form an appraisal team, typically the immediate supervisor and three or four other supervisors who have knowledge of the work being evaluated. Each person does an independent evaluation and then the results are combined.
	The second form may be used as a supplement to a supervisor's evaluation. Members of a team evaluate one another and team members' evaluations are included in the final evaluation. All persons use exactly the same job-based criteria for their evaluations.

The Appraisal Interview

The interview associated with the performance evaluation should occur in a timely fashion, be held in a setting that provides for privacy, and have a constructive focus. The dialogue may include both positive and negative feedback. Positive feedback is information that communicates to others what they have done correctly. Negative feedback is more difficult because it identifies areas of unsatisfactory performance. Giving negative feedback takes skill and experience and is a significant part of the coaching role mentioned earlier in this chapter. Negative feedback is best provided at the time the incident occurs and should be objective and accurate. For example, if you see a nursing assistant moving from client to client without washing her hands in between contacts, you would not want to wait until the formal evaluation conference to correct the behavior. Employees usually want frequent and continuous informal appraisal or feedback on their performance and it should not be left until the formal interview.

As a new graduate working in a health care facility, you are more likely to be the one being evaluated as opposed to being the one doing the evaluation. (However, hopefully the institution provides some means by which you can evaluate your superior.) There are some steps you can take to assist with the interview aspects of this performance appraisal session.

First of all, remember that the effective performance appraisal is a two-way street. Before the interview, prepare three or four questions that you can ask during the interview session.

These might be as simple as "How do you think I am doing given the time I have been here?" or "Are there ways that you think I might organize my work more efficiently?" Both of these questions would indicate that you are eager to try to improve your performance and meet the demands of the job. Should your manager have a tendency to fill the time with friendly chit-chat, the questions will help to focus the interview.

If you believe that some of the statements made by your manager are not accurate or are broad generalizations, challenge the statements. Of course, you will want to do so in a polite and constructive manner. You will want your manager to talk about the specifics of your behavior and performance. For example, if the manager says, "You seem to have difficulty completing tasks on time," ask for an example of a particular task that should have been done more efficiently. This will bring the conversation back to specifics rather than dealing in generalities. You need to be prepared for the fact that this could result in more negative feedback than might have otherwise occurred. If you receive negative feedback, it should be accompanied with some constructive suggestions for improvement. If the suggestions are not provided, ask for guidance, such as, "Okay, what can I do to work more effectively?" Then set a time frame with your manager for the improvement. If you receive ratings that you believe are inaccurate, negotiate with the manager about the rating. If you can convince the manager that there were factors that were overlooked, he or she may be willing to change the score. It is hard to predict how the manager will react to this response, but if you truly believe the rating is not accurate, you have nothing to lose. However, you must accept those statements that are a true reflection of your performance, even though they may be negative. These behaviors will be ones you will want to work at improving.

Behaviors to Avoid in the Interview

McConnell (1993, p. 81) identifies four simple "do nots" for the appraisal interview. As you become responsible for evaluating others and then sharing this information with others, you will want to consider these "do nots."

- Do not argue with the employee. It is counterproductive and destroys communication.
- Do not scold or reprimand the employee. Behavior needing a reprimand should have been dealt with when it occurred.
- Do not dispense personally referenced advice. Providing constructive instructions is part of the evaluation and is often considered "advice" from the supervisor. It should not be confused with advice that has a personal reference rather than advice of a professional nature. Making statements such as "If I were you, I would. . ." possess a personal reference and should not be a part of the appraisal process (Fig. 13-2).
- Do not wield your authority by making statements designed to coerce, intimidate, or demonstrate your power. The employee already understands your role, and wielding authority in this way will destroy the two-way nature of the process.

Common Problems With Performance Appraisal

In the best of circumstances, performance appraisal probably falls somewhat short of accomplishing the goals for which it is intended. McConnell (1993) has identified five areas in which problems can occur. The area that creates the greatest difficulty is motivational weaknesses

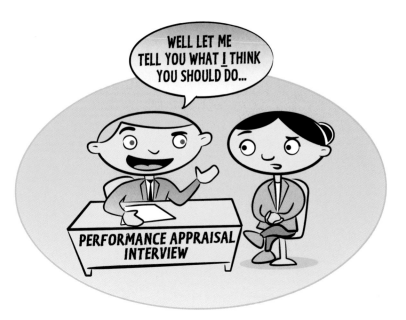

FIGURE 13-2   Personally referenced advice should not be a part of a performance appraisal interview.

and shortcomings on the part of managers who are responsible for the evaluations. Good evaluation systems require the total support of top management. All persons involved must believe in the process and its value.

The second concern cited relates to confusion as to what is being evaluated. We have already stressed the importance of evaluating performance but all too often the focus strays to personality. In fact, 15 or 20 years ago it was not uncommon for evaluation criteria to include attitude, dependability, cooperativeness, appearance, adaptability, and similar personal characteristics as areas to be evaluated. Perhaps you once had a job that included such criteria in your evaluation.

System administration barriers also can cause the evaluation process to fail. We have already stated that all persons must believe in and support the appraisal system. Often, managers find the process to be an unpleasant one and one that is very time consuming. Evaluations will be done late, hurriedly, or not at all. Systems work best when someone or some department has the responsibility for assuring that all the steps in the evaluation process are completed in a timely and appropriate manner. This includes training for those persons who will be doing the evaluations. Training in the use of the evaluation instruments and the process helps to decrease variations in rating from manager to manager and will reduce inconsistencies in application of the process.

The discomfort sometimes felt by the evaluators may also present a problem to the appraisal system. Many people dislike having to give feedback to others when it is aimed at correcting shortcomings or weaknesses. We shy away from criticizing others, especially when it is discussed face to face. As a result, one of two things may happen. The manager may tend to "gloss over" the areas that need improvement, or the manager may come down too heavily on the negative concerns. Neither approach is appropriate. Criticism, when given, needs to be assertive, constructive, and specific and relate to a particular behavior required in the job.

Display 13-5   EMPLOYEE EXPECTATIONS OF THE APPRAISAL INTERVIEW*

- A feeling that they were dealt with fairly
- An appreciation for their contribution to the organization and its goals
- Recognition of special accomplishments, efforts, or endeavors
- Some indication of how their performance can be improved, with specific recommendations on how it can be achieved
- An honest appraisal of future potential or prospects
- A sense of being fairly rewarded financially relative to others who are in the same position
- A sense that they have been allowed to contribute to the appraisal session and discussion, and that the evaluator actively listened to the comments.

Adapted from McConnell, C. R., (1993). The health care manager's guide to performance appraisal. Aspen Publishers, Inc., pp. 30–31.

The last problem area relates to fear of legal repercussions. As employee organizations have gained strength and recognition, managers have concerns that actions may be taken against them either in a legal form or in the nature of complaints, grievances, or appeals. Apprehensions of this nature are less common when all aspects of an appraisal can be backed up with specifics. When assessments are completed using specific criteria and definable measures, unsupportable judgments are less apt to occur. Maintaining consistency is as important as avoiding surprises. Evaluations should focus on what an employee does, not who the employee is.

It is important to remember that the primary objective of performance appraisal from the organization's perspective is to maintain or improve performance. However, the manner in which it is accomplished can make a significant difference. Display 13-5 identifies some of the aspects of a performance interview that we all desire. Be certain that you consider these when you are responsible for evaluating others.

Critical Thinking Activity

Think back to the last time you were involved in an evaluation interview. What were the positive aspects of that interview? Were there any negative aspects? How did you feel throughout the interview? How could the interview have been made more productive?

Evaluating Your Manager

Most organizations supportive of personnel evaluation will provide an opportunity for you to evaluate your supervisor. Therefore, we need to add a word or two about this process. First of all, be certain that you adhere to all the principles that you would want observed in your own evaluation. You should work from clearly stated job expectations, a job description, or other document outlining the standards to be observed. Deal with aspects of the position, not the personality. Word any negative comments as positively as possible. Try to form the comments into constructive criticism. Avoid the use of words like "always" and "never." Rarely are statements that include these words completely true. If you can think of some corrective action or constructive suggestion that would make the situation better, include it. Do not attempt to address areas about which you have no knowledge—just indicate that you cannot respond to those criteria. Be fair, be kind, and be honest.

TIME MANAGEMENT

As a new graduate, one of the biggest challenges you may face in your first position is organizing and using your time efficiently—a process known as **time management**. As a student, the number of patients assigned to your care was typically fewer than those you are assigned as a regular employee. In addition, you have not had time to become efficient in many of the technical procedures required in your job. Because time is finite—there are just 60 minutes in each hour and 24 hours in each day—time management skills become essential. Like many other areas you have already mastered, time management can be learned.

Principles of Time Management

As you work at learning to manage time more effectively, the following general principles will be of assistance to you. They can be applied in every setting and will facilitate your work in any role.

Understand yourself. Learning to manage your time begins as many other behavior-related concerns, with a thorough assessment of yourself. This includes giving attention to your basic physical needs and identifying things that restore and enhance your level of energy, as well as examining individual patterns of behavior. Adequate nutrition, sufficient rest, appropriate exercise, and relaxation are all part of appearing in the work environment in the best possible condition to perform. Analyze your body rhythms and determine when your energy is at it highest peak. You will want to plan activities requiring the greatest energy output and concentration to coincide with these peaks whenever possible. Are there things that boost your energy, such as a cup of tea, a break, or a power bar? Generally, it is considered unwise to skip breaks or lunch to capture more time. Your efficiency, and perhaps your disposition, will suffer. What things create the greatest stress for you? How can they be mitigated or avoided? What activities help you best deal with stress?

Take control of your own time. Responding to the requests of others results in one of the greatest expenditures of time. These requests may be for assistance or simply directed toward socialization. In either case, they can rob you of needed minutes and hours.

We recognize that it is difficult to say "no," especially when a colleague is asking for assistance. However, there are some clear-cut situations in which it is easier. The first of these occurs when you are asked to assist with something for which you lack the necessary skill. You need to honestly recognize these instances and decline involvement when they occur. For example, if a seasoned nurse on the unit asks you, as a new graduate, to watch

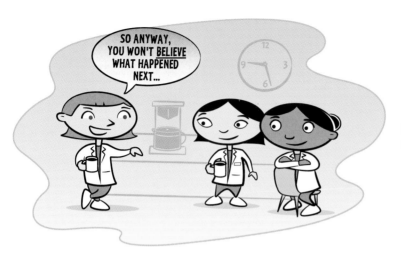

FIGURE 13-3 Perhaps the greatest time waster is social chit-chat.

a critical patient while she takes a break, and you lack the needed knowledge to safely evaluate that patient, it is essential that you refuse. You do not want to jeopardize the patient's safety.

There are times when honoring a request, although you are capable of performing the necessary actions, will make it impossible for you to complete your own assignment in a timely fashion. In such instances, it is best to be honest and say, "I'm sorry, I simply cannot take the time right now." Although this is difficult, particularly at first, it is preferable to trying to do too much.

Interruptions also rob us of valuable time. In addition to stopping an action in process, we often have to restart or reorient ourselves to the task at hand before starting again—all lengthening the time it takes for completion. You may need to be assertive with those who have a tendency to interrupt you frequently; explaining as kindly as possible that you cannot be interrupted.

Some activities, such as developing a patient's plan of care, require thoughtful attention. Seeking a quiet place where you are least apt to be disturbed will increase the efficiency with which you will be able to complete the plan. Some hospitals are now structuring units with a room located away from the major area of activity where such tasks can be carried out.

Perhaps the greatest time waster is social chit-chat. Nurses typically are a gregarious group and no one intends to waste time—it just happens. Although it is fun and interesting to learn what other team members are doing, who is dating whom, what the latest movie was about, where the hottest sale is occurring, or any of the myriad items that captures one's attention, it is easy to lose 15 to 30 minutes in such an exchange. If you find yourself frequently involved in such conversation, excuse yourself by saying, "I need to check my patient now, but can we discuss it during break time or over lunch?" If your message is communicated in a kind and genuine manner, feelings will not be hurt and people will not feel put off (Fig. 13-3).

Develop a time schedule. Developing a time schedule or a plan for how you use your time helps you to stay focused and to avoid interruptions. It also requires that you set priorities. You can do this for long-term activities as well as for those to be completed in a shorter period of time. Once you have established a basic plan, develop a to-do list and determine what activities must be done first, which second, and so on. Look at your to-do list and determine if there are any items on it that can be deleted, or if there are items that can be delegated to someone else. (Remember that you retain responsibility for professional care that is delegated.) To-do lists will help you to avoid forgetting to do something that is important. They also serve as reinforcement to many individuals who are amazed at how many items they have completed in a given period of time.

Dealing With Procrastination and Time Wasters

Two final behaviors that help manage time are related to avoiding time wasters and managing the tendency to procrastinate.

We all experience time wasters. Certain occurrences in our day-to-day existence are sure to rob us of valuable time. Mackenzie (1990) has identified a list of 20 common time wasters that include telephone interruptions, drop-in visitors, ineffective delegation, personal disorganization, socializing, attempting to do too much, poor communication, lack of self-discipline, and many other items. To some extent, time wasters are unique to each individual. One individual spends too much time on the telephone, another makes too many trips to the water fountain, while another only manages by crisis. When you complete your personal analysis suggested earlier, you will want to look at ways in which you spend your time and decide which of those activities represent time wasters. Once identified, you can make plans for eliminating or decreasing the time spent in such activity.

Some individuals are more inclined toward procrastination than others. If procrastination has been a big part of your life, avoiding it may be the most difficult of the tasks we have outlined. **Procrastination** is defined as a chronic delay in carrying out actions that are necessary to accomplish important tasks (Ellis & Hartley, 2000). Delaying a task can result in it seeming to be much larger, more time consuming, or more difficult than it actually is. Researchers include fear of failure, lack of interest, and feelings of anger or hostility among the many explanations for procrastination. Regardless of the basis of the behavior, an important step in correcting it lies in making a personal commitment to complete tasks on time. This involves establishing realistic deadlines and then adhering to them

Kanarek (1996) provides five suggestions for dealing with procrastination. First, she suggests that you start working on a project for 10 minutes and quit if tired or bored. Often, at least half an hour will pass and you will have made progress. Next, she suggests that you save the best for the last, a form of reward. Making a game out of things may also help. Challenge yourself to handle one task in less than half an hour and make a game of seeing how quickly you can complete tasks you have been putting off. She also suggests breaking tasks into smaller, more manageable units and telling others of your plans, thus putting pressure on yourself to do what you have indicated you are going to do.

Critical Thinking Activity

Identify one activity about which you procrastinated. Using the material discussed above, determine why you delayed completing the task. Does this occur frequently? What steps can you take in the future to avoid such behavior? In what ways will you benefit from avoiding procrastination?

KEY CONCEPTS

- Differences exist in how leadership and management are practiced. Management refers to activities such as planning, organizing, directing, and controlling, while leadership refers to the ability to persuade others to follow your direction, to motivate, to inspire, and to instill vision and purpose.
- Accountability and responsibility are used synonymously and refer to the obligation to answer for one's actions and to do what is promised. Authority can be defined as the power or right to give directions, take action, and make decisions.
- A number of theories exist regarding leadership. The theories can generally be classified as Trait theories, Attitudinal theories, Situational theories, and Contemporary theories.
- Three major leadership styles prevail: autocratic or authoritarian leadership, laissez-faire or permissive leadership, and democratic or participative leadership. Each is appropriate in a particular situation or setting.
- A multicratic leadership style that combines the most favorable aspects of all styles is probably most frequently used in health care.
- Theories of leadership evolve with social cultures. Currently, a leadership approach referred to as transformational leadership is advocated by many theorists. A transformational leader shares information and decision-making with all employees.
- Power refers to the ability an individual has to get things done. Empowerment refers to the process by which one individual who has power is able to share it with another. Both are essential components of effective leadership.
- For individuals to realize their full potential, they must be empowered. Empowerment occurs when information is shared, individuals are involved in goal setting and finding solutions to problems and decision-making, and when efforts are recognized.
- Leadership is a skill that can be developed. You can enhance the development of your leadership skill by continuing to learn and grow, seeking a role model or a mentor, maintaining your personal physical resources, retaining an open mind and developing flexibility, demonstrating respect and consideration for others, and believing in yourself.
- Communication is a critical part of everything we do. It is occurs at an intrapersonal, interpersonal, and group setting, and is experienced in verbal, nonverbal, and written forms that may complement or contradict one another. Therapeutic communication has purpose and direction, focuses on the needs of others, and involves active listening. Words mean different things to different individuals, and feedback allows us to know which messages are received and how they are understood. Communication is influenced by a variety of factors, and blocks to communication occur when responses are made that are not helpful. Communication is culturally sensitive and culture-bound.
- In the leadership role, communications should be clear, concise, should maintain a positive approach or perspective, should recognize and accommodate diversity, and should involve active listening.
- Performance appraisal represents a formal process by which an individual's performance is evaluated. Employees know who will be conducting the evaluation and where the records will be placed. Good performance evaluation systems are based on appropriate standards of performance, have top management support, are conducted in a timely

fashion, involve a two-way communication, and assist the employee to grow in his or her position. Evaluators have training for this responsibility.

- Effective performance appraisal interviews are a two-way communication system that recognizes an employee's accomplishments and provides direction and motivation for further growth. The interviews are conducted in a setting where privacy can be assured.
- Time management involves learning to use your time more effectively and efficiently. To accomplish this, you must understand yourself, take control of your own time, develop a time schedule, avoid procrastinating, and avoid time wasters.
- You can avoid time wasters by examining the ways in which you spend your time and then deciding which of those activities were time wasters. Once identified, they can be decreased or eliminated. Making a game of tasks that you want to delay doing can help procrastination. Breaking tasks into smaller, more manageable units can also help.

RELEVANT WEB SITES

Electronic Resource Center/Management Sciences for Health: *http://erc.msh.org/*
National Council of State Boards of Nursing: *http://www.ncsbn.org/*
National Library of Medicine: *http://nlm.nih.gov*
NursingNet: *http://www.nursingnet.org/*
Nursing World (ANA): http://www.nursingworld.org/

REFERENCES

Avolio, B. J. (1997). The great leadership migration to a full range leadership development system. KLSP: Transformational Leadership, Working Papers. Academy of Leadership Press, [On-line]. Available: *www.academy.umd.edu/scholarship/casl/klspdocs/bavol_p1.htm.* Accessed 1/09/2002.

Blake, R. R. & Mouton, J. S. (1964). *The managerial grid.* Houston: Gulf Publishing.

Blanchard, K., Carlos, J. P. & Randolph, A. (1999). *The 3 keys to empowerment.* San Francisco: Berrett-Koehler Publishers.

Burns, J. M. (1978). *Leadership.* New York: Harper & Row.

Cherry, B. & Jacob, S. R. (1999). *Contemporary nursing: Issues, trends, & management.* St. Louis: Mosby.

Dochterman, J. M. & Grace, H. K. (2001). *Current issues in nursing* (6th ed.). St. Louis: Mosby.

Ellis, J. R. & Hartley, C. L. (2000). *Managing and coordinating nursing care* (3rd ed.). Philadelphia: Lippincott Williams & Wilkins.

Fiedler, F. E. (1967). *A theory of leadership effectiveness.* New York: McGraw-Hill.

French, J. & Raven, B. (1951). The basis of social power. In Cartwright, D. & Lander, A. (Eds.), *Studies in social power* (pp. 150–167). Ann Arbor, MI: University of Michigan: Institute for Social Research.

Harari, O. (2002). Behind open doors: Colin Powell's seven laws of power. *Modern Maturity 45r*(1): 48–50.

Heineken, J. & McCloskey, J. (1985). Teaching power concepts. *Journal of Nursing Education 24*:(1): 40–42.

Herzberg, F. (1966). *Works and the nature of man*. New York: World Publishing.

Herzberg, F., Mausner, B. & Snyderman, B. B. (1959). *The motivation to work*. New York: John Wiley.

House, R. J. (1971). A path-goal theory of leadership effectiveness. *Administrative Science Quarterly,* 16: 321–338.

Kanarek, L. (1996). *Everything's organized*. Franklin Lakes, NJ: Career Press.

Lewin, K. (1951). *Field theory in social sciences*. New York: Harper & Row.

Mackenzie, A. (1990). *The time trap*. New York: American Management Association.

Maslow, A. (1954). *Motivation and personality*. New York: Harper & Row.

McConnell, C. R. (1993). *The health care manager's guide to performance appraisal*. Gaithersburg, MD: Aspen Publishers, Inc.

McGregor, D. (1966). *Leadership and motivation*. Cambridge, MA: MIT Press.

Neufeldt, V. (Ed.). (1996). *Webster's new world college dictionary* (3rd ed.). New York: Macmillan.

Ouchi, W. G. (1981). *Theory Z: How American business can meet the Japanese challenge*. Reading, MA: Addison-Wesley.

Senge, P. M., Kleiner, A., Roberts, C., Ross, R. B. & Smith, B. J. (1994). *The fifth discipline fieldbook: Strategies and tools for building a learning organization*. New York: Doubleday, a division of Bantam Doubleday Dell Publishing Group, Inc.

Swansburg, R. C. & Swansburg, R. J. (2002). *Introduction to management and leadership for nurse managers* (3rd ed.). Sudbury, MA: Jones & Bartlett Publishers.

Videbeck, S. L. (2001). *Psychiatric mental health nursing*. Philadelphia: Lippincott Williams & Wilkins.

von Pierer, H. (1994). Informatik und informationstehnik als basis industrieller innovation. *Informatik Spektrum 17*(2): 77–78.

14

Working With Others for Patient Care

LEARNING OUTCOMES

After completing this chapter, you should be able to:

1. Discuss the importance of teams in health care settings and identify key factors in effective team function.
2. Analyze the differences among multidisciplinary, interdisciplinary, and transdisciplinary health teams and describe the nurse's role on the transdisciplinary team.
3. Discuss the relationship of physicians and nurses within the health care team, and identify actions the nurse can take to facilitate positive interactions.
4. Describe the team-building process and identify some behaviors that will strengthen a team.
5. Discuss the concept of motivation and describe steps that can be taken to motivate others.
6. Explain the process of delegation and why it is necessary in today's health care environment.
7. Outline the steps to be followed for effective delegation.
8. Identify factors to be considered when care should not be delegated.
9. Describe two models of change that can be used to facilitate change and reduce resistance to it.
10. Explore your personal response to change and how you might more successfully adapt to changes in your work environment.
11. List the various sources of conflict in a health care setting.
12. Explain five strategies for managing conflict and give examples of appropriate situations for the use of each.

In all health care settings, many different health care workers provide differing skills to meet patient needs. In Chapter 1 we discussed the various health care occupations; in Chapter 12 we described patterns of care practiced in different health care settings. Here we will discuss some of the strategies for effectively working with all of the diverse group of individuals comprising the health care team, and will address some of the problems that arise between and among workers.

TRANSDISCIPLINARY HEALTH CARE

A **team** is comprised of a group of people working together for a common goal. The very nature of health care requires the development of health care teams and collaboration among all the variously prepared individuals caring for a particular patient or within a given setting. In today's health care environment, many different individuals who represent a wide variety of disciplines contribute to patient care; sometimes their roles overlap. This team could include the nurse, the physician, the pharmacist, the nutritionist, social and pastoral services, physical therapy, speech therapy, respiratory therapy, and housekeeping, just to name a few.

It is this grouping of individuals and specialties that Jean Watson (1996) describes as **transdisciplinary health care**—"relationship-centered caring and healing which transcends any one health profession." In transdisciplinary teams, team members may all be addressing the same problem, bringing different expertise, with roles that may often overlap. For example, the multiple avenues to address pain may include medicine, nursing, counseling, and activities therapy, to name just a few. All are focused on the same problem and are working together toward a similar goal. In her message to membership, Dr. Watson, who is past president of the National League for Nursing, discusses how transdisciplinary health care has evolved from **multidisciplinary health care** (where the knowledge and skills of many are used to meet the total needs

TABLE 14-1.	HEALTH CARE TEAMS
Multidisciplinary health teams	The total needs of the patient are addressed, using the skills of many disciplines. Each discipline functions somewhat independently.
Interdisciplinary health teams	The efforts of the various disciplines providing care are coordinated to provide a more therapeutic approach. Typically, the nurse coordinates the care.
Transdisciplinary health teams	Incorporates the skills of many disciplines to meet all of the patient's needs but includes the sharing of roles between some areas of care. Involves more collaborative relationships among disciplines, with bonding, interacting, and uniting occurring among members of the various disciplines.

of the patient) and **interdisciplinary health care** (which adds the concept of coordination and collaboration between disciplines that usually are considered distinct). In multidisciplinary teams, each team member focuses on different problems that relate to their own specialty in the same patient. In interdisciplinary teams, the work of the members, while focused on their own specialty, is coordinated with effective communication occurring (Table 14-1).

Teams are a naturally occurring phenomenon in health care settings. Nurses are in a pivotal position to affect how the team functions because they contact all the differing individuals who are involved in the team. The nurse, with input from other disciplines, develops the patient's plan of care. The nurse can help move the team from a multidisciplinary approach to a more interdisciplinary approach. This role requires finely tuned interpersonal and coordinating skills. Moving further to a truly transdisciplinary team requires a high degree of trust, commitment, and collaboration by all team members.

Critical Thinking Activity

Review the number and background of caregivers in the clinical area to which you are currently assigned. How many different health careers are represented? What are the primary responsibilities of each area? If there are responsibilities that overlap, what are they? Who is responsible for bringing the individuals together as a team?

Communication Within the Health Care Team

To be successful in this environment, you first must recognize the importance and contribution of each person and the necessity for teamwork. **Respect** should be the hallmark of all relationships within health care. The same characteristics that demonstrate respect toward a patient may demonstrate respect toward coworkers. From using their preferred name when you address individuals, to avoiding intrusion upon privacy, to using language that reflects courtesy and consideration (such as saying "please" when making a request), you have many opportunities to demonstrate respect for others.

Trust in the integrity and purpose of all individuals in the team creates the foundation for successful interaction and problem-solving, as well as for team building. Others must be able to trust that you will fulfill your obligations and carry through on responsibilities. They need to be able to predict your response to various situations. Conversely, you must be able to trust that they will fulfill their responsibilities. When you find yourself unable to meet commitments, you maintain trust when you are honest with others and address the issue in a straightforward manner. Letting others know that a situation has changed or that you will be unable to complete something promised is the only ethical way to handle the circumstances.

Relationships Within the Health Care Team

As in all human activities, there is a tendency for individuals to align relationships in health care settings into a hierarchical system; it is the history that has pervaded the system. Thus, some people see themselves as being of higher status or more important than others. This occurs among disciplines as well as within disciplines and translates into an expectation of more power within the system. Those in lesser-paid jobs are most often assigned lower status and typically are viewed as having less power. Often, they accept this as the expected way systems will operate. Some do not want the added responsibility that often accompanies higher-paid positions.

One of the major lessons learned (and sometimes forgotten again) by business leaders in the 1980s was of the importance of each individual. The work of W. Edwards Deming in Japan during the early 1950s, of Joseph M. Juran (who also consulted in Japan in the 1950s), and Armand V. Feigenbaum laid the foundation for quality-improvement initiatives concerned with improving the quality of the product or service. Their work was later adapted and expanded by a new wave of thinkers, including Philip B. Crosby, Tom Peters, and Claus Moller, all of whom pushed for quality improvement. Along with Dr. Kaoru Ishikawa, Dr. Genichi Taguchi, and Dr. Shigeo Shingo, all of Japan, these men are often referred to as the Quality Gurus (wise teachers) ("The Quality Gurus," 2002) because of their interest in improving quality.

Common to all thinking regarding quality control is the concept that maximum efficiency and effectiveness of an organization occurs when management begins to tap into the knowledge and skills of everyone. Those closest to the situation are often those with keen insight into how to improve processes. From this body of management work, the strategies of **total quality management (TQM)**, **continuous quality improvement (CQI)**, and **quality assurance (QA)** were developed. All of these strategies were built on basic principles of respect for everyone in the system and trust among members of the various teams.

NURSING TEAMS

Nursing teams focus on the provision of nursing care. Registered nurses (RNs), licensed practical (vocational) nurses (LP[V]Ns), nursing assistants (with various titles), as well as nursing students, may all be part of a nursing team. In most situations, it is anticipated that the RN will lead the nursing team. However, in some long-term care facilities, LPNs lead nursing teams because there are so few RNs. In that situation, however, an RN must be available for oversight of the nursing care. There are a wide variety of nursing teams in different settings. Some nursing teams are small, composed of two or three persons; other teams may be quite large.

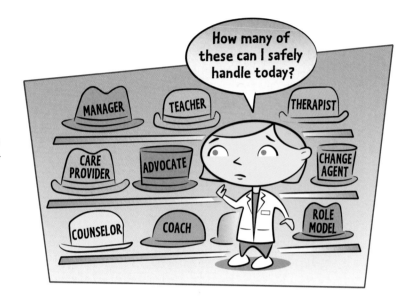

FIGURE 14-1   Often times the nurse wears more than one hat and performs several roles simultaneously.

NURSING ROLES

Traditionally, we have thought of the nursing role as being one of providing care. That certainly remains true in today's health care environment. However, the role of the nurse has expanded to include many other responsibilities and obligations. Often times the nurse wears more than one hat and performs several roles simultaneously (Fig. 14-1).

An important role filled by the nurse is that of educator. As a patient educator, the nurse is responsible for ensuring that patients and their families have a clear understanding of posthospital care, know when to take medications, are aware of side effects that need to be reported, and a host of information related to recuperation. As a leader of the nursing team, the RN plays a key role in the ongoing education of team members with lesser educational preparation. Registered nurses improve patient care through coaching and teaching staff on an ongoing basis. As a member of the community, the nurse is an informal educator, who can provide important information related to health issues for friends and others within the community. In an era when health promotion and health maintenance are emphasized, this role is more important than ever.

The nurse also fills the role of patient advocate. The health care system has become so complex (see Chapter 1) that clients may need assistance in maneuvering through it. It is often the nurse who is keenly concerned with assuring that patient's rights are not violated, that care is of the quality that it should be, and that service is provided in a timely manner.

Tied closely to the role of advocate is that of counselor. In their educational programs, nurses are provided with interpersonal knowledge and skills that allow them to assist others to express their concerns, seek alternative approaches and second opinions, and to ask questions. Through such activities the nurse is able to empower the client and family.

Nurses also occupy roles as managers and leaders of health care teams. Often this involves serving as a change agent within the health care environment. Leadership and management were discussed in Chapter 13, and we will discuss the change process later in this chapter.

The RN can fill a wide variety of other roles in health care. Two roles that we see more and more frequently relate to nursing informatics and nursing research. Information management has never been greater, and when that information relates to health care, nurses are in a unique position to take a key role in data management for decision-making. Similarly, as the profession stretches to enlarge to a body of knowledge that is uniquely nursing, the demand for nurses who will participate in research increases.

Critical Thinking Activity

You have just moved into a new position in the long-term care facility where you have been employed for 6 months. The position requires that you do more teaching and counseling of staff than you have done in the past. What resources will you tap to gain information to increase your skill in these areas? Which persons might you contact? How will you assess your new competencies? How can you be alert to personal biases?

NURSE/PHYSICIAN RELATIONSHIPS

Nurses work more closely with physicians in the acute care or long-term care setting than any other group. The relationships of nurses with physicians may be very positive, but it also results in some of the most stressful encounters for nurses. Because this stress plays a key role in job satisfaction, a number of studies have been done focusing on nurse/physician relationships. When these relationships lack respect and trust, the result is a difficult working environment and potential for ineffective patient care. Interpersonal relationships always are the result of actions by both parties, and both are responsible for their success. Here we will look at strategies the nurse can use to positively influence nurse/physician relationships.

A cardinal behavior involves treating the physician with respect and expecting respect in return. This is no different than relationships you might have with other individuals with whom you have worked and interacted. It requires that we are considerate, sensitive to factors in the environment, and respond in a manner similar to that which would be pleasing to us. Expecting to be treated with respect is the first step to receiving it.

Nurses must be mindful that they work and communicate within the scope of practice of nursing. Nurses can jeopardize their license and endanger the relationship with physicians by stepping over the boundary of nursing practice and into the role of the physician. Although a collaborative role allows for all team members to contribute ideas regarding patient welfare, it is important that nurses remain in the realm of nursing practice when making suggestions for care. For example, if a patient is not able to obtain comfort from a medication that has been ordered, it would be appropriate for the nurse to call the physician and describe the discomfort the patient is experiencing, giving full details of time of medication and response. It would not be appropriate for the nurse to say that the patient be given morphine 10 mg.

Ensuring competence and possessing excellent nursing skills fosters positive nurse/physician relationships. If procedures are not carried out correctly, if medication errors occur, if the nurse appears inept in a particular situation, it can be anticipated that the physician will be critical of the behavior.

A recent study that looked at nurse/physician relationships and how they impacted nurse satisfaction and retention (Rosenstein, 2002) identified five key circumstances or events that resulted in disruptive physician behavior. These occurred

- After placing calls to physicians
- After questioning or seeking to clarify physicians' orders
- When physicians were concerned that their orders were not being carried out correctly or in a timely manner
- After perceived delays in the delivery of care
- After sudden changes in patient status

Rosenstein (2002, p. 27) defined disruptive behavior as "any inappropriate behavior, confrontation, or conflict ranging from verbal abuse to physical and sexual harassment." Nurses can help reduce the occurrence of this disruptive behavior in several ways. When placing calls to physicians, be certain that you have all necessary information available before placing a telephone call. This is doubly important if that call is made in the middle of the night. None of us appreciate being wakened from a sound sleep, especially if we know we have a busy day to follow. If the call must be repeated because the nurse has failed to complete an assessment of the client or gather other important information, a disgruntled attitude on the part of the physician can be expected.

When it is necessary to question a physician's order, do so politely and in a considerate manner. Often it is not what is said but the manner in which it is said that will result in a positive exchange or an unpleasant one. Provide information such as assessment data that will help to substantiate your concern. Because nurses are held legally accountable if incorrect doses of a medication are administered, it is important to learn to question orders in a pleasant and polite manner.

Recognize and allow for situations in which the emergency nature of what is occurring with the client may require haste in "getting things done," and that what appears as domineering or demanding behavior on the part of the physician is part of ensuring that care is rendered quickly and efficiently. A difference exists between meeting the demands of the situation and being disruptive or rude.

Fortunately, the number of physicians who display inappropriate behavior is very small. Sometimes a physician's angry and rude response to nursing inquiries makes nurses reluctant to contact the physician when the patient needs medical care. If you are sure that you have fulfilled your nursing responsibility through appropriate assessment and communication, you should continue to seek the care the patient needs. Part of your own legal and ethical responsibility is to continue the quest for care and not be intimidated. This also is the hallmark of patient advocacy. If the physician refuses to respond, if the physician berates you instead of clarifying the medication order, or other such situations occur, contact the appropriate person in the organization. This may be the nursing supervisor, but in some instances, the head of the medical staff for the unit should be contacted. If an emergency exists, you should communicate that clearly and you may need to contact an emergency department physician or some other hospital resource.

If the situation is not urgent for the patient, you may confer with your manager and determine the best course of action. You have a right to expect that the health care agency will support an employee in situations of abusive behavior. Many health care facilities have policies, procedures, or protocols in place for dealing with such issues. Check to determine whether the institution in which you are employed has such guidelines; if so, you will want to follow them in dealing with the situation. If those in the expected chain of command do not follow through nor provide support, you may want to look for other methods to remedy the problem. You might have a union that will support a grievance or you may find support in the human resources department, where individuals are more familiar with employment laws and standards.

Critical Thinking Activity

It is 2:00 AM on a busy surgical unit. A new surgery patient, who had abdominal surgery late the previous afternoon, is experiencing a great deal of discomfort. You have administered all the medication for which orders were left. You are going to call the attending surgeon but you know that she has surgery early the next morning. What should you consider before calling? What information should you have? Are there other persons with whom you should discuss this before making the call?

TEAM BUILDING

Having looked at nursing teams and relationships among team members, let us focus our attention on activities of the nursing leader or manager regarding the team members. Five important aspects require some degree of mastery: team building, motivating others, delegating, facilitating change and managing conflict. Let's first look at **team building**.

In the late 1980s and 1990s, the concept of team building began receiving a great deal of attention in business environments as well as in health care. This can be attributed in part to the changes occurring in management strategies, as managers responded to guidelines that had evolved from recommendations designed to improve quality, as mentioned earlier in this chapter. In implementing a quality-improvement process, managers need to have a concern for the satisfaction of staff and must demonstrate respect for staff and their abilities. Without these attributes, team building will not be successful.

Team building itself sometimes seems rather nebulous. People aren't quite sure what it is. For purposes of our discussion, we will refer to our earlier definition of a team: a group of people working together towards a common goal. The goal of team building is to create a type of **synergy**, in which the effect of everyone working together toward the common goal results in a greater total effect than could be achieved by the sum of the efforts of everyone working individually. Synergy is a concept that ties closely to transdisciplinary health care models.

Teams and team building are not new. The most obvious forms of it that exist in today's world can be found in the sports arena, where teams and team functions are integral to the activities that take place. As we look at the idea of team building, we will draw some analogies between the concepts we are presenting and its implementation in athletics.

Team building begins with involving all members of the team in identifying the goal and establishing the steps that need to be taken to achieve that goal. If it is a sports team, the goal is to win the game; that is, they want to score more points than the other team. In health care, the goal is to provide the highest quality health care and patient satisfaction, measured in a wide variety of ways in today's health care environment (see Chapter 2). Teams are composed of a diverse membership, with a variety of skills and abilities represented. On a football team, for example, some block, some pass, some carry the ball, and others kick, using the skills that each brings to the game. In health care, some have special knowledge of pharmacy, some of medicine, some of respiratory therapy, some of nursing, with each member contributing to the patient's recovery. Through the process of goal setting, members of the team recognize the importance of their role in and contribution to the work of the team. All members of the team have an ownership in the process and the product.

Central to building effective teams is the belief that those who are closest to problems may be able to provide the sound solutions to the concern. All share in the problems that occur; all share in the success that is achieved. In bringing together members of the team, the manager needs to establish a working environment that recognizes and values the contribution of each individual on the team. Abilities are acknowledged.

Another part of team building relates to celebrating successes. Think of the soccer team that rejoices when a goal is scored. The efforts of the individual who scored the goal and the person who assisted are recognized and all team members share in the accomplishment. As we look at building health care teams, we need to look for opportunities to celebrate the good things that happen. This will help members appreciate one another and the effort that has been made as a group.

Leaders focus on how problems can be corrected rather than on how they occurred. Again, making a comparison with the field of athletics, if a basketball team is consistently breaking through the defense and scoring baskets, the team comes together, the plays are revised and another approach is tried. Similarly, in health care, if one approach to treatment is not providing the outcome desired, a conference is held and other strategies are discussed and decided upon. The focus centers on how things can be made better rather than on what was not working right.

Individual faultfinding is eliminated. On the volleyball court, if a team member allows a point to be scored, that member is not made to feel at fault. Rather, the team looks for ways to tighten the defense so that it is prevented in the future. In a good team-building situation, this would be the desired approach. Instead of spending valuable time discussing with a nursing assistant why the dinner trays were not promptly delivered for the evening meal, helping that individual develop an organized approach to tray distribution would have more long-lasting and better results. The role of the manager often becomes more one of "coach" than that of "boss."

Critical Thinking Activity

As a new graduate you have accepted a position on the medical unit of a community hospital. After working for 1 month, you have determined that the morale among the nurses and nursing assistants on the unit is low, that they do not function as a team, and that they don't have much team spirit. What can you do about this situation? Where would you begin? What are your limitations?

MOTIVATING OTHERS

In a sense, team building and motivating are first cousins. What team building is to a group, motivating is to an individual. Motivating others to perform at their best for the benefit of the organization is a huge task. It requires a good understanding of "people" skills, leadership, clear personal goals, and participatory supervision.

Understanding Motivation

Motivation encompasses the sum of all those individual factors that cause or impel an individual to do something. Individual factors, called **motives**, are generally referred to as extrinsic or intrinsic. Extrinsic factors include things such as salary, the work environment, and recognition by others, in other words, factors outside the individual. Intrinsic factors are much more difficult to work with because they arise from within the individual. Some would argue that all motives are intrinsic and that the most we can do is try to foster within the individual the desire to act in a certain way, to perform certain activities, or to strive for certain goals, because the motivation to do so originates from within the person who will be doing the acting. Thus, when we are talking about motivating others, it is limited to those acts of persuasion that will fire the inner desire within another individual to take the desired action.

Why do some individuals strive for grades of "A" while others are satisfied with a "C"? Why do some seek leadership roles within organizations while others prefer positions that may capture a lower salary but be less stressful? Why do some people seek PhDs, while others believe a high school diploma will provide them with all the education they need? A lot of study and a number of theories have been set forth to explain why people make the choices they do from among a variety of possible behaviors.

You may already have learned about human needs as motivation and that needs appear in a hierarchy, with unmet needs creating motivation (Maslow, 1954). Another approach to motivation suggests that some people are motivated by a desire for achievement, others by a desire for relationships, and still others by a desire for power (McClelland, 1953, 1961). McGregor (1966) suggested that some managers operate as if people are motivated only by fear of the manager's displeasure or the potential for a concrete reward, such as pay. He recommended another approach to managing people that started from the viewpoint that most people want to do well and that tapping into this basic tendency was the way to motivate people. A central concept is that different factors can motivate different people and that one individual might be motivated by one factor at one point in life but by another factor at a different time. Keeping a broad view of what might motivate others will enable you to work more effectively to motivate nursing staff.

Developing Your Ability to Motivate Others

As a team leader, how will you be able to motivate others? What behaviors on your part will encourage others to perform at their best? What people skills can you develop that will assist you in working with others? A key aspect of being successful in this area relates to your ability to develop the kind and quality of relationships with others that will positively influence the way they perform. It is important to get to know the people with whom you work. As discussed above, different things motivate different people. Personal praise may result in outstanding performance in one individual; another may respond best when given new responsibilities or challenging assignments. You will want to know your team members well enough to know what things you can do that will bring out the best in them.

As you examine the personal behaviors that will help you motivate others, you will want to give serious consideration to the things that people do to inspire trust and confidence in others. This helps you to be a credible person, one that others can count on to do what you say you are going to do, when you say you are going to do it. You are predictable, you exercise good judgment, and you are knowledgeable about procedures, policies, and protocols. You are even-tempered and patient, even in stressful situations. Having these qualities will result in your being the type of individual others will look up to, a person from whom others will seek answers and directions.

You will want to role-model the behaviors you want to see in others. In doing so you set the pace for your team. When you are energized, others also will be energized. When you respond to others in a positive way, it becomes contagious and others respond positively. Foster all opportunities to take pride in the accomplishments of the team and share ideas for improvement. Avoid any behaviors that would undermine a team member's motivation, such as being arrogant, showing favoritism, telling jokes that put down others, making racist statements, or issuing threats. Find ways to let your team members know you care about them as individuals. Show a genuine interest in things that are important to them. Be sensitive to problems they may be encountering away from the workplace as well as within. Learn what their personal goals and aspirations are and encourage activities that will help them to reach those goals.

Receiving recognition for things done well helps motivate many people. Even those that answer shyly, "It was nothing" appreciate having their efforts acknowledged. Giving praise for accomplishments also means that you will be working closely with individuals, so that you know when they have done something well. Praise and recognition, even in the form of "thank you," serve as great reinforcers and encourage people to keep trying. Most individuals seek to please others by their performance and need to know when that has been achieved. If you can offer this praise in public, it will reap even greater rewards. You have heard before that we praise publicly and correct privately. This is certainly true when trying to motivate others to do their best.

Another aspect of encouraging individuals to perform at their best focuses on having them know that their opinion is wanted and valued. This means involving them in decision-making. We have talked earlier in this chapter and in Chapter 13 about involving those closest to the action in the decision-making process. People perform better when they believe they are important and contributing to the team effort—that they are valued. You can provide the opportunity for others to have input into decisions and to articulate their thoughts and opinions. When you initially try this, you may run into resistance. When encouraging others to participate in decision-making, you may get the response, "That's what they pay you for." If this occurs, continue to offer opportunities for input. If this is a new experience for the team member, that individual may doubt your sincerity. Developing a genuine approach when working with others is important.

When working with others, it is important that you maintain your sense of humor. Being able to laugh at things that go awry or fail to meet our expectations helps to decrease the discomfort of the situation. By contrast, becoming upset or angry if something is done incorrectly will only cause your team members to avoid you during this time. They will consider you unapproachable and communication will decrease. The opportunity to build the strength of the team will be missed.

A final word should be said about redirecting the efforts of others. Especially when working with unlicensed assistive personnel, you may identify techniques that are incorrect or approaches to client care that need improvement. When this occurs, always focus your comments on the observed behavior you believe needs to be changed, not on the individual's personal characteristics. For example, if the nursing assistant fails to protect a patient's modesty, you would say, "I noticed that you did not pull the curtain when you were assisting the resident to the commode. Our residents have to be provided modesty and privacy. You must remember to pull the curtain before providing care." You would avoid making general statements such as, "You are inconsiderate and careless of the modesty of our residents." When you observe the corrected behavior, be certain to positively comment about it.

DELEGATING

When you first began your clinical experience, you may have felt that you and your classmates were the only people who needed to be directed in what to do. As you progressed, you may have become aware that staff nurses were directing the actions of all the individuals on the nursing team. In today's health care environment, all RNs have the responsibility for supervising the activities of those who have lesser educational preparation than they. It is possible that you have already had to provide direction to a nursing assistant or an LPN.

Delegation is the process by which one individual is able to accomplish necessary tasks with and through others. It is an important management process and allows organizations to function effectively and efficiently. The American Nurses Association (ANA) (1997) defined delegation as "the transfer of responsibility for the performance of an activity from one individual to another while retaining accountability for the outcome." An example would be the RN asking that a nursing assistant to help a client ambulate in the hall. The nursing assistant assists the client to walk; the RN is still responsible for seeing that the client ambulates, and that it is completed safely and is documented in the client's record.

In today's health care environment, which uses a wide variety of variously prepared caregivers, the importance of being able to effectively delegate responsibilities is critical. Nurses would not be able to complete their duties, tasks, and responsibilities without the ability to delegate some nursing activities. Delegating effectively requires that you have skill in the ability to guide, teach, and direct others. And like other skills you have mastered, it can be learned.

The ANA (1997) also has made a distinction between the delegation and assignment of tasks. They have defined **assignment** as "the downward or lateral transfer of both the responsibility and accountability of an activity from one individual to another." It is intended that the assignment would be made to an individual of skill, knowledge, and judgment. The two critical elements of this distinction are the accountability for actions when delegating to another and the skill, knowledge and judgment of the person to whom tasks are assigned. Assignments given to assistive personnel may involve making beds, passing water, answering lights, and taking specimens to the lab. In the clinical environment, tasks for which the nursing assistant is accountable (an assignment) and tasks that are delegated both may be referred to as an "assignment." This causes some confusion in discussions. For practical purposes, you should keep in mind that the nursing assistant can be accountable for some routine tasks, but that accountability for outcomes for patient care remains with the RN who is supervising the nursing assistant.

Reasons to Delegate

There are a number of reasons that we delegate certain tasks to others. Primary among these is the current trend in health care facilities to cut costs by hiring **unlicensed assistive personnel (UAP)** to perform those tasks that they can perform safely, thus allowing the RN more time for critical aspects of care. At one time in nursing, a primary care model of care delivery was popular in which the RN performed all nursing care activities for a group of patients (see Chapter 12). Although this was a desirable approach from a patient care standpoint, it was very costly. In an effort to contain costs, hospitals restructured and redesigned staffing patterns to change the "skill mix" of employees who provided care. In other words, staffing patterns decreased the number of RNs and included caregivers with lesser educational preparation to provide certain aspects of care. This change was predicated on the assumption that many tasks occurring on a nursing unit do not require the skills of an RN. Individuals with lesser educational preparation can carry out certain aspects of care such as taking vital signs, ambulating, transporting clients, and performing basic procedures. This allows the RN to focus on activities such as client assessment, care coordination, and teaching. In this way, delegating provides for effective time management.

Critical Aspects of Effective Delegation

For delegation to be effective and to assure that the quality of patient care remains high, a number of factors must be considered. You will want to review these before you begin delegating task to others.

It is critical to remember that although you have asked someone else to carry out a nursing task, you are still **accountable** for the care that is given (see the discussion of accountability in Chapter 13). You need to be able to ensure that the task will be completed in compliance with accepted standards, in a timely fashion, and that the activity, along with the patient's response, if appropriate, is adequately documented.

KNOWING WHEN NOT TO DELEGATE

Are there tasks that should not be delegated? When should I not delegate a task? What are the situations in which I should retain responsibility for doing the task? How will I know the difference? These are questions frequently asked by the nurse who is just moving into the role of managing the activities of others.

Certain tasks cannot be delegated. Any activity that requires knowledge and judgment that is unique to the function of an RN cannot be delegated to others. Thus, you would not ask or expect a UAP to do assessments or evaluations or make decisions that required nursing judgment.

You may not delegate responsibilities that call for professional judgment, skill, or decision-making ability. An RN must complete all assessments of the client and client needs. Information from the assessment that is important to the client's care then needs to be communicated to any person to whom care is delegated. The ability to do a thorough assessment and to not overlook some critical need is part of the nursing judgment acquired through your education. Someone

Display 14-1   **SITUATIONS IN WHICH DELEGATION IS INAPPROPRIATE**

- When the activities to be delegated fall outside the scope of practice of the person to whom they would be delegated. You cannot delegate something the individual is not allowed to do.
- When the activities to be delegated require independent, specialized nursing knowledge and judgment. This protects the safety of the client.
- When the activities to be delegated fall within job description and role of the registered nurse and delegating it would erode that role. This would apply to situations in which the nurse is responsible for evaluating the performance of others.
- When the work situation will not allow time for adequate supervision of those to whom tasks are delegated. Delegated tasks must be supported and supervised at all times.

with lesser preparation might overlook that need. For example, if you admit to your unit a new patient with head trauma, the assessment of that patient cannot be delegated.

You may not delegate roles that are limited to licensed individuals in the nursing licensure laws. For example, giving medications cannot be delegated because medication administration involves assessment, understanding of appropriate procedural safeguards, knowledge of pharmacology, and the ability to evaluate the effectiveness of the medication. Because of this, the law limits who may administer medications. Display 14-1 summarizes information on what should not be delegated.

IDENTIFYING TO WHOM TO DELEGATE

You can delegate only to a person who is competent to perform the task delegated. The nurse who is delegating tasks must know and understand the level of care that can be performed by the person to whom the task is being delegated. In other words, you need to understand that person's competency level or, if they are licensed, their **scope of practice**—what activities a person with a particular license may legally perform. The scope of practice for RNs and for LP(V)Ns is outlined in state practice acts and may vary from state to state (see Chapter 7). You will want to be familiar with the practice acts of the state in which you are employed. When working with someone who is not licensed, you will want to be knowledgeable about job descriptions, specific competencies, and agency policies and protocols.

DETERMINING WHAT TO DELEGATE

The tasks delegated to assistive personnel should not require nursing judgment while being carried out. This implies that the tasks should be routine in nature, ones that can be performed according to certain exact standards, and that the client's condition be relatively stable. We have said it before, but it bears repeating—activities that require specialized nursing skill, knowledge, or experience cannot be delegated. It is the use of this specialized nursing judgment that constitutes the heart of professional nursing.

The anticipated outcome of the care that is being delegated should be reasonably predictable. For example, if the responsibility for checking the vital signs of a patient is assigned to an LPN, the result will be the accurate assessment and recording of the patient's vital signs.

Tasks associated with any situation requiring ongoing assessment, complex observations, additional instructions, or critical decisions should not be delegated. Again, these activities require the use of nursing judgment and, therefore, should be completed by the RN. This would apply to any situation in which a client's condition is unstable, changing, or whose acuity level is high.

SUPERVISING DELEGATED TASKS

The supervision of delegated activities is essential. ANA (1997) defines supervision as "the active process of directing, guiding and influencing the outcome of an individual's performance of an activity." This means that an individual with greater skill and education is available, usually in person, but occasionally through various means, such as written or verbal communications, to give directions and assure that activities are being carried out properly. For delegation to be successful, there must be sufficient personnel and adequate time to provide the needed supervision and follow up. If either of these is missing, problems may result.

MATCHING THE TASK TO THE PERSON TO WHOM IT IS DELEGATED

When delegating, you have the responsibility for assuring that a "match" exists between what care the client needs to have performed and the level of competence and understanding of the person being asked to provide that care. In this way, you are assured that the tasks that are delegated are not beyond the ability of the individual asked to do them. This can be an important consideration in situations where an RN is floated into a special care unit to assist during especially busy times. Aspects of care in that unit that are "specialized" should not be delegated to someone who has not had the necessary additional training and education required to render safe care, even if that person has the RN license. Rather, the floated nurse should be asked to perform those aspects of care with which he or she is familiar.

The Five Rights of Successful Delegation

If you have followed all the above guidelines when delegating responsibilities to others, in all likelihood you will have also followed the five rights of successful delegation. The National Council of State Boards of Nursing (NCSBN) issued these five rights in 1995, when changes in delivery of patient care first included use of UAP and similar care providers. (Typically, this includes positions with job titles such as nurse aides, certified nurse assistants, nurse technicians, patient care technicians, personal care attendant, or unit assistants.) The Five Rights as identified by the NCSBN are found in Display 14-2.

Display 14-2   **THE FIVE RIGHTS OF DELEGATION**

Right Task	Right Direction/Communication
Right Circumstances	Right Supervision/Evaluation
Right Person	

Suggestions for Successful Delegation

A number of elements can result in delegation either enhancing or compromising patient care. Following the steps in the nursing process will help ensure the best outcomes.

ASSESS THE SITUATION

Before you decide which aspects of care you can ask others to do and which you should complete yourself, you will want to be certain that a complete assessment of the client has been done. You will want to know what that individual's needs involve, what priorities have been set, the goals of care, the time you have to accomplish the care, and other factors that impinge on the situation.

If you are to make a good "match" between the skills of the person to whom you delegate responsibilities and the complexity of the task, you must know the abilities of the person to whom you will delegate tasks. This can sometimes be determined through hospital protocols that establish the competencies of various levels of caregivers or via job descriptions that define what an individual in a certain job category is capable of performing. If the individual is licensed, you can be guided by what that category of worker can legally do. The length of time they have worked in that position or on that unit can also give some guidance. The best way to understand what individuals can and cannot do is to have worked with them for a sufficient period of time. If you are unfamiliar with the skills of a particular worker, you will need to provide greater supervision as you begin working with that person.

Initially, you will want to delegate only those tasks that have the highest level of predictive outcome, that is, those that are routine and standard. In so doing, you are also considering the potential for harm to the client and how difficult a particular task is to perform. You will note that your process of assessment has broadened to include the patient, members of your team, and the work situation.

PLAN YOUR ACTIONS

At this point, you will need to compare in your mind the information you have about the skill level of your team and the nursing care activities to be accomplished. Using the information you have gleaned in your assessment, you will then identify the specific persons to whom you may delegate the various tasks. You will want to plan the time to give them their assignments to assure that you have adequate opportunity to clearly communicate your expectations. You will also want to plan time for them to ask any questions they may have regarding the assignment.

You will also want to think about the situations that may require you to provide teaching and guidance to your team members. You will want to create an environment in which those you direct feel comfortable asking for assistance or instruction regarding procedures and skills with which they are less familiar. This could include the actual skill itself, but areas such as communication, priority setting, and critical thinking should not be forgotten.

IMPLEMENT YOUR PLAN

As you begin to direct the activities of others, your directions and instructions should be complete, easily understood, and able to be followed correctly. What activities need to be completed immediately? Which ones can be done later in the shift? How should time be organized? What are the expected outcomes? If you are working with an individual who has English as a

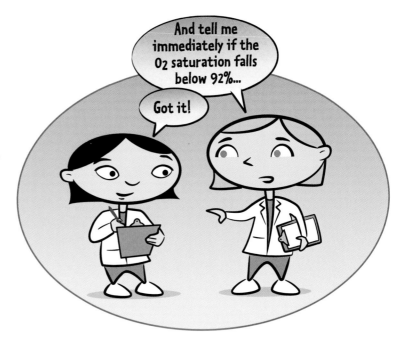

FIGURE 14-2   Good communications skills are critical to delegating tasks, setting down expectations, and providing ongoing evaluation.

second language, this may take more time (see "Communicating Effectively" in Chapter 13). Be certain that the assistants know what to report back to you and when you want to receive that information. What information can be left until the end of the shift? What data should be shared immediately? (Fig. 14-2) Listening carefully to their response to your instructions will help you to know that they have understood what you want accomplished. Watch for both verbal and nonverbal cues to their comprehension of your expectations. Ask them to repeat back to you what they plan to do and when. Ask if they have any questions before beginning their work. Tell them where you will be if they need assistance.

Supervising care constitutes an essential part of delegation. Supervising care means that you know what is occurring with the patients and the staff, what has been accomplished, what remains to be done, and what problems may have occurred in the process. This requires that you check with individuals throughout the day to determine how they are progressing, what problems they may be having, or what assistance or instruction they may need. Asking questions such as, "How are you progressing with your task?" or, "Are you having any difficulties with care?" or, "Is there anything with which you need help?" will provide opportunity for feedback. If you find that a team member is behind in the tasks you have delegated, you will want to plan adjustments that will allow completion of the care. You many need to help the individual set new priorities, or you may need to find another person to assist with the completion of care if you are unable to do so yourself.

Sometimes the individual who is a novice in the supervising role finds it difficult to know when to step in and assist and when to step back. Initially, you may be so concerned about doing a good job that the situation is overly controlled. When you delegate responsibilities, you will want to provide an appropriate amount of autonomy for the person to decide how to accomplish the work. Generally speaking, once you delegate a task you should not take it back. If your assistance is required, provide just that—assistance—rather than taking over the situation. You want to develop team members who have confidence in their own abilities and who feel they are valued members of the team.

EVALUATE THE RESULTS

When you are responsible for the activities of others, evaluating the outcomes of care is more important than ever. Remember, the fact that you have delegated part of it to another person does not absolve you of the responsibility of seeing that it is completed according to established standards and in a timely manner. You will want to evaluate all patients in your care and determine that their needs have been met to the highest degree possible. You will want to be certain that all documentation is complete and done according to standards. You will want to talk with members of your team to obtain needed information about the care they gave and any observations they made in the process of providing that care. Asking questions such as, "Did any problems arise while care was being given?" or "How did Mr. Drummer respond to the range of motion you performed?" or, "Did Mrs. Winston seem comfortable when you finished?" or, "Did Julie drink all of her apple juice?" will help elicit responses.

If, in your evaluation, you believe there is some aspect of care that has been done well, do not fail to comment on it. We all like to know our efforts are appreciated and to receive recognition for a job well done. Positive feedback is a powerful motivator. A pat on the back along with a few positive words lets people know their work is appreciated. On the other hand, if corrections need to be made in the care, be certain that such conversations occur in private and in a supportive manner. Display 14-3 summarizes suggestions for delegating successfully.

Blocks to Effective Delegation

Situations exist in today's health care environment that result in blocks or barriers to effective delegation. If these blocks can be eliminated or reduced, delegation will be more satisfying to all who are involved.

Display 14-3 **SUGGESTIONS FOR EFFECTIVE DELEGATION**

- Know what your team members are able to do, including their scope of practice and educational preparation.
- Plan ahead to avoid problems, decide what tasks to delegate.
- Match the task to be accomplished with the abilities of the individual to whom you are assigning the task.
- Communicate clearly the task you are delegating and your expected outcomes.
- Provide the necessary authority and responsibility to accomplish the task to the individual to whom you are delegating.
- Monitor and assess the performance of the task.
- Provide positive feedback as is appropriate; take corrective action when necessary.

LACK OF JOB DESCRIPTIONS

The first serious block to good delegation is the lack of current and complete job descriptions for all employees within the institution. As mentioned earlier, the RN must know the abilities and competency of members of the nursing team. These are most commonly found in the job descriptions of the institution. As new positions are created, management should form and distribute clear job descriptions. Communicating the content of the job descriptions is just as important as developing the documents. This will help assure that the individual responsible for delegating tasks has access to the information and can use it for decision-making. Similar to this problem is that of job descriptions that are not kept current. Jobs may be changed and tasks redistributed, but job descriptions reflecting these changes may not be completed. Thus, those needing the information find themselves having to make decisions without being fully informed.

TIME REQUIRED TO DELEGATE AND SUPERVISE

A second concern rests with the time required to effectively delegate and supervise. Many nurses believe they do not have enough time to spend with their patients. Time that is taken to plan, implement, supervise, teach, coach, and evaluate activities delegated to others may be viewed as taking even more time away from that spent at the bedside. This is especially true when working with inexperienced UAP, who may require a lot of teaching and support. The high rate of turnover in UAP positions heightens the frustration. There are no simple answers to this problem. To some extent, these are system problems that need to be addressed at a level higher than the individual nursing unit. The best action you can take in such situations may be to let your supervisor know that the problem exists. Perhaps longer periods of orientation can be planned for the assistants or better screening in the hiring process.

INADEQUATE TRAINING

A final block to effective delegation rests with inadequate training both for those who will be involved in patient care and for those who are moving into management positions. Formal orientations to the facility and to on-the-job type skills for the position the employee will fill help ease new employees into their roles. This is also true for those who will be responsible for supervising the new employees or who are new to the management role. It is one thing to know how to provide quality care to a small group of patients and quite another to oversee the activities of a team who are caring for a large group of patients. As with other situations in nursing, you will develop greater skill with experience.

MANAGING CHANGE

The one most constant feature of today's health care environment is the inevitability of change. To **change** means simply to alter, become different, or to transform. As an individual who will have the responsibility for managing others, you need to know how to deal with change yourself and how to help others deal with the change process.

Origins of Change

Typically, change occurs because of either internal or external forces that are brought to bear on the individual or the organization. External forces are those that originate outside the entity experiencing the change. Internal forces are those forces that come from within the individual or the individual organization

Aspects of health care change because of external factors such as new technology, new legislation, new standards, economic constraints, and changing population demographics of the people served. For example, accreditation standards may be revised, insurance companies may mandate different procedures, companies that have provided services may close or be purchased by another group, and legislation may require additional considerations, to name but a few situations that result in the need to change. The Americans with Disabilities Act was responsible for many changes, not only in health care facilities but also in many other places that serve the public. Health care agencies currently are experiencing changes mandated by the Health Insurance Portability and Accountability Act (HIPAA) related to patient's privacy. As we move closer to a national position on patient's rights, we will experience change that legislation requires.

Forces within the individual may be in response to a desire to advance oneself, to retire, to marry, to find a more challenging job, and so forth. Other internal factors, such as a desire for more efficiency, new ideas of management and staff, and education that give individuals greater knowledge, also create change. Within organizations, you might identify a new system of nursing care delivery, changes in the way pharmacy will dispense medications, the opening of new units, and myriads of other events. Whether the change is internal or external, you will want to be able to work with the change and, if in the position of providing leadership to others, to assist them in the process.

The Change Agent

The person who is responsible for facilitating the change process with others is known as a **change agent**. This may be an individual within the organization who is particularly knowledgeable about theories of change and skilled in assisting people in the process of change, or it may be someone hired from outside the organization who has those skills to bring about the process. On occasion, teams are established to bring about a change. In organizations that have adopted continuous quality improvement (CQI), the change agent is often referred to as the "champion." Within that system, anyone could have an idea for improvement of the organization.

Theories of Change

A noted authority on the subject of change is Kurt Lewin (1951) whose theory of change had three stages: the unfreezing stage, the moving stage, and the refreezing stage. According to Lewin, the unfreezing stage occurs when some individual is motivated by the need to create a change. That individual "unfreezes" or loosens the resistance to change or selects someone else to do it. This person becomes a change agent. Having gathered data, identified the problem, and decided that change is needed, the change agent sets about making others aware of the need for change. Those who will be affected by the situation requiring change are notified about it and become discontent with the status quo. The problem is then diagnosed and the best solution selected. Thus, those who will be involved begin to see the need for the change. If successful change is to occur, people must believe that it is necessary. It avoids having individuals "blind-sided" by conditions that will affect their way of operating. It enlists their cooperation.

The second phase of Lewin's theory is called the movement phase. During the movement phase, the person planning the change identifies, plans, and implements strategies that will facilitate the change.

In the final phase, refreezing, the change agent helps to stabilize the change that has been made in the organization so that it becomes part of everyday operation. Most changes need between 3 and 6 months before being totally accepted. During this time, the change agent supports those affected by the change and helps them adapt to it.

Lewin also described driving and restraining forces that affect change. Driving forces are those which push a system toward change; restraining forces pull the system away from change. Systems maintain equilibrium through the interaction of the two forces. For change to occur, the balance between the two must be altered so that the driving forces outweigh the restraining forces.

A number of other individuals have set forth theories related to change. Each of these explores a different aspect of change or addresses change from a different framework. Each might have value in differing situations. Lippitt, Watson, and Westley's (1958) theory begins by recognizing and diagnosing the problem, determining the ability to change, selecting the change, planning, implementing and evaluating the change, and then stabilizing afterward. This may sound very much like the problem-solving methods with which you are already familiar. Rogers and Shoemaker (1971) identified five factors that determined successful planned change: relative advantage, compatibility, complexity, divisibility, and communicability. Havelock (1973) identified six elements leading to the accomplishment of planned change. Asprec (1975) described four ways in which one can recognize resistance to change. In 1990, Perlmam and Takacs listed 10 emotional phases that are experienced throughout the change process. As you work with change, you may wish to explore some of these ideas more fully.

Developing Strategies for Change

Along with the theories that have been developed to explain and facilitate the change process, strategies for change have also been identified. We will discuss some of the most commonly recognized strategies for change.

EMPIRICAL–RATIONAL STRATEGY

The empirica–rational strategy suggests that individuals will follow their rational self-interest once it is revealed to them (Benne et al, 1976). This means that people will accept change when they see it as desirable and when it fits with their personal interests. This strategy is based on reason and knowledge and is often used to implement technologic changes. This strategy might be useful in helping to shift from paper documentation of care at the nurse's station to one using a computer at the bedside. When individuals understood how much easier and accurate computer charting would be, they would be more eager to learn how to use it and would learn the process more quickly.

POWER-COERCIVE STRATEGY

A power-coercive strategy is in use when a leader orders change and those with less power or position comply (Benne, Bennis, & Chin, 1976). The use of this strategy requires that the change agent have official authority to mandate the change. The compliance of those affected rests in their desire to please or with their fear of the sanctions that might accompany non-compliance – such things as loss of employment, rewards, advancement or other benefits. We may see this strategy used when new laws are enforced such as occurred when the minimum data set (MDS) was mandated for use in long-term care.

NORMATIVE-REEDUCATIVE STRATEGY

The normative-reeducative approach to change states that change will take place only after changes have occurred in values, attitudes, skills, and significant relationships (Benne et al, 1976). To accomplish this, those that will be involved in the change must necessarily be included in working out the plans for the change. Mutual trust and collaboration are hallmarks of the process. If conflict occurs, the process of change must be delayed until the conflict is resolved.

Facilitating Change

Because making a change will require that we alter the way we have been doing things, most people are initially resistant to change. We become comfortable with the way that things have been done and may be apprehensive of new approaches that require us to change established patterns of behavior. The new approaches may take additional time to learn or may be threatening to us if they involve skills with which we are not entirely familiar. Resistance to change may be the basis of sayings such as, "If it's not broken, don't fix it." One of the roles of the change agent is to overcome resistance to change.

Most authorities on change agree that change is most easily implemented when it is the result of a collaborative process (the normative-reeducative approach). This means involving everyone who is going to be affected by the change. All persons involved need a good understanding of the change, why it is necessary, how it is to be accomplished, and what will be the benefits. If possible, suggestions from those affected by the change need to be built into the change model. Mutual trust and respect must exist between all persons working with the change.

Communications should remain open throughout the entire process. When questions arise, they should be answered in an honest and straightforward manner. Often during the change process, rumors will begin to circulate. These rumors need to be addressed as quickly as possible and facts supplied where perceptions are incorrect.

Successful change is well thought out and planned. A process similar to that which you have used in the application of the nursing process provides good guidance. First of all, once a problem that might benefit from change has been identified, data need to be gathered that will assist with the diagnosis of the problem. Is it a problem? Why is it a problem? Who does it affect? How are they affected? Might there be a better way to approach the situation? What would the costs be in terms of time? What would be the personal cost to those affected? What would be the effects of not addressing the problem? Should we move forward with the change or look for other solutions?

Once as much data has been gathered as is reasonable, planning needs to begin. Who needs to be involved? How might the change best be implemented? What would be the best timing? Who should be the key players? What resources will be needed? What needs to be done to help those affected "unfreeze"? What needs to be built into the plan that will help to assure that the changes remain in place? What additional training and education will be necessary?

Early in this process, those who are going to be affected by the change need to be included. They need to be informed of intentions to make changes and be brought into the collaborative process for planning. Mutual objective-setting will help motivate others toward change. Smith (1996) includes, as one of his management principles related to change, ensuring that each person always knows why his or her performance and change matters to the purpose and results of the whole organization. Providing maximum information is important, as is calming concerns about the personal effects of the change. Those who will be affected need to realize how they can benefit from the change. Positive relationships must be built between the change agent and those experiencing the change.

Once plans are well formulated and people who will be affected have full information and a role in the process, the change needs to be implemented. Establishing a timetable is often useful. Celebrating milestones of accomplishment throughout the entire process can generate team spirit. It is unwise to change dates or to postpone actions once they have been announced because people will become suspicious and/or critical of the process. If delays are necessary, full explanation of the reason(s) for the delay need to be shared. This is a continuation of the open communication process mentioned earlier. Positive efforts toward making a change need to be recognized and praised.

The change process should be monitored throughout its implementation and evaluated after it is completed. This will provide the information that will indicate whether the change is accomplishing what was desired. Did it do what it was supposed to do? Evaluation provides information about how people are adjusting to the change and how satisfied they are with it—data that is crucial to sustaining the change.

For a change to be sustained, it must be standardized and refined. The change agent, if outside the usual staff, needs to transfer responsibility for the continuance of the project to the participants in the change. If the change requires changes in policies or protocols, those need to be written and incorporated in organizational manuals. People who have made notable contributions need to be recognized for their efforts.

It is through careful planning, implementation, and follow-up that successful change occurs. Flexibility in addressing and adjusting problems that arise is important. Interpersonal relationships need to be given high priority during this time.

Spencer Johnson, in his book *Who Moved My Cheese?* (1998), reminds us that change is a part of life and encourages us to enjoy change, to savor the adventure, and enjoy the aspects of the new approach. He also reminds us that we need to be ready to change again and enjoy it.

Responding to Change

As a new graduate, it is most likely that you will be one of the individuals affected by the change rather than the one trying to implement the change. How will you react if a change must occur on the unit to which you are assigned? Will you drag your feet and be one of the last to accept the change or will you be one of the first the join the change team? How can you be an effective participant?

First of all, you will want to take all opportunities to learn about the anticipated changes. Attend any scheduled meetings; read all announcements that are circulated. If there are matters that seem unclear to you, ask questions at the appropriate time. Learn what the benefits will be for you and for others. Discuss your thoughts and findings with others and share any suggestions you have. If you have concerns, express those also and listen carefully to any responses that are provided to your concerns. You will find that if you actively participate in the change, it will be much easier to move into the new behaviors it may require. Change can be energizing for some individuals. It often opens the door for new opportunities. It can provide empowerment and enjoyment if managed correctly.

Critical Thinking Activity

You have just learned that a new form of charting is being initiated on your unit. As a new employee, you have just become comfortable with the current system, which was quite different from anything you used as a student. You are dismayed that you will now need to learn a new system. What steps can you take to participate effectively in this change? How can you develop a more positive attitude toward this change? What will facilitate the process for you? What role do you see for yourself in the change process? If you become really frustrated during the change process, to whom will you speak?

MANAGING CONFLICT

We have talked about collaboration and collaborative relationships throughout this chapter. Some would propose that the opposite of collaboration is conflict. Let's now look at how one might deal with conflict.

Certainly conflict is not a new topic to you. You have dealt with it from the time you were a child. It is a part of everyday living. The very nature of conflict is what keeps attorneys, marriage counselors, mediators, and arbitrators in business. Our ability to work positively with conflict may determine our success in today's world.

Conflict and Nursing

Conflict, broadly defined, results when people with differing values, interests, goals, needs, or approaches come together to address a common concern. Because people view things from different perspectives and bring different values to the situation, incompatible ideas, approaches, or resolutions can occur. The settling of a conflict is known as **conflict resolution**. The process through which the conflict is recognized and resolved is called **conflict management**. The critical element is not that conflicts come about—the important aspect is how we deal with them.

In this chapter we discussed the conflict that can occur between physicians and nurses. In Chapter 12 we discussed collective bargaining, a major area in which there can be discord. As nurses exercise professional judgment, differences of opinion may arise regarding the best approach to treatment for a client. There may be disagreements about staffing patterns, particularly during the holidays. Overlapping roles can result in conflict, and not having sufficient resources can cause discord.

These represent just a few of the many situations in nursing in which disagreements can happen. Phyllis Kritek (2001), author of *Negotiating at an Uneven Table*, reflects on nurses and conflict, noting that conflict is pervasive in nursing, endemic and integral to the role. She questions why this is so and asks if it is because most "nurses are women, or because they are socialized to be conflict-aversive, or essentially conservative, or primarily healers, or inherently nurturant" (p. 474). Regardless of the answer, all nurses must be skillful in dealing with conflict.

The Positive Side of Conflict

It should be noted that conflict can have positive aspects; not all conflict is serious, ominous, or intimidating. Conflict can result in personal growth and development. We learn by contrasting our values and beliefs with those of others. As we learn about others, we learn about ourselves.

Conflict can provide the impetus for change. Conflict can contribute to innovation and creativity. When conflict is a major part of any operation, reasons for its presence must be sought and alternatives set forth. Thus, new approaches are tried. For example, conflict over the use of completing morning baths during busy and rushed morning hours could result in a more flexible bathing routine for patients that schedules some baths for the evening.

Conflict also assists employees of an organization to have a better understanding of one another's jobs and responsibilities. As health care becomes more and more specialized, differences become greater and give rise to conflict. Conflict may result in people from different areas sitting down and talking to resolve the problem (Fig. 14-3). As talk continues, a greater appreciation for others can develop, thus creating unification within the organization.

Conflict can also open new channels of communication. As efforts are made to eliminate sources of conflict, new approaches and avenues may evolve. Similarly, conflict may serve to energize people. A good disagreement has the potential to sharpen people's awareness, to get them thinking, and to put new spark into their work.

Types of Conflict

Conflict can be looked at from a number of perspectives and can be broken into several categories. Your approach to dealing with the conflict may vary depending on the type of conflict that exists.

INTRAPERSONAL, INTERPERSONAL, AND INTERGROUP CONFLICT

Intrapersonal conflict occurs within one's self in circumstances in which a choice must be made between two alternatives. Choosing one alternative means that you cannot have the other. An example would be a situation in which the nurse must decide whether to participate

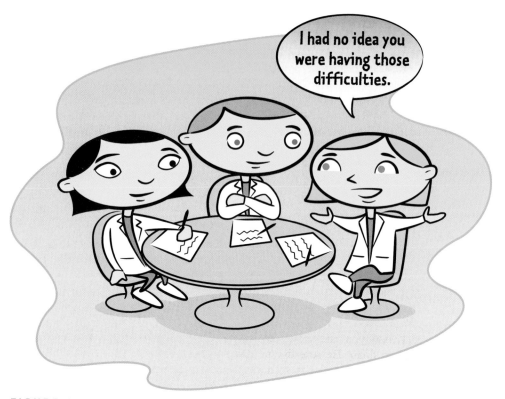

FIGURE 14-3   When people from different areas sit down to talk to resolve a problem, they often gain a greater appreciation for one another.

in a committee on nursing practice that will take time away from direct patient care or choose to decline the opportunity in order to spend more time with patients. Either choice has some benefits and some drawbacks. The conflict that occurs is within the nurse who must decide which is more important personally.

Interpersonal conflict occurs between or among individuals. This is where differences in values, ideas, perceptions, and goals play an important role. If one nurse believes that the most important aspect of care is that every patient has a complete bath every day, and another nurse believes that having all patients ambulate is more critical and there is not time for both, an interpersonal conflict results. The basis of the conflict is the difference in what each perceives as the first priority in nursing care.

Intergroup conflict is seen when two or more groups of people or departments struggle for power, authority, territory, or resources. Each group tends to perceive the situation only as it affects that group. Each group acknowledges only its own value and positive aspects, attributing negative aspects to the other group. Negative stereotypes form, hostility develops, and communication deteriorates. Intergroup conflicts can occur between those who work on different shifts of a nursing unit—the evening shift personnel critical of the day shift and the day shift people believing that their job is harder than that of the evening shift. Intergroup conflicts might also occur between the nursing staff and the housekeeping staff over setting priorities for cleaning rooms and preparing them for new admissions. The housekeeping staff may have a set of priorities based on how personnel are distributed, while the nursing staff may want the priorities to change and flex based on their perceptions of patient needs. Inter-group conflicts can be increased when those in one group spend time recounting to others within their group all the perceived inadequacies of the other group. As they do this, they may gather additional anecdotes to support their own perceptions. Thus the conflict is maintained and spread.

ORGANIZATIONAL CONFLICT

Some conflicts originate within the structure and function of an organization; typically, the style of management being used, policies, procedures, channels of communication generate them, and similar factors related to organizational operations. These are termed **organizational conflict**. In organizational conflict, the leader's role and behavior are particularly important to both the origin of the conflict and to the resolution of issues.

Role ambiguity and **role conflict** are one major cause of organizational conflict. Role ambiguity refers to a situation in which the role is not clearly defined. Role conflict occurs when two or more individuals have role descriptions that overlap. This frequently occurs because of the lack of good job descriptions and clear communications regarding what is expected. An example of role conflict could be seen in the provision of discharge planning. Both the RN and the social worker clearly may view this as an important aspect of their professional responsibilities, and the job descriptions of both may include this aspect of patient care.

The structure of the organization may also lead to conflict. The term "turf" refers to the territory that one or one's group controls. "Turf battles" are not uncommon in organizations, with various individuals within the system attempting to protect, expand, or advance the area for which they are responsible. Again, good job descriptions, organizational charts, and communications will minimize the advent of this type of problem.

Conflict within an organization also can arise when a scarcity of resources exists. Scarcity of resources refers not only to money but also to supplies, equipment, space, personnel, and similar necessities. As nursing moves into one of the greatest shortages experienced in recent years, conflicts related to securing and retaining adequate nurse staffing can be anticipated.

Strategies for Coping With Conflict

The approach that you use to deal with conflict will depend on a number of factors. The investment you have in the situation will be one major consideration—there is an old adage that advises us to pick our battles carefully. This suggests that not all differences or conflicts are worth the effort of resolving them. The nature of the conflict, the individuals that are involved, your ability to influence the outcome, and the possibility of retribution are all elements that will affect the situation. Thus, a wide variety of approaches to the management of conflict exists, which tend to fall into one of five categories.

WITHDRAWING FROM OR AVOIDING CONFLICT

You employ the strategy of avoiding or withdrawing from the conflict when you choose not to address the issue at hand. Some would also refer to this as denying the existence of the conflict, sometimes with the hope that if it is ignored it will go away. There are many times when this approach is appropriate. This would include situations in which the conflict clearly is not your problem, when there is little or nothing that you can do about it, when there is more to lose than to be gained by becoming involved, when you lack sufficient information about the conflict and its cause, or when the problem will straighten itself out if given time.

Although appropriate at times, this strategy is often preferred by people who are very uncomfortable with conflict situations, and it may not be the best approach. In a competitive society, individuals who will back away from a conflict can be taken advantage of. It is important to learn to advocate for yourself as well as for your clients. An example might be a situation in which both you and another nurse want to be off duty on Halloween evening so that you can participate in your children's trick-or-treat activities. Although the other nurse enjoyed that evening off last year, you again concede to her request because you do not want to deal with her comments and criticisms if you are awarded the evening off.

SMOOTHING, SUPPRESSING, OR ACCOMMODATING

Smoothing, suppressing, or accommodating conflict involves trying to relieve feelings associated with conflict without solving the underlying problem. It may involve apologizing for something that is not one's fault, stating agreement with a position with which one does not truly agree, or taking action that one does not really support to stop the feelings of conflict occurring. Similar to avoidance of the issue, smoothing, suppressing, or accommodating may also be referred to as surrendering to the conflict. In such situations, it is easier not to address the issue and to deal with feelings of anger or expressions of difference than it is to deal with the conflict.

We see this approach used by individuals with a strong need to be liked or those who are overly concerned with the welfare of others. They would prefer a "martyr" or self-sacrificing approach that will result in a peaceful environment. An individual who wishes to preserve harmony or build up social credits may employ this technique.

There are times when smoothing, suppressing, or accommodating is appropriate. It may be the best approach if the conflict and anger that accompanies it disrupts the work situation or interferes with the immediate needs of the patients. In such situations, harmony and constancy are important. If the outcome does not matter to you or if you obviously are wrong, this is a good approach. If you have little chance to win or if this represents a situation in which you can lose the battle but win the war, it is appropriate.

FORCING THE ISSUES, FIGHTING, OR COMPETING

Competing, forcing the issue, or fighting in a conflict situation means you are working exclusively for your own solution to the problem. You may have taken this approach because you believe you know more about the issues involved than others or when your values will allow no other compromise. It is an aggressive approach that could result in retaliation at another time. It might be the best approach if you observe a violation of ethical or legal standards.

NEGOTIATING AND COMPROMISING

Compromising and negotiating involve give and take; one factor is balanced against another. It is the approach to the conflict seen in collective bargaining. It serves to minimize the losses for all parties while allowing each to realize some gains. It may be the approach of choice if the opposing goals are so incompatible that no resolution can be reached and discussion has stalled. It would also be appropriate if an immediate settlement to the issue were needed due to time constraints or other factors.

PROBLEM-SOLVING AND COLLABORATING

Although problem-solving or collaborating to achieve a mutually agreed-upon plan of action may be the most difficult to achieve, many believe this to be the best approach to conflict. It encourages participants in the conflict to work towards common goals and to work toward consensus. The process can be very time consuming and requires that all persons involved come to the table willing to examine and discuss issues openly and honestly. If effective in resolving the conflict, it is viewed as a win–win situation for everyone.

Personal Preparation for Conflict

If you find yourself in a conflict situation, you will want to be as prepared as possible to deal with the conditions at hand. This is often hard to do at the time the conflict occurs. Like your preparation for carrying out nursing procedures, you can take steps before needing the skill to prepare you to perform more adequately. You may need to confront another person with the reality of the conflict and the necessity for resolution.

One of the best techniques is to practice for the situation. Rehearse what you will say. Think about the tone of your voice, the speed with which to talk, and your body language. Think positively about yourself. Be confident. Visualize what a successful interaction would be like.

When engaged in the confrontation, do not interrupt others. Give them an opportunity to express their position. Practice good listening skills when they are talking. Insist that you are given the same courtesy of uninterrupted explanation.

Be clear and concise in presenting your point of view. Long, complicated presentations lose everyone's interest. Be assertive but considerate of others.

If you find that you are involved in conflict situations more frequently than most other individuals, a personal inventory is appropriate. Questions you should ask yourself might include:

- Do I have good relationships with most of my coworkers?
- How do I manage stress in other situations?
- Do I have the proper balance between work and relaxation?
- Do I feel competent in this situation?
- Do I hold personal biases that are interfering with my interactions with others?
- What else is going on in my life?

If after completing this inventory you find there are areas that give you concern, then they can be addressed in an appropriate manner. Clearly, if you are experiencing high levels of stress in any area of life, you may find yourself more easily in conflict with others and less able to manage that conflict effectively. Therefore, if there is a lack of opportunity for relaxation in your life, you can adjust your schedule so that you maximize the time you spend on things that result in leisure and rest. If you are feeling less than competent regarding the expectations of the job you are doing, some continuing education, reading, or research may be helpful. Seeking and working with a mentor may also bring positive results.

If your relationships with other coworkers or in your private life are lacking, seeking the help of a qualified counselor may be the best approach.

KEY CONCEPTS

- A team is comprised of a group of people working together for a common goal. Because of the diverse disciplines that are now involved in health care, the effective functioning of the health care team is critical to the provision of quality health care. Trust and respect of others are key ingredients in team function.
- Health care teams have moved from being multidisciplinary to interdisciplinary to transdisciplinary. Transdisciplinary teams involve role sharing among the various disciplines that provide care. Transdisciplinary health teams have more collaborative relationships, with much interacting and bonding occurring among team members. The nurse has a key role in coordinating the efforts of the team.
- Nurses and physicians fill key positions on the health care team. The relationship between these two care providers must be symbolized by mutual respect and consideration. Nurses can take positive actions to help assure that this occurs.
- Many leaders in health care are using team-building techniques to strengthen the functioning of their teams. Team building involves setting common goals, recognizing the contribution each person makes to the team, involving others in decision-making, focusing on problems rather than individuals associated with the problem, and sharing in accomplishments.
- Motivation encompasses the sum of all the factors that cause an individual to do something. To motivate individuals, the leader must understand personal behaviors and role model those that are desired in others.
- Delegation is the process by which one individual is able to accomplish necessary tasks with and through others. It is an important management process and allows the health care system to function efficiently. Nurses remain accountable for all nursing care that is provided. It is important to follow the guidelines for effective delegation and know which aspects of care can never be delegated.
- The five rights of successful delegation include the right task, the right circumstances, the right person, the right direction and communication, and the right supervision and evaluation.
- Nurses cannot delegate aspects of care that require nursing judgment, including such activities as patient assessment.
- Change is inevitable in today's health care environment. Individuals tend to resist change, and leaders must become familiar with the steps that will facilitate the change process.
- A number of theories of change have been developed. Many of them describe processes to facilitate change, including helping others see the need for change, involving those who will be affected by the change in the process, and stabilizing the change once it is in place.
- You will experience change as a new employee. You can make the process more positive by learning all that you can about the anticipated changes, understanding the benefits, asking appropriate questions of the right individuals, and expressing any concerns you may have respectfully and to the right people.

- Conflict occurs in all aspects of our lives. Conflict can be intrapersonal, interpersonal, intergroup, or organizational.
- Strategies for dealing with conflict include withdrawing or avoiding the conflict; smoothing, suppressing or accommodating to the conflict; forcing, fighting, or competing; negotiating or compromising; and problem-solving or collaborating. There is a proper time and circumstance for the use of each strategy.
- Conflict can have positive aspects. It can provide an impetus for change, it can energize individuals, it can help persons in different roles understand one another better, and it can facilitate communication.
- If you find yourself in conflict more than is desirable, a self-inventory can be helpful. Asking yourself a variety of questions may help identify the actions you will want to take.

RELEVANT WEB SITES

Conflict management: Conflict Management Guidebook: *http//www.usbr.gov/hr/conflict/* Provides links to other conflict management sites.

Delegation: National Council of State Boards of Nursing: *http//www.ncsbn.org*. Type "delegation" into search box for a list of references.

Information about change: Change Management: A Primer. Available at *http//home.att.net/~nickols/change.htm*

Information on change and team building: *http//www.squarewheels.com*

REFERENCES

American Nurses Association. (1997). Attachment I: Definitions related to ANA 1992 Position Statements on Unlicensed Assistive Personnel. Kansas City, MO: Author.

Asprec, E. (1975). The process of change. *Supervisor Nurse*, 6:15–24.

Benne, K. D., Bennis, G. & Chin, R. (1976). Planned change in American. In W. G. Bennis, K. D. Benne, R. Chin, & K. E. Corey (Eds.), *The planning of change*. New York: Holt, Rinehart and Winston.

Havelock, R. (1973). *The change agent's guide to innovation in education*. Englewood Cliffs, NJ: Educational Technology Publications.

Johnson, S. (1998). *Who moved my cheese?* New York: G. P. Putnam's Sons.

Kritek, P. B. (2001). Some reflections on conflict resolution in nursing: The implications of negotiating at an uneven table. In J. M. Dochterman & H. K. Grace, *Current issues in nursing* (6th ed.) (pp. 473–478). St. Louis: Mosby.

Lewin, K. (1951). *Field theory in social service: Selected theoretical papers*. New York: Harper Brothers.

Lippitt, R., Watson, J. & Westley, B. (1958). *The dynamic of planned change*. New York: Harcourt, Brace & World.

Maslow, A. (1954). *Motivation and personality*. New York: Harper & Row.

McClelland, D. (1961). *The achieving society*. Princeton, NJ: Van Nostrand.

McClelland, D. (1953). *The achievement motive*. Norwalk, CT: Appleton-Century-Crofts.

McGregor, D. (1966). *Leadership and motivation*. Cambridge, MA: MIT Press.

National Council of State Boards of Nursing. (1995). *Delegation: Concepts and decision-making process*. Chicago: Author.

Perlman, D. & Takacs, G. J. (1990). The ten stages of change. *Nursing management 212*(4):33–38.

Rogers, E. & Shoemaker, F. (1971). *Communication of innovations: A cross cultural approach*. New York: Free Press.

Rosenstein, A. H. (2002). Nurse–physician relationships: Impact on nurse satisfaction and retention. *AJN 102*(6):26–34.

Smith, D. K. (1996). *Taking charge of change: Ten principles for managing people and performance*. Menlo Park: Addison-Wesley.

"The Quality Gurus." (2002). [On-line]. Available at *http//www.simplesystemsintl.com/quality_gurus.htm*.

Watson, M. J. (1996). NLN perspective president's message: From discipline specific to "inter" to multi" to "transdisciplinary" health care, education, and practice. *Journal of Nursing & Health Care: Perspectives on Community* 17:2.

Commonly Used Acronyms

AACN	American Association of Colleges of Nursing
AACN	American Association of Critical-Care Nurses
AAN	American Academy of Nursing
ABNS	American Board of Nursing Specialties
AD	Associate degree
ADA	Americans with Disabilities Act
ADEA	Age Discrimination and Employment Act
ADN	Associate degree nursing
AHA	American Hospital Association
AHCPR	Agency for Health Care Policy and Research (now the AHRQ)
AHRQ	Agency for Health Care Research and Quality (formerly the Agency for Health Care Policy and Research—AHCPR)
AMA	American Medical Association
ANA	American Nurses Association
ANA—PAC	American Nurses Association Political Action Committee
ANCC	American Nurses Credentialing Center
ANF	American Nurses Foundation
APIC	Association for Professionals in Infection Control
APN	Advanced practice nurse
BSN	Bachelor of science in nursing
CADP	Council of Associate Degree Programs of the NLN
CAT	Computer adaptive testing
CBHDP	Council of Baccalaureate and Higher Degree Programs of the NLN
CCNE	Commission on Collegiate Nursing Education (related to American Association of Colleges of Nursing)
CDC	Centers for Disease Control and Prevention
CDPN	Council of Diploma Programs in Nursing of the NLN
CE	Continuing education
CEU	Continuing education unit
CHAP	Community Health Accreditation Program
CINAHL	Cumulative Index to Nursing and Allied Health Literature
CNA	Canadian Nurses Association

CNPE	Congress on Nursing Practice and Economics of the ANA
CNS	Clinical nurse specialist
CPNP	Council of Practical Nursing Programs of the NLN
CQI	Continuous quality improvement
DHHS	Department of Health and Human Services
DOE	Department of Education
DRG	Diagnosis-related group
EEOC	Equal Employment Opportunity Commission
EPO	Exclusive Provider Organization
FAQs	Frequently asked questions
FDA	Food and Drug Administration
FTE	Full-time equivalent
HCFA	Health Care Financing Administration
HEDIS	Health Plan Employer Data and Information Set
HGP	Human Genome Project
HHS	Health and Human Services
HIPPA	Health Insurance Portability Act
HMO	Health maintenance organization
HPPO	Hours per patient day
ICN	International Council of Nurses
IOM	Institute of Medicine
JCAHO	Joint Commission on Accreditation of Healthcare Organizations
LP(V)N	Licensed Practical (Vocational) Nurse
MBO	Managed by objectives
MCO	Managed Care Organizations
MSN	Master's of science in nursing
NANDA	North American Nursing Diagnosis Association
NAPNES	National Association for Practical Nurse Education and Service
NCH	Nursing Care Hours
NCLEX–PN	National Council Licensing Examination for Practical Nursing
NCLEX–RN	National Council Licensing Examination for Registered Nursing
NCQA	National Committee for Quality Assurance
NCSBN	National Council of State Boards of Nursing
NFLPN	National Federation of Licensed Practical Nurses
NFSNO	National Federation for Specialty Nursing Organizations
NIC	Nursing Interventions Classifications
NIH	National Institutes of Health
NINR	National Institute of Nursing Research
NIOSH	National Institute of Occupational Safety and Health
NLM	National Library of Medicine
NLN	National League for Nursing
NLNAC	National League for Nursing Accrediting Commission (related to the National League for Nursing)
NLRA	National Labor Relations Act
NLRB	National Labor Relations Board

NOADN	National Organization for Associate Degree Nursing
NOC	Nursing Outcomes Classification
NP	Nurse practitioner
NSNA	National Student Nurse Association
NSNCO	National Specialty Nursing Certifying Organization
OASIS	Outcomes and Assessment Information Set
OBRA	Omnibus Budget Reconciliation Act
OSHA	Occupational Health and Safety Administration
PA	Physician assistant
PN	Practical nurse
PPOs	Preferred provider organizations
PPS	Prospective payment system
PSRO	Professional Standards Review Organizations
QA	Quality assurance
QAI	Quality assessment and improvement
RN	Registered Nurse
RUGs	Resource utilization groups
SBNs	State Boards of Nursing
SEIU	Service Employees International Union
TQM	Total quality management
UAP	Unlicensed assistive personnel
VN	Vocational nurse
WHO	World Health Organization
WWW	World Wide Web

Index

Page numbers followed by d indicate displays; those followed by f indicate figures; those followed by t indicate tables.